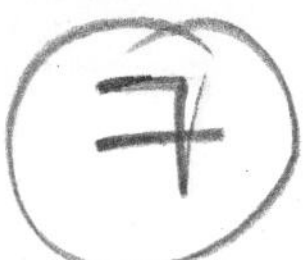

VACCINE MANUAL

The Production and Quality Control of Veterinary Vaccines for use in Developing Countries

Noel Mowat
and
Mark Rweyemamu

1999
Reprinted by arrangement with the
Food and Agriculture Organization of the United Nations

by
Daya Publishing House
A Division of
Astral International Pvt Ltd
New Delhi - 110 002

"This book was originally published by the Food and Agriculture Organization of the United Nations (FAO) as Vaccine Manual, FAO Animal Production and Health Series No. 35".

"The designations employed and the presentation of material in this publication do not imply the expression of any opinion, whatsoever on the part of the Food and Agriculture Organization of the United Nations concerning the legal status of any country, territory, city or area or of its authorities, or concerning the delimitations of its frontiers or boundaries."

'The designations 'developed' and 'developing' economies are intended for statistical convenience and do not necessarily express a judgment about the stage reached by a particular country, territory or area in the development process.'

First Indian Edition, 1998
ISBN: 978-81-7035-217-4

Published by : **Daya Publishing House**
A Division of
Astral International Pvt Ltd
4736/23, Ansari Road
Darya Ganj, New Delhi - 110002
Phone: 011-43549197
Email: info@astralint.com
Web: www.astralint.com

Printed at : **Chawla Offset Printers,**
Delhi-110 052

Contents

Introduction

In December 1991 at FAO headquarters in Rome, the Animal Production and Health Division held an Expert Consultation on the Quality Control of Veterinary Vaccines in Developing Countries.[1]

The purpose of the consultation was to bring together experts in various aspects of vaccine production and quality control to consider present problems and likely future developments in the application of vaccines for the control of animal disease and to make recommendations for further improvements in this important field.

One of the most important conclusions reached at the end of the consultation was: "Discussions at this meeting have repeatedly highlighted duplication of recommendations and procedures from international organizations. WHO, OIE and FAO have previously prepared guidelines and recommendations for various aspects of animal vaccine preparation and quality control. There appears to be a lack of coordination or cooperation in undertaking these activities."

As a consequence of this, the following general recommendation was made: "This meeting recommends that a closer cooperation be established with other international organizations to develop a more coherent approach on guidelines for vaccine quality control and to this end *urges FAO to take the initiative*." This manual represents one of FAO's responses to that recommendation.

FAO has been very fortunate in obtaining contributions from some of the best recognized international experts in the field of veterinary vaccine development, both at the theoretical and the "hands on" practical level. In producing this manual, the intention has been to compile the latest information on all aspects of the production and quality control of vaccines which are primarily intended for use in domestic livestock and, where appropriate, to take into consideration the particular conditions of production and application in the developing countries.

While it is principally concerned with providing guidelines and recommendations for the application of modern methods of vaccine production and evaluation (and as such can have no *mandatory* significance), the manual attempts to bring together information on the state of the art in veterinary vaccine development, with some of the chapters presenting a "definitive" text on certain topics.

It is hoped that the Overview will prove to be of exceptional interest to the majority of readers. Many of the contributions in this section indicate the remarkable impact that modern biotechnology is having on a wide range of topics related to veterinary vaccines. They include work on understanding the mechanisms of immunity and protection against disease, as well as the exploitation of genetic engineering and molecular biology for the development of more effective vaccines, and also cover the particular problems and practical aspects of vaccines for fish and those required for the control of multicellular parasites. There is also a very useful contribution from the Office international des Épizooties (OIE) summarizing its functions and activities to promote the standardization of vaccine quality at the international level.

[1] For the proceedings of the expert consultation, see: FAO. 1993. *Quality control of veterinary vaccines in developing countries.* Animal Production and Health Paper No. 116. Rome.

Part 2 of the manual deals with the planning and management aspects of vaccine production and control. Under present-day conditions of financial constraint and limited budgets, efficient planning and management of resources according to modern practice is of paramount importance – and nowhere is this more relevant than in the developing countries. This section is therefore concerned with the design and maintenance of production facilities and equipment, the principles of financial management, the registration and licensing of veterinary immunoprophylactics, the logistics of vaccine manufacture as related to working in the developing countries, and the pros and cons of one solution to setting up vaccine production under such conditions, namely the role of private industry in transferring modern vaccine technology to developing countries.

The next section, Part 3, is devoted to the practical aspects of vaccine production and covers the basic laboratory facilities and services necessary, the application of modern fermentation technology, the preparation of inactivated antigens, the freeze-drying of vaccines, the need for adjuvants in modern vaccines and the requirements for the bottling, packing and distribution of the final product. All of these chapters provide much of the "hard" practical information necessary for running an efficient vaccine production unit.

The final section, Part 4, deals with the major topics of quality assurance and quality control. Chapters cover good laboratory and manufacturing practice, the essential documentation required of a modern unit, the assessment of the safety and potency of vaccines and the statistical interpretation of the results of those tests. There is also a useful chapter on the role and contribution made by the internationally recognized regional laboratories which have responsibilities for the diagnosis and characterization of the causative organisms of disease outbreaks of major economic importance, such as foot-and-mouth disease, and also the provision of advice on the most appropriate vaccines and the required standards of efficacy.

At present, animal husbandry and production industries, particularly in the developing countries, are attempting to meet the demands for increased food production from expanding human populations with expectations of higher standards of living.

Infectious disease is a major constraint to the development of improved livestock production, to which the solution for many of the developing countries must be prevention by means of efficient immunization programmes. In a frequently changing environment in which the conditions favour the rapid spread of disease and the possible emergence of new strains of organisms, greater dependence has to be placed on the use of modern biological science to counter these threats. More effective vaccines, produced by up-to-date methods as economically as possible, can make a significant contribution to the control of animal disease. By bringing together some of the latest information and guidelines on modern vaccine technology, this manual is intended to help achieve these aims.

PART 1

Overview: the present state of veterinary vaccine development

The induction of immunity by veterinary immunoprophylactics

W.I. Morrison

Infectious disease continues to be one of the most important constraints on the efficient production of farm livestock in both developing and developed countries. While vaccination and the therapeutic or prophylactic use of drugs both play an important role in animal disease control, vaccination is increasingly being viewed as the more sustainable option. This view is influenced not only by the potential that vaccination offers for greater economic efficiency but also by the concerns that have been raised about the selection of drug-resistant pathogens and the potential harmful effects of drug residues in animal products and the environment. Vaccination has had a major impact on the control of epidemic viral diseases of livestock such as foot-and-mouth disease and rinderpest. However, there are many other important diseases for which efforts to develop effective methods of vaccination have been unsuccessful.

The advent of recombinant DNA technology in the early 1980s created exciting new opportunities to produce vaccines based on the use of expressed products of cloned genes. However, only a few such vaccines have been successfully developed. In retrospect, it can be seen that the immediate expectations of the new technology were unrealistically high, given the limited knowledge of the immunology of many of the target diseases and of how antigens are processed and recognized by the immune system. In the intervening decade there have been major advances in immunology which, coupled with further developments in the application of DNA technology, now provide a strong conceptual framework for the rational development of new vaccines.

This chapter will consider recent developments in immunology that are pertinent to understanding how the immune system controls infections and will discuss their implications for contemporary approaches to vaccine development.

APPROACHES TO VACCINE DEVELOPMENT

Most of the current veterinary vaccines are based on the use of either killed organisms or their products or live attenuated organisms. The development of these vaccines has not relied on knowledge of the immune responses that mediate immunity. Significant advances have been made primarily by the development of new culture techniques, improved attenuation procedures and better adjuvants. While there is some scope for further efforts to develop vaccines along these lines, there are many diseases for which the more empirical methods are unlikely to be successful.

Two main approaches to vaccine design can be considered using modern molecular technologies, namely the production of attenuated mutant organisms by deliberate molecular manipulation and the identification of antigenic components of pathogens that can be used to induce protective immune responses (these components are known as subunit vaccines). Unlike the traditional vaccine strategies, the ability to exploit these new approaches to vaccine development is dependent on an intimate knowledge of the molecular structure of the target pathogens and an understanding of the mechanisms of immunity.

PROCESSING AND RECOGNITION OF ANTIGENS

Immune effector mechanisms

Studies in laboratory animal model systems have demonstrated that the immune system can respond in a number of different ways to control an infection. The type of response elicited by a pathogen depends largely on the nature of the organism and its site of replication within the host. In general, organisms that establish systemic infections and replicate extracellularly are controlled by antibody responses.

Secretory antibody responses also play an important role in the control of infections at mucosal surfaces. By contrast, cell-mediated immune responses are generally more important in controlling organisms which replicate intracellularly. The T lymphocytes that participate in cell-mediated immune responses may exert their effector function in a number of different ways. They may kill infected cells or release cytokines, which inhibit growth of intracellular organisms or which recruit and activate accessory cells such as macrophages, to perform these functions. Indeed, a number of different mechanisms may operate against the same organism. Stimulation of T lymphocyte responses is also essential to provide help, again in the form of cytokines, for the production of antibody by B lymphocytes. Hence, T lymphocytes have a pivotal role in the induction of virtually all specific immune responses. The way in which antigen is processed and recognized by the immune system determines the type of T cell response that is induced.

Recognition of antigen by B and T lymphocytes

The antigen recognition structures on B and T lymphocytes, namely immunoglobulin (Ig) and the T cell receptor (TCR) are both generated by a process of gene rearrangement whereby each of the two chains that make up the molecules is produced by bringing together two or three variable sequences, from a pre-existing library of variable genes, with a constant sequence to form a functional gene (Cooper and Burrows, 1989; Davis and Bjorkman, 1988). This mechanism, together with the further diversity created by a combination of different variable regions in Ig heavy and light chains and TCR alpha and beta chains facilitates the generation of a very large repertoire of B lymphocytes and T lymphocytes, each with a unique antigen recognition specificity.

Despite the similarity in structure of Ig and TCR molecules, B and T lymphocytes differ fundamentally in the way they recognize antigen. Immunoglobulins, whether on the surface of B lymphocytes or as secreted antibodies interact directly with foreign antigen, usually in the form in which it is initially encountered by the host, i.e. as an intact organism or as molecules released from the organism. Recognition of antigens by antibody is, therefore, often dependent on the conformational integrity of the molecules. By contrast, T lymphocytes only recognize antigens after they have been degraded and presented on the surface of other cells (Brodsky and Guagliardi, 1991). These antigen-bearing cells may be cells infected with foreign organisms or "professional" antigen-presenting cells, such as macrophages and dendritic cells, which have ingested antigen. The processed antigen, which is in the form of short peptides of less than 20 amino acids, is associated with major histocompatibility complex (MHC) molecules on the surface of the antigen-presenting cell (Bodmer, 1984). The T cell receptor does not react with antigen alone but rather recognizes a combination of the antigenic peptide and the associated MHC molecule (Townsend and Bodmer, 1989).

The special role of MHC molecules

The MHC consists of a set of closely linked genes, many of which encode molecules involved in antigen processing and presentation (Trowsdale, 1993). There are two main types of MHC molecules, namely class I and class II. The most striking feature of these MHC molecules is the high degree of polymorphism they display among individuals of a species (Bodmer, 1984; Trowsdale, 1993). Class I molecules are heterodimers composed of a polymorphic heavy chain and a non-polymorphic light chain (β_2-microglobulin), the latter encoded outside the MHC. They are expressed on most cells of the body. Class II molecules are also heterodimers, both polypeptides being encoded within the MHC, but their expression in healthy animals is confined mainly to "professional" antigen-presenting cells, namely macrophages, dendritic cells and B lymphocytes. In most mammalian species examined, each class is encoded by two gene loci and, in each instance, both alleles are expressed.

While it has been recognized since the early 1970s that class I and class II molecules are involved in presenting antigen to T cells, the precise molecular and structural basis of presentation was not elucidated until the late 1980s. A key event was the resolution of the structure of class I molecules by X-ray crystallography (Bjorkman *et al.*, 1987). This revealed a prominent cleft in the membrane-distal part of the molecule, which subsequent studies have shown to be the site of antigen binding. A similar structure has been described for class II MHC molecules (Brown *et al.*, 1993; Stern *et al.*, 1994) although the antigenic peptides that associate with class II are longer (13 to 17 amino acids) than those bound to class I (eight to ten amino acids). Much of the sequence polymorphism in MHC molecules occurs in and around the peptide-binding region and, although this variation does not affect the overall structure of the peptide-binding groove, it results in subtle differences that influence the nature of the peptides that each molecule will bind. Thus, each individual class I molecule tends to bind a different repertoire of peptides (Sette *et al.*, 1987; Rothbard and Gefter, 1991), so that T cells from animals expressing different MHC molecules will often recognize different epitopes from the same pathogen, and in some cases these epitopes may be on different proteins.

Although this variation might be expected to result in quantitative differences in the immune response to pathogens, and hence differences in susceptibility to disease, there are relatively few well-documented examples of strong associations of MHC with susceptibility to infectious disease in outbred species. This probably reflects the large number of potential T cell epitopes in most pathogens and the fact that most animals in an outbred population will be heterozygous and therefore will express several class I or class II molecules. Variations in the epitopes that are selected in individual animals may, however, affect the strain specificity of the T cell response if some of the epitopes vary between pathogen strains (Vitiello and Sherman, 1983).

As already indicated, the TCR recognizes a combination of self MHC molecule and bound peptide. Since the region of the MHC molecule recognized by the TCR, i.e. the peptide-binding groove, is polymorphic, each T cell will only recognize an antigenic peptide associated with a particular MHC molecule. This phenomenon, known as MHC-restriction (Doherty, Blanden and Zinkernagel, 1976), has important practical implications for studies of T cell responses in outbred animals; T cells from one animal will recognize antigen presented on the animal's own antigen-presenting cells but will not recognize the same antigen on presenting cells from another animal of a different MHC phenotype.

Until recently, the capacity of a given MHC molecule to bind a large number of different antigenic peptides was difficult to explain. However, studies carried out over the last four years, involving the isolation and sequencing of peptides bound to class I molecules, have helped to resolve this issue. The heterogeneous mixture of peptides isolated from an individual class I molecule were found to be conserved at one or two residues, usually at positions 2 and 9, and these conserved amino acids were shown to be essential for binding the peptides to the respective MHC molecule (Matsumura *et al.*, 1992; Rammensee, Falk and Rotzschke, 1993). Thus, the amino acids at these positions represent an MHC binding motif, the antigenic specificity of the peptide being determined by amino acids at other positions. Information on the binding motif of a particular MHC molecule can be used to predict possible T cell epitopes within proteins of known amino acid sequences. There is some evidence that similar characteristics determine the binding of peptides to class II molecules (Rudensky *et al.*, 1992) although this has proved difficult to substantiate.

T cell subpopulations recognize antigen processed in different subcellular compartments

The identification of the cell surface molecules, CD4 and CD8, as markers for the two major subpopulations of T cells in mammals was followed by the demonstration that $CD4^+$ T cells recognize antigen presented by class II MHC molecules whereas $CD8^+$ T cells recognize antigen presented by class I MHC molecules. These interactions are accompanied by binding of the CD4 and CD8 molecules to conserved regions on the presenting class II and class I MHC molecules, respectively. $CD4^+$ T cells were shown to mediate help for B cell responses and delayed-type hypersensitivity reactions whereas $CD8^+$ T cells were responsible for cell-mediated cytotoxicity of virus-infected cells. However, for some time the factors that determined whether an antigen was presented by class I or class II MHC molecules were unclear. This was resolved by studies which showed that class I and class II molecules bind peptides generated within different subcellular compartments of antigen-presenting cells. Antigens derived from organisms that replicate in the cytoplasm of cells are degraded by proteases within the cytosol and the resultant antigenic peptides are transported into the endoplasmic reticulum where they associate with newly synthesized class I MHC molecules destined for the cell surface (van Bleek and Nathenson, 1992). By contrast, organisms or proteins taken into antigen-presenting cells by phagocytosis or endocytosis undergo enzymatic degradation within endosomes and associate within an endosomal compartment with newly synthesised class II MHC molecules transported from the Golgi apparatus before being expressed on the cell surface (Brodsky, 1992; Unanue, 1992).

These alternative routes of antigen processing are known as the endogenous and exogenous pathways, respectively. Clearly, processing of antigens by the endogenous pathway and presentation by class I will be confined to organisms, such as viruses and some bacteria and protozoa, that replicate intracellularly (in the cytoplasm). The killing of such infected cells by CD8⁺ T lymphocytes can occur early in the replication cycle and thus represents an effective means of limiting multiplication of the pathogens.

Heterogeneity of CD4⁺ T lymphocyte function

Mosmanm *et al.* (1986), working with mouse T cell clones, described two types of CD4⁺ T cell, termed Th1 and Th2, that were distinguished by the cytokines they produced. This and subsequent studies established that activated Th1 cells secrete interleukin 2 (IL-2) and interferon-γ (IFN-γ) but not IL-4, IL-5, IL-10 and IL-13, whereas the converse applies to activated Th2 cells (Mosmann and Coffman, 1989). A similar dichotomy has been reported for human T cells (Weiranga *et al.*, 1990).

Studies of murine models of parasitic infections have proved invaluable in elucidating the biological significance of the differences in Th1 and Th2 cells. Infection of mice with *Leishmania major*, or immunization with *Leishmania* antigens, can induce either Th1 or Th2 T cell responses, depending on the strain of mouse and route of immunization. Th1 responses result in the control of infection and immunity, whereas Th2 responses lead to enhanced disease (Liew, 1990). This is just one of a growing number of examples in which the outcome of infection is strongly influenced by the cytokine profile of the responding T cells. The induction of Th1 responses in mice is associated with the activation of macrophages, the production of antibody of the IgG_{2a} isotype and the detection of delayed-type hypersensitivity reactions, while Th2 responses give rise to eosinophilia and production of antibody of the IgG_1 and IgE isotypes. The latter characteristics feature prominently in many helminth infections and there is evidence that Th2 responses are beneficial for the control of enteric nematode infections (Else and Grencis, 1991; Urban *et al.*, 1992).

Studies of the biological activities of the cytokines produced by Th1 and Th2 cells have demonstrated strong cross-regulation operating between the subsets: IFN-γ produced by Th1 cells inhibits the induction of Th2 responses and both IL-4 and IL-10 have inhibitory effects on the induction of Th1 responses (Mosmann *et al.*, 1991; Fitch *et al.*, 1993). Thus, the initial induction of a strong Th1 or Th2 response will tend to inhibit responses by the reciprocal subset. Nevertheless, in some infections, notably *Schistosoma mansoni* in mice, an initial Th1 response is followed by a switch to a Th2 response (Pearce *et al.*, 1991). The switch is believed to reflect the presence of antigens in the parasite eggs with a strong propensity for inducing Th2 responses. This may represent a deliberate strategy by the parasite to favour survival of the adult worms. The parameters that determine whether an antigen will stimulate a strong Th1 or Th2 response are poorly understood. However, there is evidence that the biochemical nature of the antigen and the type of antigen-presenting cell in which it is presented to T cells are important contributory factors.

IMPLICATIONS FOR VACCINE DEVELOPMENT

Induction of antibody responses

In the early 1980s, a series of studies demonstrated that antibodies raised against intact proteins recognized short peptide fragments of the proteins (Geyson, Meloen and Barteling, 1984). These observations encouraged the belief that it would be possible to use synthetic peptides for vaccination. A large number of studies aimed at stimulating immunity with peptides were undertaken, in which animals were immunized with synthetic peptides representing B cell epitopes, conjugated either to other peptides from the same pathogen or to unrelated proteins, to provide the necessary T helper cell epitopes. With a few exceptions, these attempts at immunization were unsuccessful. In many instances, the synthetic peptides completely failed to induce antibodies against the parent protein or organism while, in other cases, antibody responses did occur but were at best only partially effective.

Subsequent studies of protein structure have highlighted the fact that so-called linear epitopes have a degree of conformation and that this conformation may differ subtly from that adopted by the respective synthetic peptides. The process of conjugating a peptide to a carrier molecule may also affect the conformation of the peptide, resulting in antibodies of low avidity for the pathogen in question.

One pathogen for which a degree of success has been achieved by immunization with a synthetic peptide is foot-and-mouth disease virus. Immunization with a peptide consisting of two linked peptide sequences representing residues 141-158 and 200-213 of the VP1 capsid protein resulted in a proportion of immunized cattle (Di Marchi *et al.*, 1986). Structural studies of the virus demonstrated that the 141-158 component of the peptide corresponds to a superficial loop on the surface of the virus particle (Acharya *et al.*, 1989) and suggested that the peptide successfully reproduces this loop structure. Nevertheless, it is still unclear whether the failure to achieve protection in all animals immunized with the peptide was due to subtle conformational differences in the antibody recognition site or to inadequacies in the helper T cell response.

Another factor that may limit the success of immunization with peptides is the use of an unrelated carrier protein to stimulate T cell help for antibody production. No anamnestic T cell response will occur following the challenge of immunized animals with the pathogen, and immunity will therefore rely largely on the pre-existing antibody induced by vaccination.

The use of intact, purified or recombinant proteins for immunization can overcome some of the problems associated with immunization with peptides. Such proteins are likely to contain several T cell epitopes and, if appropriately produced, should have the correct conformation for recognition by antibodies. However, the latter is not always true. For example, the integrity of antibody epitopes on individual viral capsid proteins may be dependent on the structural interaction with other protein components of the capsid. This is the case for several of the neutralizing epitopes on the surface of foot-and-mouth disease virus; of the three capsid proteins only one (VP1) retains any immunogenicity following purification, and it is much less immunogenic than killed intact virus (Bachrach *et al.*, 1975).

The methods by which recombinant proteins are produced can also affect the integrity of epitopes recognized by antibodies. Thus, if glycosylation is required for antibody recognition, production of the proteins in bacteria will be inappropriate and proteins produced in insect cells may be defective because of differences in the sugar side chains added by these cells compared with mammalian cells. Differences in the folding of proteins produced in bacteria may also result in the disruption of some B cell epitopes.

The need for multiple T cell epitopes

Since T lymphocytes recognize small processed fragments of antigens, the conformational structure of antigens is generally not a constraint for the induction of T cell responses. However, because T cells from animals of different MHC types tend to recognize different peptide sequences within an antigen, immunization with short polypeptides containing only one or two potential T cell epitopes is likely to induce a response in only a proportion of animals. This will be true both for T helper cell responses for antibody production and for effector T cell responses. This further strengthens the argument for using one or more intact proteins in subunit vaccines so that there will be sufficient numbers of potential T cell epitopes to ensure that the majority of individuals within an outbred population will respond to the antigens. In some circumstances, there may be a case for excluding particular T cell epitopes from a vaccine construct. For example, if an antigen contains a particularly dominant T cell epitope that is variable between strains of a pathogen, exclusion of such an epitope might result in a response that is less strain-specific.

Constraints on stimulation of $CD8^+$ T cell responses

Because of the need for antigen to be processed by the endogenous pathway for recognition by $CD8^+$ T cells, the immunization of animals with killed organisms or their component proteins generally fails to induce $CD8^+$ T cell responses. Therefore, alternative antigen delivery systems must be considered when developing subunit vaccines required to stimulate $CD8^+$ T cell responses. These could include the use of virus vectors or vaccination with "naked" DNA, both of which result in the expression of proteins within the cell cytosol. Recent studies have also provided evidence that the active component of the adjuvant saponin, when used to prepare antigen-complexed structures known as immunostimulating complexes (ISCOMs), facilitates the transfer of antigen across cell membranes and the induction of $CD8^+$ T cell responses (Takahashi *et al.*, 1990).

Influencing the cytokine response

The recognition that the cytokines produced by $CD4^+$ T cells to a large extent determine their function and that antigenic stimulation may result in the activation of T cells producing different patterns of cytokines is of major importance when considering immunization strategies. It is, therefore, desirable to know whether the protective responses against the target pathogens involve Th1 or Th2 $CD4^+$ T cell responses. However, since the early events in antigen processing that result in a bias to Th1 or Th2 responses are still incompletely understood, strategies for preferential induction of one or other response are not yet well established. The use of adjuvants that give a bias in the response, for example the induction of Th1 responses by mycobacteria, is one approach that can be pursued. Experiments in mice involving administration of recombinant cytokines or cytokine-specific antibodies at the time of immunization have implicated IL-4 and IL-12 as promoters of Th2 or Th1 cell responses, respectively (Swain *et al.*, 1991; Locksley, 1993). These findings indicate that, by administering cytokines with antigen or by including cytokine genes in molecular vaccine constructs, it may be possible to influence the cytokine profile of T cell responses.

More than one mechanism of immunity

It is becoming increasingly apparent that immunity against a given pathogen may be achieved by alternative immune mechanisms. This is clearly the case with complex protozoan parasites which undergo differentiation through several developmental stages that differ antigenically and replicate in different cell types. Thus, with malaria parasites, antibody against the infective sporozoite stage can block infection, class I MHC-restricted cytotoxic T cell responses are generated against the hepatic intracellular stages and other, as yet poorly understood, cell-mediated mechanisms operate against the intra-erythrocytic stages.

Similarly, different mechanisms may operate against migratory helminth parasites. However, there is also evidence that more than one immune mechanism may be effective in the control of virus infections. For example, it is well established that maternally derived antibody protects offspring from infection with the morbilliviruses (measles, rinderpest) and also interferes with vaccination (Albrecht *et al.*, 1977). Yet a proportion of cattle successfully immunized against rinderpest virus with a recombinant vaccinia virus expressing the F glycoprotein were found to produce little or no rinderpest-specific antibody (Yilma *et al.*, 1988; Belsham *et al.*, 1989), indicating that immunity must have been mediated by T cell responses. Similar results have been obtained with infectious bursal disease virus in chickens, using a recombinant avipox virus expressing the VP2 protein, although the immunity achieved with the recombinant was incomplete (Bayliss *et al.*, 1991).

Clearly, if sufficient antibody of appropriate specificity and biological activity is present in an immunized animal to prevent infection with the respective virus, cell-mediated effector mechanisms will not be required for protection. However, if some of the challenge virus escapes initial neutralization by antibody, it is likely that cell-mediated immune responses will be beneficial, if not essential, for clearance of the infection. This will be particularly true for viruses that spread by cell to cell contact. There may also be some flexibility in the type of T cell response that is employed. In mice immunized against influenza A virus, the transfer of either $CD4^+$ or $CD8^+$ T cells into native recipients resulted in the clearance of challenge virus, the important common feature being the cytokines produced by the two cell types (Lukacher *et al.*, 1986). With viruses such as that which causes foot-and-mouth disease, and for which antibody responses are undoubtedly of major importance in mediating immunity, T cell-mediated responses may provide an additional mechanism for clearing the virus. Yet the role of T cell effector mechanisms in foot-and-mouth disease has been largely ignored.

These observations indicate that the induction of highly effective immunity with subunit vaccines may necessitate the inclusion of more than one antigenic component in a vaccine and the use of an antigen delivery system that is effective at inducing both humoral and cell-mediated immune responses. The poor efficacy of some of the currently used killed vaccines may be due in part to their limited ability to stimulate T cell-mediated components of the protective immune responses.

Pathogens that subvert host immune responses

A common objective in the development of a vaccine is to mimic the immune responses that occur during recovery from natural infection. While this is an appropriate approach for many pathogens, some organisms have evolved stratagems for modifying host immune responses in order to establish persistent infections. Helminth and protozoan parasites have been particularly adept at developing a variety of escape mechanisms. One of the strategies employed by parasites such as *Leishmania* sp. and *Schistosoma* sp. is to direct the T cell response to produce cytokines that are inappropriate for parasite clearance (Sher *et al.*, 1992). In the case of *Sehistosoma mansoni*, this results in the development of characteristic egg granulomas that are responsible for clinical disease. Nevertheless, schistosome-infected (SCID) mice, which are unable to mount a granulomatous response, develop severe hepatitis that is believed to be due to release the of parasite proteases (Amira *et al.*, 1993). Thus, the "deviated" immune response not only favours parasite persistence but may also have a role in protecting and ensuring the survival of the host, albeit with some pathology. Any approach to designing a vaccine for such parasites must be based on an understanding of which components of the host's immune response are responsible for protection as well as on ensuring the avoidance of immune responses that potentiate disease.

Bloodsucking ectoparasites have developed a number of mechanisms to avoid the clotting of imbibed blood and to minimize adverse effects of inflammatory mediators released at the site of feeding. In the case of ticks, which feed continuously for several days, significant hypersensitivity reactions are induced by salivary proteins. While in previously exposed animals this results in a reduction in the number of ticks that engorge, such animals still carry significant tick burdens (Willadsen, 1980). Over the last ten years, researchers in Australia have developed an alternative strategy for vaccination against the one-host tick *Boophilus microplus* based on immunization with proteins from the tick gut, to which the host is not normally exposed (Willadsen, McKenna and Riding, 1988; Willadsen *et al.*, 1989). Antibody induced by these "concealed" antigens, when ingested by the tick, causes damage to the gut wall and results not only in tick mortality but also in a markedly reduced fecundity of surviving ticks. A similar approach is also being pursued for vaccination against the bloodsucking nematode *Haemonchus contortus*.

Several of the large DNA viruses have evolved molecular mechanisms that could potentially modify antiviral immune responses. The vaccinia virus genome contains a number of genes with homology to host receptors for the cytokines IL-1, IL-6 and IFN-γ. Some of these genes are expressed as soluble proteins (virokines) that are able to bind the respective cytokines (Smith, 1993). There is also evidence that serine protease inhibitors expressed by vaccinia may inhibit intracytosolic processing of antigens destined for association with class I MHC (Townsend *et al.*, 1988). Several of the herpesviruses and adenoviruses have been shown to express genes that inhibit the assembly of class I MHC molecules (Lippé *et al.*, 1991; Hill *et al.*, 1994). Identification of the precise role of these genes in determining the virulence of the viruses and their immunogenicity is relevant not only for understanding the pathogenesis of disease caused by the viruses but also in considering the use of animal poxviruses and herpesviruses as vaccine vectors.

NEW APPROACHES TO VACCINE DESIGN

Molecularly defined attenuation

The simplest way of producing a vaccine that mimics the immune responses induced by natural infection is to select an attenuated mutant. The use of live organisms also has the advantage of providing longer-lasting immunity than can be attained with killed antigen. Many of the traditional vaccines are based on the use of attenuated organisms that were either identified by chance or selected by the prolonged culture of the organisms. Advances in knowledge of the molecular structure of viruses and of the function of individual genes in replication and assembly now provide the opportunity to produce targeted mutations that result in altered virulence. The deletion of whole genes negates the possibility of reversion to virulence as a consequence of point mutations. Moreover, viruses with mutations in several genes can be produced. A strain of pseudorabies virus (Aujeszky's disease virus), in which the genes encoding the GI glycoprotein and thymidine kinase have been disrupted, has been shown to be avirulent and to stimulate immunity against challenge with native virus (Moormann *et al.*, 1990). This virus is being marketed as an attenuated vaccine.

A similar approach is being used with bacteria by targeting genes involved in bacterial metabolism. The most thoroughly investigated system is *Salmonella* spp., in which mutation of a number of genes has been shown to result in attenuated organisms that retain immunogenicity (Dougan, Hormaeche and Maskell, 1987). Again, the incorporation of double or triple mutations minimizes the risk of reversion to virulence. The best characterized of these are the *aro* mutants (Dougan *et al.*, 1988), in which the mutations interrupt the pathway for biosynthesis of aromatic metabolites resulting in organisms that are dependent on nutritional elements not available in mammalian tissues. Such *aro* mutants have been used successfully to vaccinate calves against *Salmonella typhimurium* (Jones *et al.*, 1991).

Immunization with recombinant proteins

The use of purified recombinant proteins for vaccination can be considered where specific antigens have been identified as the targets for protective antibody and/or $CD4^+$ T cell responses. However, as already indicated, the expression system used to produce the protein should not alter important antibody recognition sites on the protein. Generally, recombinant proteins need to be administered in a potent adjuvant.

The human hepatitis B vaccine, which consists of recombinant viral core protein, is the most notable success in this area (McAleer *et al.*, 1984); immunity has been achieved with antigen produced in *Escherichia coli* or in yeast. Recently, a vaccine for *Boophilus microplus* tick infestation in cattle, based on the production in *E. coli* of an antigen that is normally expressed in the tick gut, has been put into commercial production in Australia (Willadsen *et al.*, 1989; Rand *et al.*, 1989). A recombinant protein from the tapeworm *Taenia ovis* has been shown to be effective at immunizing sheep against tapeworm infestation (Johnson *et al.*, 1989), and immunization of cattle with a recombinant sporozoite surface antigen from *Theileria parva* has been found to protect a proportion of animals against experimental challenge (Musoke *et al.*, 1992).

Production of virus capsids

The capacity of the hepatitis B core protein to assemble spontaneously into virus-like particles (McAleer *et al.*, 1984) may partly account for the success of this vaccine, since assembly should allow the protein to adopt a conformation similar to that of the native virus particle.

In the case of non-enveloped viruses in which the capsid is composed of several proteins, the surface conformation adopted by each protein in the virus particle is dependent on interactions with the other proteins. Thus, the isolated proteins are often poorly immunogenic. This problem may be overcome if non-infectious viral capsids can be produced by expressing all of the capsid proteins in a single construct. This has been achieved with bluetongue virus (Roy, 1992). Bluetongue virus, the prototype of the orbiviruses, is made up of seven proteins, three of which are within an inner core surrounded by two concentric protein layers formed by VP3 and VP7. The remaining two proteins, VP2 and VP5, are attached to the outer VP7 layer. Empty virus-like particles have been produced by expressing the four main structural proteins (VP2, VP3, VP5 and VP7) in a single recombinant baculovirus. These particles closely resemble native virus particles in structure. Immunization experiments in sheep have shown that they protect against challenge with bluetongue virus of the homologous serotype and that they are much more immunogenic than purified VP2 or VP5 proteins (Roy, French and Erasmus, 1992).

Similar studies are under way with foot-and-mouth disease virus.

Live vectors

The potential use of viruses or bacteria as live vectors for vaccination has been a major focus of experimental investigation over the last ten years. Vectors may be naturally occurring apathogenic organisms or attenuated mutants produced by genetic manipulation. Such vectors offer many of the advantages of live vaccines and can potentially be used to express antigens from more than one pathogen. The virus vectors in particular provide a means of inducing $CD8^+$ T cell responses, which are not readily generated by killed vaccines.

Initial studies of virus vectors were focused on vaccinia, which had already been used with great success in smallpox vaccination programmes and was known to have a wide host range (Mackett and Smith, 1986). Being a poxvirus, it also had a large genome in which non-essential regions could be identified for the insertion of foreign genes. Recombinant vaccinia viruses expressing viral genes have been used successfully in experimental studies to immunize cattle against rinderpest and vesicular stomatitis and dogs and foxes against rabies (Yilma *et al.*, 1988; Belsham *et al.*, 1989; Blancou *et al.*, 1986). Field vaccination of foxes against rabies, using baits containing a vaccinia recombinant, has also been successful. Despite these successes and the demonstrated safety of the vaccines employed, concern has been expressed about the widespread release of vaccinia now that smallpox vaccination has stopped. Consequently, attention has turned to animal poxviruses.

Capripox virus, which infects cattle, sheep and goats, is found throughout large areas of Asia and Africa where it causes sporadic outbreaks of disease. An attenuated strain of the virus that had been used locally in Africa to vaccinate against the disease (Kitching, Hammond and Taylor, 1987) has been developed as a vector, and recombinant viruses expressing rinderpest virus glycoproteins have been shown to protect cattle against challenge with rinderpest virus (Romero *et al.*, 1993). A disadvantage of the capripox virus is that it cannot be used outside the areas where infection is endemic owing to its notifiable status. Nevertheless, there are many potential applications of this vector in Africa and Asia.

Avipox and canarypox viruses have been developed as potential vaccine vectors and the former has been used successfully to vaccinate chickens against Newcastle disease and infectious bursal disease (Boursnell *et al.*, 1990a and 1990b; Bayliss *et al.*, 1991). These viruses can also be considered as vectors for mammals, since they produce abortive infections in mammalian cells, i.e. the synthesis of virus proteins occurs but no infectious virus is produced; there is therefore no risk of the virus spreading to other animals.

The herpesviruses have large genomes which, like that of the poxviruses, can accommodate large inserts of foreign DNA. The potential of a number of animal herpesviruses to serve as vaccine vectors is currently being explored. These include pseudorabies virus, bovine herpesvirus 1, equine herpesvirus 1 and turkey herpesvirus. Adenoviruses are also being investigated, particularly in the context of delivering antigens to mucosal surfaces.

The coexpression of cytokine genes and foreign antigens in virus vectors offers a potential means of enhancing or modulating immune responses to the expressed antigens. Experiments with vaccinia virus in mice have yielded promising results with a number of cytokines (Ramshaw *et al.*, 1992). This approach may be of particular value in providing a bias towards Th1 or Th2 T cell responses.

Attenuated mutant strains of several different *Salmonella* species have been studied extensively for their potential as vaccine vectors (Dougan, Hormaeche and Maskell, 1987; Dougan *et al.*, 1988). Foreign antigens can be expressed from plasmids or following the integration of the genes into the bacterial genome. Much of this work has been carried out in mice and has focused on the induction of immune responses to other bacterial antigens and on the capacity to stimulate immunity at gut mucosal surfaces. Mice immunized with a *Salmonella* recombinant expressing a malaria circumsporozoite antigen were found to be protected against malaria in the absence of antibodies (Sadoff *et al.*, 1988). Since this immunity is mediated by $CD8^+$ T cells, this finding suggests that *Salmonella* spp. may be able to introduce antigens into the endogenous processing pathway.

A variety of other bacteria are being investigated as potential vaccine vectors. Because of its potent capacity to stimulate Th1 T cell responses, the mycobacterium bacillus Calmette-Guérin (BCG) may have particular utility as a vector. A recombinant BCG expressing a surface antigen from the protozoan parasite *Leishmania major* has been shown to protect mice against cutaneous leishmaniasis (Connell *et al.*, 1993), a disease that is known to require Th1 responses for immunity.

Immunization with nucleic acids

The recent discovery that the injection of DNA into animals can result in immune responses to proteins encoded by the DNA has opened up a completely new approach to the development of subunit vaccines. Vaccination of mice with plasmids containing the influenza haemagglutinin gene has been shown to result in protection against virus challenge (Ulmer *et al.*, 1993; Fynan *et al.*, 1993). The injected genes appear to be expressed within host cells without integration of plasmid into chromosomal DNA. While studies of the transfection efficiency of injected DNA have shown that muscle is 100 to 1 000 times more permissive than other tissues, protection has also been achieved following inoculation by the intravenous, intranasal and intratracheal routes and by delivering the DNA intradermally using a "gene gun". The immunization of mice with DNA induces antibody responses as well as $CD4^+$ and $CD8^+$ T cell responses. The induction of immune responses to bovine herpesvirus 1 in cattle has been investigated in one study (Cox, Zamb and Babiuk, 1993); a plasmid containing the gII viral gene stimulated neutralizing antibodies and resulted in a marked reduction in nasal shedding of the virus following challenge.

Targeting of antigen at mucosal surfaces

The stimulation of protective immune responses at mucosal surfaces presents a particularly challenging problem because of the requirement for such responses to be induced locally. Non-viable antigen administered orally is susceptible to proteolytic degradation and is absorbed in only small amounts through the gut wall. Moreover, such "dietary" antigens tend to induce tolerance rather than an active immune response. One way of overcoming this problem is to use bacterial or viral vectors, such as *Salmonella* spp. or adenovirus, which replicate in the alimentary tract.

Other strategies that facilitate the uptake of protein in the gut and the induction of an active response are currently being investigated. One of these involves the use of cholera toxin, which is a multimeric protein composed of a single A subunit and a pentameric B subunit; binding to epithelial cells occurs by interaction of the B subunit with GM_1-gangliosides while toxicity is mediated by ADP-ribosyl-transferase activity of the A subunit (Spangler, 1992). Oral administration of either subpathogenic doses of intact toxin or purified B subunits results in induction of a specific immune response. Moreover, protein antigens administered along with, or covalently linked to, the toxin or its B subunit elicit strong antibody and $CD4^+$ T cell responses (Dertzbaugh and Elson, 1993). Whether or not the B subunit retains the full adjuvant activity of the intact toxin has not been fully resolved.

Another approach to delivering antigens to the gut is to encapsulate antigen in microspheres with an outer biodegradable polymer coat that protects the antigen against rapid enzymatic degradation. Microspheres with a diameter of 5 to 10 µm have been shown to be taken up efficiently by the Peyer's patches and to induce IgG and IgA antibody responses in mice.

CONCLUDING REMARKS

In the last decade, a clear picture has emerged of how antigens are processed and recognized by the immune system and significant progress has been made in understanding the immune mechanisms that operate against different types of pathogens. This new knowledge, together with further advances in technologies for genetic manipulation, has led to a variety of new approaches to the attenuation of pathogenic organisms and to the design of antigen delivery systems appropriate for inducing particular immune responses. There has also been progress in other areas of research, not discussed here, such as the targeting of antigens at particular cell types in the immune system and studies to develop new adjuvants and understand their mode of action. These developments offer exciting potential for the production of a new generation of vaccines.

BIBLIOGRAPHY

Acharya, R., Fry, E., Stuart, D., Fox, G., Rowlands, D. & Brown, F. 1989. The three-dimensional structure of foot-and-mouth disease virus at 2.9 Å resolution. *Nature,* 337: 709-716.

Albrecht, P., Ennis, F.A., Saltzman, E.J. & Krugman, S. 1977. Persistence of internal antibody in infants beyond 12 months: mechanism of measles vaccine failure. *J. Paediat.,* 91: 715-719.

Amira, F., Locksley, R.M., Parslow, T., Sadick, M., Rector, E., Ritter, D. & McKerrow, J. 1993. Tumour necrosis factor-γ restores granulomas and induces egg laying in schistosome-infected (SCID) mice. *Nature,* 356 :604-607.

Bachrach, H.L., Moore, D.M., McKercher, P.D. & Polatnick, J. 1975. Immune and antibody responses to an isolated capsid protein of foot-and-mouth disease virus. *J. Immunol.,* 115: 1636-1641.

Bayliss, C.D., Peters, R.W., Cook, J.K.A., Reece, R.L., Howes, K., Binns, M.M. & Boursnell, M.E.G. 1991. A recombinant fowlpox virus that expresses the VP2 antigen of infectious bursal disease virus induces protection against mortality caused by the virus. *Arch. Virol.,* 120: 193-205.

Belsham, G.J., Anderson, E.C., Murray, P.K., Anderson, J. & Barrett, T. 1989. Immune response and protection of cattle and pigs generated by a vaccine virus recombinant expressing the F protein of rinderpest virus. *Vet. Rec.,* 124: 655-658.

Bjorkman, P.J., Saper, M.A., Samraoui, B., Bennett, W.S., Strominger, J.L. & Wiley, D.C. 1987. The foreign antigen site and T cell recognition regions of class I histocompatibility antigens. *Nature,* 329: 512-518.

Blancou, J., Kieny, M.P., Lathe, R., Lecocq, J.P., Pastoret, P.P., Soulebot, J.P. & Desmettre, P. 1986. Oral vaccination of the fox against rabies using a live recombinant vaccinia virus. *Nature,* 322: 373-375.

Bodmer, W. 1984. The major histocompatibility system: structure and function: summary and synthesis. *In* Y. Yamamura & T. Tada, eds. *Progress in Immunology V. Fifth Int. Congr. Immunology,* p. 959-970. Tokyo, Academic Press Japan.

Boursnell, M.E.G., Green, P.F., Campbell, J.I.A., Deuter, A., Peters, R.W., Tomley, F.M., Samson, A.C.R., Emmerson, P.T. & Binns, M.M. 1990a. A fowlpox virus vaccine vector with insertion sites in the terminal repeats: demonstration of its efficacy using a fusion gene of Newcastle disease virus. *Vet. Microbiol.,* 23: 305-316.

Boursnell, M.E.G., Green, P.F., Campbell, J.I.A., Deuter, A., Peters, R.W., Tomley, F.M., Samson, A.C.R., Chambers, P., Emmerson, P.T. & Binns, M.M. 1990b. Insertion of the fusion gene from Newcastle disease virus into a non-essential region in the terminal repeats of fowlpox virus and demonstration of protective immunity induced by the recombinant. *J. Gen. Virol.,* 71: 621-628.

Brodsky, F.M. 1992. Antigen processing and presentation: close encounters in the endocytic pathway. *Trends Cell Biol.,* 2: 109-115.

Brodsky, F.M. & Guagliardi, L.E. 1991. The cell biology of antigen processing and presentation. *Annu. Rev. Immunol.,* 9: 707-744.

Brown, J.H., Jardetzky, T.S., Gorga, J.C., Stern, L.J., Urban, R.G., Strominger, J.L. & Wiley, D.C. 1993. Three-dimensional structure of the human class II histocompatibility antigen HLA-DR1. *Nature,* 364: 33-39.

Connell, N.D., Medina-Acosta, E., McMaster, W.R., Bloom, B.R. & Russell, D.G. 1993. Effective immunization against cutaneous leishmaniasis with recombinant bacille Calmette-Guérin expressing the *Leishmania* surface proteinase gp63. *Proc. Natl Acad. Sci. USA,* 90: 11473-11477.

Cooper, M.D. & Burrows, P.D. 1989. B cell differentiation. *In* T. Honjo, F.W. Alt & T.H. Rabbits, eds. *Immunoglobulin genes,* p. 1-21. San Diego, Calif., USA, Academic.

Cox, J.M., Zamb, T.J. & Babiuk, L.A. 1993. Bovine herpesvirus 1: immune responses in mice and cattle injected with plasmid DNA. *J. Virol.,* 67(9): 5664-5667.

Davis, M.M. & Bjorkman, P.J. 1988. T-cell antigen receptor genes and T cell recognition. *Nature,* 334: 395-401.

Dertzbaugh, M.T. & Elson, C.O. 1993. Comparative effectiveness of cholera toxin B subunit and alkaline phosphatase as carriers for oral vaccines. *Infect. Immunol.,* 61: 48-55.

Di Marchi, R., Brooke, G., Gale, C., Cracknell, V., Doel, T. & Mowat, N. 1986. Protection of cattle against foot-and-mouth disease by a synthetic peptide. *Science,* 232: 639-641.

Doherty, P.C., Blanden, R.V. & Zinkernagel, R.M. 1976. Specificity of virus-immune effector T cells for H-2K and H-2D compatible interactions: implications for H-antigen diversity. *Transplant. Rev.,* 29: 89-124.

Dougan, G., Hormaeche, C.E. & Maskell, D.J. 1987. Live oral *Salmonella* vaccines: potential use of attenuated strains as carriers of heterologous antigens to the immune system. *Parasite Immunol.,* 9: 151-160.

Dougan, G., Chatfield, S., Pickard, D., Bester, J., O'Callaghan, D. & Maskell, D.J. 1988. Construction and characterisation of vaccine strains of *Salmonella* harbouring mutations in two different *aro* genes. *J. Inf. Dis.,* 158: 1329-1335.

Else, K.J. & Grencis, R.K. 1991. Cellular immune responses to the murine nematode parasite *Trichuris muris.* I. Differential cytokine production during acute or chronic infection. *Immunology,* 72: 508-513.

Fitch, F.W., McKisic, M.D., Lancki, D.W. & Gajewski, T.F. 1993. Differential regulation of murine lymphocyte subsets. *Annu. Rev. Immunol.*, 11: 29-48.

Fynan, E.F., Webster, R.G., Fuller, D.H., Haynes, J.R., Santoro, J.C. & Robinson, H.L. 1993. DNA vaccines: protective immunizations by parenteral, mucosal, and gene-gun inoculations. *Proc. Natl Acad. Sci. USA*, 90: 11478-11482.

Geyson, H.M., Meloen, R.H. & Barteling, S.J. 1984. Use of peptide synthesis to probe viral antigens for epitopes to a resolution of a single amino acid. *Proc. Natl Acad. Sci. USA*, 81: 3998-4002.

Hill, A.B., Barnett, B.C., McMichael, A.J. & McGeoch, D.J. 1994. HLA class I molecules are not transported to the cell surface in cells infected with herpes simplex virus types 1 and 2. *J. Immunol.*, 152: 2736-2741.

Johnson, K.S., Harrison, G.B.L., Lightowlers, M.W., O'Hoy, K.L., Cougle, W.G., Dempster, R.P., Lawrence, S.B., Vinton, J.G., Heath, D.D. & Rickard, M.D. 1989. Vaccination against ovine cysticerosis using a defined recombinant antigen. *Nature*, 338: 585-587.

Jones, P.W., Dougan, G., Hayward, N., MacKenzie, N., Collins, P. & Chatfield, S.N. 1991. Oral vaccination of calves against experimental salmonellosis using a double *aro* mutant of *Salmonella typhimurium*. *Vaccine*, 9: 29-34.

Kitching, R.P., Hammond, J.M. & Taylor, W.P. 1987. A single vaccine for the control of capripox infection in sheep and goats. *Res. Vet. Sci.*, 42: 53-60.

Liew, F.Y. 1990. Regulation of cell-mediated immunity to leishmaniasis. *In* S.H.E. Kaufmann, ed. T-cell paradigms in parasitic and bacterial infections. *Curr. Top. Microbiol. Immunol.*, 155: 53-64.

Lippé, R., Luke, E., Kuah, Y.T., Lomas, C. & Jefferies, W.A. 1991. Adenovirus infection inhibits the phosphorylation of major histocompatibility complex class I proteins. *J. Exp. Med.*, 174: 1159-1166.

Locksley, R. 1993. Interleukin 12 in host defense against microbial pathogens. *Proc. Natl Acad. Sci. USA*, 90: 5879-5880.

Lukacher, A.E., Morrison, L.A., Braciale, V.L. & Braciale, T.J. 1986. T lymphocyte function in recovery from experimental viral infection: the influenza model. *In* R.M. Steinman & R.J. North, eds. *Mechanisms of Host Resistance to Infectious Agents, Tumours and Allografts: A Conference in Recognition of the Trudeau Institute Centenial*, p. 233-254. New York, The Rockefeller University Press.

Mackett, M. & Smith, G.L. 1986. Vaccinia virus expression vectors. *J. Gen. Virol.*, 67: 2067-2082.

Matsumura, M., Fremont, D.H., Peterson, P.A. & Wilson, I.A. 1992. Emerging principles for the recognition of peptide antigens by MHC class I molecules. *Science*, 257: 927-934.

McAleer, W.J., Buynak, E.B., Margetter, R.Z., Wampler, E. & Miller, W.J. 1984. Human hepatitis B vaccines from recombinant yeast. *Nature*, 307: 178-180.

Moormann, R.J.M., de Rover, T., Briaire, J., Peeters, B.P.H., Gielkens, A.L.J. & van Oirschot, J.T. 1990. Inactivation of the thymidine kinase gene of a gI deletion mutant of pseudorabies virus generates a safe but still highly immunogenic vaccine strain. *J. Gen. Virol.*, 71: 1591-1595.

Mosmann, T.R. & Coffman, R.L. 1989. Th1 or Th2 cells: different patterns of lymphokine secretion lead to different functional properties. *Annu. Rev. Immunol.*, 7: 45-173.

Mosmann, T.R., Cherwinski, H., Bond, M.W., Giedlin, M.A. & Coffman, R.L. 1986. Two types of murine helper T cell clone. I. Definition according to profiles of lymphokine activities and secreted proteins. *J. Immunol.*, 136: 2348-2357.

Mosmann, T.R., Schumacher, J.H., Street, N.F., Budd, R., O'Garra, A., Fong, T.A.T., Bond, M.W., Moore, K.W.M., Sher, A. & Fiorentino, D.F. 1991. Diversity of cytokine synthesis and function of mouse CD4+ T cells. *Immunol. Rev.*, 123: 209-229.

Musoke, A.J., Morzaria, S., Nkonge, C., Jones, E. & Nene, V. 1992. A recombinant sporozoite surface antigen of *Theileria parva* induces protection in cattle. *Proc. Natl Acad. Sci. USA*, 89: 514-518.

Pearce, E.J., Caspar, P., Grzych, J.-M., Lewis, F.A. & Sher, A. 1991. Downregulation of Th1 cytokine production accompanies induction of Th2 responses by a parasitic helminth, *Schistosoma mansoni*. *J. Exp. Med.*, 173: 159-166.

Rammensee, H.-G., Falk, K. & Rotzschke, O. 1993. Peptides naturally presented by MHC class I molecules. *Annu. Rev. Immunol.*, 11: 213-244.

Ramshaw, I., Ruby, J., Ramsay, A., Ada, G. & Karupiah, G. 1992. Expression of cytokines by recombinant vaccinia viruses: a model for studying cytokines in virus infections *in vivo*. *Immunol. Rev.*, 127: 157-182.

Rand, K.N., Moore, T., Sriskantha, A., Spring, K., Tellam, R., Willadsen, P. & Cobon, G.S. 1989. Cloning and expression of a protective antigen from the cattle tick *Boophilus microplus*. *Proc. Natl Acad. Sci. USA*, 86: 9657-9661.

Romero, C.H., Barrett, T., Evans, S.A., Kitching, R.P., Gershon, P.D., Bostock, C. & Black, D.N. 1993. A single capripox recombinant vaccine for the protection of cattle against rinderpest and lumpy skin disease. *Vaccine*, 11: 732-742.

Rothbard, J.B. & Gefter, M.L. 1991. Interactions between immunogenic peptides and MHC proteins. *Annu. Rev. Immunol.*, 9: 527-565.

Roy, P. 1992. Bluetongue virus proteins. *J. Gen. Virol.*, 73: 3051-3064.

Roy, P., French, T.J. & Erasmus, B.J. 1992. Protective efficacy of virus-like particles for bluetongue disease. *Vaccine*, 10: 28-32.

Rudensky, A.Y., Preston-Hurlburt, P., Al-Ramadi, B.K., Rothbard, J. & Janeway Jr, C.A. 1992. Truncation variants of peptides isolated from MHC class II molecules suggest sequence motifs. *Nature*, 359: 429-431.

Sadoff, J.C., Ballou, W.R., Baron, L.S., Majarian, W.R., Brey, R.N., Hockmeyer, W.T., Young, J.F., Cryz, S.J., Ou, J., Lowell, G.H. & Chulay, J.D. 1988. Oral *Salmonella typhimurium* vaccine expressing circumsporozoite protein protects against malaria. *Science*, 240: 336-338.

Sette, A., Buus, S., Colon, S., Smith, J.A., Miles, C. & Grey, H.M. 1987. Structural characteristics of an antigen required for its interaction with Ia and recognition by T cells. *Nature*, 328: 395-399.

Sher, A., Gazzinelli, R.T., Oswald, I.P., Clerici, M., Kullberg, M., Pearce, E.J., Berzofsky, J.A., Mosmann, T.R., James, S.L., Morse, H.C. & Shearer, G.M. 1992. Role of T-cell derived cytokines in the downregulation of immune responses in parasitic and retroviral infection. *Immunol. Rev.*, 127: 183-204.

Smith, G.L. 1993. Vaccinia virus glycoproteins and immune evasion. *J. Gen. Virol.*, 74: 1725-1740.

Spangler, B.D. 1992. Structure and function of cholers toxin and the related *Escherichia coli* heat-labile enterotoxin. *Microbiol. Rev.*, 56: 622-647.

Stern, L.J., Brown, J.H., Jardetzky, T.S., Gorga, J.C., Urban, R.G., Strominger, J.L. & Wiley D.C. 1994. Crystal structure of the human class II MHC protein HLA-DR1 complexed with an influenza virus peptide. *Nature*, 368: 215-221.

Swain, S.L., Bradley, L.M., Croft, M., Tonkonogy, S., Atkins, G., Weinberg, A.D., Duncan, D.D., Hendrick, S.M., Dutton, R.W. & Huston, G. 1991. Helper T cell subsets: phenotype function and the role of lymphokine in regulating their development. *Immunol. Rev.*, 123: 115-144.

Takahashi, H., Takeshita, T., Morein, B., Putney, S., Germain, R.N. & Berzofsky,

J.A. 1990. Induction of CD8+ cytotoxic T cells by immunisation with purified HIV-1 envelope protein in ISCOMs. *Nature,* 344: 873-875.

Townsend, A. & Bodmer, H. 1989. Antigen recognition by class I-restricted T lymphocytes. *Annu. Rev. Immunol.,* 7: 601-624.

Townsend, A., Bastin, J., Gould, K., Brownlee, G., Andrew, A., Boyle D.B., Chan, Y. & Smith, G. 1988. Defective presentation to class I-restricted cytotoxic T lymphocytes in vaccinia-infected cells is overcome by enhanced degradation of antigen. *J. Exp. Med.,* 166: 1211-1224.

Trowsdale, J. 1993. Genomic structure and function in the MHC. *Trends Gen.,* 9: 117-122.

Ulmer, J.B., Donnelly, J.J., Parker, S.E., Rhodes, G.H., Felgner, P.L., Dwarki, V.J., Gromkowski, S.H., Deck, R.R., DeWitt, C.M., Friedman, A., Hawe, L.A., Leander, K.R., Martinez, D., Perry, H.C., Shiver, J.W., Montgomery, D.L. & Liu, M.A. 1993. Heterologous protection against influenza by injection of DNA encoding a viral protein. *Science,* 259: 1745-1749.

Unanue, E.R. 1992. Cellular studies on antigen presentation by class II MHC molecules. *Curr. Opin. Immunol.,* 4: 63-69.

Urban, J., Madden, K., Svetic, A., Cheever, A., Trotta, P., Gause, W. & Finkelman, F. 1992. The importance of Th2 cytokines in protective immunity to nematodes. *Immunol. Rev.,* 127: 205-220.

van Bleek, G.M. & Nathenson, S.G. 1992. Presentation of antigenic peptides by MHC class I molecules. *Trends Cell Biol.,* 2: 202-207.

Vitiello, A. & Sherman, L.A. 1983. Recognition of influenza-infected cells by cytolytic T lymphocyte clones: determinant selection by class I restriction elements. *J. Immunol.,* 131: 1635-1640.

Weiranga, E.A., Snook, M., deGroot, C., Chretien, I., Bos, J., Jansen, H. & Kapsenberg, M. 1990. Evidence for compartmentalisation of functional subsets of CD4 T lymphocytes in atopic patients. *J. Immunol.,* 144: 4651-4656.

Willadsen, P. 1980. Immunity to ticks. *Adv. Parasitol.,* 18: 293-313.

Willadsen, P., McKenna, R.V. & Riding, G.A. 1988. Isolation from the cattle tick *Boophilus microplus* of antigenic material capable of eliciting a protective immunological response in the bovine host. *Int. J. Parasitol.,* 18: 183-191.

Willadsen, P., Riding, G.A., McKenna, R.V., Kemp, D.H., Tellam, R.L., Nielsen, J.N. Lahnstein, J., Cobon, G.S. & Gough, J.M. 1989. Immunologic control of a parasitic arthropod: identification of a protective antigen from *Boophilus microplus. J. Immunol.,* 143: 1346-1351.

Yilma, T., Hsu, D., Jones, L., Owens, S., Grubman, M., Mebus, C., Yamanaka, M. & Dale, B. 1988. Protection of cattle against rinderpest with vaccinia recombinants expressing the HA or F gene. *Science,* 242: 1058-1061.

Genetically engineered vaccines

B.W.J. Mahy

Genetic engineering is a term used to describe experimental or industrial approaches to modifying the genome of a living cell without normal sexual or asexual transmission of genetic material. In a broader sense, it is used to describe genetic manipulation of the genome of a virus and is often used synonymously with the term recombinant DNA technology. The ability to manipulate the genome of a living cell or virus was made possible by a series of discoveries made 20 to 30 years ago.

First was the recognition of bacterial restriction enzymes by Arber and Dussoix (1962). These are endonucleases that recognize specific DNA sequences and cleave the DNA only at those sites (Meselson and Yuan, 1968). Coupled with other enzymes involved in DNA synthesis such as ligases (DNA-joining enzymes), it became feasible to introduce deliberately specific foreign DNA sequences into DNA molecules which are then described as recombinant DNA. When the recombinant DNA replicates, the foreign DNA is also replicated. If the foreign DNA is inserted into a bacterial plasmid or phage DNA which undergoes rapid multiplication together with the host bacteria, it is possible to generate large quantities of the foreign DNA. This process is called molecular cloning (Sambrook, Fritsch and Maniantis, 1989).

Another crucial discovery was the existence of reverse transcriptase, an enzyme present in oncogenic RNA viruses and which converts RNA into DNA (Baltimore, 1970). This allowed the conversion of cellular or viral messenger RNAs into DNA so that they could then be molecularly cloned and expressed to produce the polypeptide or protein specified by the original messenger RNA. Bacterial plasmids can serve both as cloning and expression vectors when introduced into appropriate host cells and, in the last few years, a range of expression vectors have become available that will replicate in bacteria, yeast, insect or animal cells to produce large quantities of a desired polypeptide or protein.

Such expressed proteins can be purified to serve as a vaccine antigen, as in the highly successful vaccine against hepatitis B prepared in yeast (*Saccharomyces cerevisiae*), which was the first genetically engineered vaccine licensed for use in humans. Alternatively, if the expression vector will replicate in animal or human cells, the expressed antigen may immunize the recipient host without the need for purification. This is the basis for the development of a wide range of candidate vaccines for both human and veterinary use which depend on recombinant gene expression in an appropriate viral or bacterial vector. Such live recombinant vector vaccines offer great promise but, to date, have not been licensed for use in human subjects.

Recently, the discovery that plasmid DNA sequences can be expressed directly after injection into mouse muscle (Wolff *et al.*, 1990) without the need for a viral or bacterial expression vector has opened up an exciting range of possibilities for the design of vaccines for human or veterinary use through polynucleotide vaccination (Cohen, 1993; Ulmer *et al.*, 1993; Ulmer, Donnelly and Liu, 1994). In addition, since the encoded antigens are expressed intracellularly in the recipient host, they are introduced into class I MHC molecules and this results in the priming of cytotoxic T cells (Townsend and Bodmer, 1989; Barber and Parham, 1994) so that both cellular and humoral immune responses are stimulated (Ulmer *et al.*, 1993).

Finally, the ability to determine the nucleotide sequence of the genomes of DNA or RNA animal viruses has led to a considerable body of research on the structure of the antigens they encode. In addition to expressing the genes in various vectors, attempts have been made to synthesize *in vitro* various polypeptides which correspond to these antigenic determinants or epitopes and to use the peptides themselves as candidate immunogens. Unfortunately, this approach has had only limited practical success, but some important early work was carried out with foot-and-mouth disease (Bittle *et al.*, 1982; Di Marchi *et al.*, 1986).

In this brief overview, the development and future prospects for genetically engineered veterinary vaccines will be described. The various types of vaccine will be considered separately according to the listing given in Table 1.

TABLE 1
Prospective genetically engineered vaccine types

Type	Examples
Attenuated live	Pseudorabies (Aujeszky's disease)
Defective live	ALVAC-FL (feline leukaemia)
Chimeric live	Capripox, rinderpest, lumpy skin disease
Subunit	Bluetongue
DNA polynucleotide	Avian influenza
Polypeptide	Foot-and-mouth disease

GENETICALLY ENGINEERED ATTENUATION

Many conventional vaccines currently employed in human or veterinary medicine contain live micro-organisms or virus that has been attenuated, for example by multiple passages in cell culture, to the point that it will multiply in the recipient host but no longer induce disease. Live vaccines offer several potential advantages compared with killed vaccines in that they usually induce a rapid immune response of long duration and also induce local immunity which may be critical in providing protection against subsequent infection by virulent micro-organisms. However, conventional methods of attenuation rely on spontaneous, random mutations occurring during multiple passages, and the basis for the attenuation is usually not known. An alternative approach is to use genetic engineering to define specific genes or regions of the genome which are responsible for virulence, then delete these in order to obtain a replicating, non-pathogenic virus for use as the immunogen.

This approach has been particularly fruitful with bacteria and DNA viruses with large genomes, such as herpesviruses and poxviruses. Since this type of attenuation involves the removal of parts of the genome, such bacteria and viruses may then be used to vector genes encoding a variety of foreign antigens, creating chimeric vaccines.

The experimental protocol for gene deletion and insertion usually requires some means of identification of the progeny which contain the desired genotype. In the original experiments to develop modified poxviruses for foreign gene insertion, the thymidine kinase (TK) gene was deleted and a positive selection of progeny which lack the gene was made by growing the virus in a TK cell line (lacking a cellular thymidine kinase) using a medium containing 5-bromodeoxy-uridine (BudR). Any progeny virus which contains the TK gene will convert BudR into a phosphorylated form which is toxic to the host cell. Consequently, only recombinant viruses with the TK deletion will survive (Mackett and Smith, 1986). A similar system can be used to select herpesviruses from which the TK gene has been deleted, for example bovine herpes-virus 1 (Bello, Whitbeck and Lawrence, 1992; Kit, Kit and McConnell, 1986). A deletion mutant of pseudorabies virus (suid herpesvirus 1) has been used successfully to vaccinate pigs against Aujeszky's disease. This genetically engineered virus, strain 783, contains three deletions: one that prevents expression of pseudorabies virus glycoprotein 1 (2 055 base pairs), one that inactivates the viral thymidine kinase (19 base pairs) and one of 100 base pairs that lies in the promoter-enhancer region of the immediate early gene (Glazenburg *et al.*, 1994).

A more general method for gene deletion and the detection of progeny virus with the required genetically engineered deletions is to use a heterologous reporter gene contained in a plasmid transfer vector. The reporter gene is inserted into a plasmid between flanking sequences of the gene to be deleted. When the virus genome DNA is cotransferred into cells along with the plasmid containing the reporter gene, recombination occurs between the homologous (flanking) sequences of the genome DNA and those in the transfer vector. This yields some progeny containing substitution of the virus gene by the reporter gene, and these can be detected in a variety of ways depending on which reporter gene is used. The most convenient plasmid transfer vectors contain a chromogenic reporter such as β-galactosidase which allows an easy visual selection of plaques containing recombinant virus (Chakrabarti, Brechling and Moss, 1985).

In the early development of poxviruses as gene vectors, it was estimated that infectious virus could be produced containing at least 25 000 base pairs of foreign DNA (Smith and Moss, 1983). More recently, a highly attenuated candidate vaccinia virus vector vaccine (NYVAC) has been constructed by the deletion of 18 genes which are involved in pathogenesis and host range (Tartaglia *et al.*, 1992). The resultant virus replicates well in Vero cells or chick embryo fibroblasts but poorly in cells of human, equine, murine or swine origin, and provides a safer alternative to vaccinia virus as a potential gene vector vaccine (Tartaglia *et al.*, 1994).

The potential of NYVAC as a vector vaccine against pseudorabies virus has been demonstrated. NYVAC recombinants expressing pseudorabies virus glycoprotein gp50 protected pigs against challenge with live virulent virus (Brockmeier *et al.*, 1993).

GENETICALLY ENGINEERED DEFECTIVE VACCINES

Recently, the potential of non-replicating (defective) poxvirus as vectors for foreign genes has been explored. Avipoxviruses do not replicate when introduced into mammalian hosts, but they may still act as gene expression vectors in mammals as well as birds, since replication is blocked at a stage after early gene expression, but before DNA replication. The basis for the avian poxvirus vector was an attenuated licensed vaccine for canaries (ALVAC) (Taylor *et al.*, 1991 and 1992; Cadoz *et al.*, 1992). When the glycoprotein gene of rabies virus was introduced into ALVAC by recombination, a highly effective vaccine preparation was obtained (ALVAC-RG) which induced high levels of immunity in humans (Cadoz *et al.*, 1992) and provided a high level of protection in dogs against challenge with virulent rabies virus, even though the ALVAC-RG virus did not replicate in the dogs or human subjects (Taylor *et al.*, 1994). The use of ALVAC as a vector for the *env* and *gag* genes of feline leukaemia virus (ALVAC-FL) has also been described (Tartaglia *et al.*, 1993).

Another highly attenuated poxvirus that has been well characterized is modified vaccinia virus Ankara (MVA). This virus was passaged more than 500 times in chick embryo fibroblasts, and is unable to replicate in mammalian cells (Meyer, Sutter and Mayr, 1991). Replication is blocked at the assembly stage so that DNA replication and late protein synthesis occur and large amounts of foreign gene products are produced, similar in amount to wild-type virus (Sutter and Moss, 1992).

It is clear that such non-replicating gene expression vectors provide a safe and effective means to immunize a variety of mammalian species, including humans, since the virus cannot spread beyond the initially infected cells.

CHIMERIC LIVE VACCINES

Candidate live recombinant vaccines expressing foreign genes have been developed from a variety of poxvirus vectors as well as adenoviruses and *Salmonella* spp. For the most part, adenoviruses are currently being explored as potential vectors for human mucosal vaccination and so will not be considered further here. However, there have been some studies in animal species, especially canines, and an excellent review on the subject has been published (Graham and Prevec, 1992). By the same token, the principal interest in *Salmonella* spp. is in the development of multivalent oral vaccines for human use. Although there is also considerable potential for *Salmonella*-based vectors in veterinary medicine, particularly in poultry, the subject is still relatively unexplored. A useful review on *Salmonella*-based vaccines has appeared recently (Chatfield, Dougan and Roberts, 1994). For these reasons, the following discussion will be confined to some remarkable examples of poxvirus vectors for use in veterinary medicine. A more detailed account of the earlier studies in this area was published by Esposito and Murphy (1989).

One of the first vaccinia virus recombinants of veterinary interest to be developed was a potential vaccine against vesicular stomatitis (VSV), which is a contagious disease of horses, cattle and pigs that can cause serious economic losses in North and South America because the lesions may be confused with those of foot-and-mouth disease (FMD). Recombinant vaccinia virus was prepared which expressed the G glycoprotein of VSV at the surface of infected cells. Some protection against intralingual challenge with virulent VSV was observed in cattle 44 days after receiving the recombinant vaccine on days 1 and 29 (Yilma, 1994).

When the glycoprotein gene of another rhabdovirus, rabies, was expressed in a vaccinia virus recombinant, good protection against challenge was found in a variety of animals such as mice, rabbits, skunks, raccoons and foxes (Wiktor *et al.*, 1984; Blancou *et al.*, 1986; Rupprecht *et al.*, 1988). It was possible to immunize raccoons and foxes, but not dogs or skunks, by oral administration of the vaccinia-rabies G protein recombinant (VRG). This has led to a series of detailed studies of the potential for oral vaccination of raccoons and foxes by distribution of baits containing VRG in the wild. Considerable success has been achieved with rabies vaccination of foxes in Europe using this method, and carefully controlled studies of the use of such baits to vaccinate raccoons are under way at several sites in North America (Rupprecht *et al.*, 1988 and 1993; Rupprecht, Hanlon and Koprowski, 1992; Hanlon *et al.*, 1993). The principal concern in the use of such VRG-containing baits in the field is the possible risk to humans who might become accidentally infected with the vaccinia recombinant. In exceptional circumstances, for example if an immunocompromised person was infected, there might be a risk of a serious vaccinia infection. Alternative poxvirus vectors such as raccoon pox (Esposito, Chandler and Baer, 1989) have been used to create a potentially safer vaccine but insufficient studies have been made of its effects in other species. For this reason the current trials with VRG are being carefully monitored and the risk of human exposure appears to be extremely low. The considerable potential for poxvirus-vectored rabies vaccines to control the unprecedented rabies epidemic in raccoons in North America (Rupprecht and Smith, 1994) needs to be carefully evaluated with regard to risks and benefits. It seems likely, however, that VRG vaccines will soon be licensed for use in the United States.

Unfortunately, a VRG recombinant vaccine that had not been sanctioned by the Argentine authorities was used in Argentina in a field experiment involving cattle (Koprowski *et al.*, 1957). The potential for human exposure to vaccinia virus had not been adequately explained to those who handled the inoculated animals; for example, it is known that vaccinia virus can be isolated from the scabs present on cattle at the site of recombinant virus inoculation (Gillespie *et al.*, 1986). Even though none of the cattle handlers suffered any disease, this incident resulted in a considerable setback to the introduction of recombinant poxvirus vaccines for agricultural purposes, especially in South America (Crawford, 1987).

One of the principal advantages of vaccinia virus, which contributed to the success of the smallpox eradication campaign, is its relative stability. Vaccinia virus preparations will remain viable in conditions which would destroy the infectivity of live vaccines against morbilliviruses such as measles or rinderpest. A highly effective vaccinia recombinant virus expressing the F and H genes of rinderpest has been described for use in cattle (Giavedoni *et al.*, 1991), and this virus will also protect goats against the related morbillivirus, peste des petits ruminants (PPR) virus (Jones *et al.*, 1993). Recently, an alternative chimeric vaccine candidate was described which is based on capripoxvirus, a natural virus infection of cattle, sheep and goats. Live attenuated capripoxvirus preparations are already in use as effective vaccines against sheep and goat pox and lumpy skin disease of cattle, so they are ideal vectors for recombinant vaccines in these species. When the F gene of rinderpest virus was introduced into the capripox vaccine virus at the TK locus, the resultant recombinant virus protected cattle against rinderpest following a lethal challenge and also immunized the cattle against lumpy skin disease (Romero *et al.*, 1993).

In addition to these examples, recombinant vaccines against other bovine diseases have been described. The protection of sheep against bovine leukaemia virus using a vaccinia recombinant expressing the gp51 polypeptide has been described, and this may well be effective in cattle also (Daniel *et al.*, 1993). The use of such poxvirus-vectored rinderpest vaccines could be crucial in the campaign to eradicate this plague from the remaining pockets of disease in Africa and Asia.

The potential of fowl poxviruses as gene vectors for vaccines against a wide range of poultry diseases was recognized more than ten years ago (Boyle and Coupar, 1988). The difficulty of producing such genetically engineered vaccines at an economic cost has hindered their development, however. For vaccines to be effective in the poultry production industry, they need to be administered by one day of age using mass delivery methods, for example inclusion in the drinking water. There are numerous examples of potential recombinant vaccines against diseases such as avian influenza, Newcastle disease and Marek's disease, but all require wing-web inoculation for maximum efficacy and this may not be practical. An excellent review of potential recombinant vaccines for poultry appeared recently (Boyle and Heine, 1993).

SUBUNIT VACCINES

Live virus vaccines usually induce high levels of immunity which persist in the host. The major concern regarding their use is the possibility of reversion to virulence, and for diseases such as foot-and-mouth disease only inactivated virus is suitable for use as a vaccine. Nevertheless, problems have occurred owing to incomplete virus inactivation, with resultant outbreaks of disease.

An alternative approach is to use subviral components as immunogens in the form of subunit vaccines. Generally, the isolated components of a virus may not be effective in stimulating an appropriate immune response but, if presented in conjunction with an appropriate adjuvant such as alumina gel or 6D-stearoyL-muramyL-dipeptide, a better response can be generated. Potentiation of the vaccine by addition of cytokines or lymphokines is also being studied (Hughes and Babiuk, 1994). For membrane proteins of enveloped viruses, an immunostimulating complex (ISCOM) was developed which, when mixed with the antigen, presents it to the immune system in the form of micelles (Morein *et al.*, 1984; Morein and Simons, 1985).

The advent of expression vectors such as baculoviruses, which can produce enormous quantities of a desired protein in cell culture, has greatly enhanced the possibilities for subunit vaccine development. For example, the baculovirus *Autographa californica* has been developed to express a variety of foreign genes under control of the strong polyhedrin promoter (Miller, 1988). The polyhedrin gene is replaced by the gene encoding the desired protein, and the recombinant baculovirus-infected *Spodoptera frugiperda* cells may produce up to 50 percent of total cell protein as the foreign gene product.

This system has been used to engineer multiple-component proteins of bluetongue virus and, when produced in appropriate quantities, the proteins self-assemble to form non-infectious virus-like particles (Marshall and Roy, 1990; Pearson and Roy, 1993). A further development of this system is to introduce other virus antigens into the bluetongue virus subunits during self-assembly to create protein chimeras which will immunize against more than one disease.

This approach offers considerable potential for the future development of veterinary vaccines.

DNA POLYNUCLEOTIDE VACCINES

Wolff *et al.* (1990) reported that the direct introduction of plasmid DNA into mouse muscle resulted in expression of encoded proteins in the muscle cells. Although the exact process by which transcription occurs in this system has not been completely elucidated, it seems that muscle injection is more effective at inducing an immune response than other routes or tissues that have been tried.

Recently, the application of a biolistic gun (gene gun) that shoots gold particles coated with DNA directly into the muscle, has been described (Williams *et al.*, 1991; Fynan *et al.*, 1993).

This field is just opening up, but the effectiveness of naked DNA in provoking immunity to rabies in mice and virulent influenza in chickens has been reported (Xiang *et al.*, 1994; Robinson, Hunt and Webster, 1993). The state of the art of DNA vaccination has been well summarized by Ulmer, Donnelly and Liu (1994), Ulmer *et al.* (1993) and Cohen (1993).

POLYPEPTIDE VACCINES

When predicted amino acid sequences from a wide range of pathogenic viruses became available in the mid-1970s, the possibility of using chemically synthesized polypeptides as immunogens was explored. Previous studies on proteins such as lysozyme had established that immune responses could be elicited by short peptides containing about 20 amino acids. It was also clear that peptides corresponding to the aminoterminus or carboxyterminus were frequently antigenic (i.e. elicited antibodies that reacted with the original protein). Numerous examples of viral peptides that served as immunogens were reported (Geysen, Barteling and Meloen, 1985; Shinnick *et al.*, 1983). When it was found that guinea pigs could be protected from foot-and-mouth disease by a short peptide of 19 amino acids corresponding to a portion of the VP1 protein of the virus (Bittle *et al.*, 1982), peptides were hailed as the next generation of foot-and-mouth disease vaccines (Brown, 1985). Subsequently, Di Marchi *et al.* (1986) showed that it was possible to protect cattle from a virulent intralingual challenge with foot-and-mouth disease virus using a peptide of 42 amino acids, but very large quantities of the peptide were required. In general, the peptides were found to stimulate a remarkably strong humoral response even at low doses of peptide, but protection against challenge did not occur except at high doses (5 mg per animal).

Despite the great amount of work done in attempting to improve on these results, for example by coupling the peptide with predicted amino acid sequences designed to stimulate cell-mediated immunity, the potential for such simple peptides as vaccines has not been realized.

BIBLIOGRAPHY

Arber, W. & Dussoix, D. 1962. Host specificity of DNA produced by *Escherichia coli.* 1. Host-controlled modification of bacteriophage. *J. Mol. Biol.*, 5: 18.

Baltimore, D. 1970. RNA-dependent DNA polymerase in virions of RNA tumor viruses. *Nature*, 226: 1209-1211.

Barber, L.D. & Parham, P. 1994. The essence of epitopes. *J. Exp. Med.*, 180: 1191-1194.

Bello, L.J., Whitbeck, J.C. & Lawrence, W.C. 1992. Bovine herpesvirus 1 as a live virus vector for expression of foreign genes. *Virology*, 190: 666-673.

Bittle, J.L., Houghten, R.A., Alexander, H., Shinnick, T.M., Sutcliffe, J.G. & Lerner, R.A. 1982. Protection against foot-and-mouth disease by immunization with a chemically synthesized peptide predicted from the viral nucleotide sequence. *Nature*, 298: 30-33.

Blancou, J., Kieny, M.P., Lathe, R., Lecocq, J.P., Pastoret, P.P., Soulebot, J.P. & Desmettre, P. 1986. Oral vaccination of the fox against rabies using a live recombinant vaccinia virus. *Nature*, 322: 373-375.

Boyle, D.B. & Coupar, B.E.H. 1988. Construction of recombinant fowlpox viruses as vectors for poultry vaccines. *Virus Res.*, 10: 343-356.

Boyle, D.B. & Heine, H.G. 1993. Recombinant fowlpox virus vaccines for poultry. *Immunol. Cell Biol.*, 71: 391-397.

Brockmeier, S.L., Lager, K.M., Tartaglia, J., Riviere, M., Paoletti, E. & Mengeling, W.I. 1993. Vaccination of pigs against pseudorabies with highly attenuated vaccinia (NYVAC) recombinant viruses. *Vet. Microbiol.*, 38: 41-58.

Brown, F. 1985. Peptides as the next

generation of foot-and-mouth disease vaccines. *BioTechnology,* 3: 445-447.

Cadoz, M., Strady, A., Meigner, B., Taylor, J., Tartaglia, J., Paolelti, E. & Ploticin, S. 1992. Immunization with canarypox virus expressing the rabies glycoprotein. *Lancet,* 339: 1429-1432.

Chakrabarti, S., Brechling, K. & Moss, B. 1985. Vaccinia virus expression vector: coexpression of β-galactosidase provides visual screening of recombinant virus plaques. *Mol. Cell. Biol.,* 5: 3403-3409.

Chatfield, S.N., Dougan, G. & Roberts, M. 1994. Progress in the development of multivalent oral vaccines based on live attenuated *Salmonella. In* E. Kurstak, ed. *Modern vaccinology,* p. 55-85. New York, Plenum Medical.

Cohen, J. 1993. Naked DNA points way to vaccines. *Science,* 259: 1691-1692.

Crawford, M. 1987. Argentine experiment did not break U.S. biotechnology rules. *Science,* 235(4786): 276.

Daniel, R.C.W., Gatei, M.H., Good, M.F., Boyle, D.B. & Lavin, M.F. 1993. Recombinant viral vaccines for enzootic bovine leucosis. *Immunol. Cell Biol.,* 71: 399-404.

Di Marchi, R., Brooke, G., Gale, C., Cracknell, V., Doel, T. & Mowat, N. 1986. Protection of cattle against foot-and-mouth disease by a synthetic peptide. *Science,* 232: 639-641.

Esposito, J.J. & Murphy, F.A. 1989. Infectious recombinant vectored virus vaccines. *Adv. Vet. Sci. Comp. Med.,* 33: 195-247.

Esposito, J.J., Chandler, F.W. & Baer, G.M. 1989. Oral immunization of animals with raccoon poxvirus expressing rabies virus glycoprotein. *Vaccine,* 89: 1-6.

Fynan, E.F., Webster, R.G., Fuller, D.H., Hanes, J.R., Santoro, J.C. & Robinson, H.L. 1993. DNA vaccines: protective immunization by parenteral, mucosal and gene-gun inoculations. *PNAS,* 90: 11478-11482.

Gao, Y., Leary, T.P., Eskra, L. & Splitter, G.A. 1994. Truncated bovine herpesvirus-1 glycoprotein 1 (gp1) initiates a protective local immune response in its natural host. *Vaccine,* 12: 145-152.

Geysen, H.M., Barteling, S.J. & Meloen, R.H. 1985. Small peptides induce antibodies with a sequence and structural requirement for binding antigen comparable to antibodies raised against the native protein. *PNAS,* 82: 178-182.

Giavedoni, L., Jones, L., Mebus, C. & Yilma, T. 1991. A vaccinia virus double recombinant expressing the F and H genes of rinderpest virus protects cattle against rinderpest and causes no pock lesions. *PNAS,* 88: 8011.

Gillespie, J.H., Geissinger, C., Scott, F.W., Higgins, W.P., Holmes, D.F., Perkus, M., Mercer, S. & Paoletti, E. 1986. Response of dairy calves to vaccinia viruses that express foreign genes. *J. Clin. Microbiol.,* 23: 283-288.

Glazenburg, K.L., Elgersma-Hooisma, M., Briaire, J, Voermans, J., Kimman, T.G., Gielkens, A.L.J. & Moormann, R.J.M. 1994. Vaccine properties of pseudorabies virus strain 783 are not affected by a deletion of 71 base pairs in the promoter/enhancer region of the viral immediate early gene. *Vaccine,* 12: 1097-1101.

Graham, F.L. & Prevec, L. 1992. Adenovirus-based expression vectors and recombinant vaccines. *In* R. Ellis, ed. *Vaccines: new approaches to immunological problems,* p. 363-390. Stoneham, Mass, USA, Butterworth-Heinemann.

Hall, W.W., Kubo, T., Ijichi, S. Takahashi, H. & Zhu, S.W. 1994. Human T cell leukemia/lymphoma virus, type II (HTLV-11): emergence of an important newly recognized pathogen. *Virology,* 5: 165-178.

Hanlon, C.A., Buchanan, J.R., Nelson, E., Niu, H.S., Diehl, D. & Rupprecht, C.E. 1993. A vaccinia-vectored rabies vaccine field trial: ante- and post-mortem biomarkers. *Rev. sci. tech. Off. int. Epizoot.*, 12(1): 99-107.

Hughes, H.R.A. & Babiuk, L.A. 1994. Potentiation of vaccines through effective adjuvant fomulations and manipulation of the immune response. *In* E. Kurstak, ed. *Modern vaccinology*, p. 87-118. New York, Plenum Medical.

Jones, L., Giavedoni, L., Saliki, J.T., Brown, C., Mebus, C. & Yilma, T. 1993. Protection of goats against peste des petits ruminants with a vaccinia virus double recombinant expressing the F and H genes of rinderpest virus. *Vaccine*, 11: 961-964.

Kit, S., Kit, M. & McConnell, S. 1986. Intramuscular and intravaginal vaccination of pregnant cows with thymidine kinase-negative, temperature-resistant infectious bovine rhinotracheitis virus (bovine herpesvirus 1). *Vaccine*, 4: 55-61.

Koprowski, H., Celis, E., Curtis, P., Dietzschold, B., Rupprecht, C., Tollis, M. & Wunner, W. 1987. Rabies experiment. *Nature*, 326: 636.

Mackett, M. & Smith, G.L. 1986. Vaccinia virus expression vectors. *J. Gen. Virol.*, 67: 2067-2082.

Marshall, J.A. & Roy, P. 1990. High level expression of two outer cepside proteins of bluetongue virus serotype 10. *Virus Res.*, 15: 189-196.

Meselson, M. & Yuan, R. 1968. DNA restriction enzyme from *E. coli*. *Nature*, 217: 1110.

Meyer, H., Sutter, G. & Mayr, A. 1991. Mapping of deletions in the genome of the highly attenuated vaccinia virus MVA and their influence on virulence. *J. Gen. Virol.*, 72: 1031-1038.

Miller, L.K. 1988. Baculoviruses as gene expression vectors. *Annu. Rev. Microbiol.*, 42: 177-199.

Morein, B. & Simons, K. 1985. Subunit vaccines against enveloped viruses: virosomes, micelles and other protein complexes. *Vaccine*, 3: 83-93.

Morein, B., Sundquist, B., Höglund, S., Dalsgaard, K. & Osterhaus, A. 1984. ISCOM, a novel structure for antigenic presentation of membrane proteins from enveloped viruses. *Nature*, 308(5958): 457-460.

Moss, B. & Flexner, C. 1987. Vaccinia virus expression vectors. *Annu. Rev. Immunol.*, 5: 305-324.

Pearson, L.D. & Roy, P. 1993. Genetically engineered multi-component virus-like particles as veterinary vaccines. *Immunol. Cell Biol.*, 71: 381-389.

Pensaert, M., Gielkens, A.L.J., Lomniczi, B., Kimman, T.G., Vannier, P. & Eloit, M. 1992. Round table on control of Aujeszky's disease and vaccine development based on molecular biology. *Vet. Microbiol.*, 33: 53-67.

Robinson, H.L., Hunt, L.A. & Webster, R.G. 1993. Protection against a lethal influenza virus challenge by immunization with a haemagglutinin-expressing plasmid DNA. *Vaccine*, 11: 957-960.

Romero, C.H., Barrett, T., Evans, S.A., Kitching, R.P., Gershon, P.D., Bostock, C. & Black, D.N. 1993. Single capripoxvirus recombinant vaccine for the protection of cattle against rinderpest and lumpy skin disease. *Vaccine*, 11: 737-742.

Rupprecht, C.E. & Smith, J.S. 1994. Raccoon rabies: the emergence of an epizootic in a densely populated area. *Semin. Virol.*, 5: 155-164.

Rupprecht, C.E., Hanlon, C.A. & Koprowski, H. 1992. Oral wildlife rabies vaccination: Development of a recombinant virus vaccine. In *Trans. 57th N.A. Wildl. Nat. Res. Conf.*, p. 439-452.

Rupprecht, C.E., Hamir, A.N., Johnson, D.H. & Koprowski, H. 1988. Efficacy of a vaccinia-rabies glycoprotein recombinant virus vaccine in raccoons (*Procyon lotor*). *Rev. Inf. Dis.*, 10: 803-809.

Rupprecht, C.E., Hanlon, C.A., Cummins, L.B. & Koprowski, H. 1992. Primate responses to a vaccinia-rabies glycoprotein recombinant virus vaccine. *Vaccine,* 10: 368-374.

Rupprecht, C.E., Hanlon, C.A., Niezgoda, M., Buchanan, J.R., Diehl, D. & Koprowski, H. 1993. Recombinant rabies vaccines: efficacy assessment in free-ranging animals. *Onderstepoort J. Vet. Res.,* 60: 463-468.

Sakaguchi, M., Hirayama, Y., Maeda, H., Matsuo, K., Yamamoto, M. & Hirai, K. 1994. Construction of recombinant Marek's disease virus type 1 (MDV1) expressing the *Escherichia coli lacZ* gene as a possible live vaccine vector: the US10 gene of MDV1 as a stable insertion site. *Vaccine,* 12: 153-957.

Sambrook, J., Fritsch, E.F. & Maniantis, J. 1989. *Molecular cloning: a laboratory manual,* 2nd ed. Cold Spring Harbor, New York, Cold Spring Harbor Press.

Shinnick, T.M., Sutcliffe, J.G., Green, N. & Lerner, R.A. 1983. Synthetic peptide immunogens as vaccines. *Annu. Rev. Microbiol.,* 37: 425-426.

Smith, G.L. & Moss, B. 1983. Infectious poxvirus vectors have capacity for at least 25 000 base pairs of foreign DNA. *Gene,* 25: 21-28.

Sutter, G. & Moss, B. 1992. Non-replicating vaccinia vector efficiently expresses recombinant genes. *PNAS,* 89: 10847-10851.

Tartaglia, J., Cox, W.I., Pincus, S. & Paoletti, E. 1994. Safety and immunogenicity of recombinants based on the genetically engineered vaccine strain, NYVAC. *Dev. Biol. Stand.,* 82: 125-129.

Tartaglia, J., Jarrett, O., Neil, J.C., Desmetre, P. & Paoletti, E. 1993. Protection of cats against feline leukemia virus by vaccination with a canarypox virus recombinant, ALVAC-FL. *J. Virol.,* 67: 2370-2375.

Tartaglia, J., Perkus, M.E., Taylor, J., Norton, E.K., Audonnet, J.-C., Cos, W.I., Davis, S.W., VanderHoeven, J., Meignier, B., Riviere, M., Languet, B. & Paoletti, E. 1992. A highly attenuated strain of vaccinia virus. *Virology,* 188: 217-232.

Taylor, J., Trimarchi, C., Weinberg, R., Languet, B., Guillemin, F., Desmetre, P. & Paoletti, E. 1991. Efficacy studies on a canary-pox-rabies recombinant virus. *Vaccine,* 9: 190-193.

Taylor, J., Weinberg, R., Tartaglia, J., Richardson, C., Alkhatib, G., Briedis, D., Appel, M., Norton, E. & Paoletti, E. 1992. Non-replicating viral vectors as potential vaccines: recombinant canarypox virus expressing measles virus fusion (F) and hemagglutinin (HA) glycoproteins. *Virology,* 187: 321-328.

Taylor, J., Tartaglia, J., Riviere, M., Duret, C., Languet, B., Chappuis, G. & Paoletti, E. 1994. Applications of canarypox (ALVAC) vectors in human and veterinary vaccination. *Dev. Biol. Stand.,* 82: 131-135.

Townsend, A. & Bodmer, H. 1989. Antigen recognition by class I-restricted T lymphocytes. *Annu. Rev. Immunol.,* 7: 601-624.

Ulmer, J.B., Donnelly, J. & Liu, M.A. 1994. Vaccination with polynucleotides: a novel means of generating immunity. *In* E. Kurstak, ed. *Modern vaccinology,* p. 13-23. New York, Plenum Medical.

Ulmer, J.B., Donnelly, J.J., Parker, S.E., Rhodes, G.H., Felgner, P.L., Dwarki, V.J., Gromkowski, S.H., Deck, R.R., DeWitt, C.M., Friedman, A., Hawe, L.A., Leander, K.R., Martinez, D., Perry, H.C., Shiver, J.W., Montgomery, D.M. & Liu, M.A. 1993. Heterologous protection against influenza by injection of DNA encoding a viral protein. *Science,* 259: 1745-1749.

van Oirschot, J.T. 1994. Vaccination in food animal populations. *Vaccine,* 12: 415-418.

Vannier, P., Hutet, E., Bourgueil, E. & Cariolet, R. 1991. Level of virulent virus excreted by infected pigs previously vaccinated with different glycoprotein-deleted Aujeszky's disease vaccines. *Vet. Microbiol.*, 29: 213-223.

Wiktor, T.J., Macfarlan, R.I., Reagan, K.J., Dietzschold, B., Curtis, P.J., Wunner, W.H., Kieny, M.P., Lathe, R., Lecocq, J.P., Mackett, M., Moss, B. & Koprowski, H. 1984. Protection from rabies by a vaccinia virus recombinant containing the rabies virus glycoprotein gene. *PNAS*, 81: 7194-7198.

Williams, R.S., Johnson, S.A., Reidy, M., Devit, M.J., McElligott, S.G. & Sanford, J.C. 1991. Introduction of foreign genes into tissues of living mice by DNA-coated microprojectiles. *PNAS*, 88: 2726-2730.

Wolff, J.A., Malone R.W., Williams, P., Chong, W., Acsadi, G., Jani, A. & Felgner, P.L. 1990. Direct gene transfer into mouse muscle *in vivo*. *Science*, 247: 1465-1468.

Xiang, Z.Q., Spitalnik, S., Tran, M., Wunner, W.H.; Cheng, J. & Ertl, H.C. 1994. Vaccination with a plasmid vector carrying the rabies virus glycoprotein gene induces protective immunity against rabies virus. *Virology*, 199: 132-140.

Yilma, T. 1994. Genetically engineered vaccines for animal viral diseases. *J. Am. Vet. Med. Assoc.*, 204: 1606-1615.

Viral vaccines

F. Brown

Vaccination is a major weapon in the control of many viral diseases of humans and their domestic and pet animals. There is no doubt that vaccines have made an enormous impact on the health and consequently the productivity of the recipients. Although this chapter concentrates on vaccines which are used in domestic livestock, where necessary it draws analogies with information involving other species. In addition, an overview on the present state of vaccine development must necessarily review what has gone before and, with advantage, should also look to the future. Consequently, this chapter contains references to products that were made in the past, including the way in which they were improved to provide the vaccines in current use, and outlines the possibilities of entirely new products which molecular biology offers.

Although it is always dangerous to make predictions, one can be certain that the methods for preparing vaccines will improve. It is also possible and even likely that the methods will change radically as we learn more about the immune response at the molecular level and apply recombinant DNA technology to produce and present to the host only those parts of the virus that are required to provide protection.

BACKGROUND

Vaccination as we know it today essentially began late in the eighteenth century with the observations of Jesty (see Wallace, 1981; Jenner, 1798) and many others that milkmaids rarely contracted smallpox. The immunity was attributed to the fact that milkmaids contracted cowpox during milking which protected them against the virulent smallpox. Many of the vaccines in use at the present time are based on the same principle, namely that of a weakened or attenuated strain of a virus multiplying sufficiently in the host to elicit a protective immune response without causing clinical disease. Vaccines based on this principle are highly effective, as shown by the eradication of smallpox; the control of many human diseases such as polio myelitis, measles and mumps; and the effectiveness in domestic animals of vaccines against Marek's disease, Newcastle disease and rinderpest.

The second part of our armoury consists of inactivated vaccines, prepared by growing large amounts of the viruses in tissue culture cells or sometimes in the intact animal and then inactivating them either chemically, with agents such as formaldehyde, phenol, β-propiolactone or an imine, or physically, with ultraviolet light. Inactivated vaccines against foot-and-mouth disease, Newcastle disease, poliomyelitis and rabies have been used extensively and with great success.

Together, these vaccines have made very important contributions to animal health worldwide. One of the early vaccines used on a large scale was described by Rosenbusch, Decamps and Gelormini (1948). This vaccine, used against foot-and-mouth disease, was prepared by formaldehyde inactivation of extracts of fresh tongue lesions of artificially infected susceptible cattle. Millions of cattle were immunized with vaccines prepared by this method. It is of interest, in view of later observations and concern about the innocuity of vaccines prepared by inactivation with formaldehyde, that the authors used an alkaline glycocoll buffer. Recent studies have shown that the virus is very rapidly inactivated at pH 8. This results from the degradation of the RNA within the virus particle by the RNA polymerase (Newman *et al.*, 1994). Rabies vaccines prepared from the brains of sheep and goats artificially infected with the virus are still widely used in humans despite the evidence that such products cause encephalitic reactions.

The discovery of antibiotics in the late 1930s and early 1940s revolutionized the way in which vaccines could be prepared. Viruses had been grown outside the animal body as early as 1930 but these experiments had been done on a small scale. To expand these laboratory observations to a production scale was clearly difficult with the technology available at that time because the problem of ensuring bacteriological sterility would have been overwhelming. The discovery of antibiotics overcame the problem.

The development of large-scale *in vitro* cultivation of foot-and-mouth disease virus by Frenkel (1947) was a major technical achievement. This led to vaccination programmes which have been used to protect millions of animals (and incidentally predated the much publicized polio vaccination programmes by several years).

ATTENUATED VACCINES

Jenner's vaccine against smallpox, referred to above, was quickly applied in many countries but it was not until almost a century later, in the 1880s, that immunization against other infections began. By that time the germ theory of infection was starting to be accepted and, in rapid succession between 1880 and 1885, Pasteur and his colleagues demonstrated the efficacy of vaccines against chicken cholera, anthrax and rabies (Pasteur, 1880 and 1985; Pasteur, Chamberland and Roux, 1881). All three vaccines had been prepared by attenuating the naturally occurring wild-type agents in the laboratory.

Vaccines for several viral diseases have been prepared by growing the wild-type agents in non-natural hosts or in tissue culture cells. For success to be achieved, careful selection of appropriate strains is required. Even then, the selection has to be accompanied by an enormous amount of luck to achieve the correct balance between loss of virulence and the ability to multiply in the host without causing clinical disease. Nevertheless, highly successful vaccines against Newcastle disease and rinderpest have been prepared and used in millions of birds and animals. The selection of a naturally occurring mutant has also been successful in the case of Marek's disease. The virus infecting turkeys was found to be avirulent for chickens and has been used in millions of birds.

CURRENT METHODS OF INACTIVATION

Most inactivated vaccines are produced by reacting the viruses with formaldehyde. This reagent has been used almost exclusively for producing diphtheria and tetanus toxoids since early this century. The reagent was used by Römer in experiments to produce a vaccine against poliomyelitis as early as 1911, but without success. However, it was used successfully by Vallée, Carré and Rinjard (1925) to produce an experimental foot-and-mouth disease vaccine. These researchers, located in Paris, were probably influenced in their choice of reagent by Ramon, who was at that time director of the Pasteur Institute in that city.

Serious concerns about the use of formaldehyde to inactivate poliomyelitis virus completely were voiced following clinical trials of a polio vaccine prepared in this way by Brodie and Park (1936) in the 1930s. Similar doubts were also expressed later about the foot-and-mouth disease vaccines prepared by the same method. It was generally considered that the preliminary step of adsorbing the virus to alum before adding the formaldehyde was necessary in the inactivation procedure. In fact, the adsorption step may have been responsible for masking the fact that inactivation of the virus was incomplete.

The Cutter incident with an early polio vaccine in the mid-1950s only served to emphasize these concerns and categorical evidence that foot-and-mouth disease vaccines prepared by treatment of the virus with formaldehyde were not innocuous was provided by Brown *et al.* (1963) and Graves (1963). But it needed the outbreaks in Normandy and Brittany in France in 1981, when the causal agent was identified by molecular methods as a virus isolated 16 years previously, to convince manufacturers that formaldehyde inactivation was not safe (King *et al.*, 1981). Subsequent evidence, provided by Beck and Strohmaier (1987) using nucleic acid sequencing to identify the viruses causing several outbreaks in western Europe, pinpointed either spills from factories or vaccines inactivated with formalin as the major causes.

In view of these findings, it is somewhat perplexing, at least to the author, that alternative inactivating agents were not used more generally before these incidents. Firm laboratory evidence had been provided several years previously that acetylethyleneimine was a better inactivant (Brown and Crick, 1958; Brown *et al.*, 1963) and this had been confirmed on a large industrial scale by the Wellcome Laboratories. In recent years, bis-ethyleneimine has replaced acetylethyleneimine because it is safer to handle on a large scale (Bahnemann, 1990).

THE NEW TECHNOLOGY

During the past 40 years, the concepts of molecular biology have been embraced by the entire field of biology and medicine. This has led to a great increase in our knowledge, not only of the molecular structure of many infectious agents but also of those elements which confer protective immunity. More recently, the same concepts have been applied to studies of the immune responses which protect against infection. The objectives of this approach, while clearly of fundamental importance, also have great practical implications for vaccine production, since they will eventually provide products which are safer and more effective and which can be designed to elicit only those responses that are required for protection.

Structure of viruses

The concept that the entire organism is not required to elicit protective immunity was demonstrated a century ago when it was shown that antiserum produced in animals against the toxins secreted by the agents causing diphtheria and tetanus would passively protect against these diseases. The subsequent extension of this work, which showed that these toxins would produce active immunity after suitable inactivation, provided the first clear demonstrations that vaccination with subunits was a practical proposition (Glenn and Hopkins, 1923; Ramon, 1923).

The advances made with viruses depended in the first place on the techniques which became available to grow them in tissue culture in quantities sufficient to allow their purification and characterization. By growing the viruses in the presence of radioactive precursors of nucleic acids and proteins, the individual constituents can be labelled. These analyses have shown that there are many distinct groups of viruses, differing in size and shape, ranging from small spherical particles of 30 nm in diameter (such as those of foot-and-mouth disease and swine vesicular disease) to bullet-shaped particles measuring 140 × 70 nm (such as that causing rabies) and large spherical particles measuring 300 nm in diameter (e.g. smallpox virus).

In addition, viruses can be grouped according to whether they contain DNA or RNA and whether they possess a lipid envelope. For example, rabies virus possesses such an envelope. By dissolving this envelope in a lipid solvent or a mild detergent, subunits of the virus can be isolated and their potential for eliciting protective immunity tested. More vigorous methods are required to disrupt those viruses not possessing a lipid envelope.

During the same period, major advances were being made in our knowledge of virus multiplication. These studies have provided genetic maps of many groups of viruses, at the same time identifying the genes coding for the proteins of immunological significance. Consequently, when the methods for ligating DNA molecules were described early in the 1970s, the knowledge required for making synthetic vaccines was already available.

The steps involved in the provision of engineered vaccines are:

i) identification of the immunogenic protein;
ii) identification of the gene coding for this protein;
iii) expression of the gene in a suitable vector to provide either a live or a dead vaccine.

i) Identification of immunogenic proteins. The identification of immunogenic proteins is made by dissection of the virus into subunits which are then tested for immunogenicity. With lipid-containing viruses this is a relatively simple procedure, since the envelope can be dissolved in a solvent such as ether or chloroform or a mild detergent such as Tween, releasing the subunits without denaturing the proteins. The separated subunits are also analysed for the proteins they contain. The method which has proved most valuable for analysing proteins is polyacrylamide gel electrophoresis (PAGE), which separates them on the basis of their relative molecular weights. Coupled with examination of the biologically active subunits in the electron microscope, the architecture of a virus can be derived with this method.

ii) Identification of the gene coding for the immunogenic protein. The genome of a virus codes for several proteins in addition to the structural proteins which are involved in the immune response. The relevant gene or genes are identified by expressing the viral nucleic acid in a suitable expression system *in vitro* and then precipitating the products with neutralizing antibody. In this way, the gene coding for the product reacting with the neutralizing antibody can be identified.

iii) Expression of genes. Once a relevant gene has been identified, several vector systems are available for its expression. If the gene is part of a DNA virus genome, it can be ligated directly into the DNA of the vector. If, however, the gene is part of an RNA virus genome, it must first be transcribed into DNA before it can be inserted into the vector DNA.

Several vectors are suitable and these can be used in two ways. In the first, the relevant gene is ligated into the DNA of a bacterium or virus which has been used, or has potential for use, as an attenuated vaccine. Examples of these are the strain bacillus Calmette-Guérin (BCG) (Bloom *et al.*, 1990), avirulent strains of *Salmonella typhimurium* (Dougan and Tite, 1990), adenovirus (Graham and Prevec, 1992), the poxviruses – notably vaccinia virus (Mackett, 1990) and some members of the herpesvirus family, for example pseudorabies virus (Kit *et al.*, 1991).

Recently, this approach was adapted by Almond and Burke (1990) to make use of the attenuated strains of poliovirus, an RNA virus, taking advantage of the fact that the DNA complementary to the virus RNA is infectious (Racaniello and Baltimore, 1981). This DNA will infect cells to produce poliovirus particles. The DNA corresponding to the gene of interest is inserted into the complementary poliovirus DNA, which then replicates to produce polio virus particles containing the inserted gene product. The recombinant organisms obtained in this way have the potential to be used as live vaccines.

In the second approach, the gene is expressed in *Escherichia coli, Saccharomyces cerevisiae*, the baculovirus *Autographa californica* or in mammalian cells, and the gene product is purified for use as a killed vaccine (Brown, 1984; Matsuura *et al.*, 1987). The initial early preference for *E. coli* has been largely superseded because the bacterial vector does not glycosylate the expressed protein. Since many of the proteins of immunogenic importance are glycosylated (e.g. the surface projections of rabies virus) this was a serious and often critical disadvantage. Consequently, more recent developments have been made with eukaryotic vectors.

Recombinant attenuated vaccines

The use of attenuated viruses and bacteria that are already accepted vaccines to carry foreign genes is clearly a concept with many attributes. For example, the great advantages of vaccinia virus (Mackett, 1990) as a vector are its extensive and successful use against smallpox and in the eventual eradication of the disease, together with the fact that its DNA can accommodate several foreign genes. Similar considerations apply to BCG (Bloom *et al.*, 1990) which has been used in tuberculosis prophylaxis for many decades with an impressive safety record, even though there is some debate about its efficacy. In contrast, poliovirus, with its smaller genome and more structurally constrained particle, would be unlikely to accommodate more than one foreign gene.

The use of *Salmonella typhimurium* (Dougan and Tite, 1990) as a carrier is more debatable as it does not possess the proven track record of vaccinia virus and BCG. However, its potential for oral immunization demands that its qualities as a vector should be investigated extensively. Strains of adenovirus (Graham and Prevec, 1992) which have been used as vaccines should also prove valuable since they can be delivered orally, provided the structural constraints imposed by the architecture of the particle do not prove too stringent. Moreover, research done with pseudorabies virus (Kit *et al.*, 1991), a member of the herpesvirus family, indicates that this virus could be a valuable vector for the immunization of animals.

The vaccinia virus system has been studied more extensively than the other candidates, and field trials with the rabies virus glycoprotein recombinant have proved very successful. Of particular interest in the control of rabies has been the successful vaccination of the fox in the wild by using the recombinant vaccine in bait. Experiments with rinderpest virus recombinant in the natural host animal have also been very successful (Yilma *et al.*, 1988). A major issue of debate in the use of such recombinant, however, has been the question of their safety. The innocuity of an organism – and in this instance a new recombinant virus – for the laboratory mouse can be no guarantee of its safety for other species.

It is also well recognized that any

product which is to be inoculated into a healthy animal should ideally not cause any side effects. This position is difficult to achieve and there seems to be no ideal solution. Another issue which has caused concern is whether insertion of a foreign gene alters the tissue tropism of the organism, or even its host range. Again there seems to be no easy solution, particularly since we have little knowledge of the factors which determine host specificity.

Killed vaccines

Proteins produced in *in vitro* systems are essentially equivalent to the subunit vaccines used experimentally several years ago. The crucial problem is to present the expressed proteins to the immune system in the configuration which they have when they form part of the intact organism. Both the subunits derived from the intact organism and the corresponding genetically engineered proteins are much less immunogenic than the intact organism. This is particularly true when the subunits are derived from viruses which do not contain a lipid envelope because their release from the intact organism requires much harsher conditions.

There are, however, lessons to be learned from the experience with the hepatitis B virus surface antigen (Valenzuela *et al.*, 1983). The protein expressed in yeast cells aggregates to form particles which are similar to the 22 nm particles found in the blood of carriers of the disease. These yeast-expressed particles are much more immunogenic than the monomeric protein and they form the basis for the first genetically engineered vaccine. Other evidence also indicates that presentation of an immunogenic protein in a multimeric form on a particulate structure greatly enhances its activity.

Most proteins expressed *in vitro* have a low immunogenicity. By presenting them in a multimeric form, most clearly demonstrated by Morein's experiments with immunostimulating complexes (ISCOMs), their immunogenicity is greatly enhanced (Morein *et al.*, 1990). The principle in this presentation system is the creation of a particle comprising several copies of the protein. The particles are composed of saponin, cholesterol, phosphatidyl choline and the protein under study, the constituents being held together by hydrophobic interactions. The ISCOMS are seen as cage-like structures in the electron microscope, about 40 nm in diameter and comprising 12 nm morphological subunits. Proteins presented in this way not only elicit high levels of antibody but they also stimulate cell-mediated immunity. Moreover, preliminary results indicate that intranasal administration of ISCOMs containing influenza and measles haemagglutinins protect mice against experimental challenge.

Peptides as immunogens

Producing a protein, either *in vitro* or *in vivo*, which has the same amino acid sequence as in the parent organism does not provide any information about the epitopes or short amino acid sequences which elicit the protective immune response. Indeed, the methods which have been used so far to express immunogenic proteins do not even attempt to organize the structure of the protein into the configuration which it has on the parent organism. It is fortuitous if a vaccine produced *in vitro* or *in vivo* is effective because it is improbable that a protein produced in a foreign environment will fold in the way it does in the parent organism. All that has been done so far is to produce immunogenic proteins in a milieu which is different from the native organism. This is not to deny that this is a remarkably sophisticated biochemical achievement but it does not provide any information about how to achieve the specific immune responses we seek from rationally designed vaccines. These answers can only be obtained by further dissection of the proteins into active peptide fragments.

There are several reasons for pursuing such a strategy (Brown, 1990):

- chemical synthesis allows the production of stable products which do not have the problems associated with materials produced in cells;
- the approach offers the advantages associated with the handling of small molecules compared with much larger protein molecules;
- the information which is accumulating on the interaction of peptides with MHC molecules (Bjorkman *et al.*, 1987; J.H. Brown *et al.*, 1993) suggests that the immune response to proteins will soon be understood at the level of short amino acid sequences.

These considerations indicate that it will be possible to design peptides which will elicit the required immune responses for any pathogen. Clearly, there is still much to be learned about the components required in a totally synthetic vaccine. Immunodominance plays a major part in B cell recognition and this factor is now being seen as important in T cell recognition also. Optimal partnerships of B and T cell epitopes are the clear goal.

Genetic immunization

During the past three years, a quite revolutionary conceptual advance has been made in vaccination. It had always been held that it would be necessary to present the immunogenic protein (or carbohydrate-protein complex) to the host in order to elicit the appropriate immune response. Recent experiments with several viruses have shown that immune responses can be obtained by injecting the DNA coding for the protective antigens directly into the muscle tissue of mice (Ulmer *et al.*, 1993). In the case of influenza, protective immunity was achieved. The proteins coded by the inserted genes are expressed in the muscle and skin cells and are then presented to the immune system. It appears that most of the DNA is degraded but, nevertheless, enough remains for the expression of sufficient protein to stimulate the appropriate immune response. It would be interesting to compare the level of the immune response elicited by this method with that produced by the direct inoculation of the protein for which the DNA codes.

Unlike recombinant proteins made in test tubes, if the proteins were made directly in living animals they would not have to go through the extensive purification steps which are currently demanded. Provided the immune response is sufficient to afford protection; this method appears to provide a major step towards the provision of new vaccines.

SUMMARY

The study of vaccines and vaccination based on the concepts of molecular biology has provided the expectation that new vaccines will be produced which elicit protective immune responses without the disadvantageous side effects of the current products. As we learn more about those parts of a virus which are required to provide immunity and the way in which to present them to the host, it is anticipated that vaccines will consist of small fragments of the agent, synthesized either chemically or biochemically, without the need to grow the agent itself. More specifically, however, it must be recognized that each disease is a separate challenge and the protective immunity which each demands should be considered accordingly. The crucial issue is to identify the immune response which correlates with protection. It should not be forgotten how effective the empirical approach has been and we should not ignore the lessons that have been learned from these successes.

BIBLIOGRAPHY

Almond, J.W. & Burke, K.L. 1990. Polio virus as a vector for the presentation of foreign antigens. *Semin. Virol.*, 1: 120.

Bahnemann, H.B. 1990. Inactivation of viral antigens for vaccine preparation with particular reference to the application of binary ethylenimine. *Vaccine*, 8: 299-303.

Beck, E. & Strohmaier, K. 1987. Subtyping of European foot-and-mouth disease virus strains by nucleotide sequence determination. *J. Virol.*, 61: 1621-1629.

Bjorkman, P.J., Saper, M.A., Samraoui, B., Bennett, W.S., Strominger, J.L. & Wiley, D.C. 1987. Structure of the human class I histocompatibility antigen, HLA-A2. *Nature*, 329: 506-512.

Bloom, B.R., Snapper, S.B., Kieser, T. & Jacobs, W.R. 1990. Development of recombinant BCG vaccines. *Semin. Virol.*, 1: 21-27.

Brodie, M. & Park, W.H. 1936. Active immunisation against polio myelitis. *Am. J. Publ. Health*, 26: 119-125.

Brown, F. 1984. Synthetic viral vaccines. *Annu. Rev. Microbiol.*, 38: 221-235.

Brown, F. 1990. The potential of peptides as vaccines. *Semin. Virol.*, 1: 67-74.

Brown, F. & Crick, J. 1958. Application of agar gel diffusion analysis to a study of the antigenic structure of inactivated vaccines prepared from the virus of foot-and-mouth disease. *J. Immunol.*, 82: 444-447.

Brown, F., Hyslop, N.St.G., Crick, J. & Morrow, A.W. 1963. The use of acetylethyleneimine in the production of inactivated foot-and-mouth disease vaccines. *J. Hyg.*, 61: 337-344.

Brown, F., Dougan, G., Honey, E.M., Martin, S.J., Rima, B.K. & Trudgett, A., eds. 1993. *Vaccine design*. Chichester, UK, Wiley.

Brown, J.H., Jardetzky, T.S., Gorga, J.C., Stern, L.J., Urban, R.G., Strominger, J.L. & Wiley, D.C. 1993. Three-dimensional structure of the human class II histocompatibility antigen, HLA-DRl. *Nature*, 364: 33-39.

Dougan, G. & Tite, J. 1990. Live bacterial vaccines for delivering antigens to the mammalian immune system. *Semin. Virol.*, 1: 29-37.

Frenkel, H.S. 1947. La culture du virus de la fièvre aphteuse sur l'épithelium de la langue des bovidés. *Bull. Off. int. Epizoot.*, 28: 155-162.

Glenn, A.T. & H. kins, B.E. 1923. Diphtheria toxoid as an immunising agent. *Brit. J. Exper. Pathol.*, 4: 283-288.

Graham, F.L. & Prevec, L. 1992. Adenovirus-based expression vectors and recombinant vaccines. *In* R.W. Ellis, ed. *Vaccines: new approaches to immunological problems*, p. 363-390. Stoneham, Mass., USA, Butterworth-Heinemann.

Graves, J.H. 1963. Formaldehyde inactivation of foot-and-mouth disease virus as applied to vaccine preparation. *Am. J. Vet. Res.*, 24: 1131-1135.

Jenner, E. 1798. *An inquiry into the causes and effects of the variolae vaccine, a disease discovered in some of the western counties of England, particularly Gloucestershire, and known by the name of smallpox*. London, Samson Low.

King, A.M.Q., Underwood, B.O., McCahon, D., Newman, J.W.I. & Brown, F. 1981. Biochemical identification of viruses causing the 1981 outbreaks of foot-and-mouth disease in the U.K. *Nature*, 293: 479-480.

Kit, M., Kit, S., Little, S.,Di Marchi, R. & Gale, C. 1991. Bovine herpesvirus-1 (infectious bovine rhinotracheitis virus) based viral vector which expresses foot-and-mouth disease epitopes. *Vaccine*, 9: 564-572.

Mackett, M. 1990. Vaccinia virus as a vector for delivering foreign antigens. *Semin. Virol.*, 1: 39-47.

Matsuura, Y., Possee, R.D., Overton, H.A. & Bishop, D.H.L. 1987. Baculovirus expression vectors: the requirements for high level expression of proteins, including glycoproteins. *J. Gen. Virol.*, 68: 1233-1250.

Morein, B., Fossum, C., Lovgren, K. & Höglund, S. 1990. The ISCOM – a modern approach to vaccines. *Semin. Virol.*, 1: 49-55.

Newman, J.F.E., Piatti, P.G., Gorman, B.M., Burrage, T.C., Ryan, M.D., Flint, M. & Brown, F. 1994. Foot-and-mouth disease virus particles contain replicase protein 3D. *Proc. Natl Acad. Sci. USA*, 91: 733-737.

Pasteur, L. 1880. De l'atténuation du virus du choléra des poules. *CR Acad. Sci.*, 673-680.

Pasteur, L. 1885. Méthode pour prévenir la rage après morsure. *CR Acad. Sci.*, 765-772.

Pasteur, L., Chamberland, C.-E. & Roux, E. 1881. Sur la vaccination charbonneuse. *CR Acad. Sci.*, 92: 1378-1383.

Racaniello, V.R. & Baltimore, D. 1981. Cloned poliovirus complementary DNA is infectious in mammalian cells. *Science*, 214: 916-919.

Ramon, G. 1923. Sur le pouvoir floculant sur les propriétés immunisantes d'une toxine diphtérique, rendue anatoxique (anatoxine). *CR Acad. Sci.*, 177: 1338-1340.

Römer, P.H. 1981. *Die epidemische Kinderlähmung (Heine-Medinsche Krankheit)*, p. 49. Berlin, Germany, Springer.

Rosenbusch, C.T., Decamps, A. & Gelormini, N. 1948. Intradermal foot-and-mouth disease vaccine: results obtained from the first million head of cattle vaccinated. *J. Am. Vet. Med. Assoc.*, 112: 45-47.

Ulmer, J.B., Donnelly, J.J., Parker, S.E., Rhodes, G.H., Felgner, P.L., Dwarki, V.J., Gromkowski, S.H., Deck, R.R., DeWitt, C.M., Friedman, A., Hawe, L.A., Leander, K.R., Martinez, D., Perry, H.C., Shiver, J.W., Montgomery, D.L. & Liu, M.A. 1993. Heterologous protection against influenza in injection of DNA encoding a viral protein. *Science*, 259: 1745-1749.

Valenzuela, P., Medina, A., Rutter, W.J., Ammerer, G. & Hall, B.D. 1983. Synthesis and assembly of hepatitis B virus surface antigen particles in yeast. *Nature*, 298: 347-350.

Vallée, H., Carré, H. & Rinjard, R. 1925. On immunisation against foot-and-mouth disease. *Rech. Med. vet.*, 101: 297-299.

Wallace, E.M. 1981. *The first vaccinator: Benjamin Jesty of Yetminster and Worth Matravers and his family*. Wareham, Dorset, UK, Anglebury Bartlett.

Yilma, T., Hsu, D., Jones, L., Owens, S., Grubman, M., Mebus, C., Yamanaka, M. & Dale, B. 1988. Protection of cattle against rinderpest with vaccinia virus recombinants expressing the HA or F gene. *Science*, 242: 1058-1061.

Bacterial vaccines

P.D. Walker

Bacterial vaccines can be divided into two categories:

i) Inactivated vaccines which are composed of whole bacterial cells and/or their metabolic products or, alternatively, a purified fraction of the cell.

ii) Live vaccines which are composed of attenuated strains of the parent virulent organisms.

Although in the developed world, particularly with medical vaccines, purified and characterized immunogens are preferred from both a safety and quality control viewpoint (Walker, 1991), in non-domestic animals economic considerations dictate that the product, in addition to being efficacious and safe, should be cost-effective in an animal of finite worth. Under these circumstances, cruder, less purified products of proven efficacy continue to be employed. In addition, protection by vaccination is often multi-factorial, involving a number of antigens, while the use of single entities produced either by conventional purification or genetic engineering should be treated with some caution (Walker, 1992).

Both types of vaccine can either be injected parenterally or administered orally. Inactivated vaccines are invariably administered by injection, although large doses administered orally have also been used successfully. Living vaccines are administered parenterally or, where protection is against enteric diseases, orally. The use of the oral route as a means of stimulating mucosal immunity in general is being increasingly exploited, particularly using genetically engineered organisms such as the *aro* mutants of *Salmonella* spp. as cloning vectors (Hoiseth and Stocker, 1981; Hone *et al.*, 1991). Such vaccines stimulate secretory, humoral and cell-mediated responses. Vaccines are designed to stimulate the normal immunological mechanisms of the host. Following parenteral injection of vaccines, antibodies, mainly IgG, appear in the bloodstream. Vaccines administered orally stimulate local production of antibody (mainly IgA) at the mucosal surface. In general, antigenicity is a function of molecular size. For this reason, bacterial proteins are good antigens, although long chain capsular polysaccharides are also antigenic and have formed the basis of successful vaccines, for example in protection against haemorrhagic septicaemia in cattle (Nagy and Penn, 1976).

In developing a vaccine strategy for the control of disease, the vaccine manufacturer has to be mindful that there are two stages in infectious disease, i.e. establishment of the organism in the host followed by the clinical signs of infection. Although, in practice, these two stages quickly pass from one to the other, from the point of view of the vaccine manufacturer, it is useful to distinguish between them. Vaccines can be designed that either prevent establishment of the organism in the host or prevent the effects of infection. The problems posed to the manufacturer differ depending on which approach is taken (Walker and Foster, 1981).

The effects of infection are caused mainly by toxins elaborated by the organisms which have specific pharmacological effects. Indeed, the results of infection can be reproduced by injecting sterile filtrates of the organisms concerned. Bacterial toxins are usually secreted into the culture medium and the manufacturer is therefore faced with the problem of producing large quantities of toxins for further processing. These are usually separated from the bacterial cell mass.

On the other hand, if the approach is to prevent establishment of infection then it is the antigens of the bacterial cell which the manufacturer needs to consider. For example it has been shown that in many diseases adherence of the organism to epithelial tissues by specific adherence mechanisms followed by multiplication of the attached organisms is important (Walker and Nagy, 1980). In this connection, the manufacturer must identify these particular bacterial antigens and adjust the growth conditions to ensure the production of large quantities of the appropriate antigen. After inactivation, the organisms are harvested for further processing. Whole culture vaccines may stimulate both types of immunity.

This overview deals with both types of protection using illustrations from veterinary vaccines which are currently in use for sheep, cattle, pigs and dogs or which are under development. A brief section on fish vaccines is included, as aquaculture may be of increasing relevance to developing countries in the future.

PROTECTION AGAINST THE EFFECTS OF DISEASE

The classic example of the use of this type of vaccine protection is that of clostridial toxoid vaccines. The most economically important diseases in sheep, cattle and pigs are caused by clostridial infections (Sterne and Batty, 1975). As a result of the stimulus to research of the potential threat of gas gangrene during the First and Second World Wars, a vast amount of literature exists on the toxins produced by these organisms (Oakley, 1943; Oakley and Warrack, 1953; Brooks, Sterne and Warrack, 1957). The major toxins responsible for disease have been identified and the use of toxoid vaccines to control clostridial diseases is widely practised (Sterne *et al.*, 1962). Bacterial toxins are inactivated to produce bacterial toxoids in such a way that toxicity is lost but antigenicity retained. The usual method of treatment is with formaldehyde (Ramon, 1924).

Toxoids are normally adsorbed on to an adjuvant, usually a mineral salt such as aluminium hydroxide, aluminium phosphate or potassium aluminium sulphate. By far the most potent adjuvants are mineral oils or their derivatives (see Table 2), which enhance immunogenicity by at least an order of magnitude over conventional adjuvants (Freund, Casals-Ariet and Genghof, 1940). However, owing to their production of severe local reactions which may persist indefinitely, they are completely unacceptable for human vaccination and even in veterinary medicine, despite their effectiveness, their use in the developed world is severely limited owing to potential carcass blemish and its effect on the export of meat. Attempts have been made to overcome this problem, for example by the use of the interperitoneal route (Thomson *et al.*, 1969). However, in the developing world it is questionable whether these issues are important. Where production is for a domestic market, the benefits of a more effective and lasting immunity, with all the advantages of reduced handling of animals, must surely outweigh any cosmetic considerations. Furthermore, it is quite possible to identify an injection site such as behind the ear or on top of the skull which is removed at slaughter and will not affect the appearance of the meat.

Adult animals are normally given two injections of toxoid separated by at least 28

TABLE 2

Arithmetic mean antitoxin responses of lambs to 2x2 ml doses of a multicomponent clostridial vaccine precipitated with potash alum and to a I ml dose adsorbed with Freund's adjuvant

Weeks after second innoculation	Adjuvant	*Clostridium*				
		perfringens		*septicum*	*novyi*	*tetani*
		beta	epsilon			
Two	Alum	25.4	2.2	1.9	10.2	16.0
	Freund's	46.6	12.9	5.7	13.2	27.8
Ten	Alum	1.1	0.6	-	0.38	0.7
	Freund's	5.6	3.1	0.6	1.3	6.7

days for a primary immunization course. Thereafter, further boosting to the immunity can be given at critical periods of life. One such period coincides with the 14 days preceding parturition to ensure that the maximum amount of antibody is transferred from the serum via the colostrum and milk for the protection of the newborn. Following the disappearance of such protection, the young animal should undergo prophylactic vaccination.

The range of clostridial diseases against which vaccination is practised is shown in Table 3. Both single and combined vaccines are available, with individual manufacturers responding to the needs of the market place. Based on experience, manufacturers have been able to formulate multicomponent products so that there is a balanced response to all the major antigens despite antigenic competition (Table 4). It is clear from the table that, although individual antigenic responses may be lower with a multicomponent than with an equivalent monocomponent vaccine, the responses to the multicomponent vaccine are above the minimum responses required by the regulatory authorities.

In the United Kingdom, in order to provide effective and safe vaccines, manufacturers have had to comply with the conditions laid down in the British Pharmacopoeia (Veterinary) (HMSO, 1985) whose requirements have subsequently been incorporated in the European Pharmacopoeia. These regulations were originally formulated after consultation

TABLE 3

Principal *Clostridia* spp. causing diseases in animals

Species	Disease
Cl. perfringens type A	Wound infections, gangrenous mastitis, enterotoxaemia in nursing lambs in California and Oregon ("yellow lamb")
Cl. perfringens types B, C and D	Enterotoxaemias in various animals including calves, sheep, goats, piglets and foals
Cl. septicum	Malignant oedema of horses, cattle, sheep and swine
Cl. chauvoei	Blackleg in sheep and cattle
Cl. novyi type A	Gas gangrene in cattle and sheep
Cl. novyi type B	Black disease in sheep, sudden death in cattle and pigs
Cl. haemolyticum (*Cl. novyi* type D)	Bacillary haemoglobinuria in cattle
Cl. sordellii	Gas gangrene
Cl. tetani	Tetanus in all species of domestic animals
Cl. botulinum type C and D	Botulism in sheep, cattle, dogs, chickens and wild duck

TABLE 4

Arithmetic mean antitoxin response of groups of rabbits in tests on 10 consecutive batches of combined vaccines compared with tests on 12 consecutive single batches

Vaccines used	Responses in IU per ml to *Clostridium* spp.				
	Cl. welchii beta	*Cl. welchii* epsilon	*Cl. septicum*	*Cl. oedematiens*	*Cl. tetani*
Br. Vet. Codex standards	10	5	2[illegible]	10	3.5
Mean responses to 10 combined batches	55	6	9.2	16	62
Mean responses to 12 single batches	141	15	9	122	-

Note: IU = international units.

with major manufacturers who, based on their own experiences of vaccines that were effective in the field, were able to suggest consensus criteria for the release of products. In the case of clostridial vaccines, with the exception of *Clostridium chauvoei,* in order to release a product a manufacturer has to show that, after two injections given according to the recommended dosage regime in the field, groups of rabbits respond with certain minimum antitoxin titres. Subsequent formal studies have shown that vaccines producing adequate titres in rabbits produce an adequate serological response in the target species (Frerichs and Gray, 1975).

Nevertheless, these criteria have some drawbacks. For example, they only measure antibodies to the major lethal components and not to other toxins and cellular elements which may be important in protection. Thus, they do not distinguish between whole-culture and toxoid vaccines, for example. A further complication is the differences in response by individual breeds of rabbit, which can vary threefold in their response to the same vaccine preparation (Walker and Batty, 1985). In the case of *Cl. chauvoei,* groups of guinea pigs are vaccinated with two doses of the vaccine according to the recommended dosage regime and challenged with a virulent culture 14 days after the second injection. All vaccinates should survive and all controls die within 48 hours.

The problem for the manufacturer is then to produce large quantities of toxins that can be converted into toxoids and, following suitable processing, incorporated into vaccines.

Component manufacture

As a result of developments in fermenter technology, some manufacturers are able to grow clostridial species in fermentation culture to produce high yields of clostridial toxins suitable for toxoiding (Walker and Foster, 1981). Over a period of time, manufacturers have carefully selected those strains which give maximum toxin production in the growth media they have developed. They have, in effect, cloned their strains to give stable high-yielding toxin mutants which enable them to produce consistently high yields of toxins. Strain improvement by mutation and selection forms the basis of a continuing research programme by most manufacturers.

The majority of strains are stable when stored as freeze-dried cultures and this enables large batches of master seed cultures to be stored. By the use of a fresh aliquot of the master seed to prepare working seeds, any deterioration of the strain owing to passage in liquid media can be avoided. Where storage by freeze-drying is not satisfactory, cultures can be stored in liquid nitrogen and fresh ampoules opened as required.

As bacterial toxins are not generally produced in significant quantities in synthetic media, it is necessary to provide a source of peptides. The manufacturer has to select a source of protein for digestion which is readily available, for example meat, casein or soybean. Digests of meat are usually prepared with papain or trypsin and digests of casein with acid or trypsin. For maximum toxin production, digest media need to be supplemented with various amino acids and vitamins; yeast extract provides a convenient, reliable and cheap source for the latter. In the case of certain toxins, it is necessary to regulate carefully the amounts of various inorganic ions present, for example iron in tetanus toxin production (Mueller and Miller, 1954). Glucose is the normal energy source although maltose and sucrose are also used (Moore, 1968; Walker, Harris and Moore, 1971).

Manufacturers have invested heavily in developing media and growth conditions to give maximal toxin production (Thomson, 1979). Published data are available for the growth and toxin production of the Harvard strain of *Cl. tetani* using Mueller medium (Mueller and Miller, 1954). This consists of a calcium caseinate digest and acid hydrolysed casein base supplemented with bullock's heart infusion broth, glucose, vitamins, cystine and iron powder.

The oxidation-reduction potential of freshly prepared digest media after autoclaving is usually sufficiently low to permit the growth of almost all species of *Clostridia* without further additions, particularly when combined with the use of 5 to 10 percent inocula. If necessary, reducing agents such as cysteine hydrochloride can be added prior to inoculation. There is therefore no special requirement for the introduction of gases into the culture.

Clostridia spp. are for the most part saccharolytic, acid-producing organisms and automatic pH control and addition of carbohydrate results in considerable improvements in yield and reproducibility of culture. Nevertheless, it is possible to control these processes manually, albeit at the expense of some efficiency. By using bottled media and working in an incubator, it is possible to control pH and make periodic additions to containers using a pH meter and appropriate solutions. Where the costs of fermenters are unacceptable and adequate labour is available, this can be an effective method of production, particularly for developing countries.

The optimum pH range for maximum toxin production varies with the toxin concerned. For example, maximum production of epsilon toxin by *Cl. perfringens* (*welchii*) type D occurs in the alkaline range while the pH optima for other clostridial toxins are lower.

Toxin production during growth can be monitored by a variety of techniques. These include, where present, the measurement of enzymic activity, for example lecithinase, haemolysis and proteolysis or, alternatively, *in vivo* testing in guinea pigs, mice and rabbits, using death or skin lesions as the indicator. Values of toxin are expressed in terms of indicator effects, for example minimum lethal dose, minimum haemolytic dose or, alternatively, in terms of unit equivalents of standard antitoxin. The Lf dose of a toxin is that dose of toxin which, when mixed with one unit of antitoxin, flocculates in the least time, i.e. it is the first mixture to flocculate, while the L+ is the smallest dose of toxin which, mixed with one unit of antitoxin, kills 50 percent of injected mice of a designated weight within a designated time (Batty, 1971).

The length of incubation is determined by the particular toxin being produced. *Cl. perfringens* (*welchii*) beta toxin is destroyed by the proteolytic enzymes which the organism produces if incubation continues for too long while others such as epsilon toxin are much more stable.

Bacterial toxins are invariably inactivated with formaldehyde (Ramon, 1924). Although the principal action of formaldehyde on a toxin is to remove toxicity, this is only achieved at the expense of some loss of immunogenicity. For this reason, toxoids are normally standardized in terms of a total combining power (TCP) test. The TCP test involves a partial neutralization of a fixed dose of antitoxin with a series of varying doses of the toxoid being tested. The unreacted antitoxin is then mixed with a fixed dose of toxin equivalent to half the dose of antitoxin used and the whole series of mixtures are injected into mice which are observed for two days. The toxoid present in the mixture that kills half the mice into which it is injected is equivalent to the fixed dose of toxin used (Batty, 1971). This is necessary because, after inactivation, it is no longer possible to measure the activity of the toxoids in terms of indicator effects, although it is possible to carry out an Lf test with certain toxoids. Where there are no appropriate facilities to carry out such tests, developing countries may well have to rely on data from the original testing, for example minimum lethal doses.

Harvesting

For veterinary purposes, crude toxoids are normally used. Crude toxoids are good antigens and are extremely stable under a variety of environmental conditions. The preparation of such toxoids only involves separation from the bacterial cell mass by centrifugation (Walker and Foster, 1981).

Blending

Bacterial toxoids are normally blended into multicomponent vaccines. Very careful formulation is necessary if the host is to produce a balanced response against all components and the vaccine is to pass the criteria laid down by regulatory authorities. Toxoids are normally blended, based on TCP value or some equivalent, and the appropriate unit equivalents added to the final vaccine. In practice, the manufacturer will take into account the testing of the toxin before inactivation (Lf, L+, Lv, Lh, etc.) as well as the TCP and, where appropriate, the Lf of the toxoid. Bearing in mind the loss of immunogenicity on inactivation if the toxoiding process is allowed to proceed too far, the ratio of TCP to Lf declines. A fine balance has to be struck between a high TCP-Lf ratio, on the one hand, and minimum residual toxicity and freedom from any tendency to reversal, on the other.

After blending and the addition of the adjuvant, the vaccines are ready for issue when certain statutory regulatory tests have been completed.

Use of vaccines

The aim of the manufacturer is to provide protection both to the adult animal and to the offspring by the passive transfer of antibody. In the case of the adult animal, providing it has been given primary and secondary injections with appropriate booster doses, it should remain protected for life. In an adequately primed animal, any subsequent infection will result in an anamnestic response which will afford immediate protection (Chadnik, Watson and Hepple, 1959). In the case of the offspring, the length of protection will be determined by the persistence of antibody titres which will, in turn, be determined by the amount and titre of the colostral antibody ingested. As the decay of passively transferred antibodies is known (roughly 16 percent per week), it is relatively easy to predict how long protective levels are maintained. Protective antibody levels are known for several antitoxins, for example 0.1 unit for *Cl. perfringens* epsilon and tetanus and 0.5 units for *Cl. perfringens* beta. Tables 5 and 6 illustrate this by reference to two commercial vaccines, A and B.

Table 5 shows the difference between the performance of the two commercial vaccines, A and B, when the *Cl. perfringens* epsilon antitoxin titres to the first and second injections in previously unimmunized sheep are compared. It can be seen with vaccine A that after a single injection 90 percent of the animals gave a measurable titre compared with 65.5 percent with vaccine B. The group geometric mean (GMT) titre achieved after a single injection with vaccine A is about eight times that of vaccine B. These differences in the titres are also seen after the second injection (Table 5), and with vaccine B two animals still have no measurable titre. The responses in the ewes (Table 6) are reflected in the antitoxin titres obtained in the lambs subsequent to parturition and, hence, the length of protection afforded to the lambs during the early weeks of life (Table 7).

It can thus be seen that, even with two vaccine preparations released on the basis of the Codex requirements, there are differences in potential protection of both the adult and the newborn.

While toxoid vaccines are normally effective, there are examples of breakdown in the field, usually in cases where high levels of challenge lead to large quantities of toxins which overwhelm the antitoxic immunity. For this reason some manu-

TABLE 5

Distribution of *Cl. perfringens* epsilon antitoxin titres in the sera of 8-month sheep immunized with two commercial multicomponent clostridial vaccines, A and B

Serum titres (*IU ml*$^{-1}$)	No. of sera (%)	
	Vaccine A	Vaccine B
42 days after first injection		
5	13 (43)	1 (3.0)
1-5	9 (30)	8 (28.0)
0.1-1.0	5 (17)	10 (34.5)
<0.1	3 (10)	10 (34.5)
Total	30	29
Group GMT	**1.84**	**0.21**
14 days after second injection		
10	13 (43)	2 (6.5)
1-10	16 (53)	16 (59.0)
0.1-1.0	1 (4)	8 (28.0)
<0.1	0	2 (6.5)
Total	30	[illegible]
Group GMT	**9.04**	**1.39**

Note: GMT = geometric mean titre.
Source: Adapted from Kerry and Craig, 1979.

TABLE 6

Distribution of *Cl. perfringens* epsilon antitoxin titres in the sera of ewes immunized with two commercial multicomponent clostridial vaccines, A and B, following the second injection and bled 2 to 5 days after lambing

Serum titres (*IU ml*$^{-1}$)	No. of sera (%)	
	Vaccine A	Vaccine B
10	13 (38)	3 (9)
1-10	19 (56)	20 (61)
0.1-1.0	2 (6)	7 (21)
Total	34	33
Group GMT	**6.72**	**1.66**

Note: GMT = geometric mean titre.
Source: Adapted from Kerry and Craig, 1979.

TABLE 7

Distribution of *Cl. perfringens* epsilon antitoxin titres in the sera of 2- to 5-day lambs born to ewes immunized with two commercial multicomponent clostridial vaccines, A and B

Serum titres (*IU ml*$^{-1}$)	No. of sera (%)	
	Vaccine A	Vaccine B
5	19 (61)	4 (13)
2-5	6 (19)	8 (26)
1.0-2.0	4 (13)	3 (10)
0.5-1.0	1 (3)	4 (13)
<0.5	1 (3)	12 (39)
Total	31	31
Group GMT	**7.48**	**1.25**

Note: GMT = geometric mean titre.
Source: Adapted from Kerry and Craig, 1979.

facturers do not remove cells from all the components and leave them as anacultures so as to obtain both antibacterial and antitoxic immunity.

A typical example of this was seen in Denmark in vaccination against the disease piglet enteritis, caused by *Cl. perfringens* type C. This disease is a haemorrhagic necrotizing enteritis of young piglets which, over a period of ten years, has spread from small foci to cover large areas of Jutland and Zeeland. Initial studies on this disease by Hogh (1974) showed that the causative organism was *Cl. perfringens* type C and that the disease could be controlled by administration of high-titre horse antisera containing beta antitoxin and also by vaccination with vaccines containing beta toxoid. Using a vaccine which contained both cells and toxoid (Xento, Wellcome), successful protection was demonstrated (Hogh, 1974).

Some years later a combined *Escherichia coli/Cl. perfringens* type C toxoid vaccine (Xentocol, Wellcome), specifically designed for the market to control both *E. coli* diarrhoea and *Cl. perfringens* type C enteritis, was introduced. In many herds the vaccine was used successfully to control *E. coli* and piglet enteritis. However, in a number of problem herds the vaccine was totally ineffective in controlling piglet enteritis.

Table 8 shows the results of a comparative trial that was carried out using two product formulations and a control group. It can be seen that removal of the cells of *Cl. perfringens* resulted in a considerable loss of efficacy. The results indicated that, under conditions of high challenge, both antibacterial and antitoxic immunity were required to contain infection (Hogh, 1988). Electron microscopy studies on the disease showed a pattern of adhesion of *Cl. perfringens* type C to the jejunal villi in piglets identical to that of *E. coli* infection in the same species (Walker and Nagy, 1980). The initial phases of the disease were characterized by colonization of the villi owing to adhesion and multiplication of the organisms. Unlike *E. coli*, the adhesive factors are not characterized but clearly were present on the cells of *Cl. perfringens* in Xento vaccine and probably play the same role as the "K" antigens of *E. coli*.

The lessons of these results are clear. Protection is multifactorial and, under extreme conditions of challenge, vaccines based on more simplified entities break down.

The combination of *Cl. perfringens* type C and *E. coli*, i.e. a combination of anaerobic and aerobic vaccines, represents a further development in the marketplace. This is a response both to the needs of the market and the desire to obtain a competitive edge. In this respect it is worth noting two other developments in this area.

A combination clostridial and *Pasteurella* vaccine (Heptavac-P) was introduced by Hoechst (United Kingdom) to provide simultaneous protection against clostridial and respiratory diseases, particularly in young lambs. A somewhat different approach is the combination of clostridial vaccines with an anthelmintic, levamosole, introduced by the Tasman Veterinary Laboratories (New Zealand). This combination allows simultaneous protection against clostridial infections and parasites although, as dosing with anthelmintics is very dependent on the weight of the animal, dosage regimes can be difficult.

PROTECTION AGAINST ESTABLISHMENT OF INFECTION

The importance of the cellular component as a supplement in traditional toxoid vaccines has already been discussed. Cellular antigens are important in the establishment of an organism in the host. Antibodies interfering with establishment

TABLE 8

Comparison of *Cl. perfringens* beta toxoid vaccines and an identical vaccine containing *Cl. perfringens* type C cells in pigs on a problem farm in northern Jutland

Vaccine	Necrotic enteritis			
	Litters	Piglets	No. dead	%
Cl. perfringens beta toxoid	21	239	83	34.7
Cl. perfringens beta toxoid plus cells	22	249	21	6.8
Control	20	217	93	42.9

will prevent infection. In general, cellular antigens can be divided into cell-wall and capsular types. Until fairly recently, most whole-culture vaccines were relatively undefined and consisted of suitably inactivated cells standardized on the basis of cell numbers (approximately 10^{10} organisms per ml), as measured by opacity. Such vaccines undoubtedly act by stimulating bactericidal antibodies directed against the cell and, as such, tend to be sero-specific. When the number of important serotypes in a species is limited, the formulation of vaccines is relatively simple. However, in species where a large number of serotypes are important, it is necessary to blend a multiplicity of serotypes into the final vaccine.

Toxicity resulting from endotoxin components of the cell wall of Gram-negative bacteria which can result in adverse reactions in the adult and abortion in pregnant animals becomes important as the numbers of organisms are increased. In the case of *E. coli* vaccines for immunization against diarrhoea in animals, these consisted of a mixture of the predominant "O" serotypes prevalent in the disease. In the case of *Pasteurella* vaccines for the treatment of respiratory diseases, these again consisted of inactivated cells of the predominant serotypes of *Pasteurella haemolytica* and *Pasteurella multocida*.

Similar inactivated whole-culture vaccines have also been used for the control of leptospiral infections. *Leptospira* spp. are well known as causal agents of disease in the dog (Broughton and Scarnell, 1985). The importance of *Leptospira* spp. as a causative agent of disease, particularly in cattle, has been recognized in recent years. The problem has become acute owing to the transfer of leptospirosis from cattle to humans during handling. The organism is shed in urine and is a potential source of infection. Vaccines have been developed from inactivated whole cultures to prevent shedding of the organism into the environment (Broughton *et al.*, 1984). Results show that, in unvaccinated cattle, leptospiral organisms are isolated frequently from the urine whereas, in vaccinated cattle, there is virtually no excretion (Walker, 1987).

While the transfer of *E. coli* bactericidal antibodies via the colostrum and milk to the suckling animal undoubtedly affords some protection, the approach to vaccination against *E. coli* was revolutionized by the identification of the antigens responsible for adhesion of the organism to the intestinal villi. The adhesion of organisms to the intestinal villi is the first stage in *E. coli* infection and, if this stage can be blocked by antibodies, infection is prevented. K88ab and K88ac were identified as important adhesins for the disease in piglets (Smith and Lingood, 1971) and early work in pigs showed that experimental vaccines prepared from purified K88 antigens were effective in preventing disease in piglets after oral challenge (Jones and Rutter, 1972).

The first available commercial vaccines were based on partially purified K88 antigens of *E. coli* (Nagy *et al.*, 1978). During growth, the K88 antigen is secreted into the growth medium and can be selectively removed from the supernatant by adsorption on to aluminium hydroxide, leaving behind endotoxin in the supernatant.

Rather than depend on anti-adhesion alone, the early vaccines comprised cells of *E. coli* supplemented with measured quantities of K88ab and K88ac. In this way, both the anti-adhesive and bactericidal effects of antibodies were present. Sows or gilts were given two injections of the vaccine, with the second dose timed to be given two weeks prior to parturition, to achieve maximum levels of antibody in the colostrum and milk for a passive transfer to the piglets. To piglets of vaccinated gilts following oral challenge, such vaccines gave significant protection against mortality, diarrhoea and excretion (Nagy *et al.*, 1978). While a conventional *E. coli* K88-negative vaccine afforded significant protection over the controls, the vaccine supplemented with measured quantities of K88 antigen is even more significantly protective.

As time passed, further adhesins such as K99 and 987P were recognized as being important and it became necessary to formulate multicomponent vaccines (Orskov *et al.*, 1975; Moon *et al.*, 1977; Smith and Huggins, 1978). The protection afforded by such vaccines is shown in Tables 9 and 10. Experiments similar to those for the original K88 vaccines were performed and it can be seen that significant protection is afforded against mortality (Table 9) and diarrhoea (Table 10) with all four serotypes (Nagy and Walker, 1983; Nagy, Mackenzie and Painter, 1985).

The identification of the surface antigens responsible for adhesion in *E. coli* represents a move away from the traditional vaccine to a more defined product. Other envelope antigens which may be important in infection have been the subject of increasing interest.

Treponema hyodysenteriae is the aetiological agent of swine dysentery, a disease occurring in post-weaning pigs, ususally in fattening units where pigs are kept in large numbers (Alexander and Taylor, 1969; Taylor and Alexander, 1971; Harris *et al.*, 1972; Hughes, Olander and Williams, 1975). After infection with the organism, swine develop a mucohaemorrhagic diarrhoea characterized by extensive necrosis of the mucosal epithelium of the colon and caecum. This results in dehydration, emaciation and rapid weight loss followed, in severe cases, by death. Recent studies have shown that, following a single-dose parenteral immunization with an inactivated culture of *T. hyodysenteriae* emulsified in oil, swine are protected against experimental challenge.

A field trial indicated that this vaccine confers significant benefits. In one fattening unit, swine dysentery was reduced by 50 percent and the severity of infection by 50 percent, while vaccinated piglets showed a 10 percent increase in weight gain over controls in the same period after a single injection of the vaccine (Fernie, Ripley and Walker, unpublished results). As mentioned previously, there is increasing resistance to oil-based vaccines because of carcass blemish and its effect on the export of meat. For this reason, the vaccine has not been commercially developed.

To obtain further data on the protective antigens with a view to formulating a more non-reactive product, research has centred on the envelope proteins of *T. hydosyenteriae*. Using sodium dodecyl sulphate-polyacrylamide gel electrophoresis (SDS-PAGE) and immunoblotting, it has been shown that polypeptides with a molecular weight of between 30 000 and 36 000 were the predominant ones detected by porcine immune serum and were not present on non-pathogenic strains of this organism. These unique antigens may play a role in the virulence of *T. hyodysenteriae* and form the basis of a new effective non-oil-based vaccine (Chatfield *et al.*, 1988).

A similar outer membrane protein (68 kDa) was demonstrated to be an important antigen in protection against atrophic rhinitis in pigs caused by *Bordetella bronchiseptica*. There is a strong correlation between antibody titres to this antigen and protection in pigs. The antigen is present in virulent strains of *B. bronchiseptica* but absent in non-virulent strains. Monoclonal antibody produced against this antigen passively protects mice from aerosol challenge with the organism (Montaraz, Novotny and Ivanyi, 1985; Kobisch and Novotny, 1990).

TABLE 9

Mortality rates 24 hours after challenge in litters from vaccinated and non-vaccinated gilts after orogastric challenge with 10^{10} *Escherichia coli* plus types 24 hours after birth

Vaccine	*E. coli* challenge cultures			
	K88ab	K88ac *(died/challenged) (%)*	K99	987P
None	19/36 (53) (n=5)[a]	38/53 (66) (n=10)	10/34 (29) (n=5)	33/41 (80) (n=7)
5:1[b]	0/39 (0) (n=5)	3/36 (8) (n=5)	2/37 (5) (n=5)	3/35 (9) (n=5)
Reduction in mortality rates (%)	100	88	83	90

[a]n = number of litters used.
[b]Vaccine 5:1; partially purified K88ab, K88ac, K99, 987P of *E. coli* (100 units each).

TABLE 10

Diarrhoea rates 24 hours after challenge in litters from vaccinated and non-vaccinated gilts after orogastric challenge with 10^{10} *Escherichia coli* plus types 24 hours after birth

Vaccine	*E. coli* challenge cultures			
	K88ab	K88ac *(diarrhoea/challenged) (%)*	K99	987P
None	46/54 (85) (n=7)[a]	47/58 (81) (n=10)	34/54 (62.9) (n=8)	50/52 (96) (n=9)
5:1[b]	1/51 (1.9) (n=7)	2/53 (3.7) (n=7)	20/57 (35.1) (n=7)	22/48 (46) (n=7)
Reduction in diarrhoea (%)	97.8	95.4	44.	52.1

[a]n = number of litters used.
[b]Vaccine 5:1; partially purified K88ab, K88ac, K99, 987P of *E. coli* (100 units each).

In an attempt to improve the performance of *Pasteurella* vaccines, considerable work has been carried out using the specific pathogen-free (SPF) lamb model developed at the Mordun Institute (Gilmour *et al.*, 1975). Such lambs are highly susceptible to challenge with *Pasteurella* spp. when given in conjunction with PI 3 virus. Even in the absence of death, lung lesions develop after a few days and can be scored at post mortem examination.

For a number of the A biotypes, significant protection has been shown in this model using heat-killed cells or sodium salicylate extracts of the organisms as vaccines. However, vaccines containing extracts or heat-killed cells of serotype A2, which is responsible for the majority of outbreaks in sheep, have been less effective (Gilmour *et al.*, 1983; Donachie *et al.*, 1986).

Studies have indicated that organisms grown *in vivo* produce additional antigens to those grown *in vitro*. *Pasteurella haemolytica* A2 cells recovered from the pleural fluid of lambs with pasteurellosis were found to express previously unidentified proteins, and two of these with molecular weights of 70 and 100 kilodaltons (kDa) could be induced *in vitro* by restricting iron availability in the growth medium.

It was subsequently shown that significant protection against *P. haemolytica* A2 infection was conferred on SPF lambs by a vaccine containing extracts of *P. haemolytica* A2 cells grown under iron restriction, compared with a vaccine made in exactly the same way from cells grown in an iron-replete medium. This was confirmed by comparing the antibody responses seen previously in SPF lambs which were immune after recovery from A2 infection. Using immunoblotting, it was demonstrated that there were strong responses to iron-limiting proteins of 70 and 35 kDa and a weaker response at 100 kDa (Gilmour *et al.*, 1991).

In the case of *Pasteurella multocida,* an alternative approach has been to concentrate on the toxins produced by the organism. Some success has been reported in immunizing pigs against experimentally induced progressive atrophic rhinitis caused by this organism, using a formalin-detoxified purified toxin. This approach may well be valid for control of disease in lambs (Chantler, Rutter and Mackenzie, 1986; Fogel, Neilsen and Joral, 1989).

Surface appendages known as pili (fimbria) have also been shown to be important in the pathogenesis and protection against ovine footrot. Ovine footrot results in separation of the horn from the underlying soft tissues of the foot (Beveridge, 1941). Separation of the horn leads to abscess formation and an extremely painful condition in which the sheep have difficulty in walking and grazing. Although the flora of the foot is very complex, it has been shown that the key triggering organism for infection is *Bacteroides nodosus* (Egerton, Roberts and Parsonson, 1969). A culture of scrapings from the infected area reveals a very distinctive rhizoidal colony (Thorley, 1976), the growth of which is highly pilated. On subculture in the laboratory a number of non-pilated smooth colonies are generated, and it has been demonstrated that the most effective vaccines are those made from pilated cultures (Egerton and Thorley, 1981; Thorley and Egerton, 1981). The organism is divisible into a number of serotypes based on pili agglutination and, in Australia, a number of serotypes have been identified as being important (Claxton, 1981). Multivalent vaccines incorporating whole cultures of a mixture of serotypes have been shown to be highly effective both in experiments involving challenge and in the field.

In summary, progress has been made in recent years to identify those antigens which are important in the pathogenic process and to ensure that, under fermentation conditions, these antigens are produced for vaccine production. During production, in addition to controlling pH and temperature, it is necessary to be able to measure and control aeration of the culture. The degree of aeration is dependent on the growth rate of the organism. The growth of *E. coli* strains requires high rates of oxygenation whereas strains of *Leptospira* spp., which grow much more slowly, have relatively low oxygen requirements. For several species, it is necessary to supplement the air or oxygen with carbon dioxide. Provision must be made for the sterilization of the incoming air and outgoing effluent; the latter presents a number of problems when high aeration rates are necessary.

The majority of these problems are minimized by growing the organism on solid surfaces, although this is achieved only at the expense of efficiency as compared with fermenter-grown material.

Individual bottles of nutrient agar are inoculated with the appropriate organism and incubated for one to three days. Following incubation and growth, the organisms can be removed from the surface of the culture and put into a resuspending fluid by agitation. Where the antigens are secreted into the supernatant fluid, there has been some attempt to purify them but the marketplace does not allow the extensive purification required for its human counterpart.

LIVE VACCINES

For many diseases, investigators believe that cell-mediated immunity (CMI) is necessary to provide solid long-term protection against infection. This has led to the use of live attenuated strains as vaccines because, by comparison, killed vaccines generally do not elicit such strong CMI responses.

Live attenuated vaccines in the veterinary field include *Salmonella dublin, S. cholera suis, Brucella abortus* and anthrax spore vaccine. The attenuated *S. dublin* and *S. cholera suis* strains are avirulent rough variants of the smooth virulent strain and, as such, are unable to synthesize a number of polysaccharide side chains required for virulence. However, in the present climate of legislation, a more rationally modified strain harbouring well-defined, attenuating genetic lesions is to be preferred. Examples of the latter are strains harbouring defined mutations in genes in the prechorismate pathway rendering them deficient in the ability to synthesize certain essential aromatic compounds. In addition, it is preferable that strains used for live vaccines should harbour at least two stable attenuating mutations which map for separate regions of the chromosome, thus limiting the danger of reversion to virulence. It has been shown that such strains, for example *aroA, aroC* or *aroD*, are admirably suitable for this purpose (Hoiseth and Stocker, 1981; Hone *et al.*, 1991).

In the case of enteric pathogens, mucosal immunity is regarded as an important factor in protection. In this respect, orally delivered vaccines are superior and the use of live oral vaccines to protect against salmonellosis in cattle provides a good example of modern developments.

Using a double *aro* mutant of *Salmonella typhimurium* to immunize cattle orally, it has been shown that there is significant protection against a live challenge with this organism. Of eight cattle immunized orally with approximately 10^{10} of the mutant seven days after birth using an antacid mixture, seven were completely protected against a challenge of approximately 10^{8} organisms three weeks later. All four controls showed significant symptoms and, along with the remaining vaccinate, had to be killed (Jones *et al.*, 1991).

More recently, this approach has been extended to the use of *S. typhimurium* G30 as a vector to express the fimbrial antigens K88 and K99 of enterotoxigenic *E. coli* (Stevenson and Manning, 1985; Attridge *et al.*, 1988). Oral administration of 10^{11} vaccine organisms to adult pigs elicited significant serum antibody responses to the respective fimbrial antigens (Morana *et al.*, 1994).

Live attenuated organisms have also been used in the case of *Pasteurella* spp. Passaged in the laboratory, cultures of *Pasteurella* spp. disassociate, throwing off mutants that have lost their ability to produce capsular polysaccharides. Such mutants are non-pathogenic but highly immunogenic when injected subcutaneously into the animal. Combined vaccines comprising mixtures of the living attenuated strains can be formulated and are highly effective against challenge in the SPF lamb model (Walker, 1987). Again, these studies are limited by the use of a naturally occurring avirulent strain. Such strains will not be favoured because of potential reversion and it will be necessary to develop rationally attenuated strains harbouring well-defined attenuating genetic lesions such as the *aro* mutants for *Salmonella* spp.

Although reservations regarding the use of naturally occurring mutants or strains attenuated in the laboratory as vaccines have been stressed, the contribution that such vaccines have made in controlling economically important diseases in the field should not be forgotten. In the case of anthrax, the live attenuated spore vaccine derived from an avirulent non-capsulated variant of *Bacillus anthracis* has had a pronounced effect in limiting economic losses resulting from anthrax and an indirect effect in reducing human incidence (Sterne, Nichol and Lambrechts, 1942; Turnbull, 1991). Similarly, the *B. abortus* S19 strain attenuated by temperature has been highly effective in controlling brucellosis.

BIBLIOGRAPHY

Alexander, T.J.L. & Taylor, D.J. 1969. The clinical signs, diagnosis and control of swine dysentery. *Vet. Rec.*, 85: 59-63.

Attridge, S.R., Hackett, J., Morana, R. & Whyte, P. 1988. Towards a live oral vaccine against enterotoxigenic *Escherichia coli* of swine. *Vaccine*, 6: 387-389.

Batty, I. 1971. *In* J.R. Norris & D.W. Ribbons, eds. *Toxin-antitoxin assay: methods in microbiology, Vol. 5A*, p. 255-280. London, Academic.

Beveridge, W.I.B. 1941. Footrot in sheep: a transmissible disease due to infection with *Fusiformis nodosus*. Studies on its cause, epidemiology and control. *Commonwealth Aust. Council Sci. Ind. Res. Bull.*, 140: 1-56.

Brooks, M.E., Sterne, M. & Warrack, G.H. 1957. A re-assessment of the criteria used for type differentiation of *Clostridium perfringens*. *J. Pathol. Bacteriol.*, 74: 185-195.

Broughton, E.S. & Scarnell, J. 1985. Prevention of renal carriage of leptospirosis in dogs by vaccination. *Vet. Rec.*, 117: 307-311.

Broughton, E.S., Marshall, R.B., Little, T.W.A., Hathaway, S.C., Mackintosh, C.G. & Hellstrom, J.S. 1984. *Leptospira interrogans* serovar. Hardjo vaccines in cattle: immunogenicity of vaccines prepared from cultures grown in a protein-free medium. *Preventive Vet. Med.*, 2: 423-433.

Chadnik, K.S., Watson, A.R.A. & Hepple, J.R. 1959. Active immunisation of sheep and horses against tetanus with aluminium hydroxide adsorbed toxin. *Vet. Rec.*, 43: 904-909.

Chantler, N., Rutter, J.M. & Mackenzie, A. 1986. Partial purification of an oesteolytic toxin from *Pasteurella multocida*. *J. Gen. Microbiol.*, 32: 1089-1097.

Chatfield, S.N., Fernie, D.S., Penn, C. & Dougan, G. 1988. Identification of the major antigens of *Treponema hyodysenteriae* and comparison with those of *Treponema innocens*. *Infect. Immunol.*, 56: 1070-1075.

Claxton, P.D. 1981. Studies on *Bacteroides nodosus* vaccines with particular reference to factors associated with their efficacy in protecting against ovine virulent footrot. University of Sydney, Australia. (Ph.D. thesis)

Donachie, W., Burrells, C., Sutherland, A.D., Gilmour, J.S. & Gilmour, N.J.L. 1986. Immunity of specific pathogen-free lambs to challenge with an aerosol of *Pasteurella haemolytic* biotype A serotype 2. Pulmonary antibody and cell response to primary and secondary infections. *Vet. Immunol. Immunopathol.*, 11: 265-279.

Egerton, J.R. & Thorley, C.M. 1981. Effect of alum-precipitated or oil adjuvant *Bacteroides nodosus* vaccines on the resistance of sheep to experimental footrot. *Res. Vet. Sci.*, 30: 28-31.

Egerton, J.R., Roberts, E.S. & Parsonson, I.M. 1969. The aetiology and pathogenesis of ovine footrot, I. A histological study of the bacterial invasion. *J. Comp. Pathol.*, 79: 207-216.

Fernie, D.S., Ripley, P.H. & Walker, P.D. 1983. Swine dysentery: Protection against experimental challenge following single dose, parenteral immunisation with inactivated *Treponema hyodysenteriae*. *Res. Vet. Sci.*, 35: 217- 221.

Fogel, N.T., Neilsen, J.P. & Joral, S.E. 1989. Protection against atrophic rhinitis by vaccination with *Pasteurella multocida* toxin purified by monoclonal antibodies. *Vet. Rec.*, 125: 7-11.

Frerichs, G.N. & Gray, A.K. 1975. The relation between the rabbit potency test and the response of sheep to sheep clostridial vaccines. *Res. Vet. Sci.*, 18: 70-75.

Freund, J., Casals-Ariet, J. & Genghof, D.S. 1940. The synergistic effect of paraffin-oil combined with heat-killed tubercle bacilli. *J. Immunol.*, 38: 67-79.

Gilmour, N.J.L., Thomson, D.A., Smith, W.D. & Angus, K.W. 1975. Experimental infection of lambs with an aerosol of *Pasteurella haemolytica*. *Res. Vet. Sci.*, 18: 340-341.

Gilmour, N.J.L., Martin, W.B., Sharp, J.M., Thomson, D.A., Wells, P.W. & Donachie, W. 1983. Experimental immunisation of lambs against pneumonic pasteurellosis. *Res. Vet. Sci.*, 35: 80-86.

Gilmour, N.J.L., Donachie, W., Sutherland, A.D., Gilmour, J.S., Jones, G.E. & Quirie, M. 1991. Vaccine containing iron-regulated proteins of *Pasteurella haemolytica* A2 enhances protection against experimental pasteurellosis in lambs. *Vaccine*, 9: 137-140.

Harris, D.L., Glock, R.D., Christensen, C.R. & Kinyon, J.M. 1972. Swine dysentery: inoculation of pigs with *Treponema hyodysenteriae* (new species) and reproduction of the disease. *Vet. Med. Small Anim. Clin.*, 67: 61-64.

HMSO. 1985. *British Pharmacopoeia* (Veterinary). London.

Hogh, P. 1974. Porcine infectious enteritis caused by *Clostridium perfringens*. Royal Veterinary and Agriculture University, Copenhagen. (dissertation)

Hogh, P. 1988. Vaccinationsforsog med fire forskellige tarmbrandsvacciner. *Dansk Vet. Tidsskr.*, 71: 1-9.

Hoiseth, S.K. & Stocker, B.A.D. 1981. Aromatic-dependent *Salmonella typhimurium* are non-virulent and effective as live vaccines. *Nature*, 291: 238.

Hone, D.M., Harris, A.M., Chatfield, S., Dougan, G. & Levine, M.M. 1991. Construction of genetically defined double *aro* mutants of *Salmonella typhi*. *Vaccine*, 9: 810-816.

Hughes, R., Olander, H.J. & Williams, C.B. 1975. Swine dysentery: pathogenicity of *Treponema hyodysenteriae*. *Am. J. Vet. Res.*, 36: 971-977.

Jones, G.W. & Rutter, J.M. 1972. Role of K88 antigen in the pathogenesis of neonatal diarrhoea caused by *Escherichia coli* in piglets. *Infect. Immunol.*,6,918-927.

Jones, P.W., Dougan, G., Hayward, C., Mackensie, N., Collins, P. & Chatfield, S.N. 1991. Oral vaccination of calves against experimental salmonellosis using a double *aro* mutant of *Salmonella typhimurium*. *Vaccine*, 9: 29-36.

Kerry, J.B. & Craig, G.R. 1979. Field studies in sheep with multicomponent clostridial vaccines. *Vet. Rec.*, 105: 551-554.

Kobisch, M. & Novotny, P. 1990. Identification of a 68-kilodalton outer membrane protein as the major protective antigen of *Bordetella bronchiseptica* by using specific pathogen-free piglets. *Infect. Immunol.*, 58: 352.

Montaraz, J.A., Novotny, P. & Ivanyi, J. 1985. Identification of a 68 kilodalton protective protein antigen from *Bordetella bronchiseptica*. *Infect. Immunol.*, 47: 744-751.

Moon, H.W., Nagy, B., Isaacson, R.E. &

Orskov, I. 1977. Occurrence of K99 antigen on *Escherichia coli* isolated from pigs and colonisation of pig ileum by K99 and enterotoxigenic *E. coli* from calves and pigs. *Infect. Immunol.,* 15: 614-620.

Moore, W.B. 1968. Solidified media suitable for the cultivation of *Clostridium novyi* type B. *J. Gen. Microbiol.,* 53: 415-423.

Morana, R., Morana, J.K., Cosidine, J.A., Hackett, L., van den Bosch Beyer, L. & Attridge, S.R. 1994. Construction of K88 and K99 expressing clones of *Salmonella typhimurium* G30: immunogenicity following oral administration to pigs. *Vaccine,* 12: 513-517.

Mueller, J.H. & Miller, P.A. 1954. Variable factors influencing the production of tetanus toxin. *J. Bacteriol.,* 67: 271-277.

Nagy, L.K. & Penn, W. 1976. Protection of cattle against experimental haemorrhagic septicaemia by the capsular antigens of *Pasteurella multocida* types B and E. *Res. Vet. Sci.,* 20: 249-253.

Nagy, L.K. & Walker, P.D. 1983. Multi-adhesin vaccine for the protection of the neonatal piglet against *E. coli* infections. Proc. Int. Symp. Enteric Infections in Man and Animals: Standard of Immunology, Dublin, Ireland. *Dev. Biol. Stand.,* 53: 189-197.

Nagy, L.K., Mackenzie, T. & Painter, K.R. 1985. Protection of the nursing pig against experimentally induced enteric colibacillosis by vaccination of the dam with fimbrial antigens of *E. coli* (K88, K99, 987P). *Vet. Rec.,* 117: 408-413.

Nagy, L.K., Walker, P.D., Bhogal, B.S. & Mackenzie, T. 1978. Evaluation of *Escherichia coli* vaccines against experimental enteric colibacillosis. *Res. Vet. Sci.,* 24: 39-45.

Oakley, C.L. 1943. The toxins of *Clostridium welchii. Bull. Hyg.,* 18: 781-806.

Oakley, C.L. & Warrack, G.H. 1953. Routine typing of *Cl. welchii. J. Hyg.,* 51: 102-108.

Orskov, I., Orskov, F., Smith, H.W. & Sojka, W.J. 1975. The establishment of K99, a thermolabile transmissible *Escherichia coli* K antigen previously called "KCO" possessed by calf and lamb entero-pathogenic strains. *Acta Pathol. Microbiol. Scand.,* 83B: 31-36.

Ramon, G. 1924. Sur la toxine et sur l'anatoxine diphtériques. *Annu. Inst. Pasteur,* 38: 1-10.

Smith, H.W. & Huggins, M.B. 1978. The influence of plasmid-determined and other characteristics of entero-pathogenic *Escherichia coli* on their ability to proliferate on the alimentary tract of piglets, calves and lambs. *J. Med. Microbiol.,* 11: 471-492.

Smith, H.W. & Lingood, M.A. 1971. Observations on the pathogenic properties of the K88 and ENT plasmids of *Escherichia.coli* with particular reference to porcine diarrhoea. *J. Med. Microbiol.,* 4: 467-485.

Sterne, M. & Batty, I. 1975. *Pathogenic* Clostridia. London, Butterworth.

Sterne, M., Nichol, J. & Lambrechts, M.C. 1942. The effect of large-scale active immunisation against anthrax. *J. S. Afr. Vet. Med. Assoc.,* 13: 53-63.

Sterne, M., Batty, I., Thomson, A. & Robertson, J.M. 1962. Immunisation of sheep with multicomponent clostridial vaccines. *Vet. Rec.,* 74: 909-913.

Stevenson, G. & Manning, P.A. 1985. Galactose epimeraseless (Gal E) mutant G30 of *Salmonella typhimurium* is a good live oral vaccine carrier for fimbrial antigens. *FEMS Microbiol. Lett.,* 28: 317-321.

Taylor, D.J. & Alexander, I.J.L. 1971. The production of dysentery in swine by feeding cultures containing a spirochaete. *Br. Vet. J.,* 127: 58-61.

Thomson, R.O. 1979. Secondary products of metabolism. *In* A.H. Rose, ed. *Bacterial toxins economic microbiology,* Vol. 3, p. 435-466. London, Academic.

Thomson, R.O., Batty, I., Thomson, A.,

Kerry, J.B., Epps, H.B.G. & Foster, W.H. 1969. The immunogenicity of a multi-component clostridial oil emulsion vaccine in sheep. *Vet. Rec.*, 85: 81.

Thorley, C.M. 1976. A simplified method for the isolation of *Bacteroides nodosus* from ovine footrot and studies on its colonial morphology and serology. *J. Appl. Bacteriol.*, 40: 301-309.

Thorley, C.M. & Egerton, J.R. 1981. Comparison of alum-absorbed oil emulsion vaccines containing either pilate or non-pilate *Bacteroides nodosus* cells in inducing and maintaining resistance of sheep to experimental footrot. *Res. Vet. Sci.*, 30: 32-37.

Turnbull, P.C.B. 1991. Anthrax vaccines: past, present and future. *Vaccine*, 9: 533-539.

Walker, P.D. 1987. Current trends and advances in bacterial vaccines today. *J. Appl. Bacteriol.*, 62: 1-23.

Walker, P.D. 1991. Editorial: Proceedings of the International Conference on Prevention of Hib Meningitis in the 1990s. *Vaccine*, 9 (Suppl.) S.3.

Walker, P.D. 1992. Bacterial vaccines: old and new, veterinary and medical. *Vaccine*, 10: 977-986.

Walker, P.D. & Batty, I. 1985. The use and standardisation of multicomponent veterinary vaccines in 1986. Proc. IABS Congr. Use and Standardisation of Combined Vaccines, Amsterdam, the Netherlands. *Dev. Biol. Stand.*, 65: 227-236.

Walker, P.D. & Foster, W.H. 1981. Bacterial vaccine production. *In* J.R. Norris & M.H. Richmond, eds. *Essays in applied microbiology*. Chichester, UK, Wiley.

Walker, P.D. & Nagy, L.K. 1980. Adhesion of organisms to animal tissues. *In* R.C.W. Berkeley, J.M. Lynch, J. Melling, P.R. Rutter & B. Vincent, eds. *Microbial adhesion to surfaces*, p. 473-494. Chichester, UK, Ellis Horwood.

Walker, P.D., Harris, E. & Moore, W.B. 1971. The isolation of *Clostridia* from animal tissues – isolation of anaerobes. *In* D.A. Shapton & R.G. Board, eds. *Soc. Appl. Bacteriol. Tech. Series No. 5*, p. 25-38. London, Academic.

Mycoplasmal vaccines

A. Provost

Compared with other sectors of microbiology, it is unfortunate to have to admit that the range of available vaccines for mycoplasmal diseases does not provide entire satisfaction for a number of reasons, among which are their poor safety record for recipient animals and a weak, short-lived resistance to natural disease after vaccination.

This disappointing situation can be explained on the following grounds:

- Imprecise knowledge of the actual pathogenic processes in mycoplasmal diseases.
- Insufficient knowledge of the precise role of the different antigens present in the mycoplasmal organism in both the pathogenesis and immune mechanisms; for example, in the case of *Mycoplasma mycoides* subsp. *mycoides SC*,[1] the function of galactan, the polyosidic outer capsule, is unclear.
- A lack of progress in developing simple, cheap and reliable potency tests for vaccines, taking account of the strong host species specificity of the mycoplasms.
- An almost total ignorance of the nature of the protective mechanisms in resistant animals, either after recovery from the natural disease or after vaccination. In no case is there a strict correlation between protection and the presence of circulating antibodies. The situation in contagious bovine pleuropneumonia (CBPP) is such that complement fixing, agglutinating, growth and/or metabolism inhibiting antibodies to *M. mycoides* are no proof of resistance to a challenge. Conversely, resistance can occur without them. The same events exist in enzootic pneumonia of pigs, owing to *M. hyopneumoniae*, and in *M. gallisepticum* infection of poultry. A possible exception, found in humans, is the presence of growth-inhibiting antibodies to mycoplasms in bronchial washings. This is an avenue which should be pursued in animal mycoplasmosis. Cellular-type immunity proves equally ineffective for any correlation with protection.
- Only partial protection against natural or experimental challenge can be induced – partial being understood in two ways: either only a reduced proportion of the total number of animals are protected, or the protection leads to an abortive or less severe disease. This occurrence may happen frequently following the use of inactivated vaccines but is also encountered with live vaccines.
- Unforeseeable reactions following vaccination, either locally at the site of injection (called Willem's reaction in the case of CBPP live vaccine) or by the potentiation of other diseases after the use of an inactivated vaccine (as observed in human primary atypical pneumonia and in enzootic pneumonia of pigs).

In the field of animal diseases, there is only one condition for which vaccination

[1] In this document, *Mycoplasma mycoides* subsp. *mycoides* (SC_1 bovine biotype) will be referred to as *Mycoplasma mycoides* (abbreviated as *M. mycoides*).

is currently in use, namely CBPP. Experimental vaccines have been produced against swine pneumonia but other strategies are also used to control the disease. An inactivated vaccine against contagious caprine pleuropneumonia (CCPP) has been studied in Kenya and is reported to have given valuable results in the field; it is not known, however, whether it is produced on a large scale. Live vaccines have been developed for avian mycoplasmosis and have been produced commercially on a temporary basis but, owing to some disappointments (including a lack of safety for non-vaccinated birds), their use tends to be ignored and control is confined to a combination of means centred on the treatment of fertile eggs (dipping, heating) to evade vertical transmission of the agent.

CBPP VACCINE: GENERAL CONSIDERATIONS

Types of vaccine

Vaccination against CBPP has been implemented by the following methods:

- *Willem's method,* using the pleuritic or pulmonary "lymph", or the secondary lymph resulting from a subcutaneous Willem's reaction induced artificially. The traditional African procedure (subcutaneous inoculation of a macerated lung lesion into the nasal mucosa) is an improvised and related variation of the procedure rediscovered in Europe in the 1850s.
- *Vaccines prepared from broth cultures of naturally attenuated strains* (e.g. the Australian strain V_5 and the Sudanese strain F), some of which are freeze-dried.
- *Cultures of* M. mycoides *attenuated by subculture,* varying in number of serial passages according to the virulence of the original strain, the culture medium, the sensitivity of local cattle and the inoculation site. These vaccines have been called incorrectly "Bennett vaccines". At present, strain T_1 is one of the two available. There have been recent advances in freeze-drying, prolonging the storage life of vaccine and facilitating its distribution in the field.
- *Egg culture vaccines,* employed successfully during the 1960s on account of their good immunogenicity and availability in a freeze-dried form. However, they have been held responsible for pulmonary complications in certain circumstances and have now been abandoned.

Inactivated vaccines of various types are of only poor immunogenicity or lead to an unacceptable reaction at the site of inoculation.

Fundamental rules

Vaccines against CBPP need to comply with three fundamental rules, derived from experience:

- *Viability.* Only vaccines prepared from the specific live mycoplasma possess adequate immunogenicity, engendering a resistance of the premunition type. The vaccine strain can be recovered from lymph nodes several months after vaccination and antigens may persist for up to 204 days.
- *Virulence.* Following the observations of scientists working in 1906, which were confirmed in Kenya in 1921 and a few years later in the Sudan in 1929, subcultures in broth lead to a certain decrease in the pathogenicity of *M. mycoides.* For any given strain, there are a certain number of *in vitro* subcultures which will attenuate the culture.
- Attenuation is characterized by the ability of the particular strain to produce at the site of injection only a minor reaction (localized oedema, which heals spontaneously) after subcutaneous or intradermal inoculation.

The actual technique of inoculation varies from one laboratory to another. This attenuation is not fixed, for further subcultures lead to a progressive decrease in virulence, with the disappearance of immunogenic properties. Therefore, it is necessary to reach a delicate compromise between retention of immunogenicity and minimal local reactions acceptable to cattle owners. Subculturing should be avoided.

- The attenuation of cultures to a greater or lesser extent by *in vitro* subculturing has provided the foundation for vaccination policy during the past 80 years. It is only the approach to the problem that has varied.
- *Vaccination route.* It is usual to follow the rule of the permissible or acceptable vaccination site. This requires dense connective tissue of a low reactivity to limit adverse local and generalized reactions which may sometimes be fatal. For this reason, it has long been advisable for the vaccine to be inoculated into the skin or the subcutaneous tissue of the tip of the tail. Nevertheless, for practical purposes and to avoid loss of the tail after a severe reaction to the vaccine, the current method is to inoculate the vaccine subcutaneously on the flank posterior to the shoulder blade, necessarily using a vaccine of acceptable or no residual virulence.

Occurrence of local postvaccinal reactions

At the end of the last century it was believed that, for a vaccination to be effective, a local lesion was needed – a circumscribed Willem's reaction. It was then thought inevitable that there would be a certain number of vaccination complications, ranging from extensive postvaccinal swelling to death, which could affect 2 to 3 percent of the vaccinated animals.

Towards 1930, scientists first started to claim that there was no relationship between the residual pathogenicity of a vaccine strain of *M. mycoides* and its immunogenicity. The years that followed seemed to disprove this. Most researchers and field observers shared the view that protection was transient and weak in the absence of a local postvaccinal reaction.

This fact was widely recognized at the time, but was difficult to explain. Among the factors involved might have been poor cultures, faulty storage of vaccine and only partial vaccination in a heavily contaminated herd. The local reaction was proof of the viability of the vaccine and, in its absence, there were doubts about the vaccine's efficacy. To this may be added the lack of uniformity in methods of experimental infection of cattle, leading to differing evaluations of the resistance conferred by one or other of the various procedures.

However, research conducted in Australia between 1960 and 1970 clearly demonstrated that there was no correlation between the intensity of the vaccinal reaction and the quality of protection. Excellent resistance to experimental infection developed without any local reaction provided that the minimum required number of live mycoplasmas were inoculated (10^7 per dose for strain T_1)

If untoward local reactions of the Willem's type occur (i.e. extensive oedema starting 10 to 12 days after vaccination) antibiotic treatment (spiramycine, tylosin, tilmicosin) can be advocated.

General vaccination precautions

Vaccination against CBPP is never harmless. Apart from the local, and even generalized, reactions which may be produced, vaccination may potentiate latent infections or infestations in cattle existing under the precarious physiological balance prevalent in tropical conditions (e.g. trypanosomiasis and piroplasmosis).

Factors to take into account:

- *Breed* (where the term "breed" is often used incorrectly for species). In general, cattle breeds are more susceptible to vaccination accidents than zebu, at least in Africa. Dairy breeds are usually more susceptible than beef breeds but exceptions occur in both cases.
- *Group*. Within the same species and same breed, there are individual variations in sensitivity to vaccination (and also to infection). Such variations are a hindrance to vaccination campaigns because of possible unpredictable reactions.
- *Sex*. Pregnant females in the terminal stage of gestation should not be vaccinated.
- *Age*. The inoculation of calves under three months is usually followed by insignificant local reactions but such animals may develop arthritis, synovitis and heart valve lesions which can be fatal, at least with the most virulent strains. In practice, calves should not be vaccinated under six to eight months of age.

The level of protection induced

The vaccination of cattle against CBPP usually elicits temporary serological conversion, detectable by various standard serological tests. It takes approximately six to eight weeks to return to a serologically negative level.

The establishment of resistance is slow, at three to four weeks, and the level of resistance conferred by a CBPP vaccine can be demonstrated by testing a group of animals but not individuals. The effect of vaccination is to raise and consolidate the average level of resistance in a herd rather than to provide individual protection. Clearly, it cannot protect 100 percent of vaccinated animals. Among those vaccinated, there is a variation in resistance to infection, ranging from excellent immunity (mycoplasmocidal antibodies) to simple clinical resistance accompanied by encapsulated lung lesions from which *M. mycoides* can be recovered.

With any CBPP vaccination, there is the risk of creating semi-resistant cattle which can become chronic carriers following natural infection, thus promoting the continuance of the disease. Hence the importance of the rule of disease control which states that CBPP vaccination *must be extensive in an area and continuous in time* to be effective. By contrast, partial and unrenewed vaccination of a susceptible herd may simply maintain the disease at a low level. Failure to observe this rule has resulted in numerous disappointments in the past.

In practice, there is considerable discrepancy between resistance as assessed in the laboratory and that which operates in the field. A vaccine capable of protecting only 70 percent of cattle experimentally may still give excellent results in the field.

CBPP VACCINE: GENERAL MANUFACTURING AND CONTROL PROCEDURES

Source materials

***Strain of* M. mycoides.** The strains of *M. mycoides* used for vaccine production are identified by documents which provide information on their origin and the manipulations they have undergone. The strain selected must have been shown to be suitable for the region and the type of bovines for which it is intended, when administered by the inoculation route prescribed by the manufacturer. Before use, the strain must first have been tested to show that the resulting vaccine is safe and confers a protection lasting at least one year in cattle. One such vaccine with these characteristics is the strain T_1-44.

Strain T_1 was isolated in 1961 at the East African Veterinary Research Organisation, from a clinical case of CBPP in what is now the United Republic of Tanzania. From the outset, it appeared to be of only moderate virulence. It has been cultured in embryonated hens' eggs, first on the chorio-allantoic membrane for six passages and then in the yolk sac. Attenuated from the ninth egg passage, it has been used mainly in East Africa for preparing freeze-dried egg culture vaccines with good immunogenic qualities.

Unfortunately, following the use of egg culture vaccines there were a number of cases of postvaccinal lung lesions and numerous local reactions, leading to the suspicion that such vaccines may be dangerous. Their use was therefore suspended in 1962. Since then, it has been shown that the lung lesions may have been caused by biologically active substances present in the egg material. The intrinsic qualities of strain T_1 were not doubted, however, so it was decided to prepare liquid vaccines from broth cultures of the 44th egg passage of the strain. This material is stored in freeze-dried form.

In parallel with these studies, the possibility of combining the strain T_1 with cell-culture rinderpest vaccine to obtain a combined vaccine has also been investigated. Mutants of the strain T_1-44 that are resistant to streptomycin (present in the culture fluid of rinderpest virus) have been developed at the Institut d'Elevage et de Médecine Vétérinaire des Pays Tropicaux (IEMVT) Laboratory at Maisons-Alfort in France and the Farcha Laboratory in Chad. The Maisons-Alfort mutant (T_1-SR), obtained by three passages in a liquid medium containing increasing concentrations of streptomycin, has been studied under experimental conditions at Dakar, Senegal, for its immunogenic properties.

Thus, two lines of T_1 are now available: the original strain T_1-44 and the strain T_1-SR, which has undergone some additional passages in broth. Streptomycin appears to act as a growth factor for the latter strain, although there is no question of streptomycin-dependence. The immunogenic properties of both strains are identical, but the strain T_1-SR has produced fewer local postvaccinal reactions in humpless cattle breeds.

Both strains may be obtained from the Director of CIRAD-IEMVT, 10 rue Pierre Curie, 94704 Maisons-Alfort, Cedex, France. This is the FAO reference centre for mycoplasmas of ruminants.

Culture medium. The culture medium used contains serum or some other product of animal origin, which must be:

- either heated at 56°C for at least 30 minutes before being added to the medium, or treated by some other procedure that is equally effective in destroying contaminant microbial agents;
- submitted to appropriate tests to show that the material is free from contaminants.

In general, culture media contain:

- a basic medium consisting of meat extract (e.g. infusion or papain digest of beef heart) and / or peptone (trypose, tryptone);
- an extract or autolysate of brewer's yeast (commercially available or prepared on the spot), which provides growth factors (group B vitamins);
- glycerol, oleic acid, palmitic acid, glucose, sometimes a buffering system, a small amount of DNA and, if the vaccine is produced in a fermenter, also an antifoaming agent;
- 10 percent blood serum, preferably from adult horses, which must comply with the standard mentioned above.

If the strain T_1-SR is used, streptomycin is added at 200 mg per litre of medium. The final pH is adjusted to 8.1. A satisfactory formulation is Medium F-66 of the Farcha Laboratory.

After clarification, it is advisable to sterilize the medium by membrane filtration rather than by autoclaving. It should be used as soon as possible after pre-incubation for 24 hours at 37°C to verify the absence of bacterial contamination.

Seed lot system. Vaccine production is founded on a seed lot system. A seed lot may be part of a culture which has served for vaccine production, has been shown to be safe for cattle when administered under natural conditions and is capable of conferring an immunity that lasts for at least a year. A seed lot obtained from such a culture must not be submitted to more than three additional passages.

Seed lots[2] are freeze-dried and stored at a temperature not higher than -20°C.

Tests on seed lots. Each seed lot must be free from extraneous agents and must satisfy the standards of identity and safety in laboratory animals. In addition, a vaccine prepared from the seed lot must be tested for safety and efficacy in cattle.

Cattle used for this testing must be representative of the cattle to be vaccinated; they must come from an area free from CBPP and must be at least 24 months old and in good health. The cattle should be identified in an indelible manner and kept in quarantine under veterinary supervision for at least four months. If any clinical signs of disease are present, the animal concerned should not be used until the cause of the abnormality has been determined and recognized as having no effect on the correct conduct of the tests. Serum should be taken from each animal at the start and end of the quarantine period to be tested for CBPP antibodies. Only serologically negative cattle should be used.

- *Safety testing.* A quantity of vaccine containing at least ten times the number of mycoplasmas present in a recommended dose should be inoculated subcutaneously on the flank posterior to the scapula in each of at least ten cattle. The seed batch is satisfactory if the cattle fail to develop any unexpected clinical reaction during a period of observation lasting for at least four weeks and if no lung lesion is found on post mortem examination at the end of this period.
- *Efficacy testing.* A quantity of vaccine containing the same number of bacteria as the recommended dose should be inoculated subcutaneously on the flank posterior to the scapula in each of at least ten cattle. A similar number of cattle should be kept as a control group. After a minimum of two months have elapsed, all cattle should be submitted to challenge infection by contact with infected cattle (i.e. cattle infected by the introduction of lung lesion homogenate through an endobronchial tube). At least one infected animal should be used for each group of three cattle under test. The duration of the test is three months and any donor animal infected by intubation that dies during this period must be replaced. The seed batch passes the test if the animals inoculated with vaccine prepared from the batch do not develop a clinical or a serological reaction (i.e. an anamnestic response), post challenge, if they are free from lesions of pleuropneumonia at slaughter and if the tracheobronchial lymph nodes are free from *M. mycoides*. At least 80 percent of the unvaccinated control animals should have typical lesions at post mortem examination.

Production precautions

Inoculation and culture. The sample of the vaccine strain used for inoculating the culture vessels or the fermenter should not

[2] A seed lot prepared jointly by the IEMVT and the Pan African Veterinary Vaccine Centre (PANVAC) is now stored at both centres for free distribution to vaccine manufacturers.

have been submitted to more than two passages in broth from the seed lot.

It is best to inoculate the production medium, pre-incubated at 37°C, with a culture of the vaccine strain in the logarithmic phase of growth (36 to 40 hours culture from agitated medium), using one part of culture to ten parts of the culture medium.

After a stationary phase of incubation at 37°C, the medium is aerated (by a magnetic stirrer if flasks are used, or by injection of air if a fermenter is used).

The culture is stopped at peak growth, usually at 65 to 77 hours after inoculation. This time has to be determined precisely by each producing laboratory, with regard to local conditions, by establishing a growth curve for a culture of the vaccine strain in medium and with vessels identical to those used for production. This recommendation is important because continuation of culture after the growth peak leads to a considerable fall in pH and a diminished number of live mycoplasma.

Harvesting and freeze-drying. After a culture has been stopped, it is essential to harvest immediately, add stabilizer (for the preparation of the final product in bulk), fill the final containers and freeze-dry the product. Storage of the harvest or the final product in bulk, even in a cold chamber, has an adverse effect on the number of live mycoplasma in the vaccine. These operations are depicted in Figure 1.

The bulk suspension is prepared from a single harvest. Once transferred to the tank from which the final containers are filled, it becomes the final product in bulk. This final product is transferred quickly to the final containers and prepared for freeze-drying. At this point it becomes a batch of vaccine.

Distribution into the final containers and the subsequent freeze-drying must be done as soon as possible after the final bulk product has been prepared. After freeze-drying of the vaccine, the containers are hermetically sealed under vacuum or under dry nitrogen free from oxygen. In case of failure, all containers sealed under vacuum should be tested for airtightness and any defective container rejected.

If part of a vaccine batch is to be freeze-dried at some other time, it is best to freeze the vaccine within the final containers. After freeze-drying, it should be submitted to the control tests described below.

Freeze-drying procedure. A freeze-drying process of long duration is used where the vaccine is not exposed to temperatures above 0°C while it still contains more than 3 percent residual moisture. This can only be done in freeze-driers of the shelf type, not in the centrifuge type. Under these conditions and with a satisfactory stabilizer, the loss of viable units should not exceed 1 $\log_{10}$. In other words, with a harvest containing 10^{10} viable units per ml, concentrated freeze-dried vaccines are obtained, and their storage is considerably simplified. Operating with modern freeze-driers, less than 1.5 percent residual moisture can in fact be attained.

Control tests

Samples are taken from each vaccine batch or each distribution batch for the tests given below. The tests are performed on the vaccine reconstituted to a volume which will depend on the initial concentration of the final product in bulk. After reconstitution, samples should be stored at 4°C and tested within an hour.

Identity tests. A test of identity has to be performed on at least one labelled container of each distribution batch by using a technique suitable for identifying the presence of *M. mycoides*.

A simple and satisfactory test is growth inhibition on agar gel, using filter paper

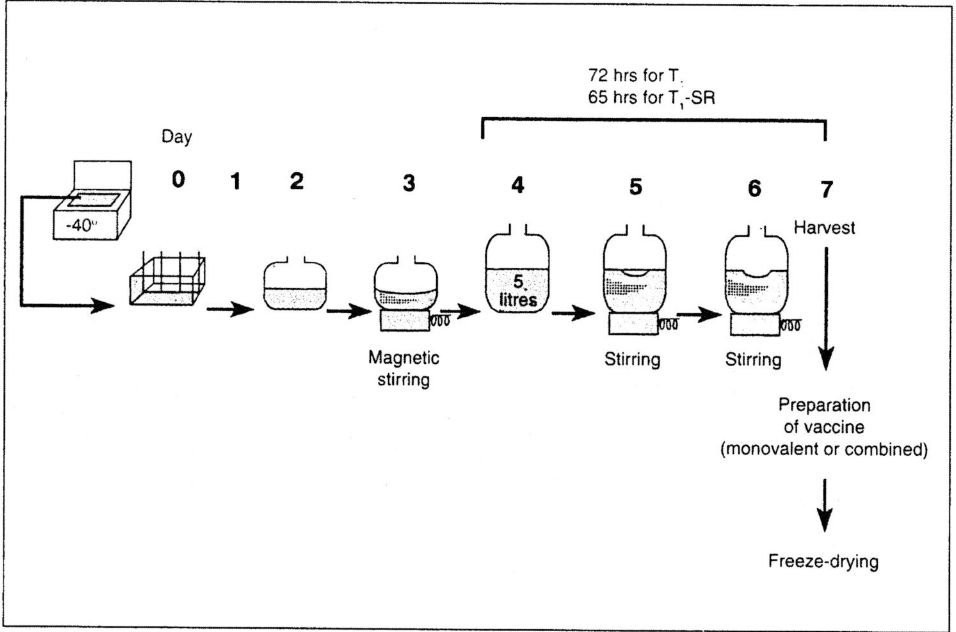

FIGURE 1
Procedure for producing CBPP vaccine from strains T_1 and T_1-SR

discs impregnated with a serum containing a high titre of antibodies to *M. mycoides* subsp. *mycoides* (SC bovine biotype). Another procedure is to place antiserum in wells punched into the agar culture. A zone of inhibition measuring at least 2 mm will be present after 48 to 72 hours of incubation. This test has the advantage of identifying other mycoplasmas (which grow within the inhibition zone) and/or bacteria present as contaminants. More refined tests (Western Blot, dot immuno-binding) can also be considered.

Sterility tests. Freedom of the vaccine from bacteria and fungi is assessed by tests made according to the recommendations of the World Health Organization's Standards for Biological Substances No. 6 (general standards concerning the sterility of biological substances).

Determination of the mycoplasma content. An organism count should be made on each batch of vaccine (or each distribution batch) to determine the number of viable *M. mycoides* per dose for cattle. This assay is done by the following procedures:

- An initial titration is performed on a mixture of at least five bottles selected at random. This mixture can also serve for testing safety and efficacy in cattle if necessary.
- Second and third titrations are each performed on the mixed contents of three bottles.
- The titre of the vaccine is the geometric mean of the three titres thus obtained.

Each titration uses a system of vaccine dilutions and the appropriate number of tubes of growth medium sufficient to estimate the 50 percent end point by a standard statistical procedure. A series of tenfold dilutions, with ten tubes of medium for each dilution, or any other dilution system which provides equal precision, is used. The tubes are incubated for at least ten days at 37°C and are shaken lightly each day to aerate the medium. The minimum titre per vaccine dose must be at least 10^7 viable mycoplasmas.

It is recommended that production laboratories take into account possible problems arising from local transport conditions and therefore supply vaccines with titres of at least 10^8 mycoplasmas per dose.

Safety tests. These tests are performed on each batch of vaccine by inoculating guinea pigs and mice. The procedure generally used consists of injecting 0.5 ml of reconstituted and undiluted vaccine intraperitoneally into each of two guinea pigs, the same dose intramuscularly into two more guinea pigs and 0.1 ml intraperitoneally into six mice. The animals are kept under observation for three weeks and then killed for examination. The batch of vaccine is considered satisfactory if the animals remain healthy and if they have no pathological lesion post mortem.

Tests for safety and efficacy in cattle. These tests are done with a mixture of vaccine from at least five bottles selected at random and as stipulated in the section Seed lot system, p. 68.

A safety test is obligatory for each vaccine batch. Because of the complexity and cost of an efficacy test, this may be performed occasionally (at least once a year) for a given batch of tested seed culture or for a vaccine derived from culture which has undergone no more than three passages from the seed culture, provided that all the arrangements for biological security of the installation and manipulations have been observed.

Stability test. It is desirable to conduct a test of stability on samples of vaccine batches to obtain experimental data to predict the effect of storage temperature and the expiry date. This data should be given on the label and in the accompanying information leaflet.

In the absence of data on long-term stability, it is recommended that accelerated degradation tests should be conducted on the vaccine to arrive at recommendations for storage conditions and expiry date. The information provided by such tests must be confirmed as soon as possible by observations on vaccine stored under the recommended conditions. Storage under these conditions must guarantee that the titre of mycoplasmas in the vaccine up to the expiry date is not less than 10^7 viable mycoplasmas per vaccine dose.

Stability tests may also be made to provide a foundation for the information accompanying each container. These tests estimate the fall in titre of mycoplasmas once the product has been reconstituted for use and after storage of the intact product under the temperature conditions which may be encountered in the field. Information should also be provided for vaccine kept in ice boxes (0° to 10°C) and vaccine kept at different ambient temperatures between 20° and 30°C (or even 40°C).

Storage conditions

While awaiting dispatch from the production establishment or storage depot, the final containers of vaccine should preferably be stored in the dark and at a temperature of -20°C or lower within rooms provided with continuous temperature-recording equipment.

During storage and transport of the vaccine, it is strongly recommended that temperature indicators be used (heat-sensitive strips or paint) to check quickly the temperature at which the vaccine has been exposed.

The expiry date should not exceed two years from the last determination of the mycoplasma count, provided that the vaccine has been stored continuously at a temperature of -20°C until delivery. Producers with large stocks of vaccine should retest the titre before extending the authorized storage period. On the other hand, no vaccine should be used later than six months after its supply by the production establishment or storage depot, and then only if the containers have been stored at temperatures of less than +10°C.

The half-life of vaccine freeze-dried to a residual moisture content of 1.5 percent is as follows:

- 4 days at 45°C;
- 1.6-2.8 weeks at 37°C;
- 2.8-4.6 weeks at 28°C;
- 30-40 weeks at 4°C.

These figures mean that, when tested during production, a vaccine that contains a concentration of 10^8 viable units per dose (which is on the low side and encountered in batches of only moderate quality) can be kept for 2 to 4 months at 28°C, 1.5 to 3 months at 37°C and 12 to 14 days at 45°C.

The storage life of reconstituted ready-to-use vaccine must not exceed the time during which the mycoplasmal count is equal to or greater than 10^7 viable organisms per vaccine dose at the specified temperatures, this having been verified experimentally.

It has been shown experimentally that reconstitution of freeze-dried vaccine in the field to give the number of doses specified by the producer is best done with a molar solution of magnesium sulphate. Under these conditions there is no fall in mycoplasma titre for four hours at 37°C. In no case should the vaccine be reconstituted with distilled water, tap water or surface water, even after boiling.

CONCLUSIONS

As stated in the introduction, any improvement in mycoplasmal vaccines is hampered by little or no information on the function of the essential immunogens of the organism, the lack of a precise understanding of the pathogenesis of mycoplasmal diseases and the insufficient knowledge of factors governing resistance to challenge or natural disease. This means that subunit vaccines, and even possibly recombinant vaccines, are still far from successful development.

Some simpler avenues appear worth exploring. New adjuvants, namely immunostimulating complexes (ISCOMs), could be studied to enhance the immunogenicity of inactivated vaccines; such steps are under way for CBPP. Another approach would be to explore the value of local immunity. In the case of CBPP, "local" means the application of the immunizing agent to the nasal mucosa by means of a vaccine spray. Preliminary tests have already been shown to be successful in some cases of enzootic pneumonia, CCPP and *M. pneumoniae* in hamsters.

Similar experiments conducted 20 years ago in Nigeria and Chad proved to be very successful with CBPP. Such an approach would now seem to be worth pursuing further.

BIBLIOGRAPHY

FAO. 1971. *Contagious bovine pleuropneumonia – a review.* FAO Agricultural Studies No. 86. Rome.

Gilbert, F.R. & Windsor, R.S. 1971. The immunising dose of T_1 strain *Mycoplasma mycoides* against contagious bovine pleuropneumonia. *Trop. Anim. Health.*, 3: 71-76.

Hudson, J.R. & Turner, A.H. 1963. Contagious bovine pleuropneumonia: a comparison of the efficacy of two types of vaccine. *Aust. Vet. J.*, 39: 373-385.

Litamoi, J., Palya, V.J., Sylla, D. & Rweyemamu, M.M. 1994. *Quality control testing of contagious bovine pleuropneumonia (CBPP) live attenuated vaccine – standard operating procedures.* Addis Ababa, PANVAC.

Office International des Epizooties. 1992. *Manual of standards for diagnostic tests and vaccines*, 2nd ed. Paris.

Provost, A., Perreau, P., Breard, A., Le Goff, C., Martel, J.L. & Cottew, G.S. 1987. Contagious bovine pleuropneumonia – a review. *Rev. sci. tech. Off. int. Epiz.*, 6(3): 625-679.

Protozoal and rickettsial vaccines

A.J. de Vos, E. Pipano, F. Musisi and W.K. Jorgensen

THE NEED FOR VACCINES

Tick-borne protozoal and rickettsial diseases affect most domestic animal species and have been a major constraint to the development of livestock industries in developing countries in the tropics and subtropics. Although tick-borne diseases (TBDs) are important in all domestic animals, this review will be concerned mainly with vaccines against the economically important tick-transmitted diseases of cattle caused by the protozoal parasites *Babesia bovis* and *Babesia bigemina* (babesiosis, red water or tick fever), *Theileria parva* (East Coast fever) and *Theileria annulata* (tropical theileriosis), as well as the rickettsial organisms *Anaplasma marginale* (anaplasmosis) and *Cowdria ruminantium* (cowdriosis, heartwater). Vaccines against coccidiosis have been reviewed by Danforth and Augustine (1989).

Babesiosis caused by *B. bovis* and *B. bigemina* is present in many countries between 40° N and 32° S (McCosker, 1981). The most important vectors are ticks of the genus *Boophilus* (Friedhoff, 1988).

East Coast fever is a disease limited to countries in eastern, central and southern Africa where the principal vector, *Rhipicephalus appendiculatus*, is present (Norval, Perry and Young, 1992). In these countries, it is of major importance because of the high morbidity and mortality it causes. Tropical theileriosis is transmitted by a number of species of the genus *Hyalomma* which have a wide distribution along the Mediterranean littoral, in the Near East and throughout Asia (Pipano, 1989).

Anaplasmosis has the widest distribution of all economically important TBDs and is transmitted biologically by at least 20 tick species. Mechanical transmission by biting flies and unsanitary veterinary practices are also important in certain areas (Palmer, 1989).

Heartwater is important in cattle and is also a major cause of losses in sheep and goats. This disease is transmitted by ticks of the genus *Amblyomma* and occurs mainly in sub-Saharan Africa, although it has also been introduced to islands in the Atlantic and Indian Oceans as well as the Caribbean. It is regarded as the most important TBD in South Africa and, next to East Coast fever, the most important one in Africa (Uilenberg, 1983; Bezuidenhout, 1989). The presence of heartwater and its vector in the Caribbean poses a threat to livestock production in the tropical and subtropical parts of the American mainland (Barre *et al.*, 1987).

Up to 500 million cattle the world over are exposed to one or more of the TBDs but this figure is not a true reflection of the number at risk to disease. Indigenous breeds of cattle often have a certain degree of natural resistance to these diseases and the consequences of infection are not as serious as when exotic *Bos taurus* breeds are involved. In addition, a state of enzootic stability frequently develops whereby local cattle become naturally infected at an early age when there is some passively acquired or innate immunity. These cattle are resistant to subsequent challenge (de Vos, 1992).

Cattle, particularly of exotic breeds, are at risk to TBDs, especially under the following circumstances.

- The importation of susceptible cattle into endemic regions. Mortality rates under these conditions can exceed 50 percent in regions endemic for babesiosis (McCosker, 1981) and the same may apply in areas infected with East Coast fever and heartwater.
- The spread of ticks and TBDs into previously uninfected areas. An example of this was the loss of over one million cattle owing to TBDs following the disruption of tick control measures in Zimbabwe (Lawrence, Foggin and Norval, 1980).
- The introduction of TBDs into a disease-free vector population – as happened when East Coast fever was introduced into southern Africa in 1896. This introduction resulted in the loss of an estimated 1.4 million cattle and took 50 years to bring under control (Lawrence, 1992).
- Increases in tick transmission rates in endemic areas caused by, among others, ecological factors. Most outbreaks of babesiosis in Australia occur in cattle bred in the endemic area (Callow and Dalgliesh, 1980).

Immunization and vector control are two options which need to be considered in all these situations. Provided there are suitable facilities and assuming commercial vaccines are not available, the local production of vaccine may be the only sustainable means of control in the country concerned.

HISTORY OF VACCINE PRODUCTION AND FUTURE PROSPECTS

B. bovis and *B. bigemina*

Methods used to immunize cattle against babesiosis have been described or reviewed (Callow and Dalgliesh, 1980; Pipano, Frank and Shkap, 1991; de Vos and Jorgensen in FAO, in press). In many countries, early attempts to vaccinate cattle against *B. bovis* and *B. bigemina* infections involved the use of blood from naturally or artificially infected carriers. This carrier-donor method, also known as premunition, has several major limitations, including unreliable potency, unpredictable reactions and the risk of contamination (Callow, 1984; de Vos and Jorgensen, 1992). During the past 30 years, more sophisticated techniques were developed to produce live vaccines from splenectomized donors, which had predicably low levels of virulence (Callow and Dalgliesh, 1980). The inherent disadvantages of vaccine containing parasites derived from the blood of animals are well documented, including the risk of reactions, contamination, sensitization against blood groups and the need for cold chain transportation (Callow and Dalgliesh, 1980; Wright, 1991). In spite of these disadvantages, virtually all operational centres producing *Babesia* vaccines are at present using variants of this technique to produce chilled or frozen live vaccines. *In vitro* culture methods reviewed by Pudney (1992) have been used to produce *B. bigemina* parasites for vaccine (Jorgensen *et al.*, 1992) and are also suitable for producing *B. bovis* parasites. However, these culture techniques are still at the developmental stage and not widely used for the production of vaccine.

Other products used in attempts to immunize cattle against babesiosis include antigens extracted from parasites or parasitized blood. Cell culture-derived exoantigens of *B. bovis* and *B. bigemina* have been extensively studied and proposed for use as vaccine in developing countries (Montenegro-James, Kakoma and Ristic, 1989). Unfortunately, the level and duration of protection conferred by these antigens against heterologous challenge are less than those of live vaccines (Timms *et al.*, 1983).

Progress to overcome the limitations of vaccines based on blood or blood extracts through the development of synthetic or recombinant *Babesia* vaccines, were reviewed by Wright *et al.* (1992) and Dalgliesh (1993). Preliminary results suggest that vaccines based on single antigens do not confer the desired level or duration of protection. It is likely that a vaccine containing several recombinant antigens will be needed to induce adequate protection (Pipano, Frank and Shkap, 1991). Even a multicomponent recombinant vaccine may not provide long-term protection against field strains of *Babesia* which have been shown to be capable of considerable genetic variation (Dalrymple *et al.*, 1992; de Vos and Jorgensen, 1992). As yet, no recombinant vaccine for bovine babesiosis has been registered for use in any country and it seems unlikely that such a vaccine will be available in the near future. When one does become available, it will almost certainly be marketed internationally and in competition with vaccines produced locally.

T. parva and *T. annulata*

As reviewed by Purnell (1977), Irvin and Morrison (1989), Pipano (1989) and Lawrence (1992), a variety of products and procedures have been or are being used to immunize cattle against East Coast fever and tropical theileriosis. Early attempts involved the use of infected blood and tissues. In the case of East Coast fever, the results were very variable but the blood of donor calves infected with low-virulence stocks of *T. annulata* was used for many years as vaccine (Pipano, 1989). Subsequently, a vaccination technique was developed which involved infecting cattle with sporozoites from ticks and then mitigating the clinical responses by chemotherapy (FAO, 1984; Irvin and Morrison, 1989; Dolan and McKeever, 1993). This "infection and treatment" method using *T. parva* sporozoites is used in some countries in East and central Africa, mainly on an experimental or field trial basis. A ground-up suspension of infected adult *R. appendiculatus* (ground-up ticks supernatant [GUTS]) is used to initiate the infection which is then controlled by treatment with oxytetracycline. Depending on the *T. parva* stocks used, sporozoite vaccine has proved effective under laboratory conditions and in field trials, providing long-lasting immunity against homologous and heterologous challenge (Burridge *et al.*, 1975a and 1975b). However, antigenic heterogeneity of *T.parva* isolates has been a major obstacle to the widespread application of this method of immunization (Irvin and Morrison, 1989). The use of a mixture of stocks is necessary to provide wide-spectrum cover against field challenge, especially where *T. parva lawrencei* is involved. In general, good protection is afforded by a vaccine made up of *T. parva* (Muguga), *T. parva* (Kiambu 5) and buffalo-derived *T. parva* (Serengeti transformed). However, because animals immunized in this way may become carriers to the infection and thus may transmit the parasite to the resident population, there is an understandable reluctance to implement immunization programmes with stocks exotic to the region or country (Irvin and Morrison, 1989).

Despite this drawback as well as the lack of attenuated, immunogenic stocks and high cost, the "infection and treatment" method is still the principal means of immunizing cattle against *T. parva*. *T. parva* (Boleni) has been used in extensive field trials in Zimbabwe. It is of low pathogenicity and treatment of reactions is rarely necessary. An application has now been made to have vaccine containing this stock registered for more general use in Zimbabwe (Pegram, personal communication, 1994). There is evidence that *T. parva* (Boleni) will also protect cattle against some highly pathogenic isolates but this feature has not been exploited in practical disease control strategies in other parts of Africa. The infection and treatment method has also been used to prepare a *T. annulata* sporozoite vaccine (Pipano, 1989) but it has not been evaluated under field conditions. Immunological differences between field isolates of *T. annulata* do not appear to be as important as in the case of *T. parva.*

In vitro techniques for the culture of schizonts of *Theileria* spp. were reviewed by Brown (1979; 1981) and Pipano (1989). *T. annulata* schizonts can readily be propagated in culture and the pathogenicity of the parasites decreases during prolonged maintenance in culture. This provided the basis for developing a safe, culture-derived vaccine for the control of tropical theileriosis (Pipano, 1989; Singh, 1990). This vaccine is currently in use or in different stages of development in several countries in Asia and around the Mediterranean (Dolan and McKeever, 1993). Unfortunately, attempts to develop a similar vaccine for *T. parva* gave disappointing results. Histocompatability is seen as one of the main obstacles to the successful transfer of *T. parva* schizonts from infected cultures to recipient hosts.

The hazards involved in using the sporozoite vaccine and the stock-specific nature of the immunity conferred have led to intensive efforts to identify parasite antigens which may be targets for protective immune responses, particularly against *T. parva* infection (Dolan and McKeever, 1993). Of sporozoite antigens identified as candidates for inclusion in a vaccine, a gene that codes for a 67 kilodalton (kDa) major surface protein has been isolated, sequenced and expressed. It provides partial protection in cattle against homologous challenge (Musoke *et al.*, 1992). Two sporozoite antigens of *T. annulata* defined by different monoclonal antibodies have also been studied as vaccine candidates. These antigens have been expressed in *Escherichia coli* and stimulate the production of neutralizing antibody in cattle (Hall and Baylis, 1993).

Anaplasma marginale

A variety of procedures have been used to immunize cattle against anaplasmosis (McHardy, 1984; Palmer, 1989). These procedures involve the use of live organisms such as attenuated *A. marginale* or *A. centrale* and killed organisms or extracts of infected blood.

A stock of *A. marginale* has been attenuated by irradiation and passage in sheep and deer (Palmer, 1989). Vaccine containing this stock was marketed as Anavac and used to immunize cattle in Latin America and the United States (Corrier, Johnson and Wagner, 1985). It provided substantial protection against challenge with most heterologous isolates. In general, use of the vaccine had no or very little clinical effect although severe morbidity and mortality have been reported, especially when older bulls and cows were immunized (Palmer, 1989). Use of attenuated *A. marginale* is the most effective means of immunization against anaplasmosis but this vaccine is apparently no longer available. Attempts to attenuate a stock of *A. marginale* by passage in sheep in Australia were unsuccessful (Jorgensen *et al.*, 1993).

Infection with *A. centrale*, an organism originally isolated in South Africa (Potgieter, 1979), provides partial cross-immunity against *A. marginale* challenge. It is usually mildly pathogenic, particularly in young animals. These features have led to the use of *A. centrale* as vaccine in a number of countries in Africa, Asia, South America and in Australia. Cross-immunity between *A. centrale* and *A. marginale* is adequate if challenge is moderate as in Australia (Callow and Dalgliesh, 1980), but may be insufficient against virulent heterologous challenge (de Vos and

Jorgensen in FAO, in press; Palmer, 1989). Despite this limitation and the risk of reactions in older animals, use of *A. centrale* appears to be the only choice available to most developing countries where anaplasmosis is endemic. An advantage of *A. centrale* is its apparent non-transmissibility by the common vectors of *A. marginale*, with the exception of the African tick *Rhipicephalus simus* (Potgieter and van Rensburg, 1987).

A non-living vaccine based on a lyophilized preparation of *A. marginale* organisms administered with adjuvant has been available for many years as Anaplaz (Fort Dodge Laboratories) in the United States and Latin America (Brock, Kliewer and Pearson, 1965). It induces partial protection against virulent heterologous challenge but the level of protection is less than that provided by live *A. marginale* vaccine (McHardy, 1984; Palmer, 1989). Neonatal iso-erythrolysis has also been reported following use of this vaccine owing to the induction of iso-antibodies to blood group antigens (Palmer, 1989). Attempts to develop a vaccine containing highly purified *Anaplasma* spp. particles have been successful (Luther *et al.*, 1989; Montenegro-James *et al.*, 1991) and a vaccine is available in Louisiana, in the United States, which does not induce sensitization against blood groups. In general, the limitations of non-living *Anaplasma* vaccines (difficulty of manufacturing them, their relative ineffectiveness and the risk of contamination with erythrocyte stroma) render production of this type of vaccine impractical in most developing countries. However, some of these vaccines are or were commercially available in Central and South American countries.

The ability to induce protective immunity with killed *Anaplasma* organisms led to further studies on purified antigens. Two surface proteins (36 and 105 kDa) induce a protective immune response in calves to homologous and heterologous challenge (Palmer, 1989; Tebele, McGuire and Palmer, 1991; McGuire *et al.*, 1992). Future work will include the evaluation of recombinants of these proteins (McGuire *et al.*, 1992).

Cowdria ruminantium

Animals which recover from heartwater acquire an immunity to the disease. This knowledge has formed the basis of an "infection and treatment" method of immunization involving the inoculation of animals with *Cowdria* sp. and treatment of ensuing reactions with tetracycline (Uilenberg, 1983). This procedure is used routinely to immunize cattle in South Africa (Oberem and Bezuidenhout, 1987; Bezuidenhout, 1989). It has been standardized to include the use of blood of sheep acutely infected with a stock of *Cowdria* sp. known to cause well-defined febrile reactions, thus allowing the optimum time of treatment to be determined. Because of the limited viability of the organisms in the unfrozen state, cryopreservation is necessary (Oberem and Bezuidenhout, 1987). The innate resistance of young animals to the clinical effects of *Cowdria* infection are well documented and have been exploited by recommending immunization at a young age. Disadvantages of this procedure include the risk of reactions in older animals, the large volume of the inoculum required (5 to 10 ml) and the need to use the intravenous route of inoculation (Uilenberg, 1983).

A supernatant of ground-up infected nymphal *Amblyomma hebraeum* ticks (GUTS) has also been used to immunize animals against *Cowdria* sp. (Oberem and Bezuidenhout, 1987; Bezuidenhout, 1989). Details of the production of this vaccine, including the infection of larval ticks, the preparation of infective nymph supernatant and the dilution and storage of the supernatant were reviewed by

Bezuidenhout (1989). The immunity conferred by this vaccine was similar to that of the blood vaccine but an unacceptably high number of animals, particularly goats, developed severe allergic or shock reactions (van der Merwe, 1987).

Considerable progress has also been made in recent years with the development of *in vitro* methods for propagating *Cowdria* sp. and a great number of stocks have been grown successfully (Bezuidenhout and Brett, 1992). One roller bottle (surface area 800 cm^2) with bovine or ovine endothelial cells can yield enough organisms to infect 20 000 animals. There is also evidence of attenuation *in vitro* without loss of immunogenicity (Jongejan, 1991). Future work will be aimed at optimizing culture conditions for organism yield, improving viability following freezing and thawing (Bezuidenhout and Brett, 1992) and overcoming the effect of antigenic differences between isolates (Jongejan *et al.*, 1993).

Attempts are being made to identify and express immunodominant *Cowdria* proteins (Barbet *et al.*, 1992). The ultimate goal of the Heartwater Research Project at the University of Florida, United States, is to develop a recombinant vaccine delivered by a live virus vector.

PRODUCTION OF VACCINES

The following methods of vaccine production are at present being used in developing countries or are likely to be within the means of countries where reliance on enzootic stability is not an option and immunization is the only viable alternative. As discussed in the previous section, the vaccines all have the drawbacks inherent in the production and use of live products.

Babesia bovis and *Babesia bigemina*

Selection, attenuation and storage of stocks. It is tempting to use *Babesia* isolates from the country in which the vaccine is to be produced. Such isolates can be obtained by feeding infected *Boophilus* spp. ticks on a susceptible bovine host or by inoculating it with blood from a long-standing carrier (Callow, 1984). The major limitation of using a carrier is the risk of contamination. Techniques for collecting, purifying and attenuating *B. bovis* and *B. bigemina* stocks have been described (de Vos and Jorgensen in FAO, in press).

Attempts to develop attenuated stocks of *B. bovis* from local isolates are not always successful (de Vos and Jorgensen, 1992). For this reason, it may be worthwhile to import a stock that is known to be protective, of low virulence and free from contaminants. Australian stocks have been shown to be protective in several countries and vaccines containing these stocks have been used with beneficial results in Africa, Asia and South America (de Vos and Jorgensen, 1992).

The attenuation of a *B. bovis* stock is usually achieved by rapid syringe passage through splenectomized calves (Callow and Dalgliesh, 1980; de Vos and Jorgensen in FAO, in press; Pipano, Frank and Shkap, 1991). The mechanism by which attenuation is achieved is not fully understood but appears to be the result of a selective enrichment of avirulent parasite subpopulations. Other methods used to attenuate *B. bovis* include irradiation (Wright, Goodger and Mahoney, 1980), *in vitro* culture techniques (Yunker, Kuttler and Johnson, 1987) and the use of alternative hosts, but these methods give less reliable results than passage in splenectomized calves. Rapid passage of *B. bigemina* in splenectomized calves is not recommended. A stock of this parasite with generally low virulence may be obtained after a series of slow passages in non-splenectomized calves (Callow and Dalgliesh, 1980).

Vaccine stocks of *B. bovis* and *B. bigemina* can be stored for lengthy periods as cryopreserved stabilates of infected blood. Dimethyl sulphoxide (DMSO) (Mellors *et al.*, 1982), glycerol (Dalgliesh, Jorgensen and de Vos, 1990) and polyvinyl pyrrolidone (PVP) (de Vos and Jorgensen in FAO, in press) have all been used successfully to cryopreserve *Babesia* spp. parasites.

Supply of infective material using donor calves. Cryopreserved master seed of an attenuated stock is used to initiate a primary infection in a susceptible, splenectomized donor. The initial *B. bovis* parasitaemia is often low but adequate to initiate a series of four to five passages, thus allowing a continuous supply of vaccine over a three- to five-week period. *B. bovis* vaccine stocks should not be passaged more than a total of 30 times to reduce the risk of losing immunogenicity (Callow and Dalgliesh, 1980; Bock *et al.*, in press; de Vos and Jorgensen, 1992). Inocula containing about 1×10^{10} parasites are ideal for passaging and will result in parasitaemias in excess of 1×10^8 per millilitre within four to five days. Up to 25 000 doses of vaccine can be obtained from a calf weighing 150 to 200 kg. *B. bigemina*-infected blood is obtained from individually infected calves; serial passing is not recommended because of possible selection for virulence.

Supply of infective material using parasites grown in vitro. Available technology allows *B. bovis* and *B. bigemina* to be maintained in continuous culture (Pudney, 1992). These culture systems have the advantage over the calf-donor system of minimizing the risk of contamination and limiting the number of animals required. A relatively robust method for producing *B. bigemina* vaccine in sealed flask suspension cultures was developed by Jorgensen *et al.* (1992) and may be a viable option in countries where insufficient numbers of donors are available for the production of vaccine *in vivo*. Some studies found that neither the virulence nor the immunogenicity of *Babesia* vaccine stocks were appreciably modified by maintenance in culture (Timms *et al.*, 1983; Jorgensen, de Vos and Dalgliesh, 1989). However, recent work using the polymerase chain reaction (PCR) of polymorphic genetic markers has shown that proportions of *B. bovis* subpopulations do change with culture *in vitro* (Bock *et al.*, in press; Lew, unpubl.).

Theileria parva

Isolation, storage and characterization of stocks. Vaccine should be prepared using master seed of well-characterized *T. parva* stocks to account for the antigenic heterogeneity of this species. If there is a requirement for local stocks, these can be obtained by using bait or naturally infected cattle or by collecting and feeding infected ticks from the field. Procedures used to isolate stocks of *T. parva* have been documented in the literature (FAO, 1984; Purnell, 1977). However, considerable expertise is required in the isolation and characterization of isolates. Species identification is based on examination of some or all of the following: geographical distribution, vector specificity, morphology, host specificity, pathogenicity, serology, cross-immunity and DNA probes. Stock characterization traditionally involves cross-immunity studies, among others. Several monoclonal antibodies and DNA probes have also been used to divide stocks of *T. parva* into groups (Minami *et al.*, 1983; Conrad *et al.*, 1987; Allsopp and Allsopp, 1988) but more work is necessary to determine whether polymorphisms detected correlate with differences in cross-protection (Irvin and Morrison, 1989).

Preparation of ground-up tick supernatant. Details of the preparation of GUTS are available in the literature (FAO, 1984). The process involves the inoculation of cattle with *T. parva* seed material. Approximately ten days after inoculation, the cattle are infested with non-infected nymphal ticks. Engorged ticks are harvested and allowed to moult. The level of infection can be determined by examining the number of infected acini in the salivary glands of some of the prefed adult ticks. The remainder of the adult ticks are fed on the ears of rabbits, detached after four days, washed, disinfected and ground up in a suitable medium. Ground-up tick tissue is centrifuged at a low speed and the supernatant collected, mixed with glycerolized medium, equilibrated and cryopreserved. One litre of frozen vaccine can be prepared from 10 000 adult ticks and this will provide 1 000 1-ml doses of vaccine.

Theileria annulata

Isolation of stocks. Isolation of *T. annulata* parasites from the field was reviewed by Pipano (1989). Isolates can be obtained by inoculating cattle with the blood of infected animals or by exposing the cattle to infected ticks. An alternative and more elegant technique is to infect peripheral blood leucocytes *in vitro* with sporozoites obtained from macerated infected ticks.

Propagation of schizonts in vitro. Techniques used to initiate and maintain *T. annulata* cultures are well documented (Brown, 1979; Pipano, 1989). Briefly, lymphocytes are collected from the blood or organs of infected cattle and grown in monolayer or suspension cultures. Alternatively, normal peripheral blood lymphocytes can be infected *in vitro* with sporozoites obtained from infected ticks (Brown, 1979). Standard culture procedures are used and a wide variety of culture media are suitable. Yields of up to 9×10^7 schizont-infected lymphocytes can be obtained from a stationary culture vessel containing 100 ml of medium, and even more from roller bottles.

Continuous propagation of *T. annulata* in lymphoid cell cultures eliminates other tick-borne agents such as *Babesia* spp., *Anaplasma* spp. and *Eperythozoon* spp. Theoretically, however, some viral infections can be introduced into cultures from ticks or cattle used as a source of infected lymphocytes.

Partial or complete attenuation of *T. annulata* is achieved by prolonged cultivation *in vitro* (Pipano, 1989). Complete attenuation (no clinical manifestation and no detectable tissue schizonts or erythrocytic merozoites) has been reported after 600 to 900 days in culture (Pipano, 1989; Singh, 1990). Partially attenuated schizonts have also been used for vaccination (Zablotsky, 1988).

When the desired degree of attenuation is reached, schizont-infected cells can be cryopreserved with a high degree of survival upon reconstitution (Wathanga, Jones and Brown, 1986). DMSO or glycerol can be used as cryopreservative. Master seed stock is usually prepared and used to initiate a series of passages in culture to yield parasites for vaccine. There is little information on the selective effect of long-term passaging of schizonts on immunogenicity but there is evidence that attenuated schizonts are less infective and less protective than virulent schizonts. Therefore, it is recommended that production cycles be restarted periodically from the same master seed (Pipano, 1989).

Anaplasma spp. using *A. centrale* as vaccine

Selection and storage of stock. Only one stock of *A. centrale* exists. The history of its isolation in South Africa in 1911 was recorded by Potgieter (1979). This stock has been used to initiate vaccine production programmes in several countries (Potgieter, 1979; Callow and Dalgliesh, 1980; Pipano *et al.*, 1986; Abdala *et al.*, 1990). Master seed of *A. centrale* is prepared and stored in the same way as that of *Babesia* spp.

Supply of infective material. Infective blood

containing suitable numbers of *A. centrale* organisms for the production of vaccine can be obtained in much the same way as *Babesia* parasites. Blood from acutely infected splenectomized calves is most suitable for the purpose although, in some laboratories, the blood of carrier-donors showing quantifiable rickettsemia is used and reported to be effective (Potgieter, 1979). *A. centrale* vaccine can be prepared in frozen or chilled forms in the same way as *Babesia* vaccines (de Vos and Jorgensen in FAO, in press). In some countries, for example Australia, mixed *Babesia/ Anaplasma* vaccines are produced (Callow and Dalgliesh, 1980).

Cowdria ruminantium

Selection and storage of stocks. The isolation and characterization of *Cowdria* stocks have been reviewed in the literature (Uilenberg, 1983; FAO, 1984; Oberem and Bezuidenhout, 1987; Bezuidenhout, 1989). Isolates can be obtained from both the vertebrate host and the tick vector by subinoculation of infected blood, organ emulsions or supernatant of ground-up, engorging *Amblyomma* ticks. Stocks vary considerably in virulence and there is some evidence of immunological differences (Jongejan *et al.*, 1993). However, immunity does not depend on the virulence of the isolate. It is important to select a stock which is as mild as possible but which shows adequate cross-protection against local isolates. Furthermore, it must also be susceptible to treatment with available anti-*Cowdria* drugs. Only one stock (Ball 3) is used in South Africa. It generally causes a marked febrile response some days before the onset of other clinical signs.

Stabilate of the stock used for production of vaccine is produced in the same way as the vaccine itself (see below) and stored at -70° or -196°C. Infective material has also been freeze-dried successfully if kept below -18°C (du Plessis *et al.*, 1990).

Production of infective material from donor sheep. The method used in South Africa has been described in some detail (FAO, 1984; Oberem and Bezuidenhout, 1987; Bezuidenhout, 1989). Briefly, susceptible sheep are inoculated with thawed stabilate and bled nine to ten days later at the height of the febrile reaction. The stabilate is usually prepared from the blood of reacting sheep but tick-derived stabilates will fulfil the same purpose. Similarly, goats and cattle can also be used as donors. Blood from reacting animals is collected directly into an equal volume of buffer to which DMSO has been added. The diluted blood is then snap-frozen and stored in liquid nitrogen. Up to 4 000 doses of vaccine can be prepared from one sheep.

VACCINE DISPENSING AND DISPATCH

Dilution of vaccine concentrate

Some vaccine starter materials, notably *Theileria* GUTS and blood infected with *Babesia* spp. and *Theileria* spp., are very concentrated and can be diluted to increase the vaccine yield. The appropriate medium to be used as diluent depends on the starter material and whether the vaccine is to be frozen or not. Details of media used in the production of TBD vaccines have been reviewed (FAO, 1984; Bezuidenhout, 1989; Pipano, 1989; de Vos and Jorgensen in FAO, in press).

Viability of *Babesia* and *Anaplasma* organisms can be maintained in chilled form by storing infected blood at 2° to 4°C. Even at this temperature, infectivity is lost exponentially, declining by about one log unit during the first week of storage (Callow, 1984). Chilled *Babesia* and *Anaplasma* vaccines usually contain 0.5 to 1×10^7 organisms per dose or about 100 times the minimum infective number required for subcutaneous inoculation. The required number of organisms is obtained by diluting the infected blood with a suitable medium. Chilled *T. annulata* vaccine can also be prepared from culture material, with the recommended number of infected cells being 0.5×10^7 (Pipano, 1989).

The minimum volume of a dose of vaccine should preferably not be less than 2 ml to allow for inaccuracies in vaccination equipment and procedures. An exeption is *T. parva* sporozoite vaccine where the recommended dose is 1 ml to allow for inoculation over the parotid lymph node.

Vaccine dispensing

Techniques for producing frozen vaccines using DMSO as a cryoprotectant were described by Mellors *et al.* (1982) and Abdala *et al.* (1990). Vaccine with glycerol as cryoprotectant has also been produced (Dalgliesh, Jorgensen and de Vos, 1990) and is known to remain viable for at least eight hours after thawing. Frozen vaccine is dispensed in cryovials suitable for low-temperature storage.

Dispatch and cold chain

The types of transport networks and their efficiency vary greatly between countries and the choice depends largely on availability. Rapid, reliable means of communication and transport are desirable for frozen vaccine and essential for chilled products. Frozen vaccine can be transported in vacuum-insulated containers with a refrigerant (liquid N_2 or solid CO_2). Vaccine should not be thawed until just before use and, once thawed, must not be refrozen. Chilled *Babesia, Anaplasma* and *Theileria* vaccines have a very short shelf-life, even when packed in ice, and may become ineffective if transport to the destination exceeds 48 hours.

QUALITY ASSURANCE

Because of the live nature of TBD vaccines, quality control is essential to ensure potency and to minimize the risk of contamination. Most of the early *Babesia* and *Anaplasma* vaccines produced by the carrier-donor method and the *T. parva* vaccines produced with tissue suspensions had variable potencies, thus bringing these vaccines into general disrepute. In some countries in the tropics and subtropics, the risk of contamination is also very real. Quality assurance therefore needs to be an integral part of any TBD vaccine production programme covering all operating procedures.

The standards of quality assurance of *Babesia, Anaplasma* and *Theileria* vaccines have been addressed by the Office internationale des épizooties (OIE, 1991). However, these standards only cover the main aspects. Quality control of *T. annulata* vaccine in Israel is based on the procedures for testing live vaccines described in the United States Code of Federal Regulations for Animals and Animal Products. In Australia, procedures for the production of *Babesia* and *Anaplasma* vaccines are being modified to comply with the Australian Code of Good Manufacturing Practice for Veterinary Preparations. Compliance with these or similar codes may not be possible in all developing countries. However, the potential consequences of providing substandard or contaminated vaccine should be considered. The contamination of one batch of *Babesia/Anaplasma* vaccine in Australia with enzootic bovine leucosis (Rogers *et al.*, 1988) resulted in the payment of US$1.5 million in compensation.

Quality control should be performed at both the preproduction and postproduction stages. Preproduction quality control is particularly important in the case of chilled vaccine but is, in itself, not adequate to guarantee potency and purity. It should include facilities, the documentation of standards and procedures for obtaining and quarantining suitable donor animals and the preproduction testing of animals, master seed and other starting materials used in the production of vaccine.

It should also include environmental monitoring to ensure that there is only a minimal risk of infectious challenge in the region where the production facility is located.

Postproduction quality control should be aimed at determining potency, purity and, where relevant, virulence. Potency and virulence are monitored by inoculating groups of susceptible cattle and then monitoring the reactions. Dalgliesh, Jorgensen and de Vos (1990) described a method for testing the potency of frozen *Babesia* vaccine. Similar procedures have been described for *Theileria* spp. (FAO, 1984) and *Cowdria* sp. (Bezuidenhout, 1989). Each batch should also be tested for freedom from contaminants, with the choice of tests depending on the diseases suspected and the type of vaccine concerned. Tick-derived sporozoite vaccines naturally do not need to be scrutinized as intensely as vaccines produced from the blood of infected animals but there is a risk of other TBDs, including Crimean Congo haemorrhagic fever.

FACTORS CRITICAL TO THE PRODUCTION OF TBD VACCINES IN DEVELOPING COUNTRIES

- Availability of stocks known to be protective against local challenge and showing other desirable traits.
- Availability of disease-free donor animals as a source of infected blood, infected ticks and other starter materials. This may require the animals to be bred under tick- and arthropod-free conditions for the specific purpose of vaccine production.
- Availability of suitable facilities to maintain disease-free animals and to perform the necessary procedures (splenectomies, feeding of ticks, collection of blood).
- Laboratory facilities and expertise to monitor donor cattle and starter materials (infected blood, culture material, infected ticks) for quality control purposes.
- Suitable laboratory facilities and services, including reliable electrical supplies and low-temperature storage facilities.
- Access to foreign capital for the purchase of equipment, reagents and other supplies needed for production and quality control.
- Access to reliable transport networks.
- A core of dedicated, trained staff.
- Access to training opportunities, procedures and proven master seed.

KEY LABORATORIES PRODUCING TBD VACCINES

The following laboratories are involved in the production of TBD vaccines and may be able to provide suitable master seed, details of production procedures and quality control as well as training opportunities.

Babesia spp.

- Tick Fever Research Centre, Wacol, Queensland, Australia
- Kimron Veterinary Institute, Bet Dagan, Israel
- Veterinary Research Institute, Onderstepoort, South Africa
- Central Veterinary Laboratory, Lilongwe, Malawi
- Instituto Nacional de Tecnologia Agropecuaria, Rafaela, Argentina
- Miguel C. Rubino Laboratory, Pando, Uruguay

Theileria parva

- Central Veterinary Laboratory, Lilongwe, Malawi
- ILRAD, Nairobi, Kenya

Theileria annulata

- Kimron Veterinary Institute, Bet Dagan, Israel
- Animal Disease Research Laboratory, NDDB, Anand, India

Anaplasma

- See *Babesia* spp. list.

Cowdria spp.

- Veterinary Research Institute, Onderstepoort, South Africa

BIBLIOGRAPHY

Abdala, A.A., Pipano, E., Aguirre, D.H., Gaido, A.B., Zurbriggen, M.A., Mangold, A.J. & Guglielmone, A.A. 1990. Frozen and fresh *Anaplasma centrale* vaccines in the protection of cattle against *Anaplasma marginale* infection. *Rev. Elevage Méd. Vét. Pays Trop.*, 43: 155-158.

Allsopp, B.A. & Allsopp, M.T.E.P. 1988. *Theileria parva*: genomic DNA studies reveal intraspecific sequence diversity. *Mol. Biochem. Parasitol.*, 28: 77-84.

Barbet, A.F., Mahan, S., Allred, D., McGuire, T.C., Palmer, G.H. & Yunker, C.E. 1992. Molecular biology of rickettsiae: gene organisation and structure in *Anaplasma marginale* and *Cowdria ruminantium*. *In* T.T. Dolan, ed. *Recent developments in the control of anaplasmosis, babesiosis and cowdriosis*, p. 87-91. Nairobi, ILRAD.

Barre, N., Uilenberg, G., Morel, P.C. & Camus, E. 1987. Danger of introducing heartwater onto the American mainland: potential role of indigenous and exotic *Amblyomma* ticks. *Onderstepoort J. Vet. Res.*, 54: 405-417.

Bezuidenhout, J.D. 1989. *Cowdria* vaccines. *In* I.G. Wright, ed. *Veterinary protozoan and hemoparasite vaccines*, p. 31-42. Boca Raton, Fla., USA, CRC.

Bezuidenhout, J.D. & Brett, S. 1992. Progress with the cultivation of *Cowdria ruminantium* in endothelial cells. *In* T.T. Dolan, ed. *Recent developments in the control of anaplasmosis, babesiosis and cowdriosis*, p. 141-147. Nairobi, ILRAD.

Bock, R.E., de Vos, A.J., Kingston, T.G., Shiels, I.A. & Dalgliesh, R.J. 1992. Investigations of breakdowns in protection provided by living *Babesia bovis* vaccine. *Vet. Parasitol.*, 43: 45-56.

Bock, R.E., de Vos, A.J., Lew, A., Kingston, T.G. & Fraser, I.R. Studies on failure of T strain live *Babesia bovis* vaccine. *Aust. Vet. J.* (in press)

Brock, W.E., Kliewer, I.O. & Pearson, C.C. 1965. A vaccine for anaplasmosis. *J. Am. Vet. Med. Assoc.*, 147: 948-951.

Brown, C.G.D. 1979. Propagation of *Theileria*. *In* K. Maramorosch & H. Hirumi, eds. *Practical tissue culture applications*, p. 223-254. New York, Academic.

Brown, C.G.D. 1981. Application of *in vitro* techniques to vaccination against theileriosis. *In* A.D. Irvin, M.P. Cunningham & A.S. Young, eds. *Advances in control of theileriosis*, p. 104-119. The Hague, Martinus Nijhoff.

Burridge, M.J., Morzaria, S.P., Cunningham, M.P. & Brown, C.G.D. 1972. Duration of immunity to East Coast fever (*Theileria parva*) infection in cattle. *Parasitol.*, 64: 511-515.

Callow, L.L. 1984. *Animal health in Australia, Vol. 5. Protozoal and rickettsial diseases*, p. 1-264. Canberra, Australian Government Publishing Service.

Callow, L.L. & Dalgliesh, R.J. 1980. The development of effective, safe vaccination against babesiosis and anaplasmosis in Australia. *In* L.A.Y. Johnston & M.G. Cooper, eds. *Ticks and tick-borne diseases*, p. 4-8. Sydney, Australian Veterinary Association.

Conrad, P.A., Iams, K., Brown, W.C., Sohanpal, B. & Ole-Moi Yoi, O. 1987. DNA probes detect genomic diversity in *Theileria parva* stocks. *Mol. Biochem. Parasitol.*, 25: 213-226.

Corrier, D.E., Johnson, J.S. & Wagner, G.G. 1985. Demonstration of vaccine-induced immunity to anaplasmosis without induction of persistent post-vaccinal complement-fixing and agglutinating antibodies in yearling steers. *Am. J. Vet. Res.*, 46: 583-586.

Dalgliesh, R.J. 1993. Immunity, immunopathology and molecular biology in babesiosis. *In* K.A. Warren & N. Agabian, eds. *Immunology and molecular biology of parasitic infections*, p. 350-381. New York, Blackwell Scientific.

Dalgliesh, R.J., Jorgensen, W.K. & de Vos, A.J. 1990. Australian frozen vaccines for the control of babesiosis and anaplasmosis in cattle – a review. *Trop. Anim. Health Prod.*, 22: 44-52.

Dalrymple, B.P., Jorgensen, W.K., de Vos, A.J. & Wright, I.G. 1992. Analysis of the composition of samples of *Babesia bovis* and the influence of different environmental conditions on genetically distinct subpopulations. *Int. J. Parasitol.*, 22: 31-737.

Danforth, H.D. & Augustine, P.C. 1989. *Coccidia* vaccines. *In* I.G. Wright, ed. *Veterinary protozoan and hemoparasite vaccines*, p. 165-175. Boca Raton, Fla., USA, CRC.

de Vos, A.J. 1992. Distribution, economic importance and control measures for *Babesia* and *Anaplasma*. *In* T.T. Dolan, ed. *Recent developments in the control of anaplasmosis, babesiosis and cowdriosis*, p. 3-12. Nairobi, ILRAD.

de Vos, A.J. & Jorgensen, W.K. 1992. Protection of cattle against babesiosis in tropical and subtropical countries with a live, frozen vaccine. *In* B.H. Fivaz, T.N. Petney & I.G. Horak, eds. *Tick vector biology – medical and veterinary aspects*, p. 159-174. Berlin, Springer.

Dolan, T.T. & McKeever, D.J. 1993. Current and future vaccines against theileriosis. *In* R. Pandey, S. Hoglund & G. Prasad, eds. *Veterinary vaccines*, p. 318-337. Berlin, Springer.

du Plessis, J.L., van Gas, L., Labuschagne, F.J. & Wijma, S. 1990. The freeze-drying of *Cowdria ruminantium*. *Onderstepoort J. Vet. Res.*, 57: 145-149.

FAO. 1984. *Tick and tick-borne disease control. A practical field manual, Vol.II. Tick-borne disease control*, p. 300-621. Rome.

FAO. *Babesia bovis, Babesia bigemina* and *Anaplasma marginale* vaccines. In *Ticks and tick-borne disease control – a practical field manual.* Rome. (in press)

Friedhoff, K.T. 1988. Transmission of *Babesia*. *In* M. Ristic, ed. *Babesiosis of domestic animals and man*, p. 23-52. Boca Raton, Fla., USA, CRC.

Hall, R. & Baylis, H.A. 1993. Tropical theileriosis. *Parasitol. Today*, 9: 310-312.

Irvin, A.D. & Morrison, W.I. 1989. Vaccines against *Theileria parva*. *In* I.G. Wright, ed. *Veterinary protozoan and hemoparasite vaccines*, p. 115-130. Boca Raton, Fla., USA, CRC.

Jongejan, F. 1991. Protective immunity to heartwater (*Cowdria ruminantium* infection) is acquired after vaccination with *in vitro* attenuated rickettsia. *Infect. Immun.*, 59: 729-731.

Jongejan, F., Vogel, S.W., Gueye, A. & Uilenberg, G. 1993). Vaccination against heartwater using *in vitro* attenuated *Cowdria ruminatium* organisms. *Rev. Elevage Méd. Vét. Pays Trop.*, 46: 223-227.

Jorgensen, W.K., de Vos, A.J. & Dalgliesh, R.J. 1989. Comparison of immunogenicity and virulence between *Babesia bigemina* parasites from continuous culture and from a splenectomized calf. *Aust. Vet. J.*, 61: 371-372.

Jorgensen, W.K., Waldron, S.J., McGrath, J., Roman, R.J., de Vos, A.J. & Williams, K.E. 1992. Growth of *Babesia bigemina* parasites in suspension cultures for vaccine production. *Parasitol. Res.*, 78: 423-426.

Jorgensen, W.K., Bock, R.E., de Vos, A.J. & Shiels, I.A. 1993. Sheep-adapted *Anaplasma marginale* maintains virulence for cattle. *Aust. Vet. J.*, 70: 192-193.

Lawrence, J.A. 1992. History of bovine theileriosis in southern Africa. *In* R.A.I. Norval, B.D. Perry & A.S. Young, eds. *The epidemiology of theileriosis in Africa*, p. 1-39. London, Academic.

Lawrence, J.A., Foggin, C.M. & Norval, R.A.I. 1980. The effects of war on the control of diseases of livestock in Rhodesia (Zimbabwe). *Vet. Rec.*, 107: 82-85.

Luther, D.G., Hart, L.T., Morris, N.G., McRae, B. & Todd, W.J. 1989. Field trial of an experimental anaplasmosis vaccine in Louisiana. *Proc. Annu. Meet. US Anim. Health Assoc.*, 93: 35-38.

McCosker, P.J. 1981. The global importance of babesiosis. *In* M. Ristic, ed. *Babesiosis*, p. 1-24. New York, Academic.

McGuire, T.C., Barbet, A.F., Tebele, N., McElwain, T.F. & Palmer, G.H. 1992. Progress in development of subunit vaccines for anaplasmosis. *In* T.T. Dolan, ed. *Recent developments in the control of anaplasmosis, babesiosis and cowdriosis*, p. 99-104. Nairobi, ILRAD.

McHardy, N. 1984. Immunisation against anaplasmosis – a review. *Prev. Vet. Med.*, 2: 135-146.

Mellors, L.T., Dalgliesh, R.J., Timms., Rodwell, B.J. & Callow, L.L. 1982. Preparation and laboratory testing of frozen vaccine containing *Babesia bovis, Babesia bigemina* and *Anaplasma centrale*. *Res. Vet. Sci.*, 32:194-197.

Minami, T., Spooner, P.R., Irvin, A.D., Ocama, J.G.R., Dobbelaere, D.A.E. & Fujinaga, T. 1983. Characterisation of stocks of *Theileria parva* by monoclonal antibody profiles. *Res. Vet. Sci.*, 35: 334-340.

Montenegro-James, S., Kakoma, I. & Ristic, M. 1989. Culture-derived *Babesia* exoantigens as immunogens. *In* I.G. Wright, ed. *Veterinary protozoan and hemoparasite vaccines*, p. 61-97. Boca Raton, Fla., USA, CRC.

Montenegro-James, S., James, M.A., Toro Benitez, M., Leon, E., Baek, B.K. & Guillen, A.T. 1991. Efficacy of purified *Anaplasma marginale* initial bodies as a vaccine against anaplasmosis. *Parasitol. Res.*, 77: 93-101.

Musoke ,A.J., Morzaria, S.P., Nkonge, C., Jones, E. & Nene, V. 1992. A recombinant sporozoite surface antigen of *Theileria parva* induces protection in cattle. *Proc. Nat. Acad. Sci. USA*, 89: 514-518.

Norval, R.A.I., Perry, B.D. & Young, A.S. 1992. *The epidemiology of theileriosis in Africa*, p. 1-481. London, Academic.

Oberem, P.T. & Bezuidenhout, J.D. 1987. The production of heartwater vaccine. *Onderstepoort J. Vet. Res.*, 54: 485-488.

OIE. 1991. *Manual of recommended diagnostic techniques and requirements for biological products, Vol. III.* Paris.

Palmer, G.H. 1989. *Anaplasma* vaccines. *In* I.G. Wright, ed. *Veterinary protozoan and hemoparasite vaccines*, p. 1-29. Boca Raton, Fla., USA, CRC.

Pipano, E. 1989. Vaccination against *Theileria annulata* theileriosis. *In* I.G. Wright, ed. Veterinary and hemoparasite vaccines, p. 203-234. Boca Raton, Fla., USA, CRC.

Pipano, E., Frank, M. & Shkap, V. 1991. Current methods for the control of tick fevers in cattle. *Is. J. Vet. Med.*, 46: 79-88.

Pipano, E., Krigel, Y., Frank, M., Markovics, A. & Mayer, E. 1986. Frozen *Anaplasma centrale* vaccine against anaplasmosis in cattle. *Br. Vet. J.*, 142: 553-556.

Potgieter, F.T. 1979. Epizootiology and control of anaplasmosis in South Africa. *J. S. Afr. Vet. Assoc.*, 50: 367-372.

Potgieter, F.T. & van Rensburg, L.T. 1987. Tick transmission of *Anaplasma centrale*. *Onderstepoort J. Vet. Res.*, 54: 5-7.

Pudney, M. 1992. Cultivation of *Babesia*. *In* T.T. Dolan, ed. *Recent developments in the control of anaplasmosis, babesiosis and cowdriosis*, p. 129-140. Nairobi, ILRAD.

Purnell, R.E. 1977. East Coast fever: some recent research in East Africa. *Adv. Parasitol.*, 15: 83-132.

Radley, D.E., Brown, C.G.D., Burridge, M.J., Cunningham, M.P., Kirimi, I.M., Purnell, R.E. & Young, A.S. 1975a. East Coast fever. 1. Chemoprophylactic immunisation of cattle against *Theileria* *parva* (Muguga) and five *Theileria* strains. *Vet. Parasitol.*, 1: 5-41.

Radley, D.E., Brown, C.G.D, Cunningham, M.P., Kimber, C.D., Musisi, F.L., Payne, R.C., Purnell, R.E. & Stagg, S.M. 1975b. East Coast fever. 3. Chemoprophylactic immunisation of cattle using oxytetracycline and a combination of *Theileria* strains. *Vet. Parasitol.*, 1: 51-60.

Rogers, R.J., Dimmock, C.K., de Vos, A.J. & Rodwell, B.J. 1988. Bovine leucosis virus contamination of a vaccine produced *in vivo* against bovine babesiosis and anaplasmosis. *Aust. Vet. J.*, 65: 285-287.

Singh, D.K. 1990. Methods currently used for the control of *Theileria annulata:* their validity and proposals for future control strategies. *Parasitologia,* 32: 33-40.

Tebele, N., McGuire, T.C. & Palmer, G.H. 1991. Induction of protective immunity using *Anaplasma marginale* initial body membranes. *Infect. Immun.*, 59: 3199-3204.

Timms, P., Dalgliesh, R.J., Barry, D.N., Dimmock, C.K. & Rodwell, B.J. 1983. *Babesia bovis*: comparison of culture-derived parasites, non-living antigen and conventional vaccine in the protection of cattle against heterologous challenge. *Aust. Vet. J.*, 60: 75-77.

Uilenberg, G. 1983. Heartwater (*Cowdria ruminantium* infection): current status. *Adv. Vet. Sci. Comp. Med.*, 27: 427-480.

van der Merwe, L. 1987. The infection and treatment method of vaccination against heartwater. *Onderstepoort J. Vet. Res.*, 54: 489-491.

Wathanga, J.M., Jones, T.W. & Brown, C.G.D. 1986. Cryopreservation of *Theileria* infected lymphoblastoid cells with functional assessment of viability. *Trop. Anim. Health Prod.*, 18: 191-197.

Wright, I.G. 1991. Towards a synthetic *Babesia* vaccine. *Int. J. Parasitol.*, 21: 156-159.

Wright, I.G., Goodger, B.V. & Mahoney, D.F. 1980. The irradiation of *Babesia bovis*. I. The difference in pathogenicity between irradiated and non-irradiated populations. *Z. Parasitol.*, 63: 47-57.

Wright, I.G., Casu, R., Commins, M.A. & Dalrymple, B.P. 1992. The development of a recombinant *Babesia* vaccine. *Vet. Parasitol.*, 44: 3-13.

Yunker, C.E., Kuttler, K.L. & Johnson, L.W. 1987. Attenuation of *Babesia bovis* by *in vitro* cultivation. *Vet. Parasitol.*, 24: 7-13.

Zablotsky, V.T. 1988. Response of cattle of different ages to *Theileria annulata* vaccine, II. Reaction and immune response of calves of different breeds to theileriosis vaccine. *Trudy Institute Eksperimental'noi Veterinarii,* 66: 62-75. (in Russian)

Multicellular parasite vaccines

J.B. McKeand and D.P. Knox

THE NECESSITY FOR ANTIPARASITE VACCINES

Diseases caused by multicellular parasites are a major cause of mortality and morbidity in humans and domestic animals throughout the world. Jenner's discovery that cowpox virus was effective in immunization against smallpox stimulated research into vaccination against most major pathogens including multicellular parasites. Unfortunately, the successes achieved against viruses and bacteria have not been paralleled in the control of diseases caused by multicellular parasites. At present these are controlled by chemotherapy, although it is now apparent that resistance is an inevitable consequence of prolonged chemical application. Anthelmintic resistance has been reported against all the broad-spectrum agents currently available (Prichard, 1990). For example, benzimidazole resistance has been found in *Haemonchus contortus*, *Ostertagia circumcincta* and *Trichostrongylus colubriformis* nematode infections in sheep and goats throughout the world, while levamisole and morantel resistance has been recorded with increasing frequency in Australasia and South Africa (Prichard, 1990; Jackson, 1993). Of concern is the fact that resistance to the relatively recently developed ivermectin has been experimentally selected in *H. contortus* (Egerton, Suhayda and Eary, 1988) and has now been reported in the field in *H. contortus* in both sheep (van Wyck and Malan, 1988) and goats (Jackson *et al.*, 1991). There is widespread acaricide resistance among the important cattle ticks, *Boophilus microplus* and *Hyalomma anatolicum anatolicum* (Wharton, 1976) and an increasing incidence of insecticide resistance is evident in the sheep blowfly, *Lucilia cuprina* (Arundel and Sutherland, 1988).

Although the rapid spread of drug resistance in parasite populations can to a degree be reduced by strategic management procedures, these can impose considerable restraints on land use, especially on marginal pastures. The cost of developing novel chemical control agents is prohibitive and considerable effort is now being directed towards prolonging the efficacy of the currently available drugs, with a particular emphasis on minimizing the effects of drug resistance. Furthermore, there is now widespread public concern regarding the effects of chemical residues in both animal products and the environment. There is clearly a requirement to develop novel control methods for parasitic disease.

Recently, biological control strategies, such as the use of nematophagous fungi, have been evaluated for the control of gastrointestinal nematodes of domestic animals (Waller and Larsen, 1993) but most research has been directed at the development of antiparasite vaccines. Despite decades of intensive work, only two commercially available multicellular parasite vaccines exist. These are based on radiation-attenuated larvae for the control of *Dictyocaulus viviparus* in cattle (Jarrett *et al.*, 1958) and *Dictyocaulus filaria* in sheep (Sharma, Bhat and Dhar, 1988). It would

The authors would like to thank Professor Andy Tait, Dr Eileen Devaney and Dr Bob Coop for their support in the preparation of this chapter.

appear that the antigenic complexity of multicellular parasites has provided an effective barrier to the development of useful vaccines. To compound this, it is often the case that protective antiparasite immune responses are absent or deficient in immature animals. The reasons for this apparent unresponsiveness are unclear but, given that production losses primarily accrue owing to the infection of young stock, studies must be undertaken to identify the cause of this and to develop vaccines which are effective in this group.

Recent advances in immunology, protein chemistry and recombinant DNA techniques have enabled a more accurate identification of potential host-protective immune responses and the parasite antigens which stimulate them. In order to understand the problems and difficulties associated with the development of vaccines against multicellular parasites, this review provides a historical account of the work that has been undertaken and then continues with a description of recent advances which suggest that the development of subunit parasite vaccines may be an achievable goal. Numerous kinds of parasite preparations have been used to immunize animals. These range from the use of attenuated whole parasites, through crude extracts of dead parasites to specific purified molecules.

VACCINATION WITH RADIATION-ATTENUATED PARASITES

Parasites attenuated by irradiation do not reach patency but can stimulate protective immune responses without significant parasite-induced pathology. Immunization with irradiated third-stage larvae (L3) of the bovine lungworm, *D. viviparus*, is a highly successful example of vaccination using this method of attenuation. Natural infection with this parasite induces high levels of resistance in calves (Poynter and Cauthen, 1942; Jarrett, McIntyre and Urquhart, 1954). Vaccination studies using two doses of 10 000 40 kilorad- (400 joules per kilogram-) irradiated L3 showed that calves could be significantly protected against challenge using attenuated larvae (Jarrett *et al.*, 1958). This vaccine was developed commercially and has been used successfully for the control of dictyocaulosis in the United Kingdom and other parts of Europe ever since. This pioneering breakthrough led to several attempts to develop similar vaccines against other important helminth species.

In India, a successful irradiated larval vaccine was developed for the control of the pathogenic ovine lungworm, *D. filaria* (Sharma, Bhat and Dhar, 1988). Vaccination of dogs against the intestinal nematode *Ancylostoma caninum* was similarly effective (Miller, 1971). Unfortunately, this vaccine failed commercially because of its respiratory side-effects, short shelf-life and, in some cases, lack of sterile immunity (Miller, 1978). *Schistosoma* spp. are trematodes of importance in humans and animals in tropical regions and successful immunization has been achieved using irradiated cercariae in laboratory models (Simpson *et al.*, 1985). Furthermore, zebu cattle were significantly protected against *S. bovis* challenge following vaccination with irradiated schistosomula or cercariae of the homologous species (Bushara *et al.*, 1978).

Other attempts to immunize animals with irradiated parasites have met with less success. Mature sheep (> six months) were protected against homologous challenge using irradiated L3 of either *H. contortus* (Urquhart *et al.*, 1966b) or *T. colubriformis* (Gregg and Dineen, 1978). However, as in natural infection, immature sheep (< three months) failed to develop immunity following vaccination (Urquhart *et al.*, 1966a; Gregg *et al.*, 1978).

VACCINATION USING MATERIAL FROM DEAD PARASITES

Attempts to vaccinate against parasitic helminths using somatic extracts from dead organisms were first made in the 1930s but achieved limited success (Chandler, 1932). However, some subsequent attempts have given protection: for example, extracts of fourth-stage larvae of *T. colubriformis* induced significant levels of protection in guinea pigs against homologous challenge (Rothwell and Love, 1974) and worm burdens in sheep immunized with sonicates of adult stage *H. contortus* were significantly lower (63 percent) than burdens found in challenge controls (Adams, 1989). Somatic extracts derived from onchospheres of the cestodes *Echinococcus* sp. and *Taenia* sp. were also found to be potent sources of host-protective antigens (Rickard and Williams, 1982; Xilinas, Papavasiliou and Marselou-Kinti, 1976). These results appear to be the exception rather than the rule, since in most other species success has been limited when somatic helminth extracts were used for immunization (Clegg and Smith, 1978).

Similar to the situation with helminths, somatic extracts of ectoparasites have induced variable degrees of protective immunity (Willadsen, 1980). Salivary gland extracts induced protective immunity to *B. microplus* (Brossard, 1976) and *Amblyomma maculatum* (McGowan *et al.*, 1981) in cattle and also in *Dermacentor andersoni* (Wikel, 1981) in guinea pigs. Subsequently, Opdebeeck *et al.* (1988) vaccinated calves with crude soluble and membrane extracts from the midgut of partially engorged female *B. microplus* and observed up to a 98 percent reduction in tick numbers following challenge. Sheep produce antibodies to *L. cuprina*, the primary agent responsible for fly strike in Australia (O'Donnell *et al.*, 1980) and vaccination of sheep with soluble extracts of third-instar larvae stimulated antibodies which inhibited larval growth and development *in vitro* (O'Donnell *et al.*, 1981). Larvae which were harvested from sheep previously vaccinated with soluble components of second-instar larvae were 58 percent smaller than larvae from control sheep (Johnston, Kemp and Pearson, 1986).

VACCINATION WITH MATERIAL FROM LIVE PARASITES

Although some studies using crude extracts of dead parasites gave protection, few of these studies were taken further owing to the difficulty in defining the protective components within these complex extracts, and attention increasingly focused on less complex parasite compartments which may comprise components essential to parasite survival within the host.

Sarles and Taliaferro (1936) first suggested that products released from helminths *in vivo* were involved in host immunity when they observed immune precipitates at the mouth, excretory pore and anus of *Nippostrongylus brasiliensis* parasites which had been incubated with serum from immune rats. It was thought that the antigen/antibody complexes formed at these parasite orifices might act by blocking the activity of secretions essential to parasite survival. Several attempts to immunize laboratory animals with these excretory-secretory (ES) antigens have produced encouraging results. For example, protective immunity was achieved in mice using the ES products of first-stage larvae of *Trichinella spiralis* (Vernes, 1976) as well as in guinea pigs using the ES products of fourth-stage *T. colubriformis* (Rothwell and Love, 1974), the ES products of third- and fourth-stage *Ascaris suum* (Stromberg and Soulsby, 1977) and the ES products of adult *D. viviparus* (McKeand *et al.*, 1995).

Immunization using ES materials has not always been successful, however, as demonstrated by Neilson (1975) who immunized lambs with the ES products of L3 and L4 *H. contortus* and found no differences in faecal egg counts or worm burdens between vaccinates and challenge controls. The lambs used in this study, however, were less than three months old and may have been immunologically unresponsive. Alternatively, the result may have reflected differences in the immunogenicity of ES in laboratory animals compared with that in natural hosts.

Materials released from ectoparasites have also been proposed as major immunogens. Fly strike is initiated by enzymes secreted by the fly larvae on to the sheep's skin and sheep exposed to several infestations strongly recognized antigens derived, and probably released from, the larval gut and salivary glands (Skelly and Howells, 1987). It has been postulated that inflammation induced by larval ES products plays a central role in wound formation and exudation and that these, in turn, may reduce larval establishment (Sandeman, 1990). More refined vaccination studies in which the potential of secreted larval enzymes as vaccine candidates have been indicated are outlined later.

Despite all these studies, until recently no one has been able to identify and isolate protective components within these fractions and incorporate them into commercially viable vaccines. With the advent of improved immunochemical methods for identifying protective antigens and the ability to produce these in large quantities using recombinant DNA technology, it now appears possible to develop subunit parasite vaccines. The likely steps in subunit parasite vaccine development are summarized (Figure 2).

DEVELOPMENT OF SUBUNIT MULTICELLULAR PARASITE VACCINES

Historically, the selection of protective antigens has been based on extracting native antigen on a small scale from parasites harvested from donor animals or from parasites maintained *in vitro*. This would clearly be unsuitable for commercial vaccine production. Emery and Wagland (1991) estimated that, to obtain sufficient nematode antigen to vaccinate one sheep, parasites would have to be harvested from three donor animals! The problem of antigen production can now be resolved by using peptide synthesis and/or recombinant DNA technology. The main challenges are to identify appropriate individual protective antigens suitable for incorporation into subunit vaccines while maintaining their immunogenicity.

Antigen selection

While many parasite proteins are antigenic, the immune responses to these antigens may not be protective (O'Donnell *et al.*, 1989). Parasite antigens can be classified as conventional or covert. Conventional antigens are recognized by the host during the course of a natural infection and, as vaccine components, would augment natural immunity. However, mutations in the genes coding for these antigens may be selected by the pressure associated with immunity in vaccinated hosts and could restrict their long-term use. On the other hand, covert antigens are hidden from the host immune system during natural infection and, in the absence of selection, are less likely to exhibit antigenic variation. The main disadvantage of using covert antigens is that repeated vaccination may be necessary as specific host immune responses would not be boosted during subsequent natural infections. However, if animals are protected during the very susceptible period in early life, as for example in haemonchosis in sheep, subsequent exposure to natural challenge may maintain protective levels of immunity.

Antigens can be selected on either an empirical or a rational basis. The empirical

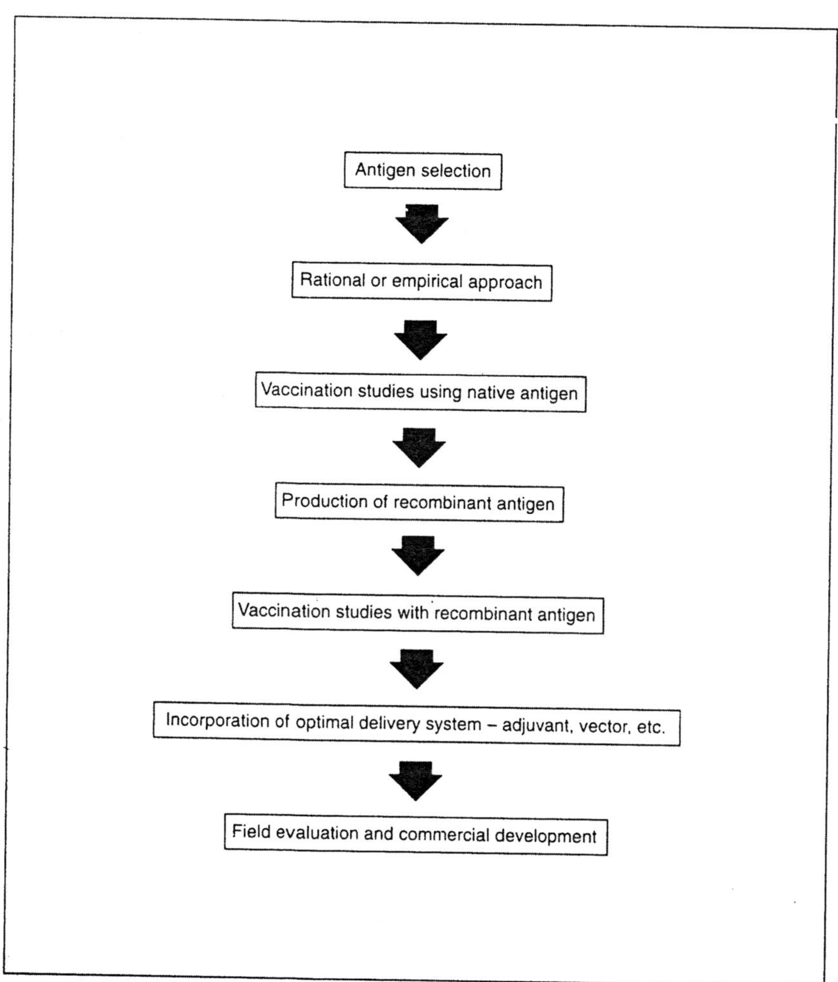

FIGURE 2
Steps in the development of subunit parasite vaccines

approach relies on the fractionation of parasite material followed by successive immunization studies. These extracts provide the starting material for progressively more refined fractionation and the ultimate definition of specific protective components. Fractionation has normally been achieved using conventional protein chemistry techniques such as gel filtration, ion exchange chromatography and polyacrylamide gel electrophoresis. Empirical evaluation is, however, extremely time-consuming and costly so a more rational approach, where molecules are selected on the basis of their contribution to parasite survival, has many advantages.

Despite its drawbacks, the empirical approach has resulted in the production of some viable vaccine candidates. For example, in Australia antigen fractionation has led to the identification of tropomyosin as a candidate antigen for stimulating protective immunity in sheep against *T. colubriformis* and *H. contortus*. Immunization with whole worm homogenates from fourth-stage larvae of *T. colubriformis* was observed to accelerate expulsion of homologous challenge in guinea pigs (Rothwell and Love, 1974; Rothwell and Griffiths, 1977; Rothwell, 1978). Subfractions of this homogenate, obtained by sodium dodecyl sulphate-polyacrylamide gel electrophoresis (SDS-PAGE), were later shown to induce host protective immunity (O'Donnell *et al.*, 1985). These subfractions, however, still comprised rather complex protein mixtures, so different extraction procedures were then evaluated to reduce their complexity (O'Donnell *et al.*, 1989). Using phosphate-buffered saline / sodium deoxycholate (PBS / NaDOC) to make somatic extracts of *T. colubriformis* larvae, a simple antigen mixture was produced which consisted of four protein components, one of which, a 41 kilodalton (kDa) protein, induced 43 to 51 percent protection in guinea pigs (O'Donnell *et al.*, 1989). Partial amino acid sequence analysis of this protein indicated that it was tropomyosin. Progress towards a recombinant vaccine based on parasite tropomyosin is outlined in the section Multicellular parasite vaccines: recent developments, p. 100.

A slightly different approach has been used to isolate protective antigen fractions from *Oesophagostomum radiatum*, a pathogenic nematode found in the large intestine of calves. Animals acquire strong resistance to reinfection (Roberts, Elek and Keith, 1962) and protective immunity was stimulated using excretory gland homogenates of adult parasites (Keith and Bremner, 1973). The adult *O. radiatum* extracts were resolved into four fractions by gel filtration (East, Berrie and Fitzgerald, 1989) and ELISA analyses showed that antibodies from naturally infected calves predominantly reacted with the void volume fraction which comprised high molecular weight components. Vaccination of calves with this fraction significantly reduced worm establishment and faecal egg output (East, Berrie and Fitzgerald, 1988). High molecular weight antigens have also been used to vaccinate against *Nematospiroides dubius* in mice (Monroy and Dobson, 1987), *T. colubriformis* (O'Donnell *et al.*, 1985) and *H. contortus* (Neilson and Van de Walle, 1987) in sheep, with varying degrees of success.

By using antibodies or cells derived from infected and / or immune animals to probe crude antigen preparations, the major immunogens can be identified. This strategy can be augmented by comparing the responses of individual hosts which are defined as susceptible or resistant to infection. Monoclonal antibodies derived from immune mice were used to define and purify the major immunogens of the small intestinal nematode, *T. spiralis*. This work led to the purification to homogeneity of the first single, protective antigen of a nematode, a 48 kDa protein (Silberstein and Despommier, 1984). Initially, three proteins were isolated from extracts of infective larvae by immuno-affinity chromatography (Silberstein and Despommier, 1984). When used to immunize mice, one of these proteins gave significant protection at very low (0.1 D1 µg) doses. Unfortunately, this protein was ineffective in the natural pig host (Gamble, Murrell and Marti, 1986).

In another study, sera from infected sheep, which were defined as resistant or susceptible to *O. circumcincta*, were used to identify a 31 kDa molecule present in Triton X-100 extracts of L3. This molecule was recognized preferentially by resistant animals as early as three weeks after experimental infection and was present in and secreted by third-stage larvae (McGillivery *et al.*, 1990). Lambs immunized with the purified protein were significantly protected against homologous challenge as judged by faecal egg counts and adult worm burdens compared with challenge controls (McGillivery *et al.*, 1992). Homologous antigens have also been identified in *T. colubriformis* and *H. contortus* (McGillivery *et al.*, 1990).

Recently, more rational approaches to vaccine design have produced encouraging results. One approach has been to identify and isolate antigens from the intestinal luminal surface of blood-feeding parasites. It has been suggested that the induction of systemic antibody responses against the gut antigens of blood-sucking parasites may cause sufficient damage to impair parasite survival. This response is "artificial" as these gut antigens are not recognized by the host during the course of natural infection, i.e. the antigens are covert. Lambs have been immunized successfully against haemonchosis, using antigens fractionated from the intestinal luminal surface of adult *H. contortus* (Munn, Greenwood and Coadwell, 1987; Munn and Smith, 1990). A major immunogen of this preparation was an integral membrane glycoprotein of molecular weight 110 kDa, termed H11 (Munn, 1988; Smith and Munn, 1990). Immunization of sheep with microgram amounts of essentially pure H11 stimulated substantial protection against challenge infection in several breeds of sheep (Munn, 1988; Tavernor *et al.*, 1992a and 1992b; Munn *et al.*, 1993a). This immunity was closely correlated with H11-specific circulating IgG levels (Munn and Smith, 1990) and vaccination was equally successful in young lambs (< two months, Tavernor *et al.*, 1992a) as in older lambs (> eight months, Tavernor *et al.*, 1992b). With respect to the age-related unresponsiveness of young lambs to vaccination with irradiated L3 (Urquhart *et al.*, 1966b), the results obtained with the H11 antigen would suggest that this would be an ideal vaccine candidate for the control of this disease. Sequence analysis of full-length cDNAs encoding H11 has shown the protein to be homologous to mammalian amino peptidases. Amino peptidase activity was subsequently found in native pure H11 and enzyme activity was inhibited by immunoglobulin from H11-vaccinated sheep (Munn *et al.*, 1993b). A full-length, enzymically active H11 cDNA has been produced in the baculovirus expression system (Munn *et al.*, 1993b) and its ability to protect lambs against haemonchosis is currently being evaluated. Recent work has indicated that integral gut membrane preparations from adult *H. contortus* contain other protective antigens apart from H11. For instance, substantial protection against *H. contortus* was induced in lambs hyperimmunized with an integral membrane extract in which the characteristic H11 doublet was not usually observed (Smith, 1993).

A similar approach has led to the

isolation of several protective antigens from blood-feeding arthropods. For example, cattle are protected against the tick *B. microplus* by using components isolated from the tick gut (Johnston, Kemp and Pearson, 1986; Kemp *et al.*, 1986; Willadsen, McKenna and Riding, 1988; Opdebeeck *et al.*, 1988). The number of ticks engorging, their average weight and egg-laying ability were all diminished in those ticks feeding from immunized cattle (Willadsen and McKenna, 1991). Triton X-100 extracts of the gut of first-instar larvae of *L. cuprina* were used to vaccinate sheep, and challenge larvae obtained from these sheep had their growth reduced by more than 40 percent when compared with larvae from challenge controls. In addition, immune sera from vaccinated sheep inhibited the growth of larvae *in vitro* by more than 50 percent indicating that the effect was antibody-mediated (East *et al.*, 1993). Gut membrane preparations have also given promising results with sucking lice, flies and mosquitoes (Schlein and Lewis, 1976).

The lumen of the blowfly gut is lined with a periotrophic membrane which, in addition to being essential to digestion, acts as a molecular sieve preventing intact antibody molecules coming into contact with underlying gut epithelial cells (East *et al.*, 1993). This range of functions, crucial to insect survival, attracted attention to the periotrophic membrane as a source of potential protective antigens. Periotrophic membranes, harvested *in vitro* from *L. cuprina* larvae, were used to immunize sheep and resulted in a 30 percent reduction in the weight of established larvae compared with those obtained from challenge control animals (East *et al.*, 1993).

Another source of potential vaccine candidates are ES products which are thought to assist in tissue invasion, parasite feeding and evasion of host effector mechanisms. ES products may be derived from the nematode cuticle or from specialized excretory-secretory organs and represent the major antigenic and functional challenge to the host (Maizels and Selkirk, 1988; Lightowlers and Rickard, 1988). In terms of so-called functional molecules, several classes of enzyme have been identified in ES products. These include proteinases which may facilitate penetration of host tissues (Matthews, 1982; Dalton and Heffernan, 1988) or act as anticoagulants (Hotez and Cerami, 1983), acetylcholinesterases (AChE) (Rhoads, 1984) and superoxide dismutases (Rhoads, 1983; Knox and Jones, 1992). Some of these have the potential to modulate host immune responses, for example secreted proteinases have been ascribed a role in cleaving surface-bound immunoglobulin in several helminth systems (Auriault *et al.*, 1981; Chapman and Mitchell, 1982; Smith *et al.*, 1993). AChE may interfere with hosts' immune mechanisms by breaking down host acetylcholine (ACh), which is known to stimulate potential effector mechanisms such as neutrophil-mediated antibody-dependent cellular cytotoxicity (Gale and Zhigelboim, 1974), neutrophil chemotaxis (Hill *et al.*, 1975) and mast cell histamine release (Kaliner and Austen, 1975). Although not an enzyme, a γ-interferon analogue has been identified in *T. colubriformis* ES products (Dopheide *et al.*, 1991). Owing to these putative functional roles, ES products have received close attention as a source of protective antigens.

Secretions produced during the moult from third- to fourth-stage larvae of *Ascaris suum* induced significant protection against challenge in guinea pigs, while soluble proteins produced during culture of L2, L3, L4 and adult worms were ineffective (Stromberg and Soulsby, 1977). Metabolites secreted by *H. contortus* during the moult from the third to fourth larval stages were also effective in sheep (Ozerol and Silverman, 1970) and the ES products of adult *D. viviparus* induced significant levels of protection in immunized guinea pigs (McKeand *et al.*, 1995).

Attention is now focusing on defining the precise nature of the polypeptides which comprise nematode ES products. The application of molecular biology and increasingly specific immunological methods to the study of parasite ES products has enabled the definition of a number of novel proteins with protective properties. Recently, the dominant glycoprotein present in ES products derived from the parasitic stages of *T. colubriformis* has been cloned and sequenced and shown to induce protective immunity and have significant homology to the porcine intestinal peptide, valosin (Savin *et al.*, 1990). Valosin can modulate several aspects of gastrointestinal function and, by secreting a homologue protein, the parasite itself may alter its local environment.

AChE is secreted by several nematode species and is immunogenic in a number of host/parasite systems (Lee, 1970; Edwards, Burt and Ogilvie, 1971; Jones and Ogilvie, 1972; Ogilvie *et al.*, 1973; McKeand *et al.*, in press). For example, sheep infected with *T. colubriformis* produce antibodies to worm AChE; however, AChE purified from this parasite failed to induce a protective immune response in vaccinated guinea pigs (Rothwell and Merritt, 1975). In the *D. viviparus* system, calves naturally or experimentally infected with this parasite also produce antibodies which bind and inhibit parasite AChE activity (McKeand *et al.*, in press) and *D. viviparus* ES preparations enriched for AChE activity protected guinea pigs against subsequent challenge compared with adjuvant controls (McKeand, 1992).

Glutathione S-transferase (GST) appears to be one of the major detoxification enzymes of parasitic helminths and has received much attention as a candidate protective antigen (Brophy and Barrett, 1990). GST is recognized by antibodies from mice infected with the trematode *Schistosoma japonicum*, and the development of protective immunity in various mice strains has been positively correlated with the levels of specific anti-GST antibody (Smith *et al.*, 1986). Recombinant GST, prepared from *S. japonicum* and *S. mansoni*, was subsequently observed to confer partial, but not significant, protection in rats and hamsters (Balloul *et al.*, 1987). However, vaccination of genetically susceptible mice with a β-galactosidase fusion protein of this enzyme gave significant protection against infection with *S. japonicum* (Smith *et al.*, 1986). Affinity-purified GST from *Fasciola hepatica* did not significantly protect rats against challenge (Howell, Board and Boray, 1988), but sheep immunized with purified GST were significantly protected (57 percent reduction in fluke numbers) (Sexton, Milner and Paraccio, 1990). The genes encoding *F. hepatica* GSTs have now been isolated with a view to testing a recombinant vaccine (Wijffels, Sexton and Salvatore, 1992). In contrast to these trematode systems, antisera raised against GST purified from adult *H. contortus*, while inhibiting enzyme activity *in vitro*, failed to affect survival of the parasite *in vivo* (Sharp *et al.*, 1991).

Proteinases are secreted by *L. cuprina* larvae on to the sheep's skin to enable the larvae to feed and it is these enzymes that are thought to initiate wound formation. It has been observed that proteinases released by these flies can be inhibited by sheep plasma proteinase inhibitors and that the proteinase inhibitors α2-macroglobulin and antithrombin III reduced larval growth *in vitro* (Bowles, Feehan and Sandeman, 1990). Furthermore, antiproteinase antibodies inhibited larval growth *in vitro* (Sandeman, 1990). In common with many helminth parasites, blowfly larvae produce a multiplicity of secreted proteinases, each of which may need to be inhibited by the host immune response to impair larval growth adequately (East and Eisemann, 1993).

Surface antigens of parasitic nematodes are often highly antigenic (Maizels and Selkirk, 1988). Cetyltrimethylammonium bromide (CTAB) surface extracts of *T. spiralis* larvae induced significant levels of protection against reinfection in mice (Grencis *et al.*, 1986). However, sheep immunized with surface extracts of *H. contortus* L3 were as susceptible as challenge control animals (Turnbull *et al.*, 1992) and cuticle collagens from the third and fourth stages of the same parasite failed to induce significant protection against homologous challenge (Boisvenue *et al.*, 1991).

MULTICELLULAR PARASITE VACCINES: RECENT DEVELOPMENTS

The isolation of protective antigens in sufficient quantities for practical use in vaccine development has, until recently, been restricted by a lack of available native parasite material. The development of recombinant DNA techniques for the *in vitro* expression of foreign genes in eukaryotic and prokaryotic cells has provided an alternative strategy which has recently stimulated extensive research into antiparasite vaccines. While there are now many examples of expression systems for parasite proteins, there are only a few reports of recombinant parasite proteins which induce significant levels of protective immunity. The steps in recombinant vaccine development are illustrated by the following successful examples.

Immunization of sheep using* T. colubriformis *tropomyosin recombinants. As discussed earlier, the *T. colubriformis* muscle protein, tropomyosin, was shown to be a potentially useful protective antigen in the guinea pig when given in native form (O'Donnell *et al.*, 1989). Using oligonucleotide probes based on partial amino acid sequence data of tropomyosin, the gene encoding this protein was isolated from a cDNA expression library prepared from fourth larval-stage mRNA (Cobon *et al.*, 1989). A 27 kDa subunit of *T. colubriformis* tropomyosin, expressed as a β-galactosidase fusion protein in *Escherichia coli*, produced accelerated worm expulsion following challenge in guinea pigs. When the *T. colubriformis* tropomyosin DNA was used as a hybridization probe, the gene encoding a related antigen was isolated from mRNA prepared from adult *H. contortus*. The expressed gene product significantly protected immunized sheep against *H. contortus* challenge (Cobon *et al.*, 1989).

Immunization of sheep with recombinants of* T. ovis *onchosphere ES antigens. A similar approach has shown promise in experiments with *Cysticercus ovis*, the intermediate stage of *T. ovis*, in sheep. Previous experiments indicated that the ES products of hatched and activated *T. ovis* onchospheres contained potent host-protective antigens. Several of the ES components, ranging from 47 to 52 kDa in size, were found to be recognized strongly by sera from resistant sheep (Rickard and Bell, 1971a and 1971b; Rickard and Adolph, 1977) and lambs immunized with a polyacrylamide gel-purified preparation of these components were significantly (98 percent) protected against challenge (Johnson *et al.*, 1989). Rabbit antibodies, specific for the 47 to 52 kDa region, were eluted from Western blots and used to probe a cDNA expression library prepared from mRNA extracted from hatched and activated onchospheres (Johnson *et al.*, 1989). β-galactosidase fusion proteins, prepared from selected immunopositives, were found to be antigenic in sheep but were not protective. Subsequently, one of the proteins was prepared as a fusion with *S. japonicum* glutathione S-transferase and was found to protect sheep significantly against challenge (Johnson *et al.*, 1989).

Recombinant proteins have also been assessed in other *Taenia* species. Three fusion proteins, derived from *T. taeniaeformis* onchosphere cDNA and expressed in a pGEX plasmid vector, gave a 95 percent reduction in total metacestode recoveries in Wistar rats (Ito *et al.*, 1991)

***Immunization of ruminants using recombinant forms of membrane gut proteins of* B. microplus.** As discussed previously, in infections in which immunity develops slowly or poorly, artificial immunization with hidden, or covert, antigens may be used to circumvent a lack of responsiveness. Recent developments using recombinant gut antigens from the bloodsucking tick *B. microplus* in cattle have been promising.

Cattle acquire limited levels of resistance following prolonged natural exposure to *B. microplus* (Wagland, 1975). Protective immunity has been achieved using antigens fractionated from gut membrane preparations of engorged female ticks (Willadsen, McKenna and Riding, 1988), and a membrane-bound glycoprotein (Bm86) expressed on the surface of tick gut digestive cells was shown to be a highly effective immunogen (Willadsen *et al.*, 1989). The gene coding for this antigen was subsequently isolated from a cDNA expression library prepared from adult *B. microplus* and a fusion comprising 599 amino acids of Bm86 and 651 amino acids of β-galactosidase was expressed in *E. coli* as inclusion bodies (Rand *et al.*, 1989). Ticks engorging on cattle vaccinated with these inclusion bodies were significantly damaged as a result of the immune response to the cloned antigen (Rand *et al.*, 1989).

The above examples have attracted considerable commercial support and are currently undergoing development.

PROBLEMS OF SUBUNIT VACCINE DEVELOPMENT

Laboratory models versus natural host/parasite systems. Potentially useful antigens are often selected on the basis of protection trials conducted in laboratory animal models. In general terms, laboratory animals expel the parasite more rapidly than does the natural host and infection is often terminated prior to patency. Protection observed in model systems is therefore often only an acceleration of an already efficient antiparasite response and does not necessarily reflect utility in the natural host. Caution must therefore be taken when extrapolating from the laboratory model to the definitive host.

Recombinants expressed in the wrong conformation. The protective properties of a recombinant protein will be influenced by the tertiary structure which can, in turn, be altered depending on the fusion partner. It also depends on whether or not the native protein is glycosylated. This cautionary note is exemplified by work on the protective onchosphere antigens of *T. ovis* in which protective immunity was only attained after expression of the recombinant molecule as a GST fusion protein (Johnson *et al.*, 1989).

Solubilization of the relevant antigens. The solvent used to extract parasite proteins can be crucial to the isolation of the appropriate protective antigens. For example, work performed on the cestode *Taenia pisiformis* indicated that sodium deoxycholate, but not PBS, extracts made from onchospheres of the parasite conferred high levels of protection to rabbits (Rajasekariah, Rickard and O'Donnell,

1985). Similarly, DOC-PAGE, but not SDS-PAGE, gel cut-outs of *T. taeniaeformis* onchosphere antigens protected mice against challenge (Lightowlers, Rickard and Mitchell, 1984). In comparison, sheep have been successfully immunized against challenge with *Echinococcus granulosus* using onchosphere antigens which had been solubilized in SDS (Dempster *et al.*, 1992) and against *T. ovis* using homogenized SDS-polyacrylamide gels containing homologous antigen (Harrison *et al.*, 1993). The variation produced by the different extraction buffers may be caused by the disruption of conformational epitopes or by the lack of solubilization of effective components.

Presence of non-peptide epitopes. B cell epitopes are often conformational and may not be peptide in nature. These epitopes will be difficult to reproduce using conventional molecular biology or peptide synthesis techniques. As the antigen binding site of an antibody molecule is complementary in physical structure to the antigen against which it is raised, the antigen binding site can, itself, be used as antigen to raise anti-idiotype antibodies which mimic the shape of the original antigen. For example, an anti-idiotype vaccine which mimics the glycan component of a 38 kDa surface component of *S. mansoni* stimulated protective immunity in rats against homologous challenge (Grzych *et al.*, 1985). This approach is very laborious, however, and would probably only be considered if the protective epitope was non-peptide or demonstrably conformational and could not be produced by the variety of recombinant DNA approaches now available. In addition to containing carbohydrate epitopes, glycosylation is also likely to affect the protective properties of proteins by modifying protein folding, so that recombinants will be more appropriately expressed in systems which glycosylate the recombinant protein such as mammalian cell lines and viral vectors.

Accessibility of antigen to the immune system. In order to have an effect on an invading parasite, host effector mechanisms must be directed against antigens which are accessible to this response. For example, *Haemonchus* spp. and *Boophilus* spp. ingest host blood so that antigens on the gut surface are bathed in blood components such as antibody. The extent to which this approach can be applied to non-bloodsucking parasites such as *Ostertagia* spp. and *Trichostrongylus* spp. remains to be defined. Furthermore, because covert antigens will not be exposed during subsequent natural infection it is presumed that booster vaccination would be required until natural immunity develops or live vaccine vectors may be used to enable persistence of the vaccine components within the host.

Genetic variation in the vaccinated population. Once a vaccine has been developed, it is essential that it is effective in most, if not all, of the target population. The major histocompatibility complex (MHC) and other, as yet undefined, background genes within a population influence the capability of individuals to respond immunologically to specific antigens. This in turn will establish the success or failure of any vaccine (Kennedy, 1990). For example, a variable responsiveness was encountered when synthetic peptides of the circumsporozoite protein of *Plasmodium falciparum* were used to vaccinate mice and it was observed that both antibody and T cell responses to this antigen were H-2^b-restricted (Del Giudice *et al.*, 1986; Togna *et al.*, 1986). Thus, it can be anticipated that subunit vaccines which stimulate elements of the natural immune response to the parasite will have to comprise a variety of peptides to maintain long-term field utility. Furthermore, the induction of natural immune responses will be profoundly influenced by the way the antigen(s) is/are presented to the immune system.

Assisting antigen presentation

The rapid developments in recombinant DNA technology and protein chemistry should provide antigens in quantity for experimental immunization studies. Individual molecules are likely to have reduced immunogenicity and will have to be presented to the host immune system in the context of an adjuvant or a live vaccine vector. Moreover, the method of antigen presentation can be optimized if the relevant effector arms of the immune response are defined.

Adjuvants

Adjuvants non-specifically stimulate immune responses to antigen. The understanding of how adjuvants work has increased rapidly and many of the adjuvants now available are recognized to stimulate different types of responses (see chapter by Bomford, Adjuvants in veterinary vaccines, p. 277, and Bomford, 1989).

Adjuvant selection, and hence vaccine efficacy, can be improved if the precise immunological mechanisms involved in parasite killing or expulsion are defined. For example, aluminium hydroxide preferentially stimulates T helper type 2 (Th_2) lymphocytes so that a humoral response, particularly IgG_1 and IgE, is favoured (Smith, 1992). In contrast, Freund's complete adjuvant, which contains bacterial components, is a strong promoter of cellular responses. Freund's incomplete adjuvant, which lacks the mycobacterial component, stimulates only a humoral response. Unfortunately, Freund's adjuvants have several adverse side-effects and are not acceptable for use in veterinary vaccines. However, because of their general efficacy, they continue to be used in experimental trials to establish antigen utility, after which less toxic adjuvant mixes may be attempted.

A novel adjuvant which is now licensed for use in domestic animals is that based on immunostimulating complexes (ISCOMs). These complexes are most readily formed with antigens which possess a hydrophobic transmembrane region (Bomford, 1989), suggesting that they may be particularly useful for the formulation of helminth vaccines based on integral membrane proteins. So far, there has been little work detailing the potential of helminth or ectoparasite subunit vaccines in the context of any novel adjuvant preparations.

Vectors and antigen delivery

The chronicity associated with many parasitic infections suggests that antigen may need to be administered over a prolonged period to stimulate protective immunity. Antigens administered orally with an avirulent virus or bacterial vector will have the potential to stimulate a vigorous cell-mediated and persistent immune response (Murray, 1989). These vectors also have the potential to stimulate IgA precursor B cells in gut-associated lymphoid tissue, a possibility for overcoming immune unresponsiveness at this site. Virus vectors, such as vaccinia and herpesviruses, have the advantage that the antigen(s) are processed in their native form (Murray, 1989). So far, vaccinia has been used successfully as a vector for a cloned 28 kDa surface antigen of *S. mansoni* (Simpson and Cioli, 1987). Enterobacteria, such as *E. coli* and *Salmonella* spp., have been used as vaccine vectors in non-parasite systems, although use of the latter may lead to public concern.

Vectors may be designed so that the antigens they encode are expressed in combination with the appropriate recombinant cytokine(s) in order to stimulate the desired immune effector arm. For gastrointestinal nematodes, antigen and cytokine genes could be expressed in parallel in a bacterial or viral vector suitable for oral vaccine delivery.

Bacterial toxins also have considerable potential for the oral presentation of antigen. For example, cholera toxin has a high affinity for specific receptors on the surface of the intestinal epithelium and stimulates both secretory IgA and serum IgG antibody responses with prolonged immunological memory (McGhee *et al.*, 1992). These responses would be appropriate in vaccination against gastrointestinal nematodes, although the problems of toxicity may have to be overcome.

CONCLUSIONS

The optimism expressed when recombinant DNA technology was first developed perhaps overestimated the capabilities of these techniques and failed to recognize the complex nature of the host-parasite interaction and the difficulty in maintaining immunogenicity. A major problem has been the inability to identify the relevant antigens from complex preparations in the face of multiple immune responses, not all of which are protective. These responses still have to be unravelled for all multicellular parasitic infections. A substantial amount of parasitological research is now directed at defining the precise immune responses relevant to the elimination, or otherwise, of parasites. Although beyond the scope of this vaccine review, it appears that, of the many immune effector mechanisms involved in the host-parasite interaction, only some are relevant to the development of protective immunity. Nearly all the studies described in this review selected antigens on the basis of humoral immunity, and there has been little detail given regarding the essential cellular arm of the immune response. In terms of vaccine development, this reflects the route that research has taken in the past. More recently, detailed analyses of the cellular responses against helminths have identified responses which are protective or those which may be immunopathological or immunorepressive (Smith, 1992). By measuring mitogen- or antigen-specific *in vitro* propagation of immune cell lines, including T cell subsets, or measuring the types of cytokines released or expresssed by these cells, cellular responses can be dissected for each parasite infection. Parasite antigens also trigger mast cell degranulation with the associated release of mast cell proteinases, histamine and various cytokines. In several cases, these responses appear to be central to worm expulsion, and assays which detect antigen-specific mast cell proteinase release may be used to identify which antigens stimlate these cells (Jones, Huntley and Emery, 1992). Thus, it can be seen that basic parasite immunology should go hand in hand with vaccine research in order to define which kind of responses should be aimed for when identifying vaccine candidates.

As outlined above, delivery systems and adjuvants can now be selected on the basis that they can optimize or augment the required effector arm of the immune system. Nevertheless, by obtaining information on putative functions for specific parasite components or realizing their contribution to parasite survival, rational subunit vaccines may be designed without the need for a full understanding of the host parasite interaction.

Pioneering advances have been made in the last decade, most notably in the definition of candidate antigens for protection against *T. ovis* and *H. contortus* in sheep, but the identification of protective antigens and evidence for their efficacy in immunization trials is only the start of the process. Field trials and the incorporation of the antigens into a commercially viable vaccine are expensive and time-consuming and will rely heavily on commitment from large pharmaceutical companies which must accept the vaccine as a potential marketable commodity. It should be noted that a vaccine which only reduces nematode egg output might reduce pasture contamination to a level where production losses are balanced by stock management savings. Thus, at least with veterinary vaccines, it may not be imperative to induce sterile immunity completely and, when considering the most appropriate vaccine development strategy, full account must be taken of the relative prevalence and epidemiology of the parasite.

BIBLIOGRAPHY

Adams, D.B. 1989. A preliminary evaluation of factors affecting an experimental system for vaccination-and-challenge with *Haemonchus contortus* in sheep. *Int. J. Parasitol.*, 19: 169-175.

Arundel, J.H. & Sutherland, A.K. 1988. Blowflies of sheep. In *Animal Health in Australia*, 10: 35-60. Canberra, Australian Government Publishing Service.

Auriault, C., Ouissi, M.A., Torpier, G., Elsen, H. & Capron, A. 1981. Proteolytic cleavage of IgG bound to the Fc receptor of *Schistosoma mansoni* schistosomula. *Parasite Immunol.*, 3: 33-44.

Balloul, J.M., Grzych, J.M., Pierce, R.J. & Capron, A. 1987. A purified 28 000 dalton protein from *Schistosoma mansoni* adult worms protects rats and mice against experimental schistosomiasis. *J. Immunol.*, 138: 3448-3453.

Boisvenue, R.J., Stiff, M.I., Tonkinson, L.V. & Cox, G.N. 1991. Protective studies in sheep immunized with cuticular collagen proteins and peptides of *Haemonchus contortus*. *Parasite Immunol.*, 13: 227-240.

Bomford, R. 1989. Adjuvants for antiparasite vaccines. *Parasitol. Today*, 5: 41-46.

Bowles, V.M., Feehan, J.P. & Sandeman, R.M. 1990. Sheep plasma proteinase inhibitors influencing activity and growth of *Lucilia cuprina* larvae *in vitro*. *Int. J. Parasitol.*, 20: 169-174.

Brophy, P.M. & Barrett, J. 1990. Glutathione transferase in helminths. *Parasitol.*, 100: 345-349.

Brossard, M. 1976. Relations immunologiques entre bovins et tiques: *Boophilus microplus*. *Acta Trop.*, 33: 15-36.

Bushara, H.O., Hussein, M.F., Saad, A.M., Taylor, M.G., Dargie, J.D., De. C. Marshall, T.F. & Nelson, G.S. 1978. Immunization of calves against *Schistosoma bovis* using irradiated cercariae or schistosomul of *S. bovis*. *Parasitol.*, 77: 303-311.

Chandler, A.C. 1932. Experiments on resistance of rats to superinfection with the nematode *Nippostrongylus muris*. *Am. J. Hyg.*, 16: 780-782.

Chapman, C.B. & Mitchell, G.F. 1982. Proteolytic cleavage of immunoglobulin by enzymes released by *Fasciola hepatica*. *Vet. Parasitol.*, 11: 165-178.

Clegg, J.A. & Smith, M.A. 1978. Prospects for the development of dead vaccines against helminths. *Adv. Parasitol.*, 16: 165-217.

Cobon, G.S., Austen, A., O'Donnell, I.J., Frenkel, M.J., Kennedy, W.P., Savin, K.W. & Wagland, B.M. 1989. Vaccines against animal parasitic nematodes. Patent: WO89/00163.

Dalton, J.P. & Heffernan, M. 1988. Thiol proteases released *in vitro* by *Fasciola hepatica*. *Mol. Biochem. Parasitol.*, 35: 161-166.

Del Giudice, G., Cooper, J.A., Merino, J., Verdini, A.S., Pessi, A., Togna, A.R., Engers, H.D., Corradin, G. & Lambert, P.-H. 1986. The antibody response in mice to carrier-free synthetic polymers of *Plasmodium falciparum* circumsporozoite repetitive epitope is I-A^b-restricted: possible implications for malaria vaccines. *J. Immunol.*, 137: 2952-2955.

Dempster, R.P., Harrison, G.B.L., Berridge, M.V. & Heath, D.D. 1992. *Echinococcus granulosus*: use of an intermediate host mouse model to evaluate sources of protective antigens and a role for antibody in the immune response. *Int. J. Parasitol.*, 22: 435-441.

Dopheide, T.A.A., Tachedjian, M., Phillips, C., Frenkel, M.J., Wagland, B.M. & Ward, C.W. 1991. Molecular characterisation of a protective, 11-kDa excretory-secretory protein from the parasitic stages of *Trichostrongylus colubriformis*. *Mol. Biochem. Parasitol.*, 45: 101-108.

East, I.J. & Eisemann, C.H. 1993. Vaccination against *Lucilia cuprina*: the causative agent of sheep blowfly strike. *Immunol. Cell Biol.*, 71: 453-462.

East, I.J., Berrie, D.A. & Fitzgerald, C.J. 1988. *Oesophagostomum radiatum*: successful vaccination of calves with an extract of *in vitro* cultured larvae. *Int. J. Parasitol.*, 18: 125-127.

East, I.J., Berrie, D.A. & Fitzgerald, C.J. 1989. *Oesophagostomum radiatum*: successful vaccination of calves with high molecular weight antigens. *Int. J. Parasitol.*, 19: 271-274.

East, I.J., Fitzgerald, C.J., Pearson, R.D., Donaldson, R.A., Vuocolo, T., Cadogan, L.C., Tellam, R.L. & Eisemann, C.H. 1993. *Lucilia cuprina*: inhibition of larval growth induced by immunization of host sheep with extracts of larval periotrophic membrane. *Int. J. Parasitol.*, 23: 221-229.

Edwards, A.J., Burt, J.S. & Ogilvie, B.M. 1971. The effect of immunity upon some enzymes of the parasitic nematode, *Nippostrongylus brasiliensis*. *Parasitol.*, 62: 339-347.

Egerton, J.S., Suhayda, D. & Eary, C.H. 1988. Laboratory selection of *Haemonchus contortus* for resistance to ivermectin. *J. Parasitol.*, 74: 614-617.

Emery, D.L. & Wagland, B.M. 1991. Vaccines against gastrointestinal parasites of ruminants. *Parasitol. Today*, 7: 347-349.

Gale, R.P. & Zighelboim, J. 1974. Modulation of polymorphonuclear leukocyte-mediated antibody-dependent cellular cytotoxicity. *J. Immunol.*, 113: 1793-1800.

Gamble, J.R., Murrell, K.D. & Marti, H.P. 1986. Inoculation of pigs against *Trichinella spiralis*, using larval excretory-secretory antigens. *Am. J. Vet. Res.*, 47: 2396-2399.

Gregg, P. & Dineen, H.P. 1978. The response of sheep vaccinated with irradiated *Trichostrongylus colubriformis* larvae. *Vet. Parasitol.*, 4: 49-53.

Gregg, P., Dineen, J.K., Rothwell, T.L.W. & Kelly, J.D. 1978. The effect of age on the response of sheep to vaccination with irradiated *Trichostrongylus colubriformis* larvae. *Vet. Parasitol.*, 4: 35-48.

Grencis, R.K., Crawford, C., Pritchard, D.I., Behnke, J.M. & Wakelin, D. 1986. Immunization of mice with surface antigens from the muscle larvae of *Trichinella spiralis*. *Parasite Immunol.*, 8: 587-596.

Gryzch, J.M., Capron, M., Lambert, P.H., Dissous, C., Torres, S. & Capron, A. 1985. An anti-idiotype vaccine against experimental schistosomiasis. *Nature*, 316: 74-76.

Harrison, G.B.L., Heath, D.D., Dempster, R.P., Lawrence, S.B., Lightowlers, M.W. & Rickard, M. 1993. Identification of host-protective antigens of *Taenia ovis* oncospheres. *Int. J. Parasitol.*, 23: 41-50.

Hill, H.R., Estensen, R.D., Quie, P.G., Hogan, N.A. & Goldberg, N.D. 1975. Modulation of human neutrophil chemotactic responses by cyclic 3', 5'-guanosine monophosphate and cyclic 3', 5'-adenosine monophosphate. *Metabolism*, 24: 447-456.

Hotez, P. & Cerami, A. 1983. Secretion of a

proteolytic anticoagulant by *Ancylostoma* hookworms. *J. Exp. Med.*, 157: 1594-1603.

Howell, M.J., Board, P.G. & Boray, J.C. 1988. Glutathione S-transferases. *J. Parasitol.*, 74: 715-718.

Ito, A., Bogh, H.O., Lightowlers, M.W., Mitchell, G.F., Takami, T., Kamiya, M., Onitake, K. & Rickard, M.D. 1991. Vaccination against *Taenia taeniaeformis* infection in rats using a recombinant protein and preliminary analysis of the induced antibody response. *Mol. Biochem. Parasitol.*, 44: 43-52.

Jackson, F. 1993. Anthelmintic resistance – the state of play. *Br. Vet. J.*, 149: 123-138.

Jackson, F., Coop, R.L., Jackson, E., Little., S. & Russell, A.J.F. 1991. Anthelmintic-resistant nematodes in goats. *Vet. Rec.*, 129: 39-40.

Jarrett, W.F.H., McIntyre, W.I.M. & Urquhart, G.M. 1954. Husk in cattle. A review of a year's work. *Vet. Rec.*, 66: 665-676.

Jarrett, W.F.H., Jennings, F.W., Martin, B., McIntyre, W.I.M., Mulligan, W., Sharp, N.C.C. & Urquhart, G.M. 1958. A field trial of a parasitic bronchitis vaccine. *Vet. Rec.*, 70: 451-454.

Johnson, K.S., Harrison, G.B.L., Lightowlers, M.W., O'Hoy, K.L., Cougle, W.G., Dempster, W.G., Lawrence, R.P., Vinton, J.G., Heath, D.D. & Rickard, M.D. 1989. Vaccination against ovine cysticercosis using a defined recombinant antigen. *Nature*, 338: 585-587.

Johnston, L.A.Y., Kemp, D.H. & Pearson, R.D. 1986. Immunisation of cattle against *Boophilus microplus* using extracts derived from adult female ticks. *Int. J. Parasitol.*, 16: 27-35.

Jones, V.E. & Ogilvie, B.M. 1972. Protective immunity to *Nippostrongylus brasiliensis* in the rat. III. Modulation of worm acetylcholinesterase by antibodies. *Immunology*, 22: 119-129.

Jones, W.O., Huntley, J.F. & Emery, D.L. 1992. Isolation and degranulation of mucosal mast cells from the small intestine of parasitised sheep. *Int. J. Parasitol.*, 22: 519-521.

Kaliner, M. & Austen, F.K. 1975. Immunologic release of chemical mediators from human tissues. *Annu. Rev. Pharmacol.*, 15: 177-189.

Keith, R.K. & Bremner, K.C. 1973. Immunisation of calves against the nodular worm *Oesophagostomum radiatum*. *Res. Vet. Sci.*, 15: 23-24.

Kemp, D.H., Agbebe, R.I.S., Johnston, L.A.Y. & Gough, J.M. 1986. Immunisation of cattle against *Boophilus microplus* using extracts derived from adult female ticks: feeding and survival of the parasite on vaccinated cattle. *Int. J. Parasitol.*, 16: 115-120.

Kennedy, M.W. 1990. Resistance to parasitic nematodes – how is the MHC involved? *Parasitol. Today*, 6: 374-375.

Knox, D.P. & Jones, D.G. 1992. A comparison of superoxide dismutase (SOD, EC:1.15.1.1) distribution in gastro-intestinal nematodes. *Int. J. Parasitol.*, 22: 209-214.

Lee, D.L. 1970. The fine structure of the excretory system in adult *Nippostrongylus brasiliensis* (Nematoda) and a suggested function for the "excretory glands". *Tissue Cell*, 2: 225-231.

Lightowlers, M.W. & Rickard, M.D. 1988. Excretory-secretory products of helminth parasites: effects on host immune responses. *Parasitol.*, 6: S123-S166.

Lightowlers, M.W., Rickard, M.D. & Mitchell, G.F. 1984. Immunization against *Taenia taeniaeformis* in mice: identification of onchospheral antigens on polyacrylamide gels by Western blotting and enzyme immunoassay. *Int. J. Parasitol.*, 4: 297-306.

Maizels, R.M. & Selkirk, M.E. 1988. Immunobiology of nematode antigens. *In* P.T. Englund & A. Sher, eds. *I: Biology of parasitism*, p. 285-308. New York, A.R. Liss.

Matthews, B.E. 1982. Skin penetration by *Necator americanus* larvae. *Z. Parasitenk.*, 68: 81-86.

McGhee, J.R., Mestecky, J., Dertxbaugh, M.T., Eldridge, J.H., Hirasawa, M. & Kiyono, H. 1992. The mucosal immune system: some fundamental concepts to vaccine development. *Vaccine*, 10: 75-89.

McGillivery, D.J., Yong, W.K., Riffkin, G.G. & Adler, B. 1990. The distribution and localisation of the stage-specific GP31 antigen from infective *Ostertagia circumcincta* larvae. *Int. J. Parasitol.*, 20: 87-93.

McGillivery, D.J., Yong, W.K., Adler, B. & Riffkin, G.G. 1992. A purified stage-specific 31 kDa antigen as a potential protective antigen against *Ostertagia circumcincta* infection in lamb. *Vaccine*, 10: 607-613.

McGowan, M.J., Barker, R.W., Homer, J.T., McNew, R. & Holscher, K.H. 1981. Success of ticks feeding on calves immunised with *Ambylomma americanum* extract. *J. Med. Entomol.*, 18: 328-332.

McKeand, J.B. 1992. Aspects of the immunobiology of *Dictyocaulus viviparus* infection. University of Glasgow, UK. (Ph.D. thesis)

McKeand, J.B., Knox, D.P., Duncan, J.L. & Kennedy, M.W. 1995. Protective immunisation of guinea pigs against *Dictyocaulus viviparus* using excretory-secretory products of adult parasites. *Int. J. Parasitol.*, 25(1): 95-104.

McKeand, J.B., Knox, D.P., Duncan, J.L. & Kennedy, M.W. The immunogenicity of the cattle lungworm, *Dictyocaulus viviparus*. *Int. J. Parasitol.* (in press)

Miller, T.A. 1971. Vaccination against the canine hookworm diseases. *Adv. Parasitol.*, 9: 153-183.

Miller, T.A. 1978. Industrial development and field use of the canine hookworm vaccine. *Adv. Parasitol.*, 16: 333-342.

Monroy, F.G. & Dobson, C. 1987. Mice vaccinated against *Nematospiroides dubius* with antigens isolated by affinity chromatography from adult worms. *Immunol. Cell Biol.*, 65: 223-230.

Munn, E.A. 1988. Production and use of anthelmintic agents and protective proteins. Patent: WO88/00835.

Munn, E.A. & Smith, T.S. 1990. Production and use of anthelmintic agents and protective proteins. Patent: WO90/11086.

Munn, E.A., Greenwood, C.A. & Coadwell, W.J. 1987. Vaccination of young lambs by means of a protein fraction extracted from adult *Haemonchus contortus*. *Parasitol.*, 94: 385-397.

Munn, E.A., Smith, T.S., Graham, M., Greenwood, C.A., Tavernor, A.S. & Coetzee, G. 1993a. Vaccination of merino lambs against haemonchosis with membrane-associated proteins from the adult parasite. *Parasitol.*, 106: 63-66.

Munn, E.A., Graham, M., Smith, T.S., Newton, S., Knox, D.P., Oliver, J. & Smith, F. 1993b. Cloning and identification of H11, a highly protective antigen from *Haemonchus contortus*. *Proc. Keystone Symp. Molecular Parasitology*, Colorado, USA.

Murray, P.K. 1989. Molecular vaccines against animal parasites. *Vaccine*, 7: 291-300.

Neilson, J.T.M. 1975. Failure to vaccinate lambs against *Haemonchus contortus* with functional metabolic antigens identified by immunoelectrophoresis. *Int. J. Parasitol.*, 5: 427-430.

Neilson, J.T.M. & van de Walle, M.J. 1987. Partial protection of lambs against *Haemonchus contortus* by vaccination with a fractionated preparation from the parasite. *Vet. Parasitol.*, 23: 211-221.

O'Donnell, I.J., Green, P.E., Connell, J.A. & Hopkins, P.S. 1980. Immunoglobulin G antibodies to the antigens of *Lucilia cuprina* in sera of fly-struck sheep. *Aust. J. Biol. Sci.*, 33: 27-34.

O'Donnell, I.J., Green, P.E., Connell, J.A. & Hopkins, P.S. 1981. Immunisation of sheep with larval antigens of *Lucilia* *cuprina*. *Aust. J. Biol. Sci.*, 34: 411-417.

O'Donnell, I.J., Dineen, J.K., Rothwell, T.L.W. & Marshall, R.C. 1985. Attempts to probe the antigens and protective immunogens of *Trichostrongylus colubriformis* in immunoblots with sera from infected and hyperimmune sheep and high and low responder guinea pigs. *Int. J. Parasitol.*, 15: 129-136.

O'Donnell, I.J., Dineen, J.K., Wagland, B.M., Letho, S., Dopheide, T.A.A., Grant, W.N. & Ward, C.W. 1989. Characterization of the major immunogen in the excretory-secretory products of exsheathed third-stage larvae of *Trichostrongylus colubriformis*. *Int. J. Parasitol.*, 19: 793-802.

Ogilvie, B.M., Rothwell, T.L.W., Bremner, K.C., Schnitzerling, H.J., Nolan, J. & Keith, R.K. 1973. Acetylcholinesterase secretion by parasitic nematodes. I. Evidence of secretion by a number of species. *Int. J. Parasitol.*, 3: 589-597.

Opdebeeck, J.P., Wong, J.Y.M., Jackson, L.A. & Dobson, C. 1988. Hereford cattle immunised and protected against *Boophilus microplus* with soluble and membrane-associated antigens from the midgut of ticks. *Parasite Immunol.*, 10: 405-410.

Ozerol, N.H. & Silverman, P.H. 1970. Further characterisation of active metabolites from histotrophic larvae of *Haemonchus contortus* cultured *in vitro*. *J. Parasitol.*, 56: 1199-1205.

Poynter, D.A. & Cauthen, G.E. 1942. Experiments on the life history of the cattle lungworm, *Dictyocaulus viviparus*. *Am. J. Vet. Res.*, 3: 395-400.

Prichard, R.K. 1990. Anthelmintic resistance in nematodes, recent understanding and future directions for research. *Int. J. Parasitol.*, 20: 515-523.

Rajasekariah, G.R., Rickard, M.D. & O'Donnell, I.J. 1985. *Taenia pisiformis*: protective immunisation of rabbits with solubilised oncosheral antigens. *Exp. Parasitol.*, 59: 321-327.

Rand, K.N., Moore, T., Sriskantha, A., Spring, K., Tellam, R., Willadsen, P. & Cobon, G.S. 1989. Cloning and expression of a protective antigen from the cattle tick *Boophilus microplus*. *Proc. Natl. Acad. Sci.*, 86: 9657-9661.

Rhoads, M.L. 1983. *Trichinella spiralis*: identification and purification of superoxide dismutase. *Exp. Parasitol.*, 56: 41-54.

Rhoads, M.L. 1984. Secretory cholinesterases of nematodes: possible functions in the host-parasite relationship. *Trop. Vet.*, 2: 3-10.

Rickard, M.D. & Adolph, A.J. 1977. Vaccination of lambs against infection with *Taenia ovis* using antigens collected during short-term *in vitro* incubation of activated oncospheres. *Parasitol.*, 75: 183-188.

Rickard, M.D. & Bell, K.J. 1971a. Induction of immunity in lambs to larval cestode antigens. *Nature*, 232: 120.

Rickard, M.D. & Bell, K.J. 1971b. Successful vaccination of lambs against infection with *Taenia ovis* using antigens produced during *in vitro* cultivation of the larval stages. *Res. Vet. Sci.*, 12: 401-402.

Rickard, M.D. & Williams, J.F. 1982. Hydatidosis/cysticercosis: immune mechanisms and immunisation against infection. *Adv. Parasitol.*, 21: 230-296.

Roberts, F.H.S., Elek, P. & Keith, R.K. 1962. Studies of resistance in calves to experimental infections with the nodular worm *Oesophagostomum radiatum*. *Aust. J. Agric. Res.*, 13: 551-573.

Rothwell, T.L.W. 1978. Vaccination against the nematode *Trichostrongylus colubriformis*. III. Some observations on factors influencing immunity to infection in vaccinated guinea pigs. *Int. J. Parasitol.*, 8: 33-37.

Rothwell, T.L.W. & Griffiths, D.A. 1977. Comparison of the kinetics of expulsion of *Trichostrongylus colubriformis* from previously uninfected, reinfected and vaccinated guinea pigs. *J. Parasitol.*, 63: 761-762.

Rothwell, T.L.W. & Love, R.J. 1974. Vaccination against the nematode *Trichostrongylus colubriformis*. I. Vaccination of guinea pigs with worm homogenates and soluble products released during *in vitro* maintenance. *Int. J. Parasitol.*, 4: 293-299.

Rothwell, T.W.L. & Merritt, G.C. 1975. Vaccination against the nematode *Trichostrongylus colubriformis*. II. Attempts to protect guinea pigs with worm acetylcholinesterase. *Int. J. Parasitol.*, 5: 453-460.

Sandeman, R.M. 1990. Prospects for the control of sheep blowfly strike by vaccination. *Int. J. Parasitol.*, 20: 537-541.

Sarles, M.P. & Taliaferro, W.A. 1936. The local points of defence and the passive transfer of acquired immunity to *Nippostrongylus brasiliensis* in rats. *J. Inf. Dis.*, 59: 207-220.

Savin, K.W., Dopheide, T.A.A., Frenkel, M.J., Wagland, B.M., Grant, W.A. & Ward, C.W. 1990. Characterization, cloning and host-protective activity of a 30-kilodalton glycoprotein secreted by the parasitic stages of *Trichostrongylus colubriformis*. *Mol. Biochem. Parasitol.*, 41: 167-176.

Schlein, Y. & Lewis, C.T. 1976. Lesions in haematophagous flies after feeding on rabbits immunised with fly tissues. *Physiol. Entomol.*, 1: 55-59.

Sexton, J.L., Milner, A.R. & Paraccio, M. 1990. Glutathione S-transferase. Novel vaccine against *Fasciola hepatica* infection in sheep. *J. Immunol.*, 145: 3905-3910.

Sharma, R.L., Bhat, T.K. & Dhar, D.N. 1988. Control of sheep lungworm in India. *Parasitol. Today*, 4: 33-36.

Sharp, P.J., Smith, D.R.T., Bach, W., Wagland, B.M. & Cobon, G.S. 1991. Purified glutathione S-transferases from parasites as candidate protective antigens. *Int. J. Parasitol.*, 21: 839-846.

Silberstein, D.S. & Despommier, D.D. 1984. Antigens from *Trichinella spiralis* that induce a protective response in the mouse. *J. Immunol.*, 132: 898-904.

Simpson, A.J.G. & Cioli, D. 1987. Progress towards a defined vaccine for schistosomiasis. *Parasitol. Today*, 3: 24-26.

Simpson, A.J.G., Hackett, F., Walker, T., De Rossi, R. & Smithers, S.R. 1985. Antibody response against schistosomulum surface antigens and protective immunity following immunization with highly irradiated cercariae of *Schistosoma mansoni*. *Parasite Immunol.*, 7: 133-152.

Skelly, P.J. & Howells, A.J. 1987. The humoral immune reponse of sheep to antigens from larvae of the sheep blowfly (*Lucilia cuprina*). *Int. J. Parasitol.*, 17: 1081-1087.

Smith, N.C. 1992. Concepts and strategies for anti-parasite immunoprophylaxis and therapy. *Int. J. Parasitol.*, 22: 1047-1082.

Smith, W.D. 1993. Protection in lambs immunised with *Haemonchus contortus* gut membrane proteins. *Res. Vet. Sci.*, 54: 94-101.

Smith, T.S. & Munn, E.A. 1990. Strategies for vaccination against gastro-intestinal nematodes. *Rev. sci. tech. Off. int. Epiz.*, 9: 577-595.

Smith, D.B., Davern, K.M., Board, P.G., Tiu, W., Garcia, E.G. & Mitchell, G.F. 1986. Mr 26000 Da antigen of *Schistosoma japonicum* recognised by WEH1 129/J mice is a gluathione S-transferase. *Proc. Natl Acad. Sci.*, 83: 8703-8707.

Smith, A.M., Dowd, A.J., McGonigle, S., Keegan, P.S., Brennan, G., Trudgett, A. & Dalton, J.P. 1993. Purification of a cathepsin L-like proteinase secreted by adult *Fasciola hepatica*. *Mol. Biochem. Parasitol.*, 62: 1-8.

Stromberg, B.E. & Soulsby, E.J.L. 1977. *Ascaris suum*: immunization with soluble antigens in the guinea pig. *Int. J. Parasitol.*, 7: 287-291.

Tavernor, A.S., Smith, T.S., Langford, C.F. Munn, E.A. & Graham, M. 1992a.

Vaccination of Dorset lambs against haemonchosis. *Parasite Immunol.*, 14: 645-655.

Tavernor, A.S., Smith, T.S., Langford, C.F., Munn, E.A. & Graham, M. 1992b. Immune reponse of Clun Forest to vaccination with membrane glycoproteins from *Haemonchus contortus*. *Parasite Immunol.*, 14: 671-675.

Togna, A.R., Del Giudice, G., Verdini, A.S., Bonelli, F., Pessi, A., Engers, H.D. & Corradin, G. 1986. Synthetic *Plasmodium falciparum* circumsporozoite peptides elicit heterogeneous L3T4$^+$ T cell proliferative responses in H-2^b mice. *J. Immunol.*, 137: 2956-2960.

Turnbull, I.F., Bowles, V.M., Wiltshire, C.J., Brandon, M.R. & Els, N.T. 1992. Systemic immunization of sheep with surface antigens from *Haemonchus contortus* larvae. *Int. J. Parasitol.*, 22: 537-540.

Urquhart, G.M., Jarrett, W.F.H., Jennings, F.W., McIntyre, W.I.M. & Mulligan, W. 1966a. Immunity to *Haemonchus contortus* infection: failure of x-irradiated larvae to immunize young lambs. *Am. J. Vet. Res.*, 27: 1641-1643.

Urquhart, G.M., Jarrett, W.F.H., Jennings, F.W., McIntyre, W.I.M. & Mulligan, W. 1966b. Immunity to *Haemonchus contortus* infection: relationship between age and successful vaccination with irradiated larvae. *Am. J. Vet. Res.*, 27: 1645-1648.

van Wyck, J.A. & Malan, F.S. 1988. Resistance of field strains of *Haemonchus contortus* to avermectin, closantel, rafoxanide and the benzimidazoles in South Africa. *Vet. Rec.*, 123: 226-228.

Vernes, A. 1976. Immunization of the mouse and guinea pig against *Trichinella spiralis*. *In* van den Bossche, ed. *Biochemistry of parasites and host/parasite relationships*, p. 319-324. Amsterdam, Elsevier/North Holland Biomedical.

Wagland, B.M. 1975. Host resistance to the cattle tick (*Boophilus microplus*) in cattle. *Aust. J. Agric. Res.*, 26: 1073-1080.

Waller, P.J. & Larsen, M. 1993. The role of nematophagous fungi in the biological control of nematode parasites of livestock. *Int. J. Parasitol.*, 23: 539-546.

Wharton, R.H. 1976. Tick-borne livestock diseases and their vectors, 5. Acaricide resistance and alternative methods of tick control. *World Anim. Rev.*, 20: 8-15.

Wijffels, G.L., Sexton, J.L. & Salvatore, L. 1992. Primary sequence heterogeneity and tissue expression of glutathione S-transferases of *Fasciola hepatica*. *Exp. Parasitol.*, 74: 87-99.

Wikel, S.K. 1981. The induction of host resistance to tick infestation with salivary gland antigen. *Am. J. Trop. Med. Hyg.*, 30: 284-288.

Willadsen, P. 1980. Immunity to ticks. *Adv. Parasitol.*, 18: 293-313.

Willadsen, P. & McKenna, R.V. 1991. Vaccination with concealed antigens: myth or reality? *Parasite Immunol.*, 13: 605-616.

Willadsen, P., McKenna, R.V. & Riding, G.A. 1988. Isolation from the cattle tick, *Boophilus microplus*, of antigenic material capable of eliciting a protective immunological response in the bovine host. *Int. J. Parasitol.*, 18: 183-189.

Willadsen, P., Riding, G.A., McKenna, R.V., Kemp, D.H., Tellam, R.L., Nielsen, J.N., Lahnstein, J., Cobon, G.S. & Gough, J.M. 1989. *J. Immunol.*, 143: 1346-1351.

Xilinas, M.E., Papavasiliou, L.T. & Marselou-Kinti, O. 1976. Active immunisation of mice against *Echinococcus granulosus*. *Hellenica Acta Microbiol.*, 21: 86-90.

Poultry vaccines (1)

Conventional vaccines

J.B. McFerran

Vaccination of poultry presents a number of special problems. The first is the limited life of the meat-producing chicken, which is often as short as 35 days from hatching to slaughter. These birds have a low individual value and any vaccine must therefore be relatively cheap. They are kept in very large numbers at a very high density. Houses often contain 10 000 to 30 000 birds and sites often have between 50 000 and one million birds. The problem is compounded because these birds have probably originated from eggs produced by a number of breeding farms. These breeding farms may well be in a different region (or even country) and may have a different antibody status and disease history. Therefore, the chickens hatching from these eggs will have considerable variations in maternal antibodies and, in some cases, chicks will have been vertically infected with viruses such as chick anaemia virus (CAV) or avian encephalomyelitis. This problem is becoming more acute as hygiene and disease precautions are increased in the breeding farms, for example to control *Salmonella* spp. If all the breeding farms are infected with a virus such as CAV before they start producing eggs, it is not a problem. However, if some are not infected, then two problems can arise: the first is if the chicks are placed in an area where CAV is endemic, in which case the susceptible chicks originating from parents without antibody become infected; the second is when one of the parent flocks becomes infected. This flock will produce infected and diseased chicks and they will infect the susceptible chicks in the hatcheries.

Poultry are infected with a number of immunosuppressive viruses, of which the most important is infectious bursal disease (IBD) virus, which has virtually a world-wide distribution. These viruses have three important effects: they can cause disease in their own right; they can compromise the birds' immunological response to other vaccines; and they can reduce the birds' resistance to other organisms so that a severe reaction to vaccination with an attenuated vaccine can occur as a result of other agents combining with the vaccine to induce disease.

The disadvantages of large-scale poultry production can in part be overcome by having an "all-in all-out" system, where a site is completely depopulated and is properly cleaned and disinfected before the next intake of day-old chicks. It is relatively easy to clean and disinfect (e.g. by formalin fumigation) environmentally controlled houses with impervious walls and concrete floors but it is virtually impossible to disinfect open-sided houses with earth floors. In addition, commercial pressures often lead to bad microbiological practices. It is not uncommon for organizations which do depopulate and clean houses to have large sites where the last houses to be depopulated are still being cleaned when chicks are filling the first houses. Even worse, in some areas litter is reused many times and young chicks are brooded in houses still containing older birds.

Most commercial poultry organizations are highly integrated with considerable movement between farms. Thus, laying flocks will have regular egg collections, with transport moving from farm to farm;

breeders and broilers are often weighed regularly by the organization's advisory staff; there is movement and contact by catching and vaccination teams, etc. While a reasonable disinfection of staff can be carried out, it is more difficult to ensure that tools and equipment (e.g. weighing scales, electrician's tools, egg trolleys) are safe. These factors make the spread of disease relatively easy.

From a disease control viewpoint there are three main types of poultry: i) commercial flocks, usually kept under intensive husbandry methods; ii) local small backyard flocks, which in most areas are unvaccinated; and iii) hobby birds. The latter range from Psittacines (especially dangerous because they can be infected with virulent Newcastle disease virus) to racing pigeons. Wild birds also pose a problem as they are capable of carrying infection long distances and may indeed be hosts of certain viruses. For instance, wild ducks are often infected with paramyxoviruses, including Newcastle disease, myxoviruses and the egg drop syndrome, adenovirus.

Humans are probably one of the most important vectors for spreading infection, second only to the bird. It is possible to reduce the risk of introducing disease by keeping all but essential people out of poultry houses and by ensuring that those who enter take precautions (e.g. by using special outer clothing kept on the farm for each essential visitor).

It is unlikely that organisms will spread from hobby birds or backyard flocks by aerial routes because the number of birds involved is too small. Some viruses can spread from commercial farm to commercial farm by wind owing to the large concentration of birds (e.g. Newcastle disease and Marek's disease viruses). Other routes are also important, such as untreated water (e.g. spreading influenza, Newcastle disease, egg drop syndrome, salmonellosis), feed (e.g. paramyxovirus type 1 [pigeon Newcastle disease], *Salmonella* spp., IBD) and transport.

Given the above considerations, it can be seen that the chances of poultry disease spreading are very high. In addition, the poultry industry is truly international, with birds (and advisory staff) moving freely between countries. The speed of the spread of "new" diseases in recent years underlines this. Diseases such as runting-stunting, egg drop syndrome, turkey rhinotracheitis virus, virulent forms of Newcastle disease, Marek's disease and IBD as well as antigenic variants of infectious bronchitis (IB) have all spread rapidly around the world. The emergence of other new diseases such as chick anaemia, may be the result of changes in management rather than the spread of virus, but this is unclear at present.

VACCINATION

Clearly, vaccination is essential to commercial poultry production. However with the birds' short life, high-density conditions and variable antibody levels, it is very difficult to achieve full protection and it is essential that every effort be made to prevent the introduction of infection or carryover of infectious agents from flock to flock. To some extent, the degree of resistance induced by any vaccine is subject to the level of challenge present and, if that challenge is great enough, vaccines are unlikely to give protection.

The ideal vaccine should:

- be able to be given by mass application;
- be cheap;
- be safe;
- be capable of inducing a strong immunity even in the presence of maternal antibody;
- be capable of inducing both local and general immunity;
- induce an immune response that can be distinguished from that induced by

infection or maternal derived antibody;
- require only one dose to give lifelong immunity;
- be packaged in different sizes (e.g. while 1 000-dose vials are appropriate for use in commercial flocks, they are not appropriate for use in a small backyard flock).

Such a vaccine does not exist at present.

Successful vaccination against many organisms depends on stimulating both local immunity at a mucosal surface and general humoral antibody. The local immunity is of major importance for those agents which affect mucosal surfaces – for example IB – and is of special importance in meat-producing birds which are housed at very high densities, have a short life span and require quick immunity.

Serology

There are a wide range of tests used to monitor vaccination and also for diagnosis. The modern tests, for example ELISA tests, are expensive and it is important to use them appropriately and not just to accumulate data. They can be used to monitor the efficiency of vaccination where immunity (general) is measured by an antibody response. Titres should not only be high but, even more important, be in a close range. It is important to remember that if 10 percent of the birds have low titres or no antibody, this can be translated into 2 000 to 3 000 birds dying in a house. There is no easy method of measuring local immunity. This is unfortunate, since local immunity is often very important, as for example in IB. Other uses for serology are to determine if a flock has been infected. Thus, if birds in the rearing period develop antibody to CAV, there is no need to vaccinate. As already discussed, it is the flocks without antibody that pose the problems.

Determination of antibody titres in breeding flocks can allow the breeding flocks to be batched into groups so that the progeny will have similar titres and, consequently, the timing of vaccination can be better judged. This has been used in the control of IBD. The difficulty is that there is often a wide variation in antibody titres in birds in any one flock.

Vaccine administration

There are a number of commonly used methods of vaccination. Meat-producing chickens are normally handled twice – at birth and at death. Therefore, vaccination is either done individually in the hatchery (e.g. Marek's vaccination) or else mass application methods are used. The easiest method is to give the vaccine in the drinking-water, yet this is most difficult to do properly. There is always a percentage of birds that will not drink. Although this percentage can be reduced by ensuring the birds are thirsty, they must not be stressed and the water must be turned on immediately afterwards, with no danger of airlocks occurring. Furthermore, the vaccine may not be uniformly available in the drinking-water because of physical problems such as uneven troughs, or vaccine may be lost as a result of adherence to rusty containers or feed which has fallen into the drinkers. Vaccine can also be inactivated by chemicals (e.g. chlorine) in the water or by heat. Such problems can in part be overcome by adding protein (e.g. dried skim milk powder) to the vaccine and by giving the vaccine in two parts (McFerran *et al.*, 1972). It is also essential to keep the birds at a comfortable air temperature. This may require raising the temperature in cold areas or vaccinating early in the morning in hot regions.

Partly to overcome the problems of water administration and partly to induce local immunity, spraying has been widely used. The use of a coarse spray (in reality a mass eye and nose drop application) to immunize day-old chicks which possess maternally derived antibody against diseases such as IB, has been routine in hatcheries in some areas for 25 years. This has given excellent immunity, lasting the life of the meat-producing chicken. Even in the case of emergency vaccinations of antibody-free chicks with Newcastle disease virus, excellent immunity was provided with acceptable side-effects (McFerran, 1992). Severe side-effects did occur when the spray was too fine and virus penetrated the lower respiratory tract. Results similar to those given by coarse spray have been obtained using the labour-intensive method of beak dipping.

Aerosols, generated using an electrically powered sprayer, or a fine spray from a hand operated pump have been used to revaccinate birds. In some instances, this has been done every 12 weeks to ensure that virtual continuous local immunity is maintained at mucosal surfaces.

One constraint on the use of spray vaccines in some areas is that other microorganisms infecting the birds, such as *Mycoplasma* spp. and *Haemophilius* spp., can produce severe side-effects. Therefore, in certain organizations or regions it is inadvisable to use spray vaccination.

In theory, the large cleft in the oral palates of fowl and turkeys should allow orally administered vaccine to come in contact with the upper respiratory tract and achieve the same results as spray vaccination. However, in practice, spray vaccination is much more effective in stimulating local immunity in the respiratory tract as well as being less labour-intensive. In part, the increased immunity following spray vaccination may be the result of stimulation of the Hardarian gland by the spray-applied vaccine.

Injection (including wing-web stabbing) is still widely used. Virtually all egg-producing birds and many meat-producing chicks are vaccinated at one day of age with Marek's vaccine. This is a quick and cheap method of application. Breakdowns occur when the vaccine is deposited in the feathers rather than under the skin in a quest for speed and when a blocked needle or bacterial contamination of the apparatus goes unnoticed.

Inactivated vaccines, often with an oil adjuvant, are widely used. They tend to be expensive to buy and deliver but have been very successful in controlling disease in adults. While they are of value in protecting chicks against disease through maternally derived antibody, recent experience has shown (as in the case of IBD) that virulent strains can break through the maternal antibody protection and active immunity must therefore be induced.

SOME CONVENTIONAL VACCINES

There are a wide variety of conventional vaccines available. Brief descriptions of some are given here, concentrating on unusual aspects or problems and potential future developments.

Marek's disease

Marek's disease has been controlled by using type 1 attenuated vaccines (either artificially attenuated or naturally occurring strains) or the type 3 turkey herpesvirus (THV). In some areas, a type 2 naturally occurring attenuated strain was necessary. In some genetic lines, if the birds are infected with both the serotype 2 and the lymphoid leukosis virus early in life, there is an enhancement of lymphoid leukosis. In the 1980s, very virulent strains of Marek's disease arose, and control was achieved using a mixture of vaccine – either types 2 and 3 or types 1 and 3. There appears to be a true synergism between different strains, especially between serotypes 2 and 3, and polyvalent vaccines have been found to provide better protection against tumour development (Witter *et al.*, 1984). However even these vaccines have not been totally successful and preliminary results suggest that, in order to ensure maximum resistance to Marek's disease, it may be necessary to select a vaccine appropriate for the predominant B-haplotype of the chicken flock (Bacon and Witter, 1993).

Infectious bronchitis

The envelope of IB virus possesses surface projections comprising two glycopolypeptides, S_1 and S_2. While both are important in the immune response, it appears that the S_1 glycopolypeptide is the major antigenic component.

Protection is given against the homologous serotype as well as, to a varying degree, against other serotypes. This has resulted in the use of a number of different attenuated vaccines in some areas. Recombination among field and vaccine strains possibly occurs and is responsible for producing new "variant" strains (Kusters *et al.*, 1990). Because of the possibility of recombination and the fact that attenuated strains can revert back to virulence, a new vaccine serotype should not be introduced into an area until there is clear evidence that its use that is essential.

There have been two approaches to immunizing egg-producing birds. The first is to prime the birds with an attenuated vaccine (around four weeks when maternal antibody levels have fallen) and then with an inactivated oil-adjuvanted vaccine or a less attenuated vaccine around 18 weeks to produce high levels of circulating humoral antibody. The second is to prime the birds and then commence spray vaccination at 18 weeks, followed thereafter every eight to ten weeks with an attenuated vaccine. The aim here is to keep a high degree of local immunity in the gut and respiratory tract.

Infectious bursal disease

Both attenuated and inactivated vaccines exist fro IBD. Attenuated vaccines have been divided into three broad categories based on virulence: i) virulent or "hot"; ii) intermediate; and iii) "mild" or avirulent. There is some discussion as to whether some of the "hot" vaccines are any more virulent than the intermediate ones. The suggestion is that some of the "hot" strains spread better between birds and can therefore infect birds that were not initially vaccinated either because they did not drink or because they have high maternal antibody levels. It has been suggested that virulent viruses can overcome virus-neutralizing antibody titres of 1.500, intermediate vaccines can overcome titres of 1.250 and avirulent viruses can overcome titres of 1.100 or less (Lukert and Saif, 1991). However, given the wide variation of titres in broiler chickens, these figures are at best only a guide as to the optimum time to vaccinate.

In view of the wide antigenic variation within IBD viruses (McFerran *et al.*, 1980) it is surprising that only one subtype vaccine (the Delaware) has been necessary. There has been a major upsurge in virulence of IBD viruses throughout the world, and the policy adapted in many areas of only vaccinating the breeders and relying on maternal antibody to protect the broilers has proved flawed. In many areas, it has been necessary to use intermediate or hot vaccines in broiler flocks to control the losses. Even when flocks are clinically normal, IBD virus can attack the bursa and cause lesions. In these circumstances, the subclinical infections can cause up to a 10 percent reduction in income (McIlroy, Goodall and McCracken, 1989).

Mycoplasma gallisepticum

Although *Mycoplasma gallisepticum* has been eradicated from commercial poultry in many areas, it is still widely distributed, especially in areas where multi-age sites and open-sided houses with earth floors make eradication very difficult. Under these conditions, vaccination of commercial egg-producing birds to control falls in egg production is indicated. Bacterins, which are inactivated suspensions of whole *M. gallisepticum* (Mg[1]) organisms in oil emulsion, are apparently effective in controlling disease but have little benefit in eliminating infection in multi-age sites. Recently, inactivated *M. gallisepticum* bacterin mixed with 0.2 percent iota carrageenan as an adjuvant induced resistance to air sacculites in chicken challenged with the virulent MGR strain (Elfaki *et al.*, 1992).

Live vaccines are also used to control *M. gallisepticum*. The F strain is a naturally occurring strain of relatively low virulence for chickens but of a higher virulence for turkeys. It will displace more virulent field strains from multi-aged sites but vaccinated birds become permanent carriers (Kleven, Khan and Yamamoto, 1990). A temperature-sensitive mutant which is avirulent has recently been described (Whithear *et al.*, 1990).

Fowl cholera

Fowl cholera is caused by *Pasteurella multocida*, which can be serologically subdivided by differences in capsular antigens and cell wall lipopolysaccharide antigens. Using a passive haemagglutinin test, five capsular serogroups (A,B,D,E and F) can be identified; however, these capsular antigens do not appear to play a role in protection. *P. multocida* can also be subdivided into 16 serotypes using a heat-stable somatic antigen (Brogdens and Rebers, 1978). Both inactivated and live *P. multocida* vaccines are available. Inactivated vaccines are whole cell products of a number of strains (often including "autogenous" local strains) emulsified in an oil adjuvant. The attenuated strains have a range of virulence, although two doses of inactivated vaccine during rearing usually provide adequate immunity as long as the appropriate strains are included in the vaccine. Attenuated vaccines are widely used in some areas, especially in meat turkeys. Live vaccines often cause chronic fowl cholera. This effect can be minimized by first giving an inactivated vaccine.

Infectious coryza

Infectious coryza is caused by *Haemophilus paragallinarum*, the isolates of which it is possible to divide into three serogroups with at least seven serovars by using the HI test (Kume *et al.*, 1983). Vaccines consist of inactivated whole-cell bacterins emulsified in oil adjuvant or absorbed on to aluminium hydroxide. The immunity induced by these vaccines is serogroup-specific. Breeders and commercial layers are routinely vaccinated in many countries, using two injections during rearing at least four weeks apart. Using chemical mutogens, Blackall *et al.*, (1993) have produced non-pathogenic mutants which may be of value as attenuated vaccines.

Coccidiosis

A widespread and serious disease caused by *Eimeria* spp. is coccidiosis. It has been controlled in the past by the continuous administration of chemotherapeutic agents to the flock's feed. However, problems with the development of resistance and the need to withdraw the agents for a specified period before slaughter have led to the development of vaccines.

At present, vaccines are used mainly in layers and breeders. They contain attenuated oocysts of multiple species of *Eimeria*. Attenuation has been achieved by a number of methods such as adaptation to growth in avian embryos or by selecting strains with a shortened prepatent period in the precocious strains.

A second approach has been to define coccidial immunogens which could be used as subunit vaccines. There are, however, many species of *Eimeria,* with little or no cross-immunity between species.

NEW TECHNICAL DEVELOPMENTS

In 1982, Sharma and Burmester inoculated embryos with THV in an attempt to circumvent the massive Marek's disease challenge that day-old chicks faced on some sites. These chickens developed a persistent THV infection and were resistant to early challenge with pathogenic Marek's disease. The vaccine was inoculated into the allantoic sac; and it was found that the best results were obtained in 17- to 18-day-old embryos. Inoculation at 18 days would coincide with the transfer of eggs from the setting to the hatching machines.

Sharma (1985) extended this work to the investigation of protection against IBD. He found that low virulent vaccine strains could induce immunity without effecting hatchability or survival of the chicks. However, maternal antibody did neutralize strains of low virulence. Recently, the use of an IBD commercial vaccine-antiserum mixture to inoculate 18-day-old embryonated eggs has been described. This preparation induced immunity in chicks produced from eggs with maternal antibody to IBD (Whitfill *et al.,* 1993). Embryos originating from specific pathogen-free (SPF) turkeys were successfully inoculated with marble spleen disease and Newcastle disease vaccines and the poults were resistant to subsequent challenge (Ahmad and Sharma, 1993).

This work has been developed commercially and an automatic egg injection system is now in operation (Marchant, 1993), injecting THV and SB-1 Marek's vaccine into embryonated chick eggs. The machine can inject 20 000 to 30 000 eggs per hour. The success of these approaches will depend on whether the economic advantages claimed are realized. This is especially true where hygiene standards are high and day-old chicks do not face a massive challenge.

One different approach to embryonated egg inoculation is to inject an immuno-stimulant containing lymphokines. It is claimed that this has enhanced the efficiency of Marek's disease vaccination and, in addition, resulted in lower mortality, reduced feed conversion and lower production costs for commercial broilers (Miles *et al.,* 1993).

Genetic engineering

Initially, organisms were modified by egg passage (e.g. IB), by cell culture passage or by identifying a naturally occurring non-pathogenic strain (e.g. Rispen's vaccine against Marek's disease). The attenuation process can be enhanced by using chemical mutagens, and mutants can be selected using a range of techniques such as plaque purification, temperature sensitivity, colony size or an appropriate monoclonal antibody. Some proteins are only expressed when bacterial cells are grown *in vivo,* and it is suggested that this is the reason why *Pasteurella multocida* grown *in vivo* gives better vaccines. An attempt to clone the genes responsible for expressing these proteins is in progress and may give rise to better inactivated or attenuated vaccines (Jost *et al.,* 1993). It is now possible to modify the genome by chemical means, as in the Aujeszky's disease vaccine virus in which the thymidine kinase gene has been deleted.

It is possible to insert genes into vectors. These vectors can be organisms which do not replicate in the host, in which case an adjuvant is indicated. Thus, a recombinant baculovirus (expressing the haemag-glutinin and neuraminidase protein of Newcastle disease virus), combined with an oil adjuvant, is effective in protecting against Newcastle disease challenge (Nagy *et al.*, 1991).

The alternative approach is to incorporate one or more genes into a vector which does replicate in the host. Avian poxviruses, avian herpesviruses (serotype 2 and turkey herpesvirus) and avian adenoviruses have been investigated. An example is the incorporation of the gene coding for the haemagglutinin of avian influenza (H5N2) into a poxvirus (Beard, Schnitzlein and Tripathy, 1991). The gene coding for the fusion protein (F) of Newcastle disease virus has also been incorporated into poxvirus (Iritani *et al.*, 1991). This gives immunity but does not give rise to H1 antibodies, thus allowing a test to detect infection by the Newcastle disease virus. Antibody to Newcastle disease did not prevent the development of immunity, but antibody to fowl pox prevented the poxvirus growing. Thus, this vaccine could be used to vaccinate ducks with maternal antibody to Newcastle disease. Similarly, a fowl poxvirus expressing the turkey rhinotracheitis fusion glycoprotein gave partial protection to challenge by turkey rhinotracheitis virus (Quinzhong *et al.*, 1993).

A promising approach is to use a turkey herpesvirus (THV) as the vector. A recombinant THV expressing the Newcastle disease virus fusion protein gave good protection against both Marek's and Newcastle diseases (Morgan *et al.*, 1992). THV is used widely to vaccinate day old chicks. It is universal and safe (unlike fowl pox which is absent in some areas and which may cause local reactions), it does not spread horizontally and, most important, it gives a persistent viraemia lasting several weeks. This approach may well overcome the problems of maternal immunity. Thus, if genes giving resistance to a number of diseases were incorporated, they could stimulate the immune response to each agent at the appropriate time as maternal antibody wanes. This would overcome the hurdle of varying levels of antibody to different viruses and also to the same virus, owing to the fact that the flock is made up of the progeny of a number of breeding flocks.

There is always the problem of the maternal antibody to the vector preventing the vector growing. In the case of THV this could be overcome by using the THV in alternate generations (it does not occur as a natural infection in chickens), as is already the practice.

While it is possible to express the genes encoding protein antigens *in vitro* for use as subunit vaccines, and also to synthesize peptide vaccines chemically, these solutions may present problems regarding the cost of production and administration of these vaccines, difficulties in obtaining the correct folding of the protein and the limited number of antigenic determinants, which could mean that strains of agents could arise which are not neutralized.

Although, in theory, anti-idiotype vaccines are possible, in practice they have been poorly immunogenic and show little immediate promise. A different approach is the use of cytokines as adjuvants. These can be incorporated in the injectible vaccine which may also include slow-release mechanisms and immunostimulating complexes (ISCOMs). Such an approach has been taken with a subunit vaccine against avian influenza in which nucleoprotein with residual haemagglutinin activity was incorporated into ISCOMs (Sivanandan *et al.*, 1993).

Liposome-adjuvanted egg drop syndrome 1976 vaccines appeared as efficacious as oil-emulsion vaccines without the side-effects of the oil (Jing-Sheng and Yi-Zhu, 1993).

Using trivalent avian influenza antigens, Fatunmbi *et al.* (1992) found that charged liposomal avridine adjuvant produced a better antibody response than other uncharged liposomal avridine or oil-emulsion adjuvants. The positively charged liposomal avridine adjuvant was superior to negatively charged adjuvant.

BIBLIOGRAPHY

Ahmad, J. & Sharma, J.M. 1993. Protection against hemorrhagic enteritis and Newcastle disease in turkeys by embryo vaccination with monovalent and bivalent vaccines. *Avian Dis.,* 37: 485-491.

Bacon, L.D. & Witter, R.C. 1993. Influence of B-haplotype on the relative efficacy of Marek's disease vaccines of different serotypes. *Avian Dis.,* 37: 53-59.

Beard, C.W., Schnitzlein, W.M. & Tripathy, D.N. 1991. Protection of chickens against highly pathogenic avian influenza virus (H5N2) by recombinant fowlpox viruses. *Avian Dis.,* 35: 356-359.

Blackall, P.J., Graydon, R.J., Rafiee, M. & Tinworth, D. 1993. Towards a live infectious coryza vaccine. In *Proc. X World Vet. Poultry Assoc. Congr.,* Sydney, Australia.

Brogdens, K.A. & Rebers, P.A. 1978. Serological examination of the Westphal-type lipopolysaccharides of *Pasteurella multocida. Am. J. Vet. Res.,* 39: 1680-1682.

Elfaki, M.G., Kleven, S.H., Jin, L.H. & Ragland, W.L. 1992. Sequential intracoelomic and intrabursal immunisation of chickens with inactivated *Mycoplasma gallisepticum* bacteria and iota carageenan adjuvant. *Vaccine,* 10: 655-662.

Fatunmbi, O.O., Newman, J.A., Sivanandan, V. & Halvorson, D.A. 1992. Enhancement of antibody response of turkeys to trivalent avian influenza vaccine by positively charged liposomal avridine adjuvant. *Vaccine,* 10: 623-626.

Iritani, Y., Aoyama, S., Takigami, S., Hayashi, Y., Ogawa, R., Yanagida, N., Saeki, S. & Kamogowa, K. 1991. Antibody response to Newcastle disease virus (NDV) by recombinant fowlpox virus (FPV) expressing a hemagglutinin-neuraminidase of NDV into chickens in the presence of antibody to NDV or FPV. *Avian Dis.,* 35: 659-661.

Jing-Sheng, L. & Yi-Zhu, W. 1993. Studies on the liposome-adjuvanted antigens of the inactivated EDS.76 virus. In *Proc. X World Vet. Poultry Assoc. Congr.,* Sydney, Australia.

Jost, H., Homchampa, P., Ruffolo, C. & Adler, B. 1993. Molecular approaches for studying the virulence genes and antigens of *P. multocida;* strategies for novel fowl cholera vaccines. In *Proc. X World Vet. Poultry Assoc. Congr.,* Sydney, Australia.

Kleven, S.H., Khan, M.I. & Yamamoto, R. 1990. Fingerprinting of *Mycoplasma gallisepticum* strains isolated from multiage layers vaccinated with live F strain. *Avian Dis.,* 34: 984-990.

Kume, K., Sawata, A., Nakai, T. & Matsumoto, M. 1983. Serological classification of *Haemophilus paragallinarum* with a hemagglutinin system. *J. Clin. Microbiol.,* 17: 958-964.

Kusters, J.G., Jager, E.J., Niesters, H.G.M. & van der Zeijst, B.A.M. 1990. Sequence evidence for RNA recombination in field isolates of avian coronavirus infectious bronchitis virus. *Vaccine,* 8: 605-608.

Lukert, P.D. & Saif, Y.M. 1991. Infectious bursal disease. *In* B.W. Calnek, ed. Diseases of poultry, p. 342-385. Ames, USA, Iowa State University Press.

Marchant, J. 1993. Embrex targeting a niche market. *Animal Pharmacol.,* 269: 14-15.

McFerran, J.B. 1992. Control of Newcastle disease in Northern Ireland (NDV vacc.). In *Proc. Workshop of Avian Paramyxoviruses,* p. 238-249. Rauischolzhasen, Germany, Commission of the European Communities

McFerran, J.B., Young, J.A., Clarke, J.K. & Wright, C.L. 1972. Observations concerning the use of living infectious bronchitis vaccine under field conditions. *Vet. Rec.,* 90: 527-530.

McFerran, J.B., McNulty, M.S., McKillop, E.R., Connor, T.J., McCracken, R.M., Collins, D.S. & Allan, G.M. 1980. Isolation and serological studies with infectious bursal disease viruses from fowl, turkeys and ducks: demonstration of a second serotype. *Avian Pathol.,* 8: 205-212.

McIlroy, S.G., Goodall, E.A. & McCracken, R.M. 1989. Economic effects of subclinical infectious bursal disease on broiler production. *Avian Pathol.,* 18: 465-473.

Miles, A.M., Doelling, V.W., Phelps, P.V., Ricks, C.A., Tyczkowski, J.K., Whitfell, C.E. & Gildersleeve, R.P. 1993. Efficacy of an immunostimulant administered *in ovo.* In *Proc. X World Vet. Poultry Assoc. Congr.,* Sydney, Australia.

Morgan, R.W., Gelb, J., Schreurs, C.S., Luttiken, D., Rosenberger, J.K. & Sandermeijer, P.J.A. 1992. Protection of chickens from Newcastle and Marek's disease with a recombinant herpesvirus of turkeys vaccine expressing the Newcastle disease fusion protein. *Avian Dis.,* 36: 858-870.

Nagy, E., Krell, P.J., Dulac, G.C. & Derbyshire, J.B. 1991. Vaccination against Newcastle disease with a recombinant baculovirus hemagglutinin-neuraminidase subunit vaccine. *Avian Dis.,* 35: 585-591.

Quinzhong, Yu., Barrett, T., Brown, D.X., Cook, J.K.A., Green, P., Skinner, M. & Cavanagh, D. 1993. Protection against turkey rhinotracheitis pneumovirus (TRT) induced by a fowl pox recombinant expressing the TRTV fusion glycoprotein (F). In *Proc. X World Vet. Poultry Assoc. Congr.,* Sydney, Australia.

Sharma, J.M. 1985. Embryo vaccination with infectious bursal disease virus alone or in combination with Marek's disease virus. *Avian Dis.,* 29: 1155-1169.

Sharma, J.M. & Burmester, B.R. 1982. Resistance to Marek's disease at hatching in chickens vaccinated as embryos with turkey herpesvirus. *Avian Dis.,* 26: 134-149.

Sivanandan, V., Kodihalli, S., Nagaraja, K.V., Halvorson, D.A. & Newman, J.A. 1993. ISCOM adjuvanted cross-protective subunit vaccine against avian influence. In *Proc. X World Vet. Poultry Assoc. Congr.,* Sydney, Australia.

Whitfill, C.E., Ricks, C.A., Haddad, E.E. & Avakian, A.P. 1993. *In ovo* administration of a novel infectious bursal disease vaccine in broiler chickens. In *Proc. X World Vet. Poultry Assoc. Congr.,* Sydney, Australia.

Whithear, K.G., Soeripto, Harrigan, K.E. & Ghiocas, E. 1990. Immunogenicity of a temperature-sensitive mutant of *Mycoplasma gallisepticum* vaccine. *Aust. Vet. J.,* 67: 168-174.

Witter, R.L., Sharma, J.M., Lee, L.F., Opitz, H.M. & Henry, C.W. 1984. Field tests to test the efficacy of polyvalent Marek's disease vaccine in broilers. *Avian Dis.,* 28: 44-60.

Poultry vaccines (2)

Special requirements for village chickens

R.P. Spradbrow

The poultry industry in developing countries, especially the village poultry industry, encounters different problems to those found in the developed countries and, consequently, the requirements for vaccine by this segment of the market are very different. Certainly, there are elements of the international commercial industry with poultry enterprises close to the larger cities in many developing countries, and these enterprises have access to international breeding stock and international expertise as well as the opportunity and funding to draw vaccines of high quality from the international market. The vaccines used on these poultry populations in a developing country will seldom have been produced in that country. Instead, they will have been produced to meet the highest standards – as discussed elsewhere in this manual – and the manufacturers will have ensured as far as possible the absolute safety and adequate efficacy of the vaccines.

Village chickens comprise the major part of the poultry industry in many developing countries. Village flocks are small, of mixed age and poorly housed or even unhoused. The chickens gain much of their nourishment by scavenging in the village environment and by consuming supplements of household scraps if these are made available. The village flocks are poorly productive, as the major call on energy is for reproduction and maintenance of the population. Extremely high mortality rates ensure that few surplus eggs and birds become available for sale, barter or consumption. Nearly all the eggs are required for brooding. Two elements responsible for these extreme mortalities have been cited. First is the high wastage that occurs during the brooding season, which is probably caused by a combination of starvation, predation and infectious disease but is indirectly the result of poor husbandry and neglect. The second cause of attrition is more directly caused by infectious disease. Outbreaks of disease causing extremely high rates of mortality in village chickens have been reported from many developing countries. Where these diseases have been identified, the major culprits are Newcastle disease and fowl cholera, which are preventable and readily controlled if effective vaccines can be applied. It is the lack of suitable vaccines and appropriate methods of application that allows Newcastle disease and fowl cholera to plunder the village flocks. If these diseases could be controlled, villagers would have the incentive to make the changes in husbandry that would control brooding losses.

Suitable vaccines are the key to a "new science" of village chicken keeping. An analysis of the special requirements of village chickens indicates that their needs are not being served by the conventional vaccines available on the international market. A start has been made on developing vaccines against Newcastle disease that are specifically suited for delivery to and use in villages, (Copland, 1987; Spradbrow, 1992 and 1993/94). However, it is important that regulatory authorities recognizse the special needs of village chickens and that well-intentioned regulations do not impose further barriers to the provision of suitable vaccines to village chickens.

Village flocks require special vaccines. The transport of vaccines to villages and their storage within these villages must usually be accomplished without refrigeration. It will still not be feasible in the forseeable future to establish adequate cold chains; therefore, the vaccines themselves must be thermostable. As long as villagers think that their flocks will survive the frequent outbreaks of infectious disease to which they are exposed, adequate housing will remain a rarity. This means catching chickens for individual vaccination will often be impossible. There seems to be no alternative to the oral application of vaccine, usually on food but also in water, in areas where the sources of drinking water can be controlled. When possible, individual applications of vaccine to the eye, nose or mouth is a more reliable method of inducing immunity with attenuated vaccines. Vaccines for use in village chickens also need to be extremely cheap. It may be necessary to reconsider some of the elements that add value to conventional vaccines – formulation, packaging, substrate, testing. Nor is it necessary to demand an extremely high degree of efficacy of a vaccine for use in village chickens. Absolute protection may require unrealistically large amounts of vaccine. The cost-effective compromise may be a moderate level of protection achieved with an inexpensive vaccine. In few places have conventional vaccines contributed to the protection of village chickens.

Many developing countries would prefer to produce their own veterinary vaccines for local use, especially the relatively simple avian vaccines that can be made in embryonated eggs. There are several reasons for this. One is the desire for national self-reliance and the belief that self-sufficiency in avian vaccines can eventually lead to independence in other areas of vaccine production. The overriding imperative is the need to conserve foreign exchange.

The purchase and transport of imported vaccines is a continuing drain on funds. On the negative side, a wasteful regional overcapacity for vaccine production can be reached, while the purchase of vaccine-producing equipment of any sophistication is also an expensive undertaking. Where vaccine is produced nationally, consideration should be given to establishing independent regional centres for testing.

Many of the standards developed for the testing of conventional avian vaccines are not appropriate for the testing of vaccines for village chickens. Tests for safety should be undertaken in local chickens and tests for efficacy should also be made locally, using indigenous chickens and challenge organisms of local origin. It should be recognized that safety and freedom from nominated adventitious agents are not synonomous. The first factor is essential, the second may be a luxury that can be postponed for vaccines for village use.

Several procedures that are used in the production of conventional vaccines might be questioned when vaccines for village chickens are being produced:

Is specific pathogen-free substrate required? Genuine specific pathogen-free flocks are not readily established in developing countries. The costs of initiation, maintenance and testing are enormous and the advantages for village-style vaccines are minimal. Some of the flocks claimed to be specific pathogen-free do not deserve that designation. Some receive live vaccines and the disease status of some is monitored only by the absence of clinical disease. Many are more realistically described as isolated flocks or minimal disease flocks. Vaccine seeds should be specific pathogen-free and production of vaccine should use a seed lot system. This will allow an eventual increase in the standards of vaccine. However, rural poultry should not at this point be deprived of vaccines because of an absence of specific pathogen-free flocks.

Is freeze-drying necessary? Most conventional attenuated vaccines produced for use in commercial poultry are lyophilized. Compared with liquid vaccines, the lyophilized product has greater stability and is more convenient to store and transport. However, freeze-drying and suitable packaging of the dried product add to the cost of a vaccine. In some developing countries, avian vaccines are produced as "wet" vaccines. This may not be a disadvantage if vaccine is to be used soon after manufacture and if local production reduces the need to transport vaccines over long distances. Nevertheless, thermostability becomes an important character of the vaccine strain.

The sophisticated packaging of conventional vaccines is not necessary for products to be used in village chickens. There are frequent calls for the production of small-dose packs because village flocks are small and the supply of vaccine in packages that contain many doses is seen to be wasteful. The conventional 1 000-dose vial is admittedly an embarrassment for the owner of a flock of 20 chickens and there is an obvious need to share vaccine among village flocks. There is also a need to develop a philosophy of overdosing, rather than discarding unused vaccine. Lentogenic Newcastle disease vaccines are not harmful to chickens when given in doses larger than those recommended by the manufacturer. The problem in villages is not the 1 000-dose content of a single vial of vaccine, rather it is that of obtaining a single vial of vaccine in systems that are designed for bulk distribution to a commercial industry.

The logistics of delivering vaccine to villages is as important a problem as developing a suitable vaccine strain. The centralized preparation of food-based vaccines and their delivery to villages are not feasible in most countries. Each chicken requires 7 tc 10 g of vaccine-coated food. In most areas, food and vaccine will need to be mixed in the villages, which will

TABLE 11

Comparison of poultry vaccine requirements for commercial and village use

	Commercial chickens	Village chickens
Place of production	Few large laboratories	Small local laboratories
Thermostability	Not essential	Very desirable
Market	International	Local
Seed material	Specific pathogen-free	Specific pathogen-free
Vaccine	Specific pathogen-free	Not necessarily specific pathogen-free
Lyophilization	Desirable	Not necessary
Efficacy	Extreme efficacy reqired	Moderate efficacy acceptable
Delivery	Individual vaccination or by aerosol, spray or drinking water	Delivery on food advantageous
Packaging units	Large dose (multidose vials)	Small-dose vials preferable

require the regular delivery of small quantities of vaccine. Recent experiments indicate that it may be possible to incorporate in a single pellet a quantity of Newcastle disease virus vaccine sufficient for a single chicken. This would help overcome the problems of central production and would ease the problem of transport.

Table 11 indicates some of the requirements that should be considered when comparing conventional vaccines and vaccines for village chickens.

BIBLIOGRAPHY

Copland, J.W., ed. 1987. *Newcastle disease in poultry. A new food pellet vaccine.* ACIAR Monograph No. 5. Canberra, Australian Centre for International Agricultural Research. 119 pp.

Spradbrow, P.B., ed. 1992. Newcastle disease in village chickens. Control with thermostable oral vaccines. In *ACIAR Proc. 39.* Canberra, Australian Centre for International Agricultural Research. 189 pp.

Spradbrow, P.B. 1993/94. Newcastle disease in village chickens. *Poultry Sci. Rev.*, 5: 57-96.

Fish vaccines

A. Adams, K.D. Thompson and R.J. Roberts[1]

With fish being the primary source of animal protein in many countries, aquaculture is growing rapidly worldwide, and stress and diseases that accompany intensive fish culture have led to treatment with antibiotics and chemicals. However, as concern over pollution associated with chemical treatments and the emergence of multiple resistance to antibiotics make the control of infections more and more difficult, the emphasis should be on disease prevention by means of optimal husbandry and biological control methods, such as vaccination and immunostimulants.

FISH DISEASES

Fish in culture suffer a variety of diseases, including bacterial, viral, parasitic and fungal infections, some of which are shown in Table 12. The majority of infections described for fish in culture are bacterial. Vibriosis, associated with a number of marine vibrios, is the most widespread worldwide and not only causes huge economic losses to the marine fish culture industry but is the main disease affecting the farming of prawns in Southeast Asia and Japan. Furunculosis, hitherto thought of as a freshwater disease of wild salmonids, is the most serious disease affecting cultured salmonids, particularly in the seawater phase. Acute furunculosis is a common problem when Atlantic salmon smolts are transferred to the sea, at which time losses of up to 30 percent of the stock may occur. The disease is often complicated by simultaneous sea lice infection and pancreatic disease. Unfortunately, once furunculosis is introduced to a site it is very difficult to eradicate and is likely to recur intermittently among the ongrowing stock. Motile aeromonads appear to be the most important bacterial pathogens of freshwater fish in tropical countries. These micro-organisms have been reported to cause mass mortality in Indian major carp and can be detected during a variety of infections, including haemorrhagic septicaemia, asymptomatic septicaemia, epizootic ulcerative disease (EUS), tail rot and fin rot.

The exact aetiology of some of the newly emerging diseases, such as EUS, have not been unequivocally determined. In the case of EUS, bacterial, viral and fungal participants are all associated with the disease complex but the principal initiating factor has yet to be determined (Roberts, Willoughby and Chinabut, 1993).

As the aquaculture industry grows and new species of fish are intensively cultured, the range of diseases and affected species is similarly expanding. For example, pasteurellosis was only recently described in Europe and rickettsiosis in Chile, Ireland and Taiwan Province of China, but now both are recognized as highly significant pathogens.

COMMERCIAL VACCINES

Of the many infectious diseases affecting fish there are to date only five for which effective commercial vaccines have been produced. Three of these are bacterial

[1] The authors wish to express their thanks to all those who provided information for this paper, in particular J. Turnbull, H. Rodger and J. McGeorge for their advice on fish diseases.

TABLE 12
Fish diseases

Disease	Causative agent	Major fish species affected	Country/region
Bacterial disease			
Enteric red mouth	*Yersinia ruckeri*	• Salmonids, primarily rainbow trout	North America, Europe, South America
Vibriosis			
- Vibriosis	*Vibrio anguillarum, V. ordalii*	• Widespread in marine fish salmonids	Worldwide, Japan, North America
- Hitra disease	*V. salmonicida*	• Atlantic salmon	Norway, Faroe Islands
Furunculosis	*Aeromonas salmonicida*	• Salmonids	Europe
Bacterial kidney disease	*Renibacterium salmoninarum*	• Salmonids	North America, Europe, Japan, Chile
Enteric septicaemia	*Edwardsiella ictaluri*	• Catfish	Southeastern United States, Canada
	E. tarda	• Eel, hirame	Japan
Motile aeromonad septicaemia	*Aeromonas hydrophila, A. caviae, A. sobria*	• Catfish, cyprinids, salmonids	Asia, Europe, United States
Pasteurellosis	*Pasteurella piscicida*	• Ayu, yellow tail, sea bream, sea bass, carp	United States, Japan, Europe, Taiwan Province of China
Bacterial cold-water disease	*L.yto psychrophilus*	• Salmonids	United States, Europe, Japan
Streptococcus infections	*Streptococcus* spp.	• Yellow tail, rainbow trout, ayu, tilapia, bass, bream	Japan, United States, Taiwan Province of China
Tuberculosis	*Mycobacterium marinum, M. fortuitum, M. chelonae*	• Snakehead, tropical aquarium fish, sea bass, wide variety of other species	Southeast Asia, Japan, Europe
Nocardiosis	*Nocardia asteroides, N. kampach*	• Tropical aquarium fish, yellow tail, rainbow trout and brook trout	Spain, Japan, Canada
Salmonid rickettsial septicaemia	*Piscirickettsia salmonis*	• Salmonids	Chile, Taiwan Province of China, Ireland
Epitheliocystis	*Chlamydia*-like organisms	• Wide variety of species	North America, Southeast Asia, Europe, South Africa
Clostridial infections	*Clostridium botulinum*	• Salmonids	Europe, United States
Columnaris disease	*Flexibacter columnaris, F. maritimus*	• All freshwater species, bream, bass, turbot, salmon	North America, Asia, Europe, Japan
Entrococcus infection	*Entrococcus serrolcida*	• Yellow tail	Japan
Bacterial gill disease	*Cytophaga* spp., *Flexibacter* spp. *Flavobacterium bronchiophilia*	• Wide variety of species	North America, Japan, Europe
Ulcerative septicaemia	*Pseudomonas* sp.	• Eels and others	Japan

(cont.)

TABLE 12 (continued)

Disease	Causative agent	Major fish species affected	Country / region
Viral diseases			
Infectious pancreatic necrosis	Birnavirus (ds RNA)	• Salmonids, sea bass, sea bream, turbot, Pacific cod	Europe
Viral haemorrhagic septicaemia	Rhabdovirus	• Salmonids	Japan, North America, Europe
Infectious haemorrhagic necrosis	Rhabdovirus	• Snakehead, carp, barbs	Japan, Taiwan Province of China, Canada, North America
Infectious salmon anaemia	Unknown (putatative virus)	• Atlantic salmon	Norway
Parasitic diseases			
Sea lice	*Lepeophtheirus salmonis*	• Marine-cultured salmonids	Northern circumpolar (Norway, Japan, Scotland, Ireland, Canada)
Proliferative kidney disease	Unidentified myxosporean extrasporgonic stage, PKX	• Freshwater salmonids	United Kingdom, Europe, United States
Costias'-	*Ichthyobodo necator*	• Freshwater, non-host-specific fingerling fish especially affected. Also a saltwater form	Worldwide, 2°-30°C
White spot	*Ichthyophthirius multifiliis*	• Freshwater, especially young fish; e.g. cyprinids, tilapiids, salmonids, Ictalurids	Worldwide, 4°-25°C
Trichodinids	*Trichodina* sp., *Tripartiella* sp. and others	• Freshwater and marine non-specific salmonids flatfish (e.g. turbot) in culture	Worldwide
Myxosporeans	A range of pathogenic species, e.g. *Myxobolus* spp., *Sphaerospora* spp., *Kudoa* spp.	• Freshwater and marine. All cultured fish	Worldwide
Microsporeans	*Pleistophora* sp., *Glugea* sp. and others	• Freshwater and marine. One reported problem in flatfish	
Fungal diseases			
Ichthyophoniasis	*Ichthyophonus* spp.	• Freshwater and marine species	Worldwide
Branchiomycosis	*Branchiomyces sanguinis, B. demigran*	• Cyprinids, eels, freshwater tench, stickleback	India, Japan, Eastern Europe
Saprolegniasis	*Saprolegnia parasitica* – diclina complex	• Cold, freshwater salmonids, catfish	Northern Europe, United States
Aspergillomycosis	*Aspergillus* spp.	• Tilapia	Worldwide
Epizootic ulcerative syndrome	Unknown (putative fungus)	• Freshwater and brackish species	Australia, Southeast Asia

diseases affecting salmonids – enteric red mouth (ERM), vibriosis and furunculosis – while the others are a bacterial disease in catfish – enteric septicaemia of catfish (ESC) and the viral infection, spring viraemia of carp (SVC), as shown in Table 13.

Fish vaccines first became available in 1976 when a commercial ERM vaccine was developed and registered in the United States (Tebbit, Erikson and Vande Water, 1981). By 1982, Busch stated that vaccination was the single most effective control for ERM. The disease is closely stress-related and the causative agent, *Yersinia ruckeri*, is an important primary pathogen for intensively cultured rainbow trout (Busch, 1982).

A commercial *Vibrio* vaccine was developed in 1980. This simple, killed whole-cell vibrio vaccine is highly effective against the marine pathogens *Vibrio anguillarum* and *Vibrio ordalii* in salmonids (Fryer, Rehovec and Garrison, 1978). The protective heat-stable lipopolysaccharide (LPS) antigens, derived from cell walls, which make the *Vibrio* vaccine so successful in salmonids have also proved effective for other farmed species, for example cod, eel, ayu (Kawai, Kusuda and Itami, 1981) with little or no modification to the vaccine's original design. More recently, with the upsurge in farming of sea bass and bream in the Mediterranean, the control of vibriosis has become important in these species too. Vaccines containing additional serotypes such as serotype III appear to be necessary for full protection (Vigneulle *et al.*, 1993). Generally, vibriosis in fish accompanies some other stress or physical trauma but some strains of *V. anguillarum* or *V. salmonicida* appear to be highly infectious primary pathogens. In Norway, where *V. salmonicida* causes Hitra disease or cold-water vibriosis, a combined vaccine is available because there is no cross-protection between the pathogens. As shown in Table 13, a triple vaccine is also available against furunculosis and the two *Vibrio* species.

Since the initial work of Duff (1942), many years of research have been dedicated to the development of a vaccine against furunculosis, the most economically important disease affecting salmonids. *Aeromonas salmonicida* is the causative agent and outbreaks of the disease are stress-associated, with high mortalities among salmon. Until recently, only limited success had been achieved with vaccination. In contrast to the early simple, killed whole-cell vaccines, the organisms for the new generation of furunculosis vaccines are cultured under iron-limited conditions which closely mimic the situation found in fish. This allows expression of the essential protective antigens, which include LPS and IROMPS (iron regulatory proteins) (Hirst and Ellis, 1994). The use of adjuvants, which enhance the immune response to the vaccine, also play an important role in the success of these vaccines while adjuvants do not appear to be necessary for the LPS-based ERM and *Vibrio* vaccines.

ESC is the major cause of mortality in farmed catfish in the southern United States and Asia. It was first identified in 1976 and is caused by the bacterium *Edwardsiella ictaluri*. The commercial vaccine available for ESC is based on a bacterin preparation and involves a two-step vaccination programme. Catfish fry (eight to ten days old) are immersed in the vaccine prior to ponding. They are then given an oral boost of vaccine 30 days before the start of the ESC season. The vaccination of fish by this method has proved effective in controlling ESC outbreaks.

The one commercial viral vaccine for SVC has been available in the Czech Republic and Slovenia since 1981 and also includes an oil-based adjuvant for administration by injection. SVC is caused

TABLE 13

Commercially available fish vaccines

Disease	Manufacturer	Country of origin	Product name/method of administration
Furunculosis	Aqua health	United Kingdom	Furogen/injection
Furunculosis	Aqua health	United Kingdom	Furogen B/immersion
Vibriosis	Aquaculture Vaccines Ltd	United Kingdom	AquaVac Vibrio/immersion
Vibriosis	Biomed Inc.	United States	Biojec 1300 injection or immersion (non-adjuvanted)
Furunculosis	Aquaculture Vaccines Ltd	United Kingdom	AquaVac Furovac-immersion/immersion
Furunculosis	Aquaculture Vaccines Ltd	United Kingdom	AquaVac Furovac-5/injection or immersion (non adjuvanted)
Furunculosis	Aquaculture Vaccines Ltd	United Kingdom	AquaVac Furovac-5/injection (oil-based adjuvant)
Furunculosis	Biomed Inc.	United States	Biojec 1500/injection
Furunculosis	Apothekernes Laboratorium	Norway	Apoject 1-Fural/injection (oil-based)
Furunculosis and cold-water vibriosis	Apothekernes Laboratorium	Norway	Apoject 2-Fural/injection (oil-based)
Furunculosis, cold-water vibriosis and vibriosis	Apothekernes Laboratorium	Norway	Apoject 3-Fural/injection (oil-based)
Cold-water vibriosis and vibriosis	Apothekernes Laboratorium	Norway	Apovax/immersion (water-based)
Furunculosis	Ewos Aqua A.S.	Norway	Lipogen Mono/injection (oil-based)
Furunculosis, cold-water vibriosis and vibriosis	Ewos Aqua A.S.	Norway	Lipogen Triple/injection (oil-based adjuvant)
Furunculosis	Ewos Aqua A.S.	Norway	Furogen/immersion (water-based)
Furunculosis	Ewos Aqua A.S.	Norway	Furogen/immersion (water-based)
Furunculosis, cold-water vibriosis and vibriosis	Ewos Aqua A.S.	Norway	Furogen B/dip (water-based)
Furunculosis	Ewos Aqua A.S.	Norway	Oravacc F Vet/Oral (water-based)
Furunculosis, cold-water vibriosis and vibriosis	Intervet Norbio A.S.	Norway	Norvax triple/injection (oil-based)
Furunculosis, cold-water vibriosis, vibriosis + infectious pancreatic necrosis	Intervet Norbio A.S.	Norway	Norvax triple + IPN/injection (oil-based)
Cold-water vibriosis and vibriosis	Intervet Norbio A.S.	Norway	Norvax vibriosis/dip (water-based)
Furunculosis, cold-water vibriosis and vibriosis	Biomed Inc.	United States	Bioject 1900/injection (oil-based adjuvant)
Enteric septicaemia of catfish	Biomed Inc.	United States	Biomed ESC/immersion (water-based)
Enteric red mouth	Biomed Inc.	United States	Bioject 1100 immersion (water-based)
Enteric red mouth	Aquaculture Vaccines Ltd	United Kingdom	Aqua Vac ERM/immersion
Enteric red mouth	Aqua health	United Kingdom	Ermogen/immersion
Spring viraemia of carp	Bioveta	Czech Republic	Injection

by *Rhabdovirus carpio* (two serotypes) and the disease is widespread in areas of carp culture.

Adjuvants

Most water-based vaccines for salmonids contain either glucan- or aluminium-based adjuvants which are partially effective and have few side-effects. The latest trend in salmonid vaccines is towards oil-based adjuvants which have been found to be more effective. These do, however, need to be injected into the fish and have many side-effects, for example suspected reduced growth rate, reduction of fertility in broodstock, reduced carcass quality owing to pigmentation at the site of injection, difficulty in administration owing to high viscosity and an increased hazard to human operators if accidentally self-injected. The use of mineral oil adjuvants has been accepted in Norway, but a licence for their use has not yet been granted in the United Kingdom.

Index of efficacy

The effectiveness of fish vaccines is calculated in terms of relative percent survival (RPS) using the following formula:

$$\mathrm{RPS} = 1 - \frac{\text{percent vaccinate mortality}}{\text{percent control mortality}} \times 100$$

Amend and Fender (1976) describe the additional considerations which need to be met.

During the development of these commercial vaccines many parameters important to the success of vaccination have been determined, for example the route of administration, the length of protection obtained, the size of the fish and the temperature dependence of the immune response (Johnson and Amend, 1983a and 1983b; Johnson, Flynn and Amend, 1982a and 1982b; Tatner and Horne, 1985).

In general, intraperitoneal injection appears to be the most effective route of vaccination, although not the most practical. Much effort is therefore being put into the development of immersion and oral vaccines.

DEVELOPMENT OF VACCINES

The primary considerations for any successful vaccine for aquaculture are cost-effectiveness and safety. To accomplish this the vaccine must provide long-term protection against the disease under the intensive rearing conditions found on commercial fish farms. Consideration must be given to all the serotypic variants of the disease agent, the time and age at which the animal is most susceptible to disease, the route of administration and the method of vaccine preparation (i.e. killed, attenuated, subunit, recombinant).

All the commercial vaccines currently available comprise *inactivated* (killed) disease agents. When that approach failed in the development of vaccines, particularly viral vaccines, live attenuated vaccines were developed.

Whenever a *live* vaccine is used there is always concern that the attenuated strain (usually the result of a gene deletion) may back-mutate and revert to the virulent wild type. Many of the successful vaccines against viral diseases of humans (e.g. rubella, measles, poliomyelitis) and in domestic animals (e.g. rabies, distemper) are attenuated organisms. The licensing of such vaccines may, however, prove to be very difficult in aquaculture. An alternative approach has been to prepare subunit vaccines using recombinant technology, where the specific components of the disease-causing agents are isolated and, following amplification, used in vaccines. To increase the amount of antigen available, amplification is acheived by cloning the genes coding for specific antigens and incorporating them into bacterial DNA, where they are expressed. Using fermentation technology for the growth of bacterial cells, expressed "foreign" proteins (antigens) can be produced in bulk.

Bacterial vaccines

Numerous fish vaccines are currently being developed, although some of them with only limited success. For example, vaccination would be an ideal approach for controlling bacterial kidney disease (BKD) because it is widespread and its control by means of chemotherapy is unsatisfactory. Experimental vaccination of coho salmon (*Oncorhynchus kisutch*) and sockeye salmon (*Oncorhynchus nerka*) indicated that agglutinating antibodies were produced but the response was slow to develop and these antibodies were not protective (Evelyn, 1971; Evelyn, Ketcheson and Prosperi-Porta, 1984; Baudin-Laurencin, Vigneulle and Mevel, 1977). Kaattari *et al.* (1987 and 1988) investigated potential BKD vaccines containing the highly immunogenic *Vibrio* vaccine components as an adjuvant; however, the results were inconsistent. Paterson, Desautels and Weber (1981) and McCarthy, Croy and Amend (1984) achieved the most promising results in Atlantic salmon and rainbow trout, where protection was conferred against a natural challenge and experimental challenge, respectively. One vaccine was adjuvanted with Freund's complete adjuvant while the other was pH-lyzed and non-adjuvanted. Other researchers (Bruno and Munro, 1984; Sakai, Atsuta and Kobayashi, 1993) have been unable to reproduce these results, and so the search for a BKD vaccine continues. The preparations tested so far appear to be inadequate. This may be because they contain inappropriate antigens and, whichever protective antigens are present, are only weakly immunogenic or responses to them are suppressed by other antigens.

It has been reported that certain components of the extracellular proteins (ECP) from *Renibacterium salmoninarum*, for example the 57 kDa protein, are immunosuppressive (Turaga, Wiens and Kaattari, 1987). These antigens must therefore be omitted (or modified) from any successful vaccine preparation. Hastings and Ellis (1988) showed that rainbow trout only responded to five out of 30 ECP components from *A. salmonicida*, while rabbits responded to 15. Thus, it is important to establish which antigens the fish respond to and whether these are protective. Current research in the United Kingdom and Canada is based on the purification of antigens from *R. salmoninarum* and its extracellular products, and includes investigation into their effects on the immune system prior to their incorporation into a recombinant vaccine.

The other vaccines currently being developed against bacterial fish pathogens include atypical *A. salmonicida*, *A. hydrophila*, *Edwardsiella ictaluri*, *Flexibacter columnaris*, *Streptococcus* sp. and *Pasteurella piscicida*.

Atypical furunculosis (caused by atypical non-pigmented *A. salmonicida*) is the main bacterial disease affecting Icelandic fish farming. An experimental vaccine given by injection has been developed (B. Gudmundsdottir, personal communication). The protective antigen was identified by passive immunization of Atlantic salmon with antisera against purified antigen raised in rainbow trout and rabbits. A method to culture the bacterium with the maximal expression of protective antigen has also been developed. The vaccine results in 70 to 100 percent RPS when administered with mineral oil as an adjuvant to Atlantic salmon parr. Protection appears to last for 12 months and there is a good correlation between antibody production and protection. Field trials have not yet been completed.

The antigenic diversity of *A. hydrophila* is the major limitation in the development of an effective vaccine and it seems likely that a polyvalent preparation will be necessary. Although there is some doubt as to whether these bacteria ever act as a primary pathogen, they do make a significant contribution to the disease process in the fish they invade. As part of the development of a vaccine, research groups in Southeast Asia are currently investigating the immune response of carp and catfish to *A. hydrophila* antigens.

Moore, Eimers and Cardell (1990) demonstrated the feasibility of immunizing channel catfish against columnaris disease by immersion vaccination with formalin-inactivated *Flexibacter columnaris*. However, a commercial vaccine has not yet been developed.

Streptococcal and *Pasteurella* spp. infections, hitherto reported principally in Japanese marine cultured fish populations, have recently become a problem in Mediterranean countries. The Japanese researchers Iida, Wakabayashi and Egusa (1982) and Sakai *et al.* (1987) reported that experimental vaccination provided protection from streptococcal infections, but a commercial vaccine is not yet available. There appear to be two serotypes. A cocktail immersion vaccine to prevent *Streptococcus* sp. and *V. anguillarum* is currently being tested in Japan and field trials are also being carried out in Italy (Ghittino, personal communication) on a potential *Streptococcus* vaccine.

Pasteurellosis has been of huge economic significance to yellow tail culture in Japan and, in 1991, was almost simultaneously reported as affecting sea bream in Italy, France and Greece. There appears to be homogeneity within this species of bacterium, although little has been published on its virulence factors and protective antigens. A *Pasteurella* vaccine is currently being field tested and researchers in Japan, the United Kingdom and Italy are continuing with development work to determine an immune response to the bacterium and investigate the pathogenesis of the disease.

Viral vaccines

The development of a successful vaccine by culturing the causative agent under defined conditions and subsequently inactivating it is not always feasible. It may be necessary to select protective antigens and engineer a recombinant vaccine genetically. This appears to be the case for most fish viral vaccines under development and requires the molecular cloning and expression of the viral genes in the bacterium *Escherichia coli* or the yeast, *Saccharomyces cerevisae.*

Viral haemorrhagic septicaemia (VHS) is a fish rhabdovirus responsible for severe losses in many continental European trout farms. It is an economically devastating disease for the aquaculture industry, since it may affect all age groups. In the past, inactivated vaccines have been developed; however, these were immunogenic only when given by injection (de Kinkelin, 1988). Following the failure of inactivated vaccines, several live vaccines were developed and appeared to provide protection against some of the serotypes. The vaccine strains were attenuated by successive passage in cell lines, but significant mortality associated with the virus was still observed and 2 to 13 percent of the fish died as a result of the vaccination alone (de Kinkelin and Bearzotti-Le Berre, 1981; Bernard, de Kinkelin and Bearzotti-Le Berre, 1983).

More recently, a subunit vaccine for VHS has been developed using recombinant DNA technology. The protective epitopes of VHS appear to be located on the surface glycoprotein of the virus, and antibody directed against the viral glycoprotein-neutralized viral infectivity (de Kinkelin,

Bernard and Hattenberger-Baudovy, 1984; Lorenzen, Oleson and Vestergaard-Jørgensen, 1990). The gene coding for the VHS glycoprotein was cloned and expressed in bacteria (Thiery *et al.*, 1990) and yeast (Lorenzen, 1991) to produce the glycoprotein inexpensively and in large quantities. Preliminary results indicate that this material induced protection following injection but no studies on immersion vaccination have been reported (Jørgensen, 1992). Thus, for VHS, a recombinant subunit vaccine may be a promising way of producing an inexpensive safe vaccine in fish.

Recent results obtained by Lecoq-Xhonneux *et al.* (1993), however, suggest that further research is needed prior to commercial exploitation, since the yield of antigens expressed was low and there was a problem with the route of delivery of the vaccine (i.e. it is only effective when introduced intraperitoneally, not orally).

Several research groups are actively developing vaccines for infectious pancreatic necrosis virus (IPN). This is a very important pathogen of farm-reared salmonids. Mortality is highest in young fish and survivors become life-long carriers, thereby maintaining the virus in the population by the continual shedding and transmission of the disease. The virus is serotypically heterogenous and has two major serotypes, the first of which comprises nine subtypes which are all pathogenic for salmonid fish.

Several inactivated IPN vaccines have been tested but only vaccine administered by injection-induced protection. The preferred route of immersion (since infected fish are usually small) was ineffective (Dorson, 1977). This was also found when individual virion polypeptides were tested. The virion proteins appeared to have lost their antigenicity following disruption with sodium dodecyl sulphate, urea and acetic acid (Hill, Dorson and Dixon, 1980).

Studies by Bootland, Dobos and Stevenson (1990) suggest that the age and size of the fish at the time of immunization are important factors in the development of protective immunity. They reported that only fry immunized at two to three weeks after hatching were protected. It appears that very young fish are capable of responding to vaccination but that growth rates must also be considered. These fish responded while in a slow weight-gaining phase.

Two attenuated IPN vaccines have also been tested and these appear to have provided protection when applied by immersion (Dorson, Castric and Torchy, 1978; McAllister, 1984). Further development was not pursued. Instead, as with other viral vaccines, many researchers are following the route of recombinant subunit vaccines for IPN (Havarstein *et al.*, 1990; Lawrence *et al.*, 1989; Hah, Park and Jeong, 1992). In these studies, the major capsid protein VP2 has been identified as the virion protein responsible for inducing protective immunity in fish.

The drawbacks of killed and attenuated vaccines (Leong, Fryer and Winton, 1988) have led research efforts to develop an effective subunit vaccine for infectious haematopoietic necrosis (IHN) virus (Leong *et al.*, 1992). During these studies, monoclonal antibodies to the virion proteins were produced, enabling characterization of the fish immune response to viral antigens and the development of *in situ* hybridization probes to detect the virus in vaccines. IHN is caused by a rhabdovirus and produces a severe disease among fry and juveniles of susceptible species of salmonid fish. Engelking and Leong (1989) demonstrated that the viral glycoprotein purified from one isolate could induce protective immunity in fish to a wide variety of IHN virus isolates from different geographical locations and different fish species. In consequence, the viral glycoprotein gene from one strain was cloned and a recombinant vaccine prepared. Further studies have identified a specific immunodominant region in the middle of the gene (Xu *et al.*, 1991; Mourich and Leong, 1991). A field trial (immersion immunization) of the IHN subunit vaccine was undertaken in Idaho, United States, and showed it to be very effective in inducing protective immunity. A commercial vaccine, however is not currently available.

Two other viral vaccines currently under development for non-salmonid species are those for SVC and channel catfish virus (CCV). Despite a commercial inactivated SVC vaccine being available in the Czech Republic and Slovenia, attenuated vaccines have also been developed (Fijan *et al.*, 1977) and appear to offer protection. However, although the live vaccine in particular provided excellent protection, the vaccinated fish appeared to become asymptomatic carriers of the virus. When these fish were reared beside unvaccinated stock, an SVC outbreak occurred. A subunit vaccine is therefore an attractive alternative. A reliable challenge model for the disease also needs to be developed so that vaccine potency testing can be performed under standard conditions.

CCV, caused by *Herpesvirus ictaluri*, is an acute, highly infectious disease of juvenile channel catfish (*Ictalurus punctatus*). The onset of the disease is sudden and 100 percent mortality can occur within ten days. Once fish are infected with the virus, survivors become carriers for their entire lives. At present, CCV outbreaks are prevented by management strategies such as the use of resistant strains of channel catfish and virus-free broodstock for the stocking of fish farms. Vaccination would seem to be the ideal strategy in areas where CCV is endemic. An attenuated live vaccine was developed by serial passage in a tissue culture cell line derived from the walking catfish (Noga and Hartman, 1981). This was protective both by injection and immersion. Booster vaccination appeared to increase the efficacy of the vaccine greatly (Walczak, Noga and Hartman, 1981). This vaccine is not available commercially and has not been licensed, probably because of concerns regarding the risk of reversion to virulence and the possible establishment of carriers among vaccinated fish. If carrier fish are generated as a result of vaccination, these fish can no longer be certified as virus-free broodstock. Attempts to develop a killed CCV vaccine have been hindered by its poor immunogenicity (Plumb, 1973). A subunit vaccine for CCV was recently developed (Awad, Nusbaum and Brady, 1989). The envelope components of the virus appear to be capable of inducing protective immunity and, once these have been determined more specifically, an effective recombinant vaccine may be possible.

Parasitic vaccines

Monoclonal antibody (MAb) probes are proving to be useful tools in the development of vaccines against sea lice (*Lepeophtheirus salmonis*) and the protozoan infection proliferative kidney disease (PKD) in salmonids. A vaccine against sea lice remains a high priority for the aquaculture industry. Monoclonal antibodies were used to produce extracts from lice and to select individual antigens from a sea louse recombinant DNA library (Andrade-Salas *et al.*, 1993). These clones form the basis of experimental vaccines which are currently under investigation in the United Kingdom.

PKD is the most economically damaging disease affecting the trout industry in Europe. MAb probes have been produced against PKX, the causative agent, in an effort to map out the antigens on the parasite's surface (Adams, Richards and Marin de Mateo, 1992) and have shown that PKX from different species of fish and different geographical locations share common antigens (Marin de Mateo *et al.*, 1993). At present, studies are under way to culture the parasite and investigate protective antigens.

A successful parasite vaccine has been described by Woo and Li (1990) working in Canada. Live attenuated *Cryptobia salmositica*, a pathogenic haemoflagellate causing cryptobiosis, was injected intraperitoneally into rainbow trout but the strategy for the delivery of the vaccine has still to be resolved.

Numerous other parasites cause significant losses to the aquaculture industry, for example *Icthyobodo necatrix*, *Ichthyopthirius multifiliis* and *Trichodina* sp., but their control by vaccination has not yet been attempted.

Future prospects

Fish vaccines have become much more sophisticated in recent years, with the trend being for the development of subunit recombinant vaccines in preference to the original killed whole-cell preparations. This has been necessary because the simpler approach did not succeed for many of the important diseases and attempts at attenuated vaccines in general have not been encouraging from a safety point of view. The cost of producing such "high-tech" vaccines must however be considered and the costs and benefits weighed up prior to commercialization.

Direct DNA vaccination has recently been successfully performed in cattle against infectious bovine rhinotracheitis virus (Cox, Zamb and Basiuk, 1993). Muscles can apparently take in naked DNA and then express it for long periods (Wolff *et al.*, 1992). DNA vaccination may prove to be a more cost-effective method of vaccinating fish against viral infections in the future.

As the range of cultured species increases, there is also a need for basic research on the immune responses of new species as well as for studies on genetically resistant species in parallel with vaccine development.

Immunostimulants. An approach recently taken by the aquaculture industry is the use of immunostimulants, either by themselves to counteract stress-induced immunosuppression in fish, or in vaccines as adjuvants. They may serve to boost the immune system in the short term and therefore have great potential. One group receiving a great deal of attention at present is the β-glucans. They apparently function as immunostimulants of the non-specific defence mechanism of fish (Robertsen, Engstad and Jørgensen, 1994).

Glucans are major structural polysaccharides from fungal and yeast cell walls, composed of glucose units which are held together through β-1,3 and β-1,6 bonds (Rosenberg, 1976; Duffus, Levi and Manners, 1982). Both soluble β-glucans (e.g. scleroglucan, schizophyllan and lentinan) and microparticulated β-glucans from yeast (M-Glucan, Macroguard®) have been shown to function as immunostimulators in fish (Robertsen, Engstad and Jørgensen, 1994). Intraperitoneal injections of glucans have resulted in enhanced disease protection of carp to *Edwardsiella tarda* infection (Yano, Mangindaan and Matsuyama, 1989; Yano, Matsuyama and Mangindaan, 1991) and yellow tail to *Streptococcus* spp. (Matsuyama, Mangindaan and Yano, 1992). Yeast glucan has been found to increase disease resistance in Atlantic salmon to *Vibrio anguillarum*, *V. salmonicida*, *Yersinia ruckeri* and *Aeromonas salmonicida* (Robertsen *et al.*, 1990; Robertsen, Engstad and Jørgensen, 1994) and in channel catfish to *Edwardsiella ictaluri* (Chen and Ainsworth, 1992).

The exact mode of action of glucans remains unclear, but enhanced protection against microbial pathogens, observed after administering glucans to fish, correlates with increased blood lysozyme and complement activities and enhanced phagocytosis and killing of bacteria by headkidney macrophages (Yano, Mangindaan and Matsuyama, 1989; Engstad, Robertsen and Frivold, 1992; Chen and Ainsworth, 1992; Matsuyama, Mangindaan and Yano, 1992; Jørgensen *et al.*, 1993). It is believed that such macrophages may have an essential role to play in immunostimulation, since it has been shown that Atlantic salmon macrophages possess receptors for β-glucan (Robertsen, Engstad and Jørgensen, 1994).

Robertsen, Engstad and Jørgensen (1994) suggested that non-specific defence may be more effective against opportunistic pathogens than specific bacteria. Glucans, therefore, probably benefit most during stress-related conditions, such as handling, transportation or smoltification, when an increased susceptibility to disease occurs. Glucan-supplemented diets and furunculosis vaccines are now commercially available. However, the dose, the type of glucan and the route of administration must all be considered when examining the effects of glucans on disease resistance (Ainsworth, Mao and Boyle, 1994). Further studies are required to standardize these parameters.

BIBLIOGRAPHY

Adams, A., Richards, R.H. & Marin de Mateo, M. 1992. Development of monoclonal antibodies to PKX, the causative agent of proliferative kidney disease. *J. Fish Dis.*, 15: 515-520.

Ainsworth, A.J., Mao, C.P. & Boyle, C.R. 1994. Immune response enhancement in channel catfish, *Ictalurus punctatus*, using β-glucan from *Schizophyllum commune*. *In* J.S. Stolen & T.C. Fletcher, eds. *Modulators of fish immune responses*, Vol. 1, p. 67-81. Fair Haven, N.J., USA, SOS Publications.

Amend, D.F. & Fender, D.C. 1976. Uptake of bovine serum albumin by rainbow trout from hyperosmotic solution: a model for vaccinating fish. *Science*, 192: 793-794.

Andrade-Salas, O., Sommerville, C., Wootten, R., Turnbull, T., Melvin, W., Amezaga, T. & Labus, M. 1993. Immunohistochemical screening and selection of monoclonal antibodies to salmon louse, *Lepeophtheirus salmonis* (Krøyer, 1837). *In* E. Boxshall & D. Defaye, eds. *Pathogens of wild farmed fish: sealice*, p. 323-331. Chichester, UK, Horwood (Ellis).

Awad, M.A., Nusbaum, K.E. & Brady, Y.J. 1989. Preliminary studies of a newly developed subunit vaccine for channel catfish disease. *J. Aquat. Anim. Health*, 1: 233-237.

Baudin-Laurencin, F., Vigneulle, M. & Mevel, M. 1977. Premières observations sur la corynebactériose des salmonides en Bretagne. *Bull. Off. int. Epiz.*, 87: 505-507.

Bernard, J., de Kinkelin, P. & Bearzotti-Le Berre, M. 1983. Viral haemorrhagic septicaemia of trout: relation between the G polypeptide, antibody production and protection of the fish following infection with the F25 attenuated variant strain. *Infect. Immun.*, 39: 7-14.

Bootland, L.M., Dobos, P. & Stevenson, R.M.W. 1990. Fry age and size effects on immersion immunization of brook trout, *Salvelinus fontalis* Michelle, against infectious pancreatic necrosis virus. *J. Fish Dis.*, 13: 113-125.

Bruno, D.W. & Munro, A.L.S. 1984. Epidemiological studies of bacterial kidney disease in Scotland. In *Int. Sem. Fish Pathology for the 20th Anniversary of the Japanese Society of Fish Pathology*, p. 57-58. Tokyo.

Busch, R.A. 1982. Enteric redmouth disease (*Yersinia ruckeri*). *In* D.P. Anderson, M. Dorson & P. Dubourget, eds. *Antigens* *of fish pathogens*, p. 201-223. Lyon, France, Marcel Merieux.

Chen, D. & Ainsworth, A.J. 1992. Glucan administration potentiates immune defence mechanisms of channel catfish, *Ictalurus punctatus*. *J. Fish Dis.*, 15: 295-304.

Cox, G.J.M., Zamb, T.J. & Basiuk, L.A. 1993. Bovine herpes virus I: immune responses in mice and cattle injected with plasmid DNA. *J. Virol.*, 67(9): 5664-5667.

de Kinkelin, P. 1988. Vaccination against viral haemorrhagic septicaemia. *In* A.E. Ellis, ed. *Fish vaccination*, p. 172-192. London, Academic

de Kinkelin, P. & Bearzotti-Le Berre, M. 1981. Immunization of rainbow trout against viral haemorrhagic septicaemia (VHS) with a thermoresistant variant of the virus. *Dev. Biol. Stand.*, 49: 431-439.

de Kinkelin, P., Bernard, J. & Hattenberger-Baudovy, A.M. 1984. *Immunization against viral diseases occurring in cold water. Symposium on Fish Vaccination*. Paris, Office International des Epizooties.

Dorson, M. 1977. Vaccination trials of rainbow trout fry against infectious pancreatic necrosis. *Bull. Off. int. Epiz.*, 57: 405-406.

Dorson, M., Castric, J. & Torchy, C. 1978. Infectious pancreatic necrosis virus of salmonids: biological and antigenic features of a pathogenic strain and a non-pathogenic variant selected in RTG-2 cells. *J. Fish Dis.*, 1: 309-320.

Duff, D.C.B. 1942. The oral immunisation of trout against *Bacterium salmonicida*. *J. Immunol.*, 44: 87-94.

Duffus, I.H., Levi, C. & Manners, D.J. 1982. Yeast cell-wall glucans. *Adv. Microbiol. Physiol.*, 23: 151-181.

Engelking, H.M. & Leong, J.C. 1989. The glycoprotein of infectious hematopoietic necrosis virus elecit neutralizing antibody and protective responses. *Virus Res.*, 13: 213-230.

Engstad, R.E., Robertsen, B. & Frivold, E. 1992. Yeast glucan induces increase in lysozyme and complement-mediated haemolytic activity in Atlantic salmon blood. *Fish Shellfish Immunol.*, 2: 287-297.

Evelyn, T.P.T. 1971. The agglutinin response in sockeye salmon vaccinated intraperitoneally with a heat-killed preparation of the bacteria responsible for salmonid kidney disease. *J. Wildl. Dis.*, 7: 328-335.

Evelyn, T.P.T., Ketcheson, J.E. & Prosperi-Porta, L. 1984. On the feasibility of vaccination as a means of controlling bacterial kidney disease in Pacific salmon. In *Abstr.: Int. Conf. Biology of Pacific Salmon*, 5-12 September 1984. Victoria / Agassiz, British Columbia, Canada.

Fijan, N., Petrinec, Z., Stanel, Z., Kezic, N. & Teskeredzic, E. 1977. Vaccination of carp against spring viraemia. Comparison of intraperitoneal and peroral application of live virus to fish kept in ponds. *Bull. Off. int. Epiz.*, 92: 1055-1068.

Fryer, J.L., Rehovec, J.S. & Garrison, R.L. 1978. Immunisation of salmonids for control of vibriosis. *Mar. Fish. Rev.*, 40: 20-23.

Hah, Y.C., Park, J.W. & Jeong, G. 1992. Neutralize epitope of DRT serotype of infectious pancreatic necrosis virus (IPNV) isolated in Korea. In *Proc. Int. Symp. Infectious Viruses in Fish*, 9-11 October 1992, p. 13-22. Seoul.

Hastings, T.S. & Ellis, A.E. 1988. The humoral immune response of rainbow trout and rabbits to *Aeromonas salmonicida* extracellular products. *J. Fish Dis.*, 11: 147-160.

Harvarstein, L.S., Kalland, K.H., Christie, K.E. & Endressen, C. 1990. Sequence of the large double-stranded RNA segment of the NI strain of infectious pancreas necrosis virus: a comparison without Birnaviridae. *J. Gen. Virol.*, 71: 299-308.

Hill, B., Dorson, M. & Dixon, P.F. 1980. Studies on immunization of trout against IPN. *In* W. Ahne, ed. *Fish diseases.* Third COPRAQ-Session, p. 29-36. Berlin, Springer.

Hirst, I.D. & Ellis, A.E. 1994. Iron-regulated outer membrane protein of *Aeromonas salmonicida* are important protective antigens in Atlantic salmon against furunculosis. *Fish Shellfish Immunol.*, 4(1): 29-46.

Iida, T., Wakabayashi, H. & Egusa, S. 1982. Vaccination for control of streptococcal disease in cultured yellowtail. *Fish Pathol.*, 16: 201-206.

Johnson, K.A. & Amend, D.F. 1983a. Efficacy of *Vibrio anguillarum* and *Yersinia ruckeri* bacterins applied by oral and anal intubation of salmonids. *J. Fish Dis.*, 6: 473-476.

Johnson, K.A. & Amend, D.F. 1983b. Comparison of efficacy of several delivery methods using *Yersinia ruckeri* bacterins on rainbow trout, *Salmo gairdneri* Richardson. *J. Fish Dis.*, 6: 331-336.

Johnson, K.A., Flynn, J.K. & Amend, D.F. 1982a. Duration of immunity in salmonids vaccinated by direct immersion with *Yersinia ruckeri* and *Vibrio anguillarum*. *J. Fish Dis.*, 5: 207-213.

Johnson, K.A., Flynn, J.K. & Amend, D.F. 1982b. Onset of immunity in salmonid fry vaccinated by direct immersion in *Vibrio anguillarum* and *Yersinia ruckeri*. *J. Fish Dis.*, 5: 197-205.

Jørgensen, P.E. 1992. Recent advances in surveillance and control of viral haemorrhagic septicaemia (VHS) in trout. *In* T. Kimura, ed. *Proc. OJI Int. Symp. Salmonid Diseases*, p. 60-71. Sapporo, Japan, Hokkaido University Press.

Jørgensen, J.B., Sharp, G.J.E., Secombes, C.J. & Robertsen, B. 1993. Effects of a yeast cell wall glucan on the bactericidal activity of rainbow trout macrophages. *Fish Shellfish Immunol.*, 3(4): 267-277.

Kaattari, S.L., Holland, N., Turaga, P. & Wiens, G. 1987. Development of a vaccine for bacterial kidney disease. Bonneville Power Administration Project 86-45. In *Annual Report 1986*. Portland, Oreg., USA, Bonneville Power Administration.

Kaattari, S.L., Chen, D., Turaga, P. & Wens, G. 1988. Development of a vaccine for bacterial kidney disease. Bonneville Power Administration Project 86-46. In *Annual Report 1987*. Portland, Oreg., USA, Bonneville Power Administration.

Karunasagar, I., Rosalind, G. & Karunasagar, I. 1991. Immunological response of the Indian major carps to *Aeromonas hydrophila* vaccine. *J. Fish Dis.*, 14: 413-417.

Kawai, K., Kusuda, R. & Itami, T. 1981. Mechanisms of protection in ayu orally vaccinated for vibriosis. *Fish Pathol.*, 15: 257-262.

Lawrence, W.R., Nagy, E., Duncan, R., Krell, P. & Dobos, P. 1989. Expression in *E. coli* of the major outer capsid protein of infectious pancreatic necrosis virus. *Gene*, 79: 369-374.

Lecoq-Xhonneux, F., Thiery, M., Dheur, I. & de Kinkelin, P. 1993. A recombinant viral haemorrhagic septicaemia virus (VHS) glycoprotein expressed in insect cells induces protective immunity in rainbow trout. Paper presented at European Association of Fish Pathologists 6th Int. Conf., Diseases of Fish and Shellfish, Brest, France.

Leong, J.C. & Fryer, J.L. 1993. Viral vaccines for aquaculture. *Ann. Rev. Fish Dis.*, p. 225-240.

Leong, J.C., Fryer, J.L. & Winton, J.R. 1988. Vaccination against infectious hemopoietic necrosis virus. *In* A.E. Ellis, ed. *Fish vaccination*, p. 193-202. London, Academic.

Leong, J.C., Anderson, E., Bootland, L., Chen, L., Drolet, B., Engelking, H.M., Mason, C., Mourich, D., Johnson, K., Trobridge, C. & Wirkkula, J. 1992. Biotechnological approaches to the development of salmonid fish vaccines. *In* T. Kimura, ed. *Proc. OJI Int. Symp. Salmonid Diseases,* p. 250-255. Sapporo, Japan, Hokkaido University Press.

Lorenzen, N. 1991. Viral haemorrhagic septicaemia virus of rainbow trout: immunological investigations in relation to vaccine development. University of Copenhagen. (Ph.D. thesis)

Lorenzen, N., Oleson, J.F. & Vestergaard-Jørgensen, P.E. 1990. Neutralisation of Egtved virus pathogenicity to cell cultures and in fish by monoclonal antibodies to the viral G protein. *J. Gen. Virol.,* 71: 561-567.

Marin de Mateo, M., Adams, A., Richards, R.H., Castagnaro, M. & Hedrick, R.P. 1993. Monoclonal antibody and lectin probes recognise developmental and sporogonic stages of PKX, the causative agent of proliferative kidney disease in European and North American salmonid fish. *Dis. Aquat. Organ.,* 15: 23-29.

Matsuyama, H., Mangindaan, R.E.P. & Yano, T. 1992. Protective effects of shizophyllan and scleroglucan against *Streptococcus* sp. infection in yellow tail (*Seriola quinqueradiata*). *Aquaculture,* 101: 197-203.

McAllister, P.E. 1984. Infectious pancreatic necrosis immunisation. (American Fisheries Society) *Fish Health Newsl.,* 12: 6.

McCarthy, D.H., Croy, T.R. & Amend, D.F. 1984. Immunisation of rainbow trout, *Salmo gairdneri* Richardson, against bacterial kidney disease: preliminary efficacy evaluation. *J. Fish Dis.,* 7: 65-71.

Moore, A.A., Eimers, M.E. & Cardell, M.A. 1990. Attempts to control *Flexibacter columnaris* epizootics in pond-reared channel catfish by vaccination. *J. Aquat. Anim. Health,* 2: 109-111.

Mourich, D.V. & Leong, J.C. 1991. Mapping of the immunogenic regions of the IHNV glycoprotein in rainbow trout and mice. In *Proc. 2nd Int. Symp. on Viruses of Lower Vertebrates,* p. 93-100. Corvallis, Oreg., USA,

Noga, E.J. & Hartman, J.X. 1981. Establishment of walking catfish (*Clarias batrachus*) cell lines and development of a channel catfish (*Ictalarus punctatus*) virus vaccine. *Cana. J. Fish. Aquat. Sci.,* 38: 925-930.

Paterson, W.D., Desautels, D. & Weber, J.M. 1981. The immune response of Atlantic salmon, *Salmo salar* L., to the causative agent of bacterial kidney disease, *Renibacterium salmoninarum. J. Fish Dis.,* 4: 99-111.

Plumb, J.A. 1973. Neutralisation of channel catfish virus by serum of channel catfish. *J. Wildl. Dis.,* 9: 324-330.

Roberts, R.J., Willoughby, L.G. & Chinabut, S. 1993. Mycotic aspects of epizootic ulcerative syndrome (EUS) of Asian fishes. *J. Fish Dis.,* 16: 169-183.

Robertsen, B., Engstad, R. & Jørgensen, J.B. 1994. β-glucans as immunostimulants in fish. *In* J.S. Stolen & T.C. Fletcher, eds. *Modulators of fish immune responses,* Vol. 1, p. 83-99. Fair Haven, N.J., USA, SOS Publications.

Robertsen, B., Rørstad, G., Engstad, R. & Raa, J. 1990. Enhancement of non-specific disease resistance in Atlantic salmon, *Salmo salar* L., by a glucan from *Saacharomyces cervisae* cell walls. *J. Fish Dis.,* 13: 391-400.

Rosenberg, R.F. 1976. The cell wall. *In* J.E. Smith & D.R. Barry, eds. *The filamentous fungi, Vol 2, Biosynthesis and metabolism,* p. 328-334. London, Arnold (Edward).

Sakai, M., Atsuta, S. & Kobayashi, M. 1993. The immune response of rainbow trout (*Oncorhynchus mykiss*) injected with five *Renibacterium salmoninarum* bacterins. *Aquaculture,* 113: 11-18.

Sakai, M., Kubota, R., Atsuta, S. & Kobayashi, M. 1987. Vaccination of rainbow trout *Salmo gairdneri* against beta-hemolytic streptococcal disease. *Nippon Suisan Gakkaishi,* 53: 1373-1376.

Tatner, M.F. & Horne, M.T. 1985. The effects of vaccine dilution length of immersion time and booster vaccinations on the protection levels induced by direct immersion, vaccination of brown trout, *Salmo trutta*, with *Yersinia ruckeri* (ERM) vaccine. *Aquaculture*, 46: 11-18.

Tebbit, G.L., Erikson, J.D. & Vande Water, R.B. 1981. Development and use of *Yersinia ruckeri* bacterins to control enteric redmouth disease. *In* W.V. Leetown, ed. *International Symposium on Fish Biologies: Serodiagnostics and Vaccines. Dev. Biol. Stand.*, 49: 395-401.

Thiery, M., Lecoq-Xhonneux, F., Dheur, I., Renard, A. & de Kinkelin, P. 1990. Molecular cloning of the mRNA coding for the G protein of the viral haemorrhagic septicaemia (VHS) of salmonids. *Vet. Microbioassay*, 23: 221-226.

Turaga, P., Wiens, G. & Kaattari, S.L. 1987. Bacterial kidney disease: the potential role of soluble protein antigen(s). *J. Fish Biol.*, 31(supplement A):191-194.

Vigneulle, M., Brevil, G., Ceschia, G. & Blanch, A. 1993. Vaccination trials of sea bass (*Dicentrarchus labrax*) against two serotypes of *Vibrio anguillarum*. European Association of Fish Pathologists 6th Int. Conf., Diseases of Fish and Shellfish, Brest, France, Abstract No. 66.

Walczak, E.M., Noga, E.J. & Hartman, J.X. 1981. Properties of a vaccine for channel catfish virus disease and a method of administration. *Dev. Biol. Stand.*, 49: 419-429.

Wolff, A., Ludtke, J.J., Acsadi, G., Williams, P. & Jani, A. 1992. *Hum. Mol. Genet.*, 1: 363-369.

Woo, P.T.K. & Li, S. 1990. *In vitro* attenuation of *Cryptobia salmositica* and its use as a live vaccine against crytobiosis in *Oncorhynchus mykiss*. *J. Parasitol.*, 76: 752-755.

Yano, T., Mangindaan, R.E.P. & Matsuyama, H. 1989. Enhancement of the resistance of carp *Cyprinus carpio* to experimental *Edwardsiella tarda* infection, by some β-1,3 glucans. *Nippon Suisan Gakkaishi*, 55: 1815-1819.

Yano, T., Matsuyama, H. & Mangindaan, R.E.P. 1991. Polysaccharide-induced protection of carp, *Cyprinus carpio* L., against bacterial infection. *J. Fish Dis.*, 14: 577-582.

Xu, L., Mourich, D.V., Engelking, H.M., Ristou, S., Arnzen, J. & Leong, J.C. 1991. Epitope mapping and characterization of the infectious hematopoietic necrosis virus glycoprotein, using fusion proteins synthesized in *Escherichia coli*. *J. Virol.*, 65: 1611-1615.

Role of the Office international des Epizooties and international organizations in vaccine quality standardization

M. Truszczynski and J. Blancou

Harmonization and standardization of requirements for veterinary vaccines have two important goals:

- to keep the quality of vaccines at a high level;
- to prevent or reduce potential trade barriers.

Specialized groups established by governments or groups of governments, such as the European Union (EU), formulate legislation and requirements on the basis of the latest technology to ensure the high quality and safety of these products.

Every new vaccine developed in a country or imported from another has to be registered according to the legislation and requirements in force in the country where the vaccine will be used.

The registration file must report on the results of experiments directly related to the product itself (Pensaert, 1992) and include:

- an analytical section, characterizing the different components and the substrates on which the antigens are produced;
- a toxico-pharmacological note, indicating the absence of remaining pathogenicity or abnormal toxicity;
- a section on the product's efficacy, describing clinically oriented experiments with relation to immunity and protection (degree, duration, etc.).

The analytical section should include the controls which have been carried out both on the product during manufacturing and on the final product. These controls are performed in the producers' laboratory or in a laboratory of their choice.

The registration files are examined by experts appointed by the ministry of health and, particularly, the national commission for veterinary drugs. The expert who examines the analytical section may require additional controls if those described in the original file are incomplete. These additional controls may have to be carried out in an officially accepted laboratory, for instance if the vaccine originates from a country for which there is little information on the quality of the local control system.

When the registration data are adequate, the commission for veterinary drugs gives a favourable assessment to the minister of health and the product is registered for marketing.

After registration, every production batch of the registered vaccine must be controlled by the producer, both during manufacturing and at the final product stage, and these controls are the responsibility of an industrial specialist. Further official controls are not required for the majority of bacterial vaccines although, in many cases, the bacterial strain used in the vaccine is controlled annually by the appropriate government institute. However, all viral vaccines and also some bacterial vaccines (e.g. for brucellosis) must undergo an official batch control by the national veterinary institute or an equivalent institution before release. Every imported vaccine must undergo an official batch control in an officially accepted laboratory chosen freely by the importer. Additionally, a control is prescribed by the national veterinary institute.

For batch controls, representative samples are collected under the responsibility of the laboratory and according to information supplied by the producer with regard to the number of doses per batch, the homogeneity of the batch, conditions of storage, etc.

In the laboratory, the samples are examined to identify the active component(s), to ascertain the absence of contaminating agents and to ensure the product's sterility, safety and potency. For these controls, the relevant monograph of the European Pharmacopoeia (see p. 149) is followed. If there is no monograph for a particular vaccine, the tests described in the original registration file must be applied. For inactivated vaccines, the potency test may be performed on the target species or on a laboratory animal species but, in the latter case, the relation between the potency in the laboratory and that in the target species must be demonstrated by the producer. For live vaccines, potency is generally limited to quantitation of the organism or of the virus, using methods described in the original registration file. If the results are satisfactory, the batch will be given an official batch number and be released on to the market.

Depending on the country or group of countries, there are varying degrees of difference in their legislation. With this in mind and in the spirit of international harmonization aimed at reducing or preventing potential trade barriers, the United States Animal Health Institute (AHI) has proposed the formation of an international working group consisting of itself, the European Federation for Animal Health (FEDESA), the EU's Committee for Veterinary Medicinal Products, the United States Department of Agriculture and international industry and government officials (Draayer, Hilsabeck and Miller, 1992; Folkers, 1992; Watson, 1992). It is suggested that annual meetings be held in conjunction with either FEDESA or AHI meetings. Issues to be dealt with include the standardization of test requirements, time-frames for implementation and other issues that could reduce or prevent trade barriers without adversely affecting product quality.

The main purpose of the working group would be to harmonize European and United States legislation as a necessary step towards international standardization and the prevention or reducion of potential trade barriers.

There are, in addition, international organizations acting in parallel – also with the goal of international harmonization and standardization of vaccines – but independently from governments and in more general terms. These organizations include the Office international des Epizooties (OIE), the World Health Organization (WHO) and the Food and Agriculture Organization of the United Nations (FAO) as well as the Pharmacopoeias (e.g. the European, United States and Japanese Pharmacopoeias).

OFFICE INTERNATIONAL DES EPIZOOTIES

The OIE, whose purpose is to harmonize and coordinate animal health activities at the international level, also contributes to the standardization of vaccine quality. The three principal aims of the OIE (Truszczynski and Blancou, 1992) are:

- The provision of information on animal health worldwide.
- International coordination of research into and control of certain animal diseases.
- The harmonization of import and export regulations for animals and

animal products at the international level.

A measure of the development and growing international recognition of the OIE is that it was established by 28 countries in 1924 while it now has 136 member countries. Seventeen are from the Americas, 42 from Africa, 43 from Europe and 34 from Asia. The OIE operates under the authority of its International Committee, formed by the delegates of the member countries, under the leadership of an elected president.

The Central Bureau, located at OIE's headquarters in Paris (12 rue de Prony), is headed by the Director-General, at present Dr J. Blancou. The Central Bureau implements decisions of the International Committee and the different Commissions.

There are five *Regional Commissions,* covering Africa, the Americas, Asia, the Far East and Oceania, Europe and the Middle East.

There are also *Specialist Commissions* for The International Animal Health Code; Standards; Foot-and-Mouth Disease and other Epizootics; and Fish Diseases, including those of crustaceans and molluscs. In addition, there are three working groups: Animal Health Information Systems, Veterinary Drug Registration and Biotechnology.

The International Animal Health Code Commission draws up animal health recommendations for the import and export of animals and animal products and contributes through the *Animal Health Code,* an important OIE publication, to international harmonization in this area. *The Standards Commission* establishes standards for diagnostic methods, including diagnostic biologicals, and for vaccines. *The Foot and Mouth Disease and other Epizootics Commission* contributes to the development and standardization of vaccines against foot-and-mouth disease and strategies for the eradication or control of this as well as other diseases. *The Fish Diseases Commission* establishes standards for diagnostic methods and vaccines for fish diseases.

From this short description it can be concluded that all the Specialist Commissions are interested in the international harmonization and standardization not only of vaccines but also of diagnostic methods, including diagnostic biologicals. These activities relate to those important diseases included in the Lists A and B prepared by the OIE (Truszczynski and Blancou, 1992).

List A includes contagious diseases which spread rapidly and the scope of which extends beyond national borders. These diseases have particularly serious socio-economic or public health consequences and are of major importance in the international trade of animals and animal products.

List B includes contagious diseases which are considered of socio-economic and/or public health importance within countries and which, naturally, are also of significance to the international trade of animals and animal products.

Among these Specialist Commissions, the one most closely connected with the standardization of diagnostic methods and vaccine quality is the Standards Commission, whose role includes participation in the standardization of biologicals, including vaccines used for prophylactic purposes for List A and B diseases.

To accomplish this goal, the Standards Commission undertakes the following activities:

- regular updating of the *OIE manual of standards for diagnostics tests and vaccines;*
- the organization of reference laboratories for several diseases in Lists A and B;
- the establishment of international standards for diagnostic tests and vaccines.

OIE manual of standards for diagnostic tests and vaccines

The purpose of the OIE manual (OIE, 1992) is to provide a uniform approach to the diagnosis of important animal diseases and to the production and control of biological products, mainly vaccines used in the control of List A and B diseases. This is implemented by the presentation in the manual of standard methods for laboratory diagnosis of diseases and for the production and control of vaccines and other biological products for veterinary use in laboratories all over the world.

The first edition of the manual was published in three volumes in 1989-1991, each covering about 30 List A or B diseases. After revision and additional editorial work, a single combined volume was published as the second edition of the manual in 1992. It contains information on 15 List A diseases and 75 List B diseases. In future, the Standards Commission plans to produce a new updated edition every four years. The 1992 edition of the manual has been distributed worldwide, recommending:

- "prescribed tests" which should be used for diagnosis; and
- requirements for vaccines, in relation to List A and B diseases.

This will undoubtedly help lead to an internationally unified approach to the diagnosis and quality control of vaccines.

Organization of OIE reference laboratories for List A and B diseases

The standardization of "prescribed tests" and the production and quality control of veterinary vaccines can only be achieved when the necessary standards are made available. The goal of standardization and availability of standards is intended to be achieved through the OIE-organized reference laboratories.

These laboratories must fulfil a specific function or range of functions at an internationally recognized level related to the standardization of diagnostic methods and vaccines applied in the prophylaxis and control of List A and B diseases, especially those of greatest importance and those causing high economic losses. The designation of these laboratories is proposed by the OIE Standards Commission and ratified by the OIE International Committee. Designation does not imply that financial support will be given by the OIE.

The functions and responsibilities of the OIE reference laboratories are as follows:

- the provision of a centre of excellence in a designated activity;
- the standardization of methodology;
- the storage and distribution of standard antisera, antigens and other important reagents;
- the development of new methods;
- the provision of consultant assistance to the OIE;
- training in a designated activity;
- the organization of scientific meetings on behalf of the OIE;
- the coordination of collaborative studies;
- the provision of assistance to the OIE in collecting and disseminating necessary information.

The Director-General of the OIE sent letters to selected laboratories around the world inviting them to become OIE reference laboratories for the more important diseases of Lists A and B. Because of the necessity of some regionalization, in several cases a number of reference laboratories for the same disease were organized in different countries or regions. At the beginning of 1994, 101 OIE reference laboratories were designated for 37 List A and B diseases or groups of diseases. The majority of these laboratories developed significant activities in accordance with their responsibilities, and this is reflected in annual reports which they submit to the OIE.

OIE requirements for vaccines

As mentioned above, these requirements are part of the OIE manual's chapters on the List A and B diseases for which vaccines are available. The chapters contain general information, indicating recommended vaccines, data on seed management (including characteristics of the vaccinal strains, culture, validation as a vaccine), manufacture, in-process control and batch control (including sterility, safety and potency tests).

The Standards Commission is aware that the manual's coverage of standards for vaccines is less comprehensive than it is of diagnostic methods. Nevertheless, some chapters are exemplary and provide a good model for others to follow in the preparation of the next edition.

The Commission will, however, avoid any involvement in product licensing procedures. It will be essential to ensure that the OIE manual keeps up to date with developments in vaccine technology through current advances in microbiology, immunology and biotechnology. Following from this, the importance of consistency between the OIE manual, EU regulations and the European Pharmacopoeia must also be emphasized.

In future, the OIE reference laboratories will prepare for distribution the standards that are essential in vaccine production and control. The present role of the OIE is, however, restricted to the distribution of information contained in the manual and which is undoubtedly contributing to international harmonization in the area of vaccine production.

OIE COOPERATION WITH OTHER INTERNATIONAL ORGANIZATIONS

FAO

FAO plays an important role in improving the quality standards of vaccines. Its main interest is in developing countries and activities are concentrated on rinderpest eradication campaigns (Pan-African Rinderpest Campaign [PARC], Western Asia Rinderpest Eradication Campaign [WAREC] and South Asia Rinderpest Eradication Campaign [SAREC]) in 53 countries on three continents; foot-and-mouth disease control in Asia, Africa and South America; and Newcastle disease of poultry in the same areas.

During the last decade, through national and regional projects, FAO has provided expertise to individual laboratories and assistance in the setting up of networks. FAO has also cooperated with international organizations (WHO, OIE) in the standardization of particular products and the holding of regional training courses on vaccines and their associated technologies.

The FAO Expert Consultation on Quality Control of Veterinary Vaccines in Developing Countries, held in Rome, Italy, in December 1991 (FAO, 1991; Rweyemamu, Sylla and Palya in FAO, 1993), recommended that closer cooperation be established with other international organizations to develop a more coherent approach on guidelines for vaccine quality control. FAO, WHO and OIE should work jointly with developing countries to agree on priorities and carry forward regional participation in standardization, including the development of appropriate laboratory facilities and post-licensing surveillance.

This should include participation at the national level as well as within regions and would require those countries with no procedures to begin standardization and regulation, unless a decision has been taken to accept standards agreed by other countries or regions. Regional repositories of master seed stocks of vaccine strains, cell lines and challenge strains should be established to aid in attaining uniform quality of vaccines.

The consultation recognized the value of the activities of the Pan African Veterinary Vaccine Centre (PANVAC) and recommended that FAO, together with the Organization of African Unity (OAU) and the Interafrican Bureau for Animal Resources (IBAR), should solicit appropriate regional and international support for the conversion of PANVAC to the status of a long-term programme institute, with appropriate facilities and support.

It was also stated that tests required by national authorities to license or release vaccines should be identical with those recommended by the appropriate international organizations. The meeting recommended the preparation of a manual on veterinary vaccines, providing guidelines for the production of veterinary vaccines in developing countries, as a project to be implemented by FAO and the other international organizations concerned.

World Health Organization

WHO, located in Geneva, Switzerland, is a specialized United Nations agency whose primary responsibility is in international and public health matters. However, it also plays an essential role in the standardization of vaccine quality.

The WHO Expert Committee on Biological Standardization is mainly responsible for human pharmaceutical products (vaccines) but also for some veterinary biologicals and products of interest to animals as well as humans. The committee has published guidelines for the preparation and establishment of reference materials and reference reagents for biological substances (WHO, 1978) and definitions of these materials and reagents have been formulated. According to these definitions, an international biological standard is a biological substance to which WHO has assigned an international unit on the basis of data obtained in a worldwide study.

The prime function of an international biological standard is to enable the activity of a sample of unknown potency to be measured in a biological system and expressed conveniently in international units. The international biological reference preparation is a biological substance which may be used for a purpose similar to that of a standard but which has been established without a full collaborative study, or after such a study has shown that it is not appropriate to establish it as an international standard.

Besides this activity, the WHO Expert Committee on Biological Standardization establishes more general requirements for biological products, among them vaccines for veterinary use. A good example is in the manufacturing and control requirements for rabies vaccines for veterinary use (WHO, 1981).

With regard to products for veterinary use or of animal origin, the committee has established requirements for tuberculins (human and bovine), anthrax spore vaccine (live vaccine for veterinary use), immune sera of animal origin, rinderpest cell culture vaccine (live) and rinderpest vaccine (live), *Brucella abortus* Strain 19 vaccine and *Brucella melitensis* Strain Rev.1 vaccine (live for veterinary use).

Requirements are revised regularly for most products as major advances in technology for manufacturing or quality control are reported and accepted by the international scientific community.

In addition to specific products, the Expert Committee on Biological Standardization also issues general recommendations on biological substances and test systems, for example on the national control of vaccines and sera and requirements for immunoassay kits. It also regularly reviews and updates the list of international biological reference preparations and reagents.

Technical units such as the Veterinary Public Health (VPH) Unit of WHO are associated with the committee's work each time a substance or a subject falling within a specific technical unit's domain of expertise comes under discussion.

European Pharmacopoeia

One effective approach to vaccine quality standardization is based on the European Pharmacopoeia (Artiges, 1992). The 19 signatory countries – the 12 (in 1992) EU Member States, countries of the European Free Trade Association (EFTA) and Cyprus – are committed to setting up common monographs and making them official in their territories. The European Pharmacopoeia has its own secretariat, administratively attached to the Council of the EU, and a laboratory, both of which are located in Strasbourg.

Monographs and general analytical methods are prepared by specialized expert groups made up of scientists from universities and national control laboratories, etc. Before their final adoption, the texts, which in most cases have been the object of interlaboratory cooperative tests, are published in public inquiry form in the European Pharmacopoeia's *Pharmeuropa*, which appears four times a year in English and French.

The close cooperation between the European Pharmacopoeia and those countries retaining their own national pharmacopoeias should be mentioned, i.e. Germany, Austria, Belgium, the United Kingdom, France, Italy, Switzerland and the Nordic countries. The latter have brought all their general methods in line with those of the European Pharmacopoeia.

To date, all general analytical methods are harmonized: there are 17 general monographs defining the main pharmaceutical forms and about 800 monographs covering starting materials and certain biological preparations such as immunosera and vaccines, both human and veterinary.

The second edition of the European Pharmacopoeia has been published since 1980 in the form of fascicles. Publication is annual (between June and September) and implementation of the standards in all member countries is effective on 1 January of the following year.

Operationally, the roles of the pharmacopoeias and the regulatory governmental agencies (mentioned earlier) are complementary:

- the regulatory agencies approve new drugs and vaccines on the basis of proven safety and efficacy and approved specifications, tests and methods of analysis for each application;
- the Pharmacopoeia establishes public standards that apply to any manufacturer of a particular drug substance or pharmaceutical product.

In Europe, there is a close legal connection between licensing systems and pharmacopoeias regarding their legal (Directive EEC/75/81/852) as well as practical aspects (shared experts and a close relationship between secretariats).

The European Pharmacopoeia provides detailed quality standards for vaccines through a series of monographs. These are assembled by an expert group and, once published, are mandatory for the member states. There are currently 33 monographs on veterinary vaccines and other biologicals. Among them are: anthrax spore live vaccine for veterinary use, avian infectious bronchitis live vaccine (freeze-dried), canine distemper live vaccine (freeze-dried), *Clostridium botulinum* vaccine for veterinary use, *C. chauvoei* vaccine for veterinary use, *C. perfringens* vaccine for veterinary use, equine influenza vaccine (inactivated), foot-and-mouth disease vaccine (inactivated), swine erysipelas vaccine (inactivated) and swine fever live vaccine (freeze-dried).

The monographs on veterinary vaccines

provide information on identification tests, testing for contaminants and storage, etc. The European Pharmacopoeia also provides a limited number of reference preparations for use as working standards – among these preparations a rabies vaccine and a bovine tuberculosis purified protein derivative (PPD). A *B. melitensis*, Rev.1 vaccine is also currently under study.

Except in the case of biotechnology products, the European Pharmacopoeia maintains only limited liaison with other major pharmacopoeias such as those of the United States and Japan. For veterinary vaccines the differences between these pharmacopoeias are of considerable significance.

In general, the European Pharmacopoeia monographs are more detailed than the OIE manual's requirements for biological products (OIE, 1992), but they only deal with vaccines of significance to Europe. Although several of these vaccines are also important to other continents, the European Pharmacopoeia may be less accessible, particularly in developing countries, than the OIE manual.

In the next edition of the OIE manual, the sections on vaccines will be revised in the full light of standards already established in the European and other major pharmacopoeias.

Pan American Health Organization

The Pan American Health Organization (PAHO) contributes towards the standardization and quality control of foot-and-mouth disease (FMD) and some other vaccines in South America (FAO, 1991). Through the work of PAHO, standards of vaccine production and quality control in particular have been significantly improved in the last decade, and vaccination campaigns against FMD are having a significant effect on the incidence of the disease.

European Union

Cooperation between OIE and the EU (DGXII – Science, Research and Development) in the control of veterinary reagents and vaccines has been initiated (Lee Aileen, 1992).

BIBLIOGRAPHY

Artiges, A. 1992. The role of the European Pharmacopoeia. *Dev. Biol. Stand.*, 79: 87-93.

Draayer, H.A., Hilsabeck, L.J. & Miller, R.H. 1992. The American manufacturer's view on the EEC texts and harmonization. *Dev. Biol. Stand.*, 79: 75-83.

FAO. 1991. Report of the FAO Expert Consultation on Quality Control of Veterinary Vaccines in Developing Countries, 2-6 December, Rome.

FAO. 1993. Regional harmonization of vaccine quality standards and stimulation of vaccine technologies in developing countries. *In* Proc. Expert Consultation. *Quality control of veterinary vaccines in developing countries*, p. 3-12. FAO Animal Production and Health Paper, No. 116. Rome.

Folkers, C. 1992. The FEDESA's point of view. *Dev. Biol. Stand.*, 79: 27-30.

Lee Aileen, M.T. 1992. Presentation of the EEC Directive/81/852 – Quality. *Dev. Biol. Stand.*, 79: 39-41.

OIE. 1992. *Manual of standards for diagnostic tests and vaccines for Lists A and B diseases of mammals, birds and bees*. Paris.

Pensaert, M. 1992. Control of product batches (before and after registration) – the Belgian approach. *Dev. Biol. Stand.*, 79: 183-186.

Truszczynski, M. & Blancou, J. 1992. The role of the Office international des Epizooties in the standardization of biologicals. *Dev. Biol. Stand.*, 79: 95-98.

Watson, J. 1992. Technical requirements of veterinary vaccines for registration –

FEDESA's point of view. *Dev. Biol. Stand.*, 79: 51-63.

WHO. 1978. *Guidelines for the preparation and establishment of reference materials and reference reagents for biological substances.* WHO Expert Committee on Biological Standardization. WHO Technical Report Series, No. 626. Geneva.

WHO. 1981. WHO Expert Committee on Biological Standardization. WHO Technical Report Series, No. 658. Geneva.

PART II

Planning and management of vaccine production

Registration, licensing, controls and practical issues related to veterinary vaccines

P. Vannier

Veterinary vaccines have to be considered as medicinal products and, therefore, should be included in a framework of regulations for marketing. Since these regulations are related to technical requirements, they alone are capable of guaranteeing to potential users the quality, safety and efficacy expected of such products.

Such a guarantee is absolutely necessary for the protection of the livestock population against infectious diseases, and also to ensure, ultimately, the high standards of hygiene required of food products that are to be marketed.

REGULATIONS FRAMEWORK

Regulations relating to veterinary vaccines have to define, as precisely as possible, the conditions required for the registration of veterinary immunobiological products, directions on how to file an application for registration of a product, the conditions under which it is permissible to manufacture a product and the issuing of marketing authorizations (licences).

The conditions under which the inspection of manufacturing premises are to be carried out need to be defined in the regulations relating to immunological veterinary medicinal products (IVMPs).

The regulations should be sufficiently precise to take into account the various standards of manufacture and methods of working with such products throughout the country concerned. Consideration has also to be given to the human and financial resources associated with the industry. If regulations demand standards that are too high – being based on theoretical considerations – and are inappropriate to the socio-economical conditions obtaining in a country, they will very probably never be applied.

Under such circumstances, it would be preferable to formulate regulations of a less demanding nature, which would therefore be more likely be recognized and would lead to improvements in the standard of IVMPs used in that country.

LICENSING AUTHORITIES AND PROCEDURES

It goes without saying that it is necessary to define the conditions and procedures which will be used by the registration authority clearly. Such definitions guarantee to national and foreign manufacturers the independence and impartiality of the registration authority.

Normally the applicant submits to the national authority (which could be the ministry of agriculture or an agency, but is always a government department), an official application to obtain a licence to market a particular IVMP. With the application, several copies of the product's documentation file, giving essential data, are also sent, to enable the authority to compile a dossier relating to that particular product. In addition, samples from typical batches of the product are sent to control laboratories for official testing. Generally, the authority acknowledges receipt of the application and allocates an official registration number to the product. Fees, which vary in amount, have to be paid.

The official registration number will later become the marketing authorization (licence) number of the registered product.

The regulations should define a time period for the examination of the application file by the official technical advisers responsible to the national authority. However, in many countries the authorization to market the product is based on an assessment made by an independent committee, working from the results of an investigation made by technical experts.

The work of the committee should be strictly confidential. Members of the committee should include representatives of the national authority and recognized experts in the field of veterinary immunobiologicals. Impartiality, objectivity, confidentiality, technical assessment and scientific competence are the essential aspects of the procedure to be followed in assessing the suitability of a product for licensing prior to marketing.

DATA TO BE INCLUDED IN AN APPLICATION (REGISTRATION) FILE

The following information is taken from European Commission Directive 81/852 (amended as 92/18 and published on 20 March 1992).

The file is composed of six sections: i) a summary, ii) expert reports, iii) analytical details, iv) descriptions and results of safety and v) efficacy (potency) trials and vi) documentation relating to safety testing and efficacy trials.

Summary of the dossier of information

The IVMP which is the subject of the application should be identified by the names of the active ingredients, together with their pharmaceutical formats and the quantities used in the product, the method and route of administration and a description of the final sales presentation of the product.

The name and address of the applicant should be given together with the name and address of the manufacturer and the sites involved in the different stages of manufacture as well as, where relevant, the name and address of the importer.

Annexed to the administrative data there should be copies of a document (e.g. a licence) showing that the manufacturer is authorized to produce IVMPs. The applicant should submit a list of countries in which such authorization has been granted. The applicant should also submit a summary of the product's characteristics.

Experts' reports

Reports must be provided on all the tests and investigations made. Each report should consist of a critical evaluation of the various tests and/or trials and should present all the relevant data for detailed evaluation. The expert(s) involved should give their opinions as to whether sufficient guarantees have been provided as to the quality, safety and efficacy of the product concerned; a brief summary is not sufficient.

Each report should be prepared by a suitably qualified and experienced person, who may be a company employee. The report should be signed and dated by the expert and should also include brief information about the educational background, training and occupational experience of the expert. The professional relationship of the expert to the applicant (i.e. the company) must be declared.

Analytical section

This section should give descriptions of all the physico-chemical, biological or microbiological tests carried out to characterize the IVMP. All test procedures used should correspond to the most up-to-date scientific methods available and should be validated procedures; results of the validation studies must be provided.

Qualitative and quantitative particulars of constituents. Qualitative particulars of all the constituents of an IVMP should give a complete description of the constituents of the final product, as administered to animals, including the designation or description of: the active ingredients; the composition and constituents of adjuvants, excipients etc. (whatever their nature); and the quantities used, including preservatives, stabilizers, emulsifiers and colouring matter.

In giving the quantitive particulars of the active ingredients of an IVMP, it is necessary to specify, wherever possible, the number of organisms, the specific protein content, the mass, the number of international units (IU) or units of biological activity (either per dosage unit or volume) and, with regard to the adjuvant and the constituents of excipients, the mass or volume of each.

Where an IU of biological activity has been defined, this should be used.

Description of the preparation of the final product. The description of the method of preparation accompanying the application for marketing authorization should be drafted in such a manner as to give an adequate description of the nature of the operation employed. This description should include the various stages of manufacture; in the case of continuous manufacture, full details concerning precautions taken to ensure the homogeneity and consistency of each batch of the finished product; and details of blending, etc.

Production and control of starting materials

The starting materials are all the components used in the production of the IVMP. It is recommended that an official monograph such as the European Pharmacopoeia should be consulted when these substances are listed.

The routine tests carried out on each batch of starting materials must be as stated in the application for a marketing licence. If tests other than those described in the pharmacopoeia are used, proof must be supplied that the starting materials meet the quality requirements of the pharmacopoeia.

In the application (registration) file, the origin and provenance of starting materials should be described and documented.

For genetically engineered starting materials, the information given should include descriptions of: the starting cells or strains, the construction of the expression vector (name, origin and function of the replicon, promoter enhancer and other regulator elements), the control of the sequence of DNA or RNA which has been inserted, oligonucleotide sequences of the plasmid vectors in cells, the plasmid used for transfection, added or deleted genes, the biological properties of the final construct and the genes expressed, copy number and genetic stability.

Information should also be provided on all the substances of biological origin used at any stage in the manufacturing procedure. Such information should include: details of the source of the materials; details of any processing, purification and inactivation applied, together with data on the validation of these processes and in-process controls; details of any tests for detecting contamination that have been carried out on each batch of the substance.

When the starting materials are not of biological origin, the information should provide a detailed description of the materials, together with their function, methods of identification and purity. A brief description should also be provided of the tests undertaken to establish the purity of each batch of the starting materials.

Control tests during production

Complete information should be provided of the control tests that are carried out on intermediate products, with a view to verifying the consistency of the production process and the final product. For inactivated or detoxified vaccines, inactivation or detoxification should be confirmed during each production run and immediately after the inactivation or detoxification process.

Control tests on the final product

The registration file should list the tests that are carried out on representative samples of each batch of the final product. The frequency of tests which are not routinely carried out on each batch should also be stated and expiry dates should be indicated.

Certain tests of the general characteristics of a product should be included among the tests of the finished product, even if they are only carried out in the course of the manufacturing process.

These tests should, wherever applicable, be concerned with establishing typical values and the maximum deviations to be expected in relation to mechanical, physical, chemical or microbiological characteristics, as well as special physical characteristics such as density, pH and refractive index. For each characteristic, average values, with appropriate confidence limits, should be established by the applicant for each particular product.

For all tests, descriptions of the techniques for assessing the final product should be set out in sufficiently precise detail, such that they can be readily reproduced.

When appropriate testing procedures are available, the quantity and nature of the adjuvant (i.e. its activity) and its constituents should be confirmed by means of tests with the final product and, when necessary, the excipient(s) used should be subject to identification tests described in detail in the file.

Safety tests prior to batch release have to be described in the registration file in addition to appropriate tests to demonstrate the absence of contamination by adventitious agents or other substances and, where applicable, a test to verify complete inactivation should be carried out on the product in its final container and the results given.

Potency tests. Potency tests also have to be described. These tests are carried out to demonstrate conformity with specifications and to ensure that the efficacy of the product is reproducible from batch to batch and is of an acceptable minimum standard.

Stability tests. A description should be given of the tests undertaken to support the shelf-life proposed by the applicant. The results of analyses, justifying the proposed shelf-life under all likely storage conditions, should also be given.

Safety tests. The particulars and documents in the registration file should include a description of all the safety tests carried out on the target species.

Laboratory tests. Trials should be undertaken in which the IVMP is administered at the recommended dose, and by each recommended route of administration, to animals of each species and category in which it is intended for use. The conditions of these trials should be described in detail together with the objective criteria to be used (such as rectal temperature and performance measurements) to assess the safety of a product. Safety tests need to be performed and the results described in terms of possible effects following:

- the administration of one dose;
- the administration of an overdose;
- the repeated administration of one dose;
- the reproducibility of the results of repeated tests.

For live vaccines, special safety tests are required to establish:

- the putative spread of the vaccine strain;
- its dissemination in the vaccinated animal;
- the possibility of reversion to virulence of attenuated vaccines;
- the biological properties of the vaccine strain (e.g. neurotropism);
- the recombination of elements of the genome and the possibility of the emergence of new strains by genomic reassortment.

Field studies. The file should include supportive data from field studies to supplement the results of laboratory studies.

Potency tests

The particulars and documents in the registration file should include descriptions of tests to demonstrate the potency (efficacy) of the product administered to each category of each target species, by the recommended route(s) and using the proposed schedule of administration.

The demonstration of potency should be undertaken under well-controlled laboratory conditions, by challenge, after administration of the IVMP to the target animal according to the recommended conditions of use. So far as possible, the conditions under which the challenge test is carried out should mimic the natural conditions for infection with regard to the number of challenge organisms and the route of administration of the challenge.

In general, detailed results of all safety and potency tests need to be presented in the file and the report of each test should include the test protocol, records of actual data, analysis of recorded results and the conclusions drawn from the data.

Controls must be included in all assays and must be clearly identified in the reports. Bibliographical references should be given where additional scientific data are required to explain some of the arguments put forward by the manufacturer in support of the product.

CONTROLS TO BE UNDERTAKEN BY NATIONAL AUTHORITIES

These controls depend on national policies and on the human and financial resources available in the country.

Controls must be carried out at the national level, by the appropriate authorities both before marketing authorization and before the release of batches.

Controls carried out before marketing authorization are not routine but may be necessary to confirm the data and results obtained by the manufacturer. These controls can be very simple, such as sterility tests and titrations of organisms, but more complex controls, such as efficacy and safety tests on target species, may also be necessary. Obviously, complex controls can only be carried out where the authorities have the technical means sufficient to obtain proper, fully validated results which cannot be contested by the manufacturer.

Efficacy and safety controls may be carried out routinely or not. In most cases, the nature of the control tests undertaken is dependent on the data given in the registration file. If some data appear unclear or insufficient, further tests may be necessary to confirm the results obtained by the manufacturer. Under these circumstances the tests undertaken are, to some extent, determined by the data produced by the manufacturer.

National authority control tests on batches prior to release are carried out on some vaccines that have strategic importance for specific vaccination or disease eradication programmes, for example rinderpest and foot-and-mouth disease vaccines. Such vaccines are produced by a public or recognized private manufacturer and batches are released only if the results of control tests carried out by the official authorities are satisfactory.

These tests are expensive in time and money and need to be carried out as quickly as possible to avoid delays in marketing the product. Such pressures can contribute to improvements in the quality of the products if the tests are carried out by an efficient and competent organization. In developing countries, it is essential to have a regional policy involving strong cooperation among countries to save resources and to promote the development of more efficient laboratories.

It may not be reasonable or possible to have one national control laboratory per country and it would be more appropriate to avoid duplication by sharing the expenses of maintaining one efficient laboratory among several countries with mutual acceptance of the results obtained by such a laboratory. In practice, however, such an approach has remained, up to now, difficult to achieve.

Official authorities should consider that in many developing countries the national laboratories are themselves producing several vaccines and, in such cases, it is essential that the laboratories in charge of production and those in charge of control tests are completely separate. If not, the independence and impartiality of the control laboratories will be compromised and disputes may arise as to the acceptability of the test results obtained.

INSPECTION

When vaccines are produced locally, the national authorities have to take measures to obtain guarantees concerning the standards of manufacturing practice. Guidelines have been established in various countries and regions such as the United States and Europe to define good manufacturing practices (GMPs). Quality assurance (QA) is increasingly defined as being all the planned and routine actions necessary to provide adequate confidence that a product or service will satisfy given requirements for quality (Soulebot, 1992) rather than demanding the overintensive testing of final products. The implication of this is that the quality of the finished product is largely determined by the quality of the raw materials and manufacturing processes used.

If, in addition to the quality of the raw materials, the various stages in the manufacturing process are controlled in an appropriate way, the probability of a defect or contamination in the finished product would be very low. The methods and standards of inspection required may be developed according to this concept.

An authorization to permit production on a trial basis, in the first instance, needs to be made by the official authorities before routine manufacturing of any product can commence and the product receive the appropriate licence. Authorization should only be given if the premises and manufacturing processes meet the technical requirements that will ensure a good-quality product. Technical requirements need to be defined at the national level (even if they have been developed and defined in other countries) and made known to manufacturers as soon as possible.

A compromise has often been made between the minimum standards required to ensure high quality of products and the economic situation of a country. Indeed, in some situations, if the national authorities intend to guarantee the quality of a particular marketed product, it may even be necessary not to authorize its manufacture in the country.

It is essential that manufacturing premises be inspected regularly but at variable and random intervals to check on the consistency of manufacturing practices.

If products are not manufactured locally, the problem becomes a little more complex because the standards required of manufacturing practices have to be the same in the exporting country as in the importing country. Inspection certificates provided by the authorities from the country of origin will be required by the authorities of the importing country and must be included in the registration file. An agreement between countries will often be necessary to ensure that the administrative and technical values of these certificates are the same. Sometimes it may be necessary to harmonize the conditions of inspection in different countries to ensure mutual recognition of certificates issued by different national authorities.

PHARMACO-VIGILANCE

It is important to set up a system which allows an exchange of information on marketed IVMPs between users and official authorities. Such an exchange of information, which may be informal, forms part of a pharmaco-vigilance network and contributes to the detection of problems in relation to the use of a marketed product. Such a system can be very useful, particularly when the economic situation does not permit important controls on finished products or routine and frequent inspections of premises. Very simple systems can be set up by authorities to inform the main users of IVMPs, for example veterinarians, including, for instance, a telephone line connected to a special unit which can give information on problems occurring after the use of certain products. The main difficulty will be to differentiate between real problems that require immediate action and occasional events in which the suspected product plays no role at all.

More complex systems can be used including a computerized database of information from users, inquiries and epidemiological surveys. At present there are very few such systems operational worldwide.

Pharmaco-vigilance is useful in assessing, in the most expeditious way, the real effects of a vaccine in the field. Side-effects and lack of efficacy can often be observed after the introduction of a new product, which may have been used under normal or abnormal field conditions. Occasionally small alterations in the manufacturing process can affect the quality of the finished product and not have been detected by tests carried out by the manufacturer and the official laboratory.

Pharmaco-vigilance is also useful for the collection of data on the effects of vaccines used under conditions that are somewhat different from those described in the registration file. In developing countries, for instance, the number of target species to which a vaccine can be administered may increase considerably. When vaccines are imported or when assays are expensive it is often difficult to carry out tests on particular species, such as camels and game animals for registration purposes and the use of vaccines may, therefore, have to be adapted to very specific and particular conditions. In such cases pharmaco-vigilance can contribute to the data required for registration files, even if it cannot provide it all because the exchange of information is insufficient and the results of serological surveys and/or clinical records are needed to provide objective and quantifiable data. In addition, when products are imported and where local conditions are not totally appropriate for the setting up of regular and important control tests on finished products, pharmaco-vigilance has an important role to play in assessing the effects of a vaccine in an animal population, particularly with regard to its efficacy.

At present, in several developing countries, there are agreements and contracts between avian and pig production cooperatives and research and control laboratories to carry out field trials for studies of, for example, the development of protective antibodies and clinical results after vaccination. Such trials make possible a better understanding of the performance of vaccines applied under specific conditions.

PRACTICAL ISSUES

To be credible, the organization set up by the national authority has to be founded on technical competence and experience. All of those involved in the different stages of the registration process have to be properly trained in the methods of official inspection, examination of data and laboratory tests. In addition, veterinary immunobiological products have certain specificities and the problems related to the manufacture and control of these products are totally different from those of chemical ones. Specialists and specialized teams are needed to manage the whole registration procedure of IVMPs. To save financial resources, it may sometimes be possible to involve the same people in the administrative procedures for the registration of both chemical and biological products but, in both cases, all technical matters have to be the responsibility of the appropriate specialists.

In developing countries, such problems often become greater because the economic situation does not permit the establishment of an operational, efficient organization. Regional cooperation among countries is therefore needed. Cooperation can include the exchange of test reagents and materials, information about the investigation of new applications for registration and the results of tests and licences which have been granted.

At present, it appears essential to develop a strong collaboration among countries based on good complementary technical competence. The poorer the financial resources of the countries in a region, the greater the need for such collaboration.

It is essential that a licensing system should be both rigorous and demanding and, at the same time, flexible and easily applicable. The system must allow an equitable treatment of all the marketable products which are to be assessed, by using the same technical criteria and standards; this is the sole guarantee for free competition among manufacturers.

If the above conditions are not in place, the system will favour the development of a black market with the opposite results to those desired. The development of a black market becomes more likely when the means and conditions for controlling the distribution of products are weak and inadequate. In all cases, the penalties imposed against those involved in black market activities should be very severe.

The national authorities may have another problem in relation to issuing licences, namely, how to define the threshold of acceptability in regard to quality, safety and efficacy, so as to be able to accept or reject a particular vaccine. In general, a vaccine will be rejected if it appears to be insufficiently safe or lacking in efficacy, there is insufficient scientific data available on file or the qualitative or quantitative composition of the vaccine at the time of testing does not correspond to the data given in the registration file.

It is impossible to generalize about all the possible cases that may justifiy the rejection of a product and, therefore, the refusal of a licence. However, national authorities have to elaborate a policy that can be properly understood and accepted by manufacturers and this policy should be founded on technical requirements and guidelines developed from present scientific understanding and from the requirements set up in other countries, adapted to local conditions.

Whatever the efforts to develop good technical guidelines, some problems will remain and, at some point, the competence and experience of the official inspectors will be required to intervene to make a decision. Under these circumstances it is essential that the legal requirements of the licensing procedure be such as to limit the subjective element in the interpretation of test results and in the judgement of inspectors on the merits of a particular application for a licence.

BIBLIOGRAPHY

Commission of the European Communities. (1992). *The rules governing medicinal products in the European Community*, Vol. V A. Directorate General for International Market and Industrial Affairs.

International Association of Biological Standardisation. 1992. *Symposium on the First Steps Towards an International Harmonization of Veterinary Biologicals: 1993 and the Free Circulation of Vaccines within the EEC.* Developments in Biological Standardisation, No. 79.

Soulebot, J.P. 1992. Fedesa's point of view: quality – application to IVMPs. *In* International Association of Biological Standardisation. *Symposium on the First Steps Towards an International Harmonisation of Veterinary Biologicals: 1993 and the Free Circulation of Vaccines within the EEC*, p. 201-211. Developments in Biological Standardisation, No. 79.

The role of private industry in the transfer of vaccine technology to developing countries

A.J.B. Haigh

VACCINE TECHNOLOGY EXPERTISE WITHIN PRIVATE INDUSTRY

Commercial vaccine producers

Companies that produce vaccine are in business to generate profit from the sale of licensed products. In certain circumstances some are prepared to sell technology transfer packages to state or parastatal bodies and deals of this nature may be financed by government or agency aid in the form of a soft loan.

In such cases it is very important that a contract is signed which clearly defines the objectives to be met by the company and the performance criteria which must be acheived for the company to discharge its obligation including a defined follow-up period of support consultancy with specified responsibilities.

A feasibility study may be necessary to establish a project outline and broad specification to facilitate a costing and the formulation of a contract that both parties can sign. The cost of the feasibility study may also be funded by government or agency soft loan.

The developing country must be satisfied that the commercial company is capable of meeting the commitments it is proposing to undertake and that it does in fact own the technology it is proposing to sell. The developing country is advised to engage an independent consultant with the appropriate technical background and expertise to advise it and act on the country's behalf in the formative, implementation, handover and support consultancy stages.

Engineering and bioengineering companies

There is a large range of engineering and bioengineering companies available – from manufacturers of equipment (e.g. pressure vessels, filters, process modules) to process development contractors. While these companies are specialists in their own specific fields, their role is really one of support and supply to the existing vaccine production and development industry; they generate solutions to engineering and/or processing problems against specifications defined by the customer.

Consultants

Consultants range from individuals with particular expertise in one or more areas of vaccine technology to consulting companies with teams of specialists constituted to meet the particular technical aspects of a project at various stages. Consulting companies are unlikely to have the required biological process technology expertise but can usually provide the other expert inputs required.

Takeovers and mergers within the pharmaceutical and veterinary biological industry have for some time resulted in the availability of a number of individuals with extensive experience in veterinary biologicals production and control who offer their services as self-employed consultants. These independent consultants have much to offer not only as noted in the section Commercial vaccine producers, above, but also as an alternative to commercial vaccine producers as a source of technology expertise.

THE PROCESS OF ACQUIRING TECHNOLOGY

Prior to contract

Regardless of the size of the proposed business, the stages to be worked through by the purchaser and vendor are similar and differ only in scale and the range of skills and specialized inputs required.

The purchaser must first define his or her needs. Ideally a document should be prepared which sets out the requirements and includes any particular conditions or constraints the purchaser may wish to impose or bring to the attention of prospective vendors. This document may be submitted to potential vendors and/or provide the supplementary information to a published tender invitation. The services and assistance of an expert consultant in preparing the basic terms of reference and in selecting the vendor are advisable.

Potential vendors should submit outline proposals and cost estimates. Then, following further evaluation and negotiation, a detailed contract should be made with a selected vendor. Depending on the size and scope of the project, vendors may need to do extensive detailed work, which may include feasibility studies, both to satisfy the purchaser and to establish detailed costings. This can be both time-consuming and costly and will not be undertaken lightly.

Ultimately the purchaser needs to know what is going to be supplied, how much it will cost and the stages at which payments are due. The vendor must be satisfied that the obligations can be discharged within the agreed time-frame and that the way of doing this has been understood and accepted by the purchaser. These points should be embodied within a contract which clearly states who will do what and by what time, what the acceptance criteria are and what will happen in the event of non-compliance. The contract should provide for binding arbitration in the event of an inability to agree. By and large the clauses in the contract which define the obligations and specify what must happen when either party fails to fulfil its obligations are the most important. While everything is going smoothly the contractual details tend to assume a lesser significance.

Post-contract

Implementation of the contract may demand nothing more than the vendor accepting a number of the purchaser's staff at the vendor's production facility and providing specified training. The terms of the agreement (contract) to do this will state how many staff, how and by whom they will be funded, for how long, the specific techniques they will be trained in, how they will be evaluated, the fee to be charged by the vendor, how many payments are to be made by the purchaser, when they are to be made, etc.

Alternatively, implementation of a contract may involve the erection of a vaccine production unit on a greenfield site and its handover in working order, fully staffed by local personnel. Obviously the scope and scale of this requires a multidisciplinary project team and dedicated project management to ensure definition of, and coordinated adherence to, the critical path.

Even large commercial vaccine companies are unlikely to have the required range of expert staff on hand to implement such an undertaking. Projects of this size are usually implemented by teams composed of experts from more than one company. The contractors may be a consortium of the key technology sources, such as process, civil and mechanical and electrical technicians, and project management may be provided from one or a combination of these, or by a consultancy group. The purchaser should insist that the managing contractor carrying overall responsibility be the vendor responsible for providing the process technology and that all other inputs, from whatever source, be arranged through subcontracts with that vendor.

Project implementation can be considered as a series of phases which overlap. The efficient management of this overlap offers savings in time which can mean a considerable saving in cost. An outline of each of the phases involved follows.

Design. A great deal of design work will have been carried out pre-contract to enable contractors to establish the financial commitments and obligations they are undertaking. This work initiates the preparation of the master design document which lays down criteria and tolerances for all aspects of the project such as technology criteria, operating methods and quality standards. An important aspect of the master design document is the setting of overall design tolerances. Biological systems are, by their nature, relatively unpredictable and very susceptible to operator error. Excess capacity above that specified by the purchaser must be "designed in" to provide the purchaser with a reasonable expectation of meeting specified capacity. This capacity is in addition to that allowed for predictable factors arising from planned maintenance, public and religious holidays, etc.

Design involves detailed drawings, isometrics, models, etc. Models not only assist in three-dimensional design but also facilitate the preliminary validation of the process operating manual. Detailed specifications for the purchase of plant and equipment are issued. The site is usually selected pre-contract since its suitability and availability and the quality of major utilities have an enormous impact on the civil and mechanical and electrical costs. Further visits to the site by design staff may be necessary depending on the quantity and quality of the data acquired previously. Evaluations of locally available equipment, materials and skills (e.g. stainless steel fabricators, welders) will be necessary. Time and money spent at this stage save far heavier costs later.

The design stage includes:

- civil design (buildings, site, etc.): plans and specifications, models;
- mechanical and electrical engineering design (air-handling and treatment, process services, effluent treatment, utilities, etc.): plans, flowsheets, layouts, models, specifications;
- process design (the biological production and handling element): preparation of operating and quality control manuals, plans, flowsheets, layouts, models, specifications;
- spares and spare parts quantification and specification;
- consumables quantification and specification;
- support and ancillaries (refrigerated trucks, regional cold stores, serum processing plants): layouts, specifications, models.

Procurement. Project management in conjunction with design will, so far as it is possible, ensure that the plant and equipment with the longest procurement lead times are specified first and placed on order as soon as possible. These key items and their place in the installation schedule have a major influence on the implemention critical path.

To minimize future problems with importation, vendors should use local sources of supply where possible. However, process plant and equipment and key mechanical and electrical plant will usually have to be imported if the vendor has to guarantee performance; biological processes are quirky and two apparently equivalent pieces of plant may not offer the same biological performances.

Ordering is phased against stated lead times to place equipment on-site adequately in advance of the needs of the installation programme.

Installation. The first element of on-site activity is site preparation and civil construction. Mechanical and electrical installation commences soon after the installation of process plant and equipment installation commences well before completion of mechanical and electrical installation. There should be "milestones" in the contract and critical path at which contractors receive a phased payment. Any training of the purchaser's staff at the vendor's facility should commence at times appropriate to returning them to the site as soon as they can usefully contribute to the completion of the project. The future site maintenance engineer should commence training as soon as the contract is signed so as to be back on-site as soon as installation starts.

Commissioning. Commissioning is the initiation of data collection for justification of handover acceptance. All items of plant and equipment are tested and operated to ensure they perform to specification. Items first undergo engineering commissioning to check that the mechanical and electrical parts function and perform within the criteria specified. These tests are certified and become a cumulative record for handover. All measuring, monitoring and control equipment is tested, calibrated and certified.

Commissioning of the air-handling and filtration system is crucial. This system is the key to biological containment and security. Its capacity to perform reliably to the specified design parameters in the face of both extreme environmental conditions and process loadings must be demonstrated. This should be the responsibility of the specialist contractor.

Finally all plant and equipment with a biological function is tested and certified for performance and, where relevant, sterilizability (e.g. filters, culture vessels, valves, transfer lines, centrifuges, autoclaves). Seed banks are set up with certified stock and scale-up cultures are established. At this point plant is ready to move to the preproduction stage.

Training. Local staff of a suitable background and education are selected very early in the project and subjected to both classroom and practical training in a working environment using the same technology as that of the project. The trainees return to the site to assist in the biological commissioning and to prepare the specific standard operating procedures for the plant to be approved by the vendor.

Preproduction. An agreed series of trial batches are prepared in the new installation by the local staff under the supervision of the vendor, to prove the operability of the plant within the performance criteria specified and, at the same time, to validate the new standard operating procedures.

Handover. The final handover of the plant is dependent on the preproduction batches meeting the target criteria.

Consultancy. Failures of plant, equipment and structures occur even in the most efficiently organized projects. Contractor indemnities for a specified period to cover such events must be written into the contracts/purchasing agreements.

Performance problems of a biological nature may be beyond local expertise. The consultancy phase is designed to place the expertise of the vendor at the disposal of the new facility for a specified period, for instance, three years. Biological technology is constantly being improved and it is very important that the original contract clearly defines the purchaser's rights with respect to improvements in the process technology being purchased, particularly over the period of the follow-up consultancy and any subsequent extension to that period. Ideally, the contract should require the vendor to notify the purchaser of improvements to the technology over this period and the purchaser should have the right of acquisition at a reasonable price.

The vendor should make an annual audit inspection of the facility and provide the purchaser with a written report together with recommendations for implementation. The inspecting team should be appropriately staffed for the target facilities to be properly inspected. Additional vendor support should be available on request. This may be provided at the vendor's facilities or on-site as appropriate for the particular problem. The formal annual inspection and recommendations should command a consultancy fee. Ad hoc support should be available on request on a time charge plus expenses basis.

The purchaser should have the option to extend the consultancy phase against renegotiated rates.

TRADITIONAL TECHNOLOGY ACQUISITION BY DEVELOPING COUNTRIES: POINTS FOR AND AGAINST

The single most quoted justification for technology acquisition by developing countries is self-sufficiency followed closely by a cheaper product which saves hard currency by avoiding the import of commercial vaccine.

Unfortunately the facts do not generally support this justification (although every individual case must be evaluated on its merits). The benefits of scale are lost. The initial capital investment is enormous and the bulk of this investment (about 70 percent) is in civil and mechanical engineering, i.e. the creation of the envelope and environment in which the process plant and associated equipment and resources are located and operated. Most of the process plant and many of the mechanical and electrical plant spares as well as many process liquor components and control reagents must still be imported, requiring hard currency. This is frequently subject to bureaucratic delay. Major utility supplies, especially water and electricity, are unreliable in developing countries, resulting in frequent production crises and disasters. The provision of effective standby sources is expensive both to provide and to operate. Trained staff salaries are rarely competitive, resulting in continuous losses of staff which further endangers production reliability. The need to operate to international good manufacturing practice (GMP), good laboratory practice (GLP), quality and environmental standards adds further to unit costs.

Self-sufficiency requires that certified quality- and potency-tested vaccine meeting the standards (with long lead times in many cases) will be available when the demand arises. The points given above are only a few of the more common causes of failure to achieve this and, unfortunately, the management of vaccine plants in developing countries is rarely sufficiently experienced or powerful in the hierarchy to influence the situation for the better.

A further consideration is that of emerging new technologies. The possibility of multiple antigen vector vaccines administered orally, possibly even via the feed, is quite real. Against such a possibility the validity of investing in traditional vaccine technology, rather than continuing to import until the position clarifies, becomes very doubtful.

The above remarks should not in any way deter those seeking to improve existing production facilities particularly with respect to meeting GMP/GLP standards or upgrading quality assurance.

General design and operating requirements for vaccine manufacturing establishments

P.J. Radlett

The design and operation of facilities suitable for the manufacture of veterinary vaccines depend on many factors, including the nature of the organisms from which the vaccines are to be prepared, the specific manufacturing processes used and the particular economic, technical and geographical situation in which the facility is to operate.

This chapter will give only a broad outline of the principles which should be borne in mind for the design and construction of new facilities or the upgrading of existing installations. Many of the design features are relatively uncomplicated and should therefore not be prohibitively expensive to incorporate into a new building design although it may be difficult and expensive to make changes to existing buildings which did not take into account these factors at the design stage. Similarly, when facilities are being upgraded or modified for other purposes, it is often appropriate to review basic design and operating parameters to ensure that, wherever possible, improvements which permit the most satisfactory functioning of the plant are incorporated.

The essential requirement for a manufacturing plant is that it should produce a sufficient quantity of good-quality, safe and effective product in an economic manner as required. The objectives of optimum plant design and the concepts of good manufacturing practice and total quality management are intended to ensure that these requirements are met on a routine basis.

In a number of countries, general guidelines for the manufacture of veterinary products have been in place for some time. In particular, manufacture within the United Kingdom has been subject to compliance with published guidelines (Sharp, 1983; Government of the United Kingdom, 1983) and a set of guidelines for the manufacture of veterinary immunological products within the European Union (EU) has also been published (Commission of the European Communities, 1992). These guidelines set out the general requirements for facilities and their operation and are based on an appreciation of the problems that can occur in the manufacture of veterinary vaccines and of how such problems can be avoided.

Although these guidelines are not mandatory in other parts of the world, most of the principles they contain are applicable to any manufacturing situation and, where they can be effectively integrated into the design and operation of other units, it is frequently advantageous to do so. Incorporation of some specific design features at the start of a project may not be practicable or cost-effective, but careful design with thought to future possible needs when setting down the basic design and layout is likely to prove worthwhile and may save expensive modification work as and when these features become important.

The following sections describe the main principles governing the general layout of laboratories, the major factors which need to be considered in their operation and the specific needs of particular manufacturing areas.

GENERAL ARRANGEMENT OF BUILDINGS

Buildings should be constructed of good-quality materials, with impervious finishes which can be easily cleaned and maintained and constructed in such a way that adjacent areas can be effectively sealed and separated from one another and from the outside. In today's manufacturing environment wood is not regarded as ideal and, where used, needs to be thoroughly painted and regularly maintained.

In many situations it will be necessary or desirable to hold individual areas under an air-pressure differential, which may be negative or positive to the outside and to adjacent areas. The materials and method of construction should be such that this can be achieved easily.

In the construction and fitting out of all manufacturing areas, consideration should be given to the avoidance of ledges and crevices and unnecessary internal protrusions such as surface water downpipes or other architectural features. Wherever possible, windows should be fitted flush to internal wall surfaces and coving used to create smooth, easily cleaned corners.

Areas where the product or its sterile constituents are directly exposed during manufacture will require greater attention to these details than those in which the product is manipulated within totally enclosed containers. However, the principal aim remains to create the cleanest possible manufacturing environment and one which is easily maintained.

Attention paid to the logistics of product and material flow and staff movements during manufacture will ensure that sequential manipulations may be carried out in adjacent areas and will promote an efficient flow of materials into and out of each area.

To maintain cleanliness and the integrity of the manufacturing environment, facilities need to be provided for the transfer of materials into and out of manufacturing areas in such a way that the environment of the room is protected and infectious agents (either to be manufactured or adventitious) are contained. In general these access points should be separate from those used for the entrance and exit of staff.

Materials, in particular live organisms, that are handled in quality control (QC) laboratories are considered by most regulatory authorities to present a risk to the manufacturing operation. Such laboratories should therefore be situated in a building separated from that used for manufacturing. Where this is not practical or feasible there should be at least a solid wall between the two different activities. Again, care taken at the design stage will ensure that features can be accommodated that will make possible the smooth flow of samples from the manufacturing areas to the QC laboratory and of the results of analyses from QC back to manufacturing.

The sizing of manufacturing facilities is a complicated operation. Areas need to be large enough for the operations which will be carried out in them but such facilities are expensive and excess space is unnecessarily costly. Conversely, as will be clear from the above, if logical flow patterns are to be established and maintained, the later expansion of individual areas may be difficult to achieve. In consequence, it is usually prudent to make allowance for any future expansion of activities while the project is still at the design stage.

EQUIPMENT

The detailed equipment requirements for a vaccine manufacturing establishment will depend on the scope and capacity of the particular unit, but some general points can be made.

Many facilities will require stainless steel fermenters, inactivation and blending vessels which may vary in volume from a few to several thousand litres. Many manufacturers can provide fermenters and other vessels of satisfactory design but it should be noted that the control package which accompanies the vessel may be much more sophisticated than is actually required – resulting in unnecessary costs. In most of the situations covered by the scope of this manual, process operations will be essentially hand controlled and, while a degree of automatic environmental control will be required, it would be wise to ensure the vessel manufacturer provides only that which the process needs and not the ultimate of which it is capable.

At the other end of the spectrum, it is sometimes considered appropriate to minimize capital costs by fitting mild steel jackets insulated with cheap lagging instead of using good-quality stainless steel. In many cases this is a false economy since, once installed, such fermenters are frequently required to function over an indefinite lifespan in a hot humid atmosphere, which soon results in deterioration of the lagging and ultimately the jacket. Effecting repairs is then difficult, disruptive and expensive.

Great care needs to be taken at the design stage to ensure that fermentation equipment is installed with due regard to both process and service flows and particularly that drainage from both vessel and pipework during steam sterilization is effective. Open drainage channels in floors are frequently considered undesirable because of the resultant contamination risk and the efficient draining of steam condensate to ensure the sterility of pipework and vessels is made considerably more complicated where valves cannot simply be purged.

In addition to fermentation equipment, the facility will need autoclaves and sterilizing ovens, designed in such a way that the minimum requirements for sterilization can easily be met (Parenteral Drug Association, 1978 and 1981), and a range of other equipment such as freeze-driers, filling machines, centrifuges, filters and antigen concentration equipment. Again, there is a wide range of sophisticated commercial equipment available from which to choose and it is important to balance the right level of sophistication against the needs of the process and the situation in which it is being operated. Simple systems are frequently more labour-intensive but tend to require less maintenance and are easier to put right when they go wrong.

AIR-HANDLING SYSTEMS

Most manufacturing facilities require a fairly sophisticated air-handling system. In the interests of the operators, their efficiency and the product itself, it will be necessary to maintain equitable temperature and humidity levels in the facility. In addition, a principal objective should be to maintain as clean a working environment as possible. This will entail segregation, both internally and externally, from other areas, which may pose some risk to the maintenance of a satisfactory manufacturing environment.

The methods normally employed to promote a clean working environment include the provision of air filtered through sterilizing high-efficiency particle adsorption (HEPA) filters and the maintenance of pressure differentials between adjacent areas. In situations where live organisms are handled within the manufacturing area there will also be a requirement to filter exhaust air. In small installations it is possible to achieve these requirements with simple individual "through the wall" fan/filter units. The balancing of such a system, however, can become an extremely complex problem, since the pressure drop across, and the flow of air through, each unit may cause detrimental effects on the atmosphere of the next one.

In practice it may prove more satisfactory to use a separate fan unit to supply each related group of rooms. The same principles apply to the extraction side of the system and great care should be taken to ensure that potentially contaminated air extracted from a unit handling live organisms cannot be recirculated into clean production areas.

The detailed airflow rates and pressure differentials required depend on the particular functions and layout of the facility. In general, a minimum pressure differential of 1.5 mm water gauge between adjacent areas is normally used. Care must be taken with the layout to ensure the cumulative effect of this does not result in very large pressures on windows and doors which connect with or are related to nearby areas. This could cause problems with the sealing of windows or the opening of doors.

For general manufacturing or enclosed processing areas, an air exchange rate of seven to eight changes per hour is usually considered adequate, but for sterile areas exchange rates of at least 20 changes per hour are required if the low particle and bacterial counts specified in the European and United States guidelines are to be met. These are undoubtedly necessary to ensure that satisfactory working conditions are maintained.

It is important that inlet and outlet ducts are carefully positioned to provide a good sweeping action in workrooms. Typically, inputs are terminally filtered into the area at a high level and balanced with low-level extractors on the opposite side of the room.

STAFFING

It is essential that any manufacturing facility should be staffed with personnel who are of the right calibre and sufficiently trained to perform the tasks required of them. This will almost invariably mean that a nucleus of qualified and/or experienced senior staff will need to implement an ongoing training programme to ensure that all staff are fully conversant with the tasks required of them. To make the latter possible all personnel will benefit from an overview of the entire facility, its functions and the rationale behind the operating regimes implemented. It must be remembered that training will need to cover not only the technical methods employed but also the basis of good manufacturing procedures, safety and quality assurance in the broadest sense.

To be confident that live agents and materials, including both those used for manufacture and the adventitious agents that are inevitably present on the site, do not gain access to manufacturing areas other than those in which they originate, it is good practice, and in many situations a mandatory requirement, to restrict the free access of staff to all areas of the site. A commonly used rule of thumb restricts operations to one type of product organism, per operator, per air space, per day. The restrictions on staff, especially the time period, will depend on the particular manufacturing operation, but such restrictions should prevent the direct movement of personnel between QC facilities and manufacturing areas and between manufacturing areas handling live organisms and those in which inactivated antigens or products are handled.

These restrictions, however desirable from the manufacturing standpoint, inevitably tend to create and amplify barriers to effective communication. This places an even greater emphasis on the importance of adequate and continuing staff training and dialogue among the various groups on site. It is essential to ensure the unit works as one and not as a series of disparate groups.

WATER

Manufacturing facilities require a reliable supply of good-quality water for general purposes and for direct use in the manufacturing process. Important factors influencing the quality of water are the microbial content and the total quantity and nature of both organic and inorganic impurities.

Traditionally, the water used in tissue culture or bacterial fermentation processes has been produced by distillation, usually following a desalting or ion-exchange purification stage. More recently, excellent results for both tissue culture and bacterial-based products have been obtained using water produced by the method of reverse osmosis instead of distillation. This is an extremely energy-efficient process and, in some situations, plants which have switched to reverse osmosis from distillation have been known to recover their capital costs in a matter of months.

Whatever the method used for the manufacture of pure water, the equipment used for its production and storage require careful management. Bacterial growth in storage tanks and purification columns, whether ion-exchange or reverse osmosis, is a constant hazard and toxins may persist even if the live contaminants are eliminated. As yet, the columns available for purification stages cannot be steam-sterilized and regular chemical disinfection must be carried out. The problem of water storage can largely be overcome by heating the storage vessel, and preferably the distribution system, to at least 65°C and maintaining that temperature until the water is required for manufacture. Careful attention needs to be paid to the layout of the distribution system itself to avoid "dead ends", poorly designed valves and other points at which water may remain stagnant.

Whatever process and procedures are adopted, the quality of both "feed" and purified water will require regular monitoring and equipment will require regular sterilization or sanitization.

LIQUID EFFLUENT

Manufacturing facilities almost inevitably produce large amounts of liquid effluent which need to be discarded in a safe and satisfactory manner. The appropriate necessary procedures depend on local regulations and the nature of the agents handled in the facility but should take into account the possible presence of live agents, their inactivation and the chemical content of the material to be discarded.

Total segregation of live from non-infective areas within the facility will minimize the volume of the more difficult materials that arise from the former areas.

Small quantities of liquid effluent can normally be rendered innocuous by autoclaving, but larger quantities require a dedicated collection and treatment facility. Heat treatment of contaminated effluent is commonly practised, either as a batch or a continuous process. Care needs to be taken to ensure that there is sufficient storage capacity for untreated material, both to balance the throughput of the sterilizer and to provide storage during equipment failures and accidents within the facility.

WASTE DISPOSAL

If the risks of environmental contamination and cross-contamination are to be avoided, solid wastes arising from areas handling live agents require decontamination prior to removal from the area in which they were generated. This can be accomplished either by fumigation (e.g. with formaldehyde) or heat-sterilization (e.g. autoclaving). This in turn requires the provision of suitable facilities for these activities at, or close to, the perimeter of the area in which the agent is handled. With careful design one sterilization/fumigation facility can serve more than one area and, depending on the nature of the agent handled, an acceptable compromise can sometimes be found by surface decontamination of materials at the time of removal from the infected area and subsequent sterilization in an adjacent facility. It should be pointed out, however, that suitable sterilization/fumigation facilities are frequently required for the transfer of materials into manufacturing areas and, where this is so, the same facilities can serve for the removal of waste materials.

Waste materials should not be allowed to accumulate on the site or to become dispersed around the site. The identification of a single deposition point at the perimeter of the site, combined with regular collections by the appropriate waste disposal authority, should serve to minimize problems with solid waste.

MANUFACTURING MATERIALS

If a high degree of assurance is to be obtained in relation to the quality of routinely manufactured products, it is important that all materials used for manufacture are of a suitable quality. This does not necessarily require the importation of expensive high-purity components, provided a reliable source of satisfactory materials can be found locally.

Where a pharmacopoeial standard for a particular component exists, there is frequently a requirement to meet it and this can be accomplished either by purchasing ready tested material or by arranging for the appropriate tests to be carried out. Where there is no requirement to meet a pharmacopoeial standard the manufacturer needs assurance that the supplier can routinely supply material which will result in the production of a satisfactory product. Such assurance needs to take into account both the satisfactory yield and the efficacy of the final product and its safety.

In many cases it is advisable to set up routine tests on batches of raw materials prior to their use for manufacturing operations. It could also be important in the subsequent investigation of production trends and in solving the inevitable production problems, which arise from time to time in all biological manufacturing operations, that the individual batches of raw materials used for each operation can be traced. It is therefore advisable to batch-label each consignment of raw materials on arrival, to introduce some formal QC release procedure to confirm that the materials are considered acceptable for use and to record the batch identification as materials are used, thus ensuring traceability throughout the production process.

SEED PRODUCTION AND STORAGE

Under most circumstances the production of seeds, including both the live agent and, where appropriate, the substrate on which it is to be grown, will require the provision of facilities for the handling of relatively small amounts of materials under conditions in which these materials are at some stage exposed to the air in the workroom or cubicle. This will necessitate close attention to the quality of the air and the maintenance of clean conditions in the room itself.

Manufacturing operations in which live agents are handled under conditions in which sterile materials are exposed, albeit transiently, to the environment, represent one of the most difficult challenges in the design of facilities which satisfy all aspects of modern manufacturing requirements. The principles described here for seed production can be modified and extended for other aspects of the manufacturing operation and will be cross-referenced in other sections of this chapter.

The European guidelines (Commission of the European Communities, 1992) recommend that sterile operations of the type described here are carried out in a laminar airflow cabinet (meeting the guidelines' Grade A classification) which has been installed in a "clean" room (meeting the guidelines' Grade B standard). Such a facility would require a supply of HEPA-filtered air, at a rate that provides at least 20 changes per hour to the room itself, and a similarly filtered extractor system. A full garment change facility for operators would also be required. This too, would need its own supply and extractor of HEPA-filtered air – providing the same level of air replacement as for the laboratory. A pressure differential of at least 1.5 mm water gauge should be maintained between the changing room and the laboratory. The laboratory will also need some form of transfer lock, preferably capable of fumigation, for the movement of materials into and out of the seed production facility.

With the introduction of appropriate quality assurance procedures and a suitable arrangement of pressure differentials between corridors, anterooms, changing rooms and laboratories, such a facility provides an effective barrier against the ingress of contamination from external sources (including the environment, the operators and materials brought into the unit) and an effective barrier ensuring containment of the live organisms handled within the facility. A convenient way of achieving this is to hold the workroom under negative pressure, make the changing room more strongly negative and provide an anteroom at a positive pressure. In this way the changing room acts as a plenum or "sink" and provides a barrier against air movements from either side.

Recently, totally enclosed isolation units have been developed, in which operators work through glove ports. The units are fitted with "pass-through" hatches, which can be fumigated, and sometimes even include environmental control facilities. Such units, although expensive, can be highly effective, enabling different organisms and/or operations to be handled in adjacent units without compromising either the environment or the operator.

A "master" seed bank should be established, based on an isolate of the material from which the vaccine is to be prepared and, in the case of viral vaccines, the substrate (or cell line) on which the agent is to be cultivated. The manufacturer will need to be assured that these materials are free from all adventitious agents which might cause contamination losses in the manufacturing process or untoward effects, or even disease, in animals on which the vaccine is subsequently used or on others which are in contact with such vaccinated animals.

In addition to an assurance of the purity of the material, the manufacturer also needs to be assured that the seed material will routinely produce high, and therefore economically acceptable, yields in the production system and that it produces a safe, reliable and effective end product. Examples of these requirements can be found in the series of documents issued by the European Union's European Committee for Veterinary Medicinal Products (EC, n.d.a and n.d.b).

Aliquots of suitable material need to be stored for long periods under conditions appropriate for the particular entity. Depending on the organism, storage over liquid nitrogen, storage at -70°C, freeze-drying or, occasionally, storage at cool-room temperatures may all be appropriate. The essential requirements are that the organism should not lose titre or undergo any change in its characteristics while in storage for long periods. From this material it is customary to set up one or a number of working seed banks, which can be stored under similar conditions to the master bank and used to initiate each production cycle or series of cycles. By careful use of the seed banks in this way the original master bank becomes almost immortal and can be used to support production over long periods without the serial passaging of the organism to a level where the characteristics of the seed material itself might become modified.

MEDIA PRODUCTION

The media used for the cultivation of the agents under manufacture can be purchased ready prepared or as sterile concentrates from reliable sources. They can also be prepared on-site from component materials. In most cases considerations of cost and the volumes required dictate that media are produced on-site.

By their very nature, the components and media used for manufacture usually tend to encourage the growth of adventitious contaminants, and care needs to be taken to ensure the components themselves and the facilities in which they are prepared are as free from such contaminants as possible. It is usual to provide a dedicated media production facility, close to but separated from other manufacturing areas on the site. This unit should be well ordered, free from materials not immediately required for the process and amenable to routine and methodical cleaning. It may be considered appropriate to provide a working environment of HEPA-filtered air and it is preferable that staff working in the area should not enter other manufacturing areas on the same day.

The components used for media production should meet the general requirements outlined in the section Manufacturing materials (p. 176) and particular care should be taken over materials of biological origin which form an essential part of many culture media. In some countries there are specific regulatory requirements governing the use and testing of such materials (Medicines Control Agency, n.d.). These are intended to ensure that no disease-causing agent is introduced to the manufacturing process and, as a minimum, the manufacturer needs to be sure that the animals from which the materials, for example serum, were obtained, were healthy and from a disease-free herd and that the method of collection and processing was unlikely to have adversely affected the quality of such materials.

Depending on the nature of the manufacturing process, once prepared, the medium may be sterilized and put into storage containers – or vice versa. Alternatively, the medium may be transferred directly into the production vessel before or after the sterilization cycle. The dispensing of sterilized media into multiple storage containers may require sterile handling facilities similar to those described in the section Seed production and storage (p. 176).

ANTIGEN PRODUCTION

The facilities required for antigen production will depend on the nature of the organisms from which the vaccine is to be prepared, the manufacturing methods to be employed and the proposed scale of the operation. Manipulations in which sterile materials are effectively exposed to the operator and/or the local environment during manufacture will require facilities that are essentially similar to, but obviously may need to be larger than, those described for the production of seed materials. In cases where the utilization of facilities (and therefore volume throughput) is low, the same unit may be used for both functions, with the provision of suitable safeguards between operations.

Where all operations are carried out within totally enclosed vessels, pumps, pipework, etc. the inside of the equipment may be considered as the manufacturing environment and a somewhat less rigorous environment is usually considered acceptable for the location of the manufacturing equipment. Nevertheless, it is important to pay attention to the design and operation of these areas in order to minimize the likelihood of adventitious contamination arising or persisting within them. Important features to consider will be: easily cleaned surface finishes, drainage, the ventilation system, the means by which materials enter and leave the area and operator access.

Where practicable it is desirable to provide enclosed processing areas with a supply of HEPA-filtered air and for antigen production (where by definition live agents are handled) it will be preferable to hold these areas at a pressure negative to the surrounding areas. As described for seed production areas, the careful planning of layouts and pressure differentials can be used to create a situation in which the work area is protected from possible external adventitious contamination, and yet there is still a containment barrier at the point of entry through the changing room.

To provide safeguards during enclosed manufacturing operations for the integrity of both the contents of the vessels and equipment and of the environment in the room, consideration should be given to the means by which samples are taken, and additions made, during processing.

Most equipment used for large-scale manufacturing operations can and should be sterilized *in situ* with steam. Equipment which cannot be steam-sterilized presents a more difficult problem, and care should be taken to ensure any procedures used for chemical sterilization are validated under the actual conditions of the operation beforehand. Assuming that facilities are available for the *in situ* steam-sterilization of major equipment, it should be a relatively simple matter to ensure that the connections used for sampling, additions and vessel-to-vessel transfers are also steam-sterilized *in situ* before and after effecting transfers.

Where some items of equipment must be chemically sterilized it is preferable to arrange the plant in such a way that as much of the equipment, pipework and valves as possible is steam-sterilized and reliance is placed on chemical sterilization only for the essential components that cannot be subjected to steam under pressure.

ANTIGEN INACTIVATION

Unless the vaccine undergoing manufacture is a live attenuated one, the next stage in vaccine preparation is inactivation of the antigen. The major dilemma in this procedure – from the viewpoint of facility design and operational convenience – is that the process, by definition, starts with live material and after the commencement of its inactivation every effort should be made to ensure there is no possibility of its being contaminated with other live material.

These constraints have implications for both the inactivation vessel and the workroom itself. To overcome the possible risk of droplets from within the inactivation vessel (which may not have come in contact with the inactivant) reinfecting the vessel contents, it is considered good practice to transfer the mixture of live antigen and inactivant to another sterile vessel after a period of mixing. These procedures are usually carried out in the area in which the antigen was produced and the closed vessel containing the inactivating material is either isolated within the facility or transferred to a separate holding room while the inactivation process is completed. During this process it is often found preferable not to sample or open the vessel for any reason. Conversely, there is a good argument for monitoring the progress of each inactivation cycle, and this can only be done by sampling. The most appropriate approach in each situation may well depend on the regulatory environment or pharmacopoeial requirement for the product in question. In either case, it would be prudent to introduce some form of formal quality assurance clearance procedure before material that has completed the inactivation cycle is transferred for downstream processing or vaccine blending.

DOWNSTREAM PROCESSING

The requirements for any downstream processing depend on whether the product is live or inactivated and on the needs of the manufacturing process itself. While inactivated, innocuity tested antigens of different types may, with reasonable safeguards, be handled in the same area, a separate area will be needed for live antigens. Different live organisms can usually be handled in the same area providing it can be cleared, cleaned and fumigated between successive production cycles. If production throughput is high, however, it may be preferable to have separate areas for different products.

The most common type of downstream processing operation is probably concentration of the antigen, but other necessary procedures may include various purification or separation stages. Wherever possible it is preferable to carry out downstream processing of inactivated products after the inactivation stage has been completed in order to avoid the complication of handling the live material. Such processing should, wherever possible, be carried out in a separate area to that in which the live material was produced. Where this is not practicable, further innocuity tests should be carried out on the completion of operations and material should not be passed on for blending until satisfactory results are obtained from these tests.

As emphasized previously, the workrooms in which inactivated antigens are handled should be free from other live organisms and preferably held under a positive overpressure of HEPA-filtered air. If the manufacturing operation necessitates transient exposure of the product to the atmosphere of the room, the room should meet the standards defined for seed production but at positive pressure in relation to its surroundings. Enclosed processing operations may be carried out in a less rigorous environment, but a positive pressure of HEPA-filtered air is desirable. The same considerations relating to cleanliness, material and operator access will apply as were indicated in the section Antigen production (p. 178).

Where live attenuated vaccines are produced, the manufacturing area should be held under negative air pressure and operations may be carried out effectively in areas similar to those described for seed and antigen production.

The equipment required for downstream processing should preferably be sterilized *in situ* by steam under pressure but, where this is not possible, chemical sterilization using a fully validated process is likely to prove satisfactory. The remarks relating to chemical sterilization in the antigen production area also apply to this situation.

Whether or not separate rooms will be required for the downstream processing stages of manufacture depends on the nature and complexity of these operations in relation to other activities. In many situations, however, it will be appropriate and sufficient to perform these stages in a part of the room used for blending the vaccine.

VACCINE BLENDING

Vaccine blending is usually a mixing operation based on the combination of one or more antigens – each of which has been shown to conform to the manufacturer's quality requirements – together with the other components of the vaccine, such as adjuvant, preservative and frequently a diluent.

The mixing operation may be simple or may involve the use of specialized mixing equipment, as for example in the preparation of oil-emulsion vaccines. Antigens for blending have a high financial value resulting from the materials and labour which have been expended in their preparation and testing. It is therefore of particular importance that all the other components used, including both additional antigens and the blending materials, are of suitable quality and integrity and will result in the production of a satisfactory, sterile, safe and effective vaccine.

The blending of vaccine will usually require the same type of facilities as are required for any of the downstream processing stages and, as indicated previously, it is frequently appropriate to carry out both activities in the same area and in some cases even to use the same equipment.

VACCINE FILLING

At each successive manufacturing stage the investment in labour and materials increases and the manufacturer should introduce safeguards to ensure that only satisfactory materials are passed on for the next stage. This is certainly true for the filling operation, where the inconvenience and loss associated with discarding final filled product is considerable.

Filling operations almost inevitably expose the final product to the atmosphere at the actual dispensing point, so these operations are best carried out under a laminar curtain of HEPA-filtered air within a sterile room. Because of the large volume and number of containers involved in most filling operations, sterile rooms of considerable size are frequently required. As has been described elsewhere in this chapter, the facility will need its own sterile changing rooms, a satisfactory means of getting sterile materials (including final containers and product) into the room and a means of moving the filled containers out of the room – all without harming the filling operation itself. The basic requirements of the filling room will be similar to those described in the preceding sections for rooms in which sterile product is transiently exposed to the atmosphere. The air pressure within the room should be either positive or negative relative to the surrounding area, depending on whether the facility is for a live or inactivated product.

Final vaccine containers which can be heat-sterilized are best introduced directly into the filling room by means of a sterilization cycle through a double-ended "pass-through" sterilizer. Other types of final container, such as those sterilized by radiation, should be sterilized double-wrapped and in such a way that the outer packaging can be removed outside the filling room and the inner wrapping surface decontaminated or fumigated in a transfer lock prior to being introduced into the filling room proper.

Removal of filled containers can be done either on a batch basis at the conclusion of filling operations or continuously throughout the process. For large batches the latter tends to be preferable and this is frequently accomplished by means of a conveyor belt. The belt should not emerge directly from the sterile room and subsequently re-enter it.

In the case of live filled products, many will require a freeze-drying stage after the filling operation. It will be very convenient if the freeze-drier can be loaded directly from the filling area. If the freeze-drier is double-ended the product may then be transferred for storage without re-entering the filling area. For single door machines, however, it will be necessary to pass the vials back into the filling facility when unloading the machine. This tends to reduce the flexibility of the filling unit which could otherwise be decontaminated and set up for processing the next batch (which could involve a different antigen).

In all cases where live products are handled it should be remembered that the filled containers may be contaminated on the outside and some form of surface decontamination will need to be considered once the final container seals have been applied.

QUALITY ASSURANCE

For the purposes of this chapter, quality assurance will be taken to encompass the elements of quality control (QC), environmental monitoring, validation and documentation leading to batch release. Each manufacturing site will require the services of a QC unit, which should preferably be located in a different building to that of the production facilities. It is highly convenient if the QC unit is situated on the manufacturing site, but specialized tests, especially those requiring sophisticated equipment, may have to be carried out by external organizations or units.

QC facilities on a manufacturing site should be operated in such a manner that the risk of agents being transmitted from the QC unit to the production facilities is minimized. This may be effected by means of the HEPA filtration of extract air from the QC unit together with restrictions on the movement of personnel and materials. Movement of samples and documentation between units may give rise to particular problems, but arrangements which permit safe and effective transfer of materials for test and the two-way transmission of appropriate documentation are not difficult to establish.

It will be important to distinguish between those test procedures that relate directly to the quality of the manufactured product (for which there should be clearly defined acceptance criteria) and those that contribute towards an overall understanding of the manufacturing process. The latter, when considered individually, would not normally be used to condemn a production batch.

Apart from both quality control and in-process tests on materials and product during the manufacturing process, the producer should also continuously monitor the manufacturing environment, in terms of both its physical and biological performances. In this way potential problems can be identified before they become critical and corrective action may be taken before production losses are experienced.

The range of environmental monitoring that might be considered is too broad to list here in detail, but it should cover at least all of the following: environmental bacterial levels in both sterile and general manufacturing areas; the quality of process fluids (particularly water); airflow pressure differentials and filter integrity; and equipment performance (particularly of sterilizers). To establish that process equipment and operating procedures are capable of performing the tasks required of them on a routine basis and under the conditions of normal use, it is necessary to have them validated. This is usually carried out as part of the initial commissioning process and, although time-consuming, thorough testing of each stage of the process at the outset can save major losses later on. Furthermore, the regular revalidation of equipment will not only increase confidence in the operation but help to identify problem areas before they become critical.

All of the above procedures should be formally documented and the documentation made available for review, so that – in considering either the factory manufacturing record or the production of an individual batch – the results of mandatory QC tests, in-process control tests, environmental and validation studies can all be taken into account. In this way, the manufacturer can have a far greater degree of confidence in the products than would otherwise be possible from the results of statutory QC tests alone and, when difficulties occur, the possible causes can more easily be identified and eliminated.

CONCLUSIONS

Careful adherence to the principles of good facility design and manufacturing practice should help to ensure that production plants function at a high level of efficiency and that losses are a rare event. Although there is undoubtedly an element of additional expenditure related to the issues raised here, much can be done without significantly increasing installation costs. Where additional expenditure is involved, the analysis should take into account the savings associated with greater production efficiency and reduced losses and also the greater confidence in the product of customers and the relevant control authorities.

In a similar way, attention should be paid to quality throughout the manufacturing operation and every effort should be made to build quality into the product, rather than relying on testing for it.

With the appropriate design of facilities, high levels of productivity can be achieved and in-process losses can be minimized. There will also be a high degree of probability that the filled vaccine will pass all required final product tests and perform in a safe and effective manner when used in the field.

BIBLIOGRAPHY

Commission of the European Communities. 1992. *The rules governing medicinal products in the European Community*, Vol. IV, *Good manufacturing practice for medicinal products*. Directorate General for International Market and Industrial Affairs.

EC. (n.d.a) *General requirements for the production and control of live mammalian bacterial and viral vaccines for veterinary use.* Committee for Veterinary Medicinal Products of the European Community.

EC. (n.d.b) *General requirements for the production and control of inactivated mammalian bacterial and viral vaccines for veterinary use.* Committee for Veterinary Medicinal Products of the European Community.

Government of the United Kingdom. 1983. *Compendium of guidelines on the quality control of veterinary immunological products.* Weybridge, UK, Biological Products and Standards Department, Central Veterinary Laboratory, Ministry of Agriculture, Fisheries and Food.

Medicines Control Agency. (n.d.) *Use of substances of animal origin in the manufacture of veterinary vaccines.* Document MAL 67. London.

Parenteral Drug Association. 1978. *Validation of steam sterilization cycles.* Technical Monograph No. 1, Philadelphia, Pa., USA.

Parenteral Drug Association. 1981. *Validation of dry heat processes used for sterilization and depyrogenization.* Technical Monograph No. 3, Philadelphia, Pa., USA.

Sharp, J.R. 1983. *Guide to good pharmaceutical manufacturing practice.* London, Her Majesty's Stationery Office.

Design, repair and maintenance of vaccine manufacturing establishments and equipment

J. Estefanell and L. Mesopir

DESIGN

During the initial stage of designing a vaccine manufacturing establishment (VME) the following factors must be taken into consideration:

- national and international legal requirements;
- site location;
- general building layout;
- utilities and services;
- building construction and finishes;
- processes;
- equipment;
- maintenance and repair of premises, plant and equipment;
- maintenance records.

NATIONAL AND INTERNATIONAL LEGAL REQUIREMENTS

A VME is obliged to comply with legal requirements which may not be the same in every country. Taking the most stringent from different countries and compiling them in a theoretical international standard requirements for VMEs gives some indication of the most severe conditions which a VME would have to comply with.

The first question to be asked is whether the VME is to supply the national or international market. The costs of construction, equipment and the manufacturing process will depend on this.

SITE LOCATION

When planning and siting a VME the following points need to be considered: altitude, accessibility, terrain, neighbours, climate, security, noise, future developments, pollution and local regulations.

Altitude

Altitude affects the efficiency of, for example, internal combustion engines, standby electricity generator sets and tractors. It also affects the boiling point of water in steam boilers, etc. Engines and boilers are normally rated at sea level, therefore it is important to know what efficiency is to be expected at different altitudes and, when commissioning such plants, this factor has to be considered.

Terrain

VMEs should be sited in areas that are free from flooding and easily accessible. The ground has to be such that the foundations of the building are on a sound solid surface. It should also be in an area where such services as drainage and sewage disposal are accessible and, in cases where these have to be discharged into the ground, the ground should be such that it can accept or absorb the effluent so disposed of.

Climate

Weather conditions influence several of the requirements to be considered in the design, with regard to the construction and use of the premises. Hot and dry weather implies that the VME has to have air-conditioning and air filters will probably be required where dust is a constant problem. With hot, wet weather, increased drying capacity will be necessary, particularly for air under pressure, and a specific type of roof and windows will have to be used.

Noise

If the VME is adjacent to such high-noise areas as major motorways, industrial sites or airports the noise level could affect the working atmosphere within the laboratory.

Pollution

The VME should be protected from the environment and the environment from the VME. It should be sited where there is no pollution from the surrounding area, but as this can never be guaranteed completely, means for water and air filtration/purification should be installed, to ensure their appropriate quality for industrial use, otherwise contamination problems may arise.

The VME itself must be designed so as to ensure that no gaseous, liquid or solid waste disposal contaminates the soil, water streams or atmosphere. A VME can cause aerial pollution by oil-fired boilers and incinerators, if these are not well maintained.

The health and safety of personnel can also be a problem unless buildings and equipment are designed to protect both the workers and the products and are well maintained to ensure that they perform to the required standards.

Local regulations

Each country has its own regulations on the construction of buildings. These requirements must conform to the published regulations pertaining to issues such as sewage and effluent discharge, the drilling of water boreholes and wells and the standard of electric installations in the establishment.

Accessibility

The site should be accessible by road and should be such that strict entry restrictions can be enforced.

Neighbours

The establishment should be located on a site where public buildings such as hospitals, farms (especially those with livestock) and factories which could cause pollution are at some distance. This is not always possible so, as noted before, the design should have provision for the installation of purification systems for air and water supplies if needed.

Security

The VME should guarantee that no disease outbreak will occur as a result of its manufacturing activities. This means the provision of adequate installations, strict adherence to good manufacturing practices (GMPs), an adequate security system for the entry and exit of personnel, staff, visitors and contractors and a good perimeter fence.

Future developments

The site should be so designed that there is room for future expansions. Buildings should be arranged so that central services such as electricity and steam generating plant and administration blocks will not be affected during future expansions.

GENERAL BUILDING LAYOUT

Consideration has first to be given to the requirements of the different areas of a VME.

General areas are those where there is no reciprocal threat between product and environment and no special requirements other than order, cleanliness (standard GMPs) and possible temperature conditioning for personnel comfort or product conservation. These are: administration offices, general stores, material washing and preparation areas and areas for labelling, packing, storage and dispatch of the final products.

Restricted areas are those where live pathogens are handled and may impose a threat to the environment. These are: laboratories where field samples are handled, areas where seeds are prepared, areas where large-scale production takes place, areas where live vaccines are freeze-dried and areas where challenge tests take place.

In all these areas, air, liquid and solid effluents must be decontaminated and personnel leaving the area must, at least, change their clothes. Depending on the pathogen handled, showering may also be required. Access should be strictly restricted to those working in the area.

Air pressure should be negative to the ambient by air extraction through absolute, high-efficiency particle adsorption (HEPA) filters. When live pathogens are handled in open processes (e.g. freeze-drying), provisions for the supply of sterile air to the area, together with the use of safety cabinets to protect the personnel and the product are important. Liquids and solids must go through chemical and / or physical decontamination processes to avoid contamination of the environment before disposal.

Clean areas where the product must be protected from the environment include: media production, inactivated antigen process and storage, inactivated vaccine blending and inactivated vaccine filling areas. The air pressure in these areas should be positive with respect to ambient and, where sterile products are handled in open processes (e.g. sterile filling), sterile ambient conditions should be provided.

During the initial stages of designing a VME, the following are some of the many factors that should be considered:

- what vaccines are required to be produced;
- what types of laboratories are required;
- what types of animal isolation units are required;
- what equipment is required for each specific task;
- how many people are required;
- what recreational facilities are required;
- are some of the employees to be accommodated on-site;
- what services are required in the whole establishment or in specific laboratories;
- how effluents are to be treated and discharged;
- what storage facilities are required.

Once agreement on these points has been established, those concerned with the design should go through every detail and consult those who are to use the facilities, so that at this initial stage nothing is omitted.

Owing to the lack of such coordination, some establishments have had problems modifying their original plans and in many cases this has resulted in more money having to be spent.

UTILITIES AND SERVICES

Essential services are understood to be: water, furnace oils, electric power, automotive fuels, air, communications, gases, effluent treatment and steam.

Water

There should be an adequate source of water for the establishment to run smoothly. In laboratories two types of water are normally used: mains water (for cooling and heating) and purified water.

The quality of mains water is very important as this will dictate the cost of running steam boilers and water distillation plant. Where mains water is soft, say up to 23 parts per million (ppm) of hardness, scaling becomes only a minor problem and the chemicals required to descale the boilers and water stills are not expensive. Where water is available from a borehole, it is usually hard. Treatment is expensive when a water-softening plant becomes necessary.

Adequate water storage is also very important. Ideally the VME would have an elevated water reservoir from which water will flow under gravity to all water points in the establishment. The reservoir should be accessible for regular cleaning. It should also be noted that it is important to check the quality of water and, if necessary, the water in the reservoir should be treated according to normal health requirements.

Mains water must be free of pathogens, pesticides and heavy metals since traces of any of these coming into contact with production material and equipment may lead to altered production conditions.

Cooling or heating water is used for culture vessels, process equipment or ambient temperature conditioning. It must be controlled to ensure that it will not impose a threat of chemical or biological contamination to the production process.

Purified water is obtained by demineralization followed by distillation or reverse osmosis. It should be sterilized and kept sterile or in such conditions (80°C) that will prevent the growth of contaminating organisms. It should be pyrogen free.

Electric power

In many developing countries the electric power supply is not reliable. There are permanent and serious electrical fluctuations which harm electrical equipment installed in the establishment. It is advisable to install voltage stabilizers to prevent the malfunctioning of sensitive electrical and electronic equipment, such as control panels and centrifuges, and also a power factor correction facility at the main power distribution point, as this will reduce electricity consumption and protect electrical equipment such as motors.

An electricity standby generator plant should be considered as a standard piece of equipment. To determine the size of the standby generator the following factors should be taken into consideration:

- the total electrical load installed;
- the type of fuel used in the generator engine;
- the essential electrical power demand in the VME, as this will indicate the minimum size of the generating plant;
- future load expansion.

The generating plant must be able to start up automatically under any of the following situations:

- there is no power from the main supply;
- phase failure;
- short circuit;
- low voltage.

AIR

A VME needs various ventilation systems. An adequate rate of ventilation is essential to protect the plant personnel and the product from solvents or fermentation gases and from particulate or biological contamination. Up to 20 air changes per hour may be required to maintain proper process conditions, under a positive or negative pressure differential with respect to ambient.

It may be necessary to sterilize the air supplied and/or extracted from a particular area or to heat, cool or dry this air, in which case energy will be saved by recycling it as much as possible. Specific exhaust systems may be necessary to remove dangerous gases (toxic, flammable, etc.) to prevent them from diffusing into the working space.

Gases

Generally, the gases used in vaccine manufacturing establishments include: air under pressure, carbon dioxide, liquid nitrogen, methane, oxygen, acetylene and refrigeration gases such as R12, R22 and R502.

The availability of these gases is important because the operations of the establishment can be seriously handicapped if they are in short supply.

Air under pressure must be obtained from a clean source, should be filtered and should be dried before and after the compression process. This will prevent rust formation and the blockage or damage of prefilters and sterilizing filters by condensates or particles of rust scale. Most other gases will probably be obtained from specialized suppliers according to specifications.

It is important to note that several refrigeration gases are being phased out because of the harm they cause to the ozone layer of the earth's atmosphere. When choosing refrigeration equipment, this point should be considered and new technologies in this area should be favoured in spite of their probable initial higher costs.

Steam

In a VME, steam is used in small amounts for heating purposes in stills, temperature conditioners for ambient air and in fermenters, and in large amounts for sterilizing purposes in autoclaves, sterile lines, fermenters, process equipment and vaccine blending and filling vessels.

Generally, saturated steam is used, overpressurized at 6 to 10 kg/cm^2 in the generator and reduced to working pressure at the points of use. Steam can be produced from individual electrically heated boilers or from a central fuel-fired steam generation plant.

The availability of electricity and oil fuel varies from country to country but, in general, fuel-fired steam generators are cheaper to run than electrical ones. The steam supplied to steam receivers should be clean (free of undesirable chemicals "dragged" from the boiler) and filtered through 0.1-micron sintered 316 grade stainless steel filters. The pipework has to be of non-corrosive material, ideally 316 grade stainless steel. Safety devices should be fitted on the receivers. Condensate from steam lines should be returned to the boiler water feed tank. Steam and condensate pipelines should be lagged (insulated). If the steam is obtained from tap or industrial water, great attention must be given to impurities in the water and added softeners. "Dragging" of water from the boiler is possible on occasions of sudden high peak demand of steam but standard procedures should minimize these peak demands, as they will also condition the size of the boiler. The use of clean steam obtained from purified water is most advisable, but its high investment cost may not be compensated by the possible improvement of performance of the process.

It is also advisable to maintain steam pressure in the system for 24 hours a day. Vibrations provoked by the steam "hammering", which occurs when steam lines are warming up, impose a great stress on the integrity of sterile process lines and equipment.

Furnace oils

Where used the reliability of supply should be considered.

Automotive fuel

This commodity is nearly always available in developing countries but at high cost. Automotive fuel is normally used on electricity standby generating sets and vehicles.

Communications

Good communications are essential for the effective operation of any enterprise.

Effluent treatment

Where disease security has to be controlled, the treatment of gaseous, liquid and solid effluents must be considered. Laboratories and animal isolation units working with high-risk pathogens (e.g. foot-and-mouth disease or anthrax vaccine) should have:

- continuous air extraction through absolute filters to maintain negative pressure with respect to ambient at all times, thus preventing the escape of contaminated air from the unit through personnel or materials entry and exit pathways;
- discharge of liquid effluents chemically treated in a confined secure area, under an absolute air extraction system (the pH of the effluent is increased to 11.5 [0.25 percent free alkali] by the addition of concentrated sodium hydroxide solution, and maintained at this level for at least 24 hours before neutralization and discharge into the normal sewage treatment) or heat-treated in a pressure vessel located below ground level (so that the effluent can flow into it by gravity). The heat treatment of the effluent should be carried out under pressure, preferably by direct injection of steam or by electric heaters. The temperature has to be held at 121°C for about two hours, depending to some extent on the volume to be treated. The treated effluent may be discharged into the main city drainage/sewage system or, in areas where this is not available, into soak pits.
- all solid materials (glassware, paper, empty containers, tools, spares, the exterior of containers of inactivated antigen, etc.) decontaminated by one of the following means: autoclaving (heating up to 121°C for 30 minutes), hypochlorite, mild acid or strong alkali soaking treatment and/or formaldehyde fumigation before leaving the restricted area.

BUILDING CONSTRUCTION AND FINISHES

The building construction and finishes should ensure protection of the vaccine during manufacture from contamination and should permit efficient cleaning and avoid the accumulation of dust and dirt.

The construction design must be such as to prevent the entry or harbouring of insects, birds or rodents. Surfaces should be smooth, robust, non-porous, easy to clean and easy to maintain. They should be free from cracks, crevices and ledges.

The finishes of walls, floors, ceilings and doors should be of good quality and should not allow the accumulation of particulate matter. There should not be recesses that cannot be cleaned.

Where floors may come in contact with chemicals such as diluted acid or alkali solutions, the floor must be protected with chemical-resistant covering. This is very important since, if it is not done in time, serious damage can be caused to the floor and consequently to the foundation of the building. Expansion joints and cracks should be sealed with a suitable resilient compound.

There have been major problems with leaking roofs in many VMEs. Most flat roofs leak and in countries where rainfall is high and climatic changes are significant it is suggested that pitched roofs are used rather than roof slabs. Sometimes flat roofs are necessary where specific equipment for supply services to the establishment has to be mounted. If this is the case, proper design should be made to cover the roof as much as possible.

The ceilings in the building should be constructed and finished so that they are solid, capable of being completely sealed and easy to clean. Doors and windows should have a smooth impervious finish and should close tightly. Where the production room is under a controlled environment, the windows should be fixed and the doors should have seals. If the building is maintained under controlled environmental conditions, say negative or positive pressure, airlocks must be provided in manufacturing areas.

The paint used on walls and ceilings should be of a quality that can be cleaned.

Where there is a lot of dust, entrances to the VME should have airlocks to minimize its entry into the building. The inlet for the supply of air to the ventilation system should be sited in a position that will minimize the amount of dust blown into the building and it should be provided with filters of a large dust-holding capacity.

Process

Work must be done according to good laboratory practices (GLPs) and good manufacturing practices (GMPs). After a thorough study of the process, the necessary equipment and procedures should be defined and validated and detailed, precise descriptions of all procedures must be written.

There is a great variety of production processes. Mammalian cells, bacterial cells (aerobic and anaerobic), mycoplasma and virus cultures all share some common requirements, but each also imposes specific conditions related to the product that has to be manufactured.

The final product may be a live or an inactivated vaccine. Inactivation can take place before or after purification steps (such as centrifugal separation, filtration, precipitation, ultrafiltration, affinity chromatography and immunoaffinity chromatography) and it is necessary to blend active components and excipients under sterile conditions, before bottling the final product.

Equipment

All the equipment used in the production process must be validated and a manual of operating procedures should be prepared. All the procedures involving the use of the process equipment have performance parameters (pressure, agitation, temperature, pH, dissolved oxygen, oxidation-reduction potential, flow control, etc.) which require monitoring/controlling equipment.

The ageing of equipment tends to increase the possibility of failure and may reduce the efficiency of the process, unless a good maintenance programme is followed.

REPAIR AND MAINTENANCE OF PREMISES, PLANT AND EQUIPMENT

Maintenance demands large resources of labour and money but it is absolutely essential if facilities such as plant, machinery, equipment and buildings are to remain in an acceptable operating condition ready for maximum utilization.

Many developing country VMEs have no maintenance facilities. This is a very important issue since, without trained maintenance personnel, the successful running of the establishment will be jeopardized. There should be a maintenance department comprising: an engineer/technician, a fitter/plumber/welder, a refrigeration mechanic, a carpenter, an electronic/electrical technician and a mason/bricklayer).

Basic tools and equipment required in a repair and maintenance workshop

The following is the recommended list of basic tools and equipment required to carry out standard repair work on process equipment, machines, buildings, etc.

Fitter/welder/plumber's tools comprising:

- various sizes of metric spanners (ring and open-ended);
- box spanners from 6 to 22 mm;
- a set of screwdrivers;
- a measuring tape;
- a brass drift;
- punches;

- a filter gauge,
- pliers;
- a ball peen hammer;
- pipe wrenches of various sizes;
- a portable electrical drill.

Refrigeration mechanic's tools comprising:
- various metric spanners (both ring and open-ended);
- a set of refrigeration spanners;
- an Avometer;
- a refrigeration charging manifold;
- a portable refrigerant cylinder;
- a set of electrical screwdrivers;
- insulated cutter pliers;
- a thermometer.

Electronic/electrical technician's tools comprising:
- a set of electrical screwdrivers;
- an Avometer;
- a diode tester;
- electronic test/check apparatus (volt-ampere meter, etc.);
- a vacuum pump.

Carpenter/mason's tools comprising:
- basic general tools.

General workshop equipment comprising:
- oxygen/acetylene welding cylinders, regulators and complete torches with hosepipes;
- a tungsten or metal inert gas arc welder;
- a pedestal drilling machine;
- a bench grinder;
- a pressure gauge testing/calibration stand;
- thread cutting tools,
- pipe vices;
- bench vices;
- a pipe bender.

When selecting equipment or machines it is important to consider their complexity of maintenance, the availability of spares and the knowledge and expertise of maintenance staff. There have been cases where a VME has acquired equipment that was so sophisticated that nobody was able either to operate or maintain it. When an establishment acquires an expensive machine or piece of equipment, it should be ensured that whoever is to take care of the machine is properly trained by the supplier or manufacturer in its operation and maintenance. Planned preventive maintenance is the best method to adopt but it requires that spares be available at all times, and this is a major problem for many VMEs in developing countries.

Preventive maintenance is carried out on plant equipment or machines to prevent breakdowns. It is done on a scheduled basis and also when required, especially if machine performance is seen to be deteriorating.

To determine when a machine should undergo preventive maintenance it is necessary to know the machine's breakdown characteristics and also to adhere to the manufacturer's recommended schedules.

The stocking of spare parts is difficult in developing countries owing to a lack of finances and spares not being available locally when required. It is advisable, therefore, that when a machine or piece of equipment is bought a reasonable number of the spares recommended by the manufacturer should be kept in stock and supplied regularly under contract, for at least three or more years, to ensure the proper operation of the equipment.

INSPECTION

Each step of the production process should have a written inspection procedure to be followed and recorded. Equipment inspections can be carried out by different individuals as long as they are all specialists for the objects of the inspection. Easy access and correct illumination are important for inspection procedures, as poor working conditions lead to careless, inefficient work.

The following tests should be performed on process or controlling equipment for validation, when the equipment is to be used for the first time, after a modification or for verification within a maintenance routine, when applicable.

Leak tests

Leak tests should be performed on culture vessels, process and blending vessels, associated pipelines and, in general, on all pressurizable equipment. Such equipment should be filled with liquid (usually water alone or with detergent to promote penetration) in order to check the integrity of the system. These tests should be carried out under both positive and negative pressure (vacuum) as leaks may show up under only one situation.

Temperature mapping

It is necessary to ensure that the sterilizing or working temperatures are achieved at all required points of the equipment and associated pipelines. Multipoint recording equipment fitted with thermocouples will facilitate this test.

The following equipment should have temperature maps to confirm that it works correctly and that the procedures achieve the results expected:

- liquid nitrogen containers for seeds or product storage (-190°C);
- deep freezes and freezers for seeds and product storage (-120°C, -80°C, -30°C, -20°C);
- refrigeration cabinet or cold rooms (4°C);
- autoclaves and ovens with different sterilizing temperatures and workload conditions;
- culture vessels, intermediate process vessels and associated pipelines for sterilizing, working and storage conditions.

Depending on the size of the equipment and process conditions, between six and 30 recorded points will provide sufficient information to assess or confirm whether the equipment is working correctly and whether the procedures followed are achieving the expected results.

Sterilization

Sterilization parameters are established according to temperature mapping and reaction times. There is a tendency to increase sterilization time to ensure that it has been effective. This is misguided; a correct procedure should sterilize for the minimum length of time required, thus prolonging the working life of sensors and equipment. If steam traps are being used, they must be periodically tested during sterilization with an external contact thermometer.

Washing

Dirt, particularly protein, must be eliminated from the process equipment and associated lines, before the next process takes place. Careless washing leads to protein coat build-up, increased contamination rates, earlier instrument and equipment deterioration and, in general, poorer process conditions. This becomes particularly critical in centrifugal separation equipment.

Membrane integrity testing

Sterilizing (HEPA) air filters for ventilation and laminar flow units (LFUs) and sterilizing air filters for process equipment should have their integrity tested regularly by means of: specific particle-size oil aerosol penetration tests (applicable to all filters); or other tests, such as the water intrusion test applicable to hydrophobic air filters, which are generally used in small filtration units installed in process equipment.

Aerosol penetration detection equipment

is expensive and a contract service with a specialized company may be the best solution to having filters tested regularly.

Process equipment

Culture vessels and associated pipelines. Usually, standard culture vessels are bought from a specialized firm, but sometimes they are built to match the required purpose. The culture vessel should be insulated (lagged) and the stirring system should be magnetically driven whenever possible – this is the most reliable, long-term, leak-proof system.

The slope (gradient) of the associated pipelines is of great importance for the proper cleaning and sterilization of the system. The system must be equipped with vent or drain valves to prevent air or condensate accumulation in piping during steam-sterilization. Special care must be given to welded joins as these may cause failure by developing minor cracks. Contact with steam or chilled water is particularly critical for welded joins. Welds may also suffer great tensile stress owing to great and sudden changes in temperature.

All drain lines should be connected to an enclosed drain system to prevent aerosol formation and increased contamination risks.

Air filters. The glass fibre "depth" type of sterilizing air filter can deal with gases at high rates of humidity, but is unable to sterilize filtered gas when it is wet and it is therefore essential to prevent the "dragging" of condensates into this type of filter which is gradually being replaced by the hydrophobic membrane type. These new filters are very reliable and resistant to sterilization. Their integrity can be tested easily by means of water intrusion tests. Hydrophobic membranes may suddenly become clogged with humidity caused by microcondensation in the vicinity of the membrane, but they do not lose their sterilizing capacity when this occurs. The working procedures must be such that the moisture saturation point is not reached, in order to have a reliable gas filtration process.

Laminar flow units. These are required whenever sterile work has to be assured in an open process. Standard LFUs may have either horizontal (100 percent of the filtered air is run to waste) or vertical airflow (100 percent of the filtered air is recycled) and are designed to protect the product. Safety or security LFUs are designed for work with pathogens and protect both the worker from the product and the product from contamination. They are fitted with a second fan for the extraction of part of the recycled air (30 to 70 percent) through HEPA filters to prevent the escape of contaminated particles from the secure environment of the LFU. The ambient air, driven by suction into the LFU, is kept away from the sterile product by the design of the cabinet and there is therefore no risk of contamination if GMP procedures are observed.

Liquid filters. These are used for coarse or fine clarification as a specific process or for prefiltration in a final sterilization process. Liquid filters must comply with the legal requirements for pharmaceuticals production. It is usually cheaper to use depth filters for prefiltration, but the sterilizing filters should be of the membrane type. The whole system should be provided with facilities for purified water washing, *in-situ* steam-sterilization, liquid displacement by sterile air or nitrogen under pressure, draining, sterile sampling ports and the means of integrity testing of the final sterilizing filters.

Valves. Diaphragm valves are the most reliable, although care must be given to the diaphragm, as its working life is reduced by overtightening of the valve. Solids such as glass fragments from a broken electrode or metal particles released from the equipment can perforate the diaphragm. If only the first layer is perforated, a dirt pocket will be created, so valves must be dismantled routinely and inspected for cuts or holes. Valves situated on horizontal pipelines should be placed at a 45° angle from the horizontal to prevent the accumulation of condensate during steam-sterilization.

Monitoring and controlling equipment

Connections for electronic equipment. Usually monitoring and controlling equipment is installed in panels located at some distance from where the sensors are installed. The sensor transmits an electric signal which is translated in terms of the required parameter (pH, redox, dissolved oxygen, temperature, pressure, etc.) in the receiving monitor / controller. Electronic connections may be welded or of the tight plug type. They must be moisture-proof. All connecting cables should be protected from external electromagnetic interference and checks should be made to ensure that no distorted signals are received by the monitor / controller.

Manometers. Manometers installed in process lines or equipment should be regularly calibrated against a standard certified manometer.

Thermometers and thermostats. Thermometers should be calibrated against a certified thermometer in a water or oil bath. If the equipment is a controller it should have a second alarm limit set at not more than 1°C above and below the standard working limits.

pH - pOR - D.O. - meters/controllers. It is very important to check the wire connections regularly and to ensure that they are in good condition. It is also essential to check the condition of the wire mesh (shield). External induction parasitic signals gain in power relatively as the specific signal weakens, owing to poor connections or a poor shield. Probes, particularly those for dissolved oxygen, should not be kept out of solution longer than is strictly necessary, as this causes rapid ageing. Electrolytic solutions must be replaced regularly.

It is important to have electronic calibration simulators to ensure that the monitor / controller is working well, but the final calibration should be made by placing the sensors in standard solutions freshly prepared for the purpose. Specialized advice should be sought from equipment suppliers, as all the particular situations that could arise cannot be covered in this chapter.

Flow meters. Flow meters for liquids and gases must be calibrated under different working conditions against certified ones. The testing process must be conducted in such a manner as to prevent breakages and operators must be protected against such accidents, particularly when working with flow meters that measure gases under pressure.

Calibration can also be done by comparing the theoretical volume that should be obtained at a fixed flow rate and time against the volume actually obtained. This has to be done at different flow rates.

Dosing equipment. If dosing is carried out with a peristaltic pump, it is important to use high-quality flexible tubing to avoid unexpected breakages.

Solution containers must not be allowed to run empty or dry out, since this will promote the formation of crystals which will cause the dosing system to wear out prematurely.

Recorders. These have to be calibrated to register precisely the figures that the monitors/controllers show. These in turn should be in strict agreement with the real figures of the process. In critical processes, inspection and manual recording of parameters must be performed at least once a day and the results noted on worksheets or on the recording chart itself where this is necessary.

Timers. These are useful pieces of equipment where reaction times are long or where it is necessary to control a lengthy process. Computer- or PLC-controlled processes have timers incorporated as standard devices.

Maintenance records. It is important to have a register of all the process equipment and machines that are looked after by the maintenance department. For each piece of equipment or machine the register should comprise:

- identification (model/make/serial number);
- modifications or repairs carried out so far;
- the location of the equipment or plant;
- the total cost of the maintenance and repairs carried out so far.

This information will assist in assessing each individual piece of equipment and in deciding whether it is worth spending more money on it or whether a replacement is required.

Each piece of equipment should have its own logbook to record every inspection, calibration, repair job or changes of defective parts. This information will be very useful in estimating the working life of the different components and will permit the implementation of a maintenance prevention routine, which will reduce production losses caused by unexpected failures of equipment.

BIBLIOGRAPHY

Barrer, P.J. 1983. Crucial factors for design of a pilot plant. *Biotechnology*, October 1983: 661-666.

Commission of the European Communities. 1992. *The rules governing medicinal products in the European Community*, Vol. IV. *Good manufacturing practice for medicinal products.* Directorate General for International Market and Industrial Affairs.

EC. (n.d.) *General requirements for the production and control of live mammalian bacterial and viral vaccines for veterinary use.* Committee for Veterinary Medicinal Products of the European Community.

EC. (n.d.) *General requirements for the production and control of inactivated mammalian bacterial and viral vaccines for veterinary use.* Committee for Veterinary Medicinal Products of the European Community.

Everett, K. 1984. Planning for a new laboratory. *Manuf. Chem.*, April 1984: 30-33.

Glacen, M.W., Fleischaker, R.J. & Sinskey, A.J. 1983. Mammalian cell culture: engineering principles and scale-up. *Trends in Biotechnol.*, 1(4): 102-108.

Ríos, S. & Chaib, M. 1993. Sistemas integrados de salas blancas o limpias para la industria farmaceutica. *Ind. Farm.*, November-December 1993: 27-42.

Sharp, J.R. 1983. *Guide to good pharmaceutical manufacturing practice.* London, Her Majesty's Stationery Office.

Aspects of financial management of veterinary vaccine manufacturing operations in developing countries

P. de Greve

Veterinary vaccine manufacturing, like any other manufacturing process, can be referred to as a product transformation process, that is a process in which a finite number of inputs (production factors) are converted into a finite number of different outputs (products) (Naylor and Vernon, 1969). An assessment of such a process of product transformation is usually based on the neoclassical production function model whereby output is considered to be a function of fixed and variable factors in the firm's production process (Naylor and Vernon, 1969). This model basically serves as a framework for the globally applied contemporary practices of cost accounting and financial management.

Veterinary vaccine manufacturers in developing countries often face a number of specific problems including: macro-economic reforms, distorted markets, government interference and a poor financial investment basis.

In addition, in many developing countries the production of veterinary vaccines takes place in laboratories that are either owned and run by government services or at least have strong controlling links with government departments. In these government-controlled veterinary laboratories, production, research and animal health control functions are intermixed. In some rare cases, separate subunits may be in charge of specific functions, for example vaccine production units are separate from serological services or research. In most cases, however, veterinary laboratories lack the necessary transparency in managerial (i.e. functional, commercial, financial and institutional) performance to allow a detailed financial analysis of specific operations and/or functions. In other words, only seldom will a veterinary laboratory in a developing country be able to indicate the unit cost of, say, producing a specific type of animal vaccine or carrying out a specific serological service.

In an era of structural adjustments in which government services are increasingly driven by the forces of market demand and supply, the management of such services requires transparent production processes that yield products that can be valued against apparent demand in the market.

This chapter aims at highlighting some of the important managerial and, more specifically, financial aspects of the veterinary vaccine manufacturing process with special emphasis on locally based, government-controlled production units in developing countries. The following discussion will be of less relevance to the production and trading of vaccines by private companies.

Obviously, it is impossible to consider in great detail the issue of financial management within the limits set for this manual. The professional literature on the topic of financial management and cost accounting is extensive but publications that discuss this topic in relation to the production of veterinary vaccines in developing countries are all but non-existent. Field experience is limited and little has been published in this regard. The reflections found in this chapter are based on a limited number of field experiences in East, southern and West Africa in combination with the overall principles of applied economics and accounting.

FINANCIAL MANAGEMENT

The management of a firm is a process of planning, controlling, organizing, communicating and motivating with the ultimate goal of attaining the organization's objectives in the most effective manner.

Financial management – which is part of the overall management task – serves three main purposes: i) stock valuation for profit measurement; ii) decision-making (including planning); and iii) control (accountability).

In the discussion of financial management, some authors distinguish between management accounting and cost accounting (Drury, 1988):

- *Cost accounting* relates to the process of calculating actual (unit) production cost for the purposes of stock valuation and profit measurement (objective i) above).
- *Management accounting* relates to the provision of information to help management make proper investment decisions (objectives ii) and, partly, iii) above).

Cost accounting makes use of historical data that are collected and categorized on a regular basis (accountancy) with the ultimate purpose of assessing the performance of a firm and ensuring that it is profitable and thus viable.

Management accounting relates to future costs (and benefits) with the aim of planning future activities and investments. Strictly speaking, historical costs are irrelevant to the decision-maker but they are used as the best available basis (although not the only one) for predicting future costs.

Business plans and financial control

Financial statements are needed to project and/or analyse the functioning of a production unit and to allow an assessment of the efficiency, creditworthiness and liquidity of the unit. For a veterinary vaccine production unit (under public-sector control) three financial statements should be made: the balance sheet, the profit and loss account and the sources and uses of funds statement, which may also be called the cash flow.

Balance sheet. Balance sheets give a view of the assets and liabilities of the processing enterprise at the end of each accounting period, which is usually 12 months (Gittinger, 1982). The balance sheet is a kind of static picture of the financial state of the enterprise at a given moment.

The format in which balance sheets are presented may vary from country to country, but the contents are always the same. Example 1 is an example of a balance sheet (United Kingdom model) of an imaginary vaccine production plant under joint project/government control, presented with equity and liabilities in the upper section and with assets given below. The figures are based on real data from an existing plant.

In the case of Example 1, it was possible to work out a balance sheet because the vaccine production unit was set up independently from other government departments. Often, however, manufacturing units are integrated in government departments that carry out various functions, some of which belong to the public-sector mandate while others may be more related to the private sector, for

EXAMPLE 1

Balance sheet for a vaccine production plant (United Kingdom model)

	31/12/1996 *(US$)*
Equity	
Share capital	-
Vested capital	7 000 000
Retained earnings	(800 000)
Liabilities	
Current	
short-term loans	50 000
suppliers' credit	50 000
taxes payable	
Long-term	
long-term loans	400 000
	8 300 000
Assets	
Fixed	
buildings and equipment at cost	5 600 000
less accumulated depreciation	(1 100 000)
construction in progress	
Current	
cash and bank balance	200 000
inventories (stocks)	3 300 000
debtors (accounts receivable)	300 000
less overdraft	-
	8 300 000

example viability testing for other manufacturers.

It follows that in those cases where governments are involved in vaccine production, certain constraints and peculiarities may affect the management of the manufacturing plant. Looking at the data above, a number of observations can be made.

Vaccine production units are often government-owned, i.e. capital is vested with the public sector and not in the hands of private-sector shareholders (whether individuals or holding companies). This is reflected in the balance sheet in Example 1 by the somewhat unusual addition of vested capital in the equity listing. Obviously, combinations of public- and private-sector ownership are possible as well. In fact, under structural adjustment or similar macroeconomic reform programmes, many developing countries try to turn their public-owned services and/or manufacturing organizations into commercially oriented companies, at least partly owned by private-sector agents or holdings.

The balance sheet in Example 1 is a "still photograph" and does not indicate exactly how capitalization of the production unit has been realized. The inclusion of long-term loans in this particular example points at a financing construction in which outside sources (development agencies in this case) have provided part of the capital base of the unit. The other part of the capitalization presumably originates from public finance sources. Various scenarios are possible whereby the financing of new investments is done from public finance sources, private investors (through the issue of new shares) or long-term financing through funding agents (such as development organizations or the banking system).

Retained earnings are a fourth important source of capital creation in a company. In the past, government-controlled vaccine production was based on policy guidelines set out by the government and often stipulating exactly what had to be produced and in what quantities – without any linkages to market forces. This kind of uninspired management practice is slowly disappearing, even in government-controlled manufacturing units. However, it may be difficult for the management of such units to convince the owners of the company (in this case, the government) of the need to retain profits (if there are any) for reinvestment in the firm.

Valuation of stocks is a crucial factor in financial management. This issue is discussed in more detail in the section Price setting and stock valuation (p. 203).

Suppliers' credit on the equity side and debtors on the liabilities side of the balance sheet refer to temporary capital creation and culmination, respectively, because of the time lags between delivery and the payment of invoices. A common concern of financial managers will be how to avoid tying up too many funds in short-term assets such as accounts receivable or inventories. Accounts receivable are often a bottleneck, notably when government services are a main customer of the firm in question. In fact, governments are often notoriously bad in paying their arrears, especially to companies or institutes which they control and own themselves. This often leads to the cash needs of such companies being seen as part of the annual operation plan approved by government and, eventually, its designated bank and not as a business-determined factor. The problem of accounts receivable from official or semi-official sources may well be the single worst bottleneck for many semi-governmental firms involved in manufacturing for service sectors such as veterinary departments. In addition, whereas private customers can be blacklisted as bad debtors, this is often impossible with governmental customers. This problem is even more acute in cases where the product concerns essential services to society – such as for vaccinations against serious contagious diseases. In the case of outbreaks of such a disease, the delivery of vaccines is expected to be immediate and frequently in relatively large volumes. Payment is often delayed because substantial amounts of money are involved, for which no allocation was made in the government's recurrent budgets.

Cash and bank balances could be negative if – as happens far too often in government-controlled organizations – operations must be financed through bank overdrafts because the government is late in channelling the necessary (and budgeted) funds to the production firm it owns and controls. Manufacturing units must therefore try to create a sufficient recurrent capital base to finance regular operations. As indicated above, there may also be the problem that too much funding is tied up in short-term assets, such as accounts receivable or inventories. If this is the case, the manager of the manufacturing plant should try to reduce the tied capital base.

Profit and loss account. The profit and loss account is the most widely used financial statement. It is also the one which is easiest to understand since it refers to the common principle of profit analysis by comparing revenue with cost. A fairly straightforward model of profit and loss accounts is shown in Example 2.

The profit and loss account is a financial report that summarizes the revenues and expenditure of an enterprise over an accounting period (usually one year)

EXAMPLE 2

Profit and loss account

	Profit and loss account 1996 *(US$)*
Revenue	
Vaccine sales	1 450 000
Antigen sales	150 000
Cattle sales	600 000
Serology services	100 000
Donor support	500 000
Miscellaneous	–
Total revenue	2 800 000
Expenditure	
Salaries	900 000
Production cost vaccines	650 000
Production antigen	50 000
Maintenance and repairs	200 000
Office, communications and utilities	100 000
Transport/travel	80 000
Depreciation	100 000
Loan repayment and interest	110 000
Interest on overdraft	–
Bank charges	10 000
Total expenditure	2 200 000
Net profit (loss)	600 000

EXAMPLE 3

Profit and loss account (revised format)

	Profit and loss account 1996 *(US$)*
Gross revenue	2 800 000
- Cash operating expenses	-1 880 000
= Gross income	920 000
- Selling and administrative costs	-100 000
= Operating income before depreciation	820 000
- Non-cash operating expenses (depreciaton)	-100 000
= Operating income (profit)	720 000
- Non-operating income and expenses (interest, taxes other than on profit, subsidies, etc.)	-120 000
= Net income (profit) before income taxes	600 000
- Income taxes	-
= Net income (profit) after taxes	600 000

(Gittinger, 1982). It shows the results of the operations of the enterprise during that period. The format shown in Example 2 is a very simple one which perfectly suits the needs of smaller manufacturing units run under government control. A more standardized model might look as in Example 3.

Revenue can come from various sources but basically relates to the sales of goods and/or services. In the case of veterinary laboratories, sales of vaccine could be a major source of revenue as shown in Example 2, but others might exist as well, for example payment for serological services, antigen slides sales, veterinary advice against payment and sales of animals. Cash operating expenditures would include all cash expenditure incurred to produce the output. Important costs in this category are labour and material inputs. Selling and administrative costs concern the so-called overheads, which also include training, ongoing research and development and training.

The non-cash operating expenses item has one major element – depreciation. Depreciation refers to the process of allocating a portion of the original cost of an asset to each accounting period so that the value is gradually used up, or written off, during the course of the useful life of the asset (Gittinger, 1982). Depreciation may allow for a "rest value" which is treated as revenue at the time of write-off of the capital item. For example, a CO_2 incubator costing US$40 000 may have an expected useful lifetime of ten years and a rest value at the end of this lifetime of US$4 000. The annual depreciation would thus be:

$$\frac{(40\,000 - 4\,000)}{10} = 3\,600$$

This amount would appear as a non-manufacturing or period cost in the financial statement and, consequently, it would be used in deriving the unit production cost in the cost accounting exercise. The US$4 000 rest value would be treated as revenue at the end of year ten.

The profit and loss account is an extremely important source of management information. Obviously, building up the database of summarized profit and loss accounts requires a breakdown of total revenue and expenditure into its constituent parts, each of which may require various subtables with their own sets of assumptions and inputs. The following annual (or possibly quarterly) statements are usually needed:

- production and sales figures including opening and closing stocks for factor inputs and product outputs with expected losses and rejections;
- total revenues based on the production,

sales and stock figures and price information;

- a detailed costing for specific (technical) cost centres, such as different production departments, research department and advisory and research department;
- a detailed costing for support centres such as farm, rabbitry, breeding units, sales and distribution, administration, garage and workshop;
- input data for depreciation – i.e. original cost, useful life and rest value;
- financial costs and bank charges;
- the capital expenditure budget (investment planning).

It is impossible to cover these input tables in any detail in the context of this brief overview so, because the key to successful financial management lies in the development of correct and proper financial statements, reference is made to handbooks on financial management and cost accounting for further information.

It should be indicated that the profit and loss account also serves to bridge the gap between subsequent balance sheets. The net income (profit) from the profit and loss account, after the payment of dividend to shareholders (if there are any) is transferred to the balance sheet as retained earning and, if positive, will thereby increase the owners' equity.

Financial indicators. The combination of profit and loss account and balance sheet allows the manager of a production unit to assess the financial viability of the plant. For this purpose, a number of financial indicators can be used. An outline of the common financial efficiency indicators follows. For further information refer to Gittinger (1982, p. 203-209).

Inventory turnover can be calculated by dividing the cost of goods sold by the value of the inventory at year end. It measures the number of times that an enterprise turns over its stocks each year and indicates the proportion of the inventory required to support regular sales levels throughout the year. This ratio also indicates the average length of time a firm keeps its products in stock. A low inventory turnover may mean difficulties in selling the product and/or poor stock control practices. Low inventory turnover also means that a relatively large amount of capital is tied up in inventories. For veterinary vaccine producers there is a specific problem of safety stocks and non-continuous production processes.

As an example, a firm that sold US$2.8 million worth of goods and was left with $3.3 million inventory at year end would have an inventory turnover of 2 800 000/ 3 300 000 = 0.85, pointing to a low turnover rate of on average around ten months before a vaccine or service is sold.

Operating ratio is calculated by dividing the operating expenses by the revenue. It is an indicator of the management's ability to control operating costs, including administrative expenses. This ratio is especially useful in a comparative framework, i.e. when comparing one company's performance over several years or the performances of different companies. A ratio that increases over time is a sign of imbalance between costs and revenues, i.e. of disproportionately rising costs or decreasing sales prices. In vaccine production, sales prices can reasonably be controlled and the operating ratio will in the first place be useful to give an indication of the relative cost of production. In addition, if a firm has made a large investment, it will need a high cash flow in order to enable repayments. This requires a low operating ratio.

In the example above the operating ratio would be:

$$\frac{(1\,880\,000 + 100\,000 + 100\,000)}{2\,800\,000} = 0.74$$

Income ratios. The viability of a firm depends greatly on its ability to generate funds to repay investments, reinvest and compensate owners for their capital contribution.

Some useful income ratios which reflect the financial viability of a firm are: the return on sales, the return on equity and the return on assets. The return on sales shows how large an operating margin the firm has on its sales. Return on sales is calculated as net income (revenue minus costs) divided by revenue. The lower the margin (and thus the return on sales) the more the firm will have to sell in order to reach an acceptable return on investment. Return on equity is the ratio of net income (after taxes) to equity and is the main guidance to owners of the firm in their investment decisions. This applies equally well where the government is the owner of the firm. Return on assets is a more theoretical income indicator reflecting the overall return of the company on all the resources it engages. This ratio is the nearest to the internal rate of return and discounted measures of project worth (Gittinger, 1982, p. 206-207).

Financial ratios. Apart from efficiency and income ratios, there is a third important class of financial indicators that reflects a manufacturing company's financial strength, i.e. the creditworthiness ratios. These ratios concern the degree of financial risk inherent in the enterprise (Gittinger, 1982). Creditworthiness indicators are the current ratio (current assets divided by current liabilities), the debt-equity ratio (long-term liabilities divided by long-term liabilities plus equity) and the debt service coverage ratio (net income plus depreciation plus interest paid, divided by interest paid plus repayment of long-term loans).

Sources and uses of funds statement. The fourth financial statement that is used to assess the operations of manufacturing units is the sources and uses of funds statement, or the cash flow table. As the latter name indicates, the cash flow table provides an overview of the total flow of financial resources into and out of an enterprise during an accounting period and is useful for determining the likely flow of financial resources in future. Reference is made to textbooks on financial management for more information.

PRICE SETTING AND STOCK VALUATION

Price setting by (government-controlled) vaccine manufacturers is a difficult issue. In theory, the market should dictate price levels but in practice it does not. Markets for veterinary vaccines are far more imperfect than those for, say, consumables or inputs such as fodder. Quantitative knowledge of "willingness to pay" by potential customers (e.g. farmers) is often scarce and unreliable, if available at all. Moreover, in a number of cases, society is willing to cover at least part of the cost price of a vaccine because of the potential disease threat to humans. In such cases, willingness to pay cannot be assessed as customers are more or less forced to accept the product and market demand cannot truly be established.

Nevertheless, the issue of price setting is closely linked to cost accounting, in that an estimation of unit output cost is a guideline in determining break-even sales price levels. In more general terms, price setting is a less central issue than is the evaluation of stocks, being the input and output factors of the product transformation process, and financial management is concerned with the determination of the cost of all single resources used in the transformation process, including non-physical resources, and the consequent value of single outputs of the process. Once these unit values are known, management can determine proper pricing policies.

Period costs and product cost

In the process of cost accounting, individual cost items that constitute the cost "chain" – from basic inputs to final product – must be identified, quantified, valued and summarized in order to arrive at a unit product cost. In this process, a distinction is made between period costs and product cost as illustrated in Figure 3.

Product costs are directly related to the manufacturing process. Their treatment in the financial statements, however, depends on whether the output produced is actually sold or not. Non-manufacturing costs are period-related costs and thus always appear in the profit and loss account as expenses. Some of the direct manufacturing costs, on the other hand, may not appear as an expense unless the product is sold. The terms product cost and period cost are thus interchangeable with direct and indirect costs.

An example (based on an example by Drury, 1988) may clarify this issue:

A vaccine manufacturing laboratory produces 50 000 units of vaccine A during year 1. The costs for year 1 were (in United States dollars):

Manufacturing costs	
Labour costs	50 000
Materials	20 000
Manufacturing overheads	30 000
Total	100 000
Non-manufacturing costs	40 000

During year 1 the laboratory sold 20 000 units for US$90 000. The remaining 30 000 units remained in stock at the end of year 1. The profit and loss account for year 1 would then look as follows:

Gross revenue (sales)	90 000
Manufacturing costs	
Labour costs	50 000
Materials	20 000
Manufacturing overheads	30 000
Total	100 000
Less closing stock	
60 percent of total	60 000
Cost of goods sold	40 000
Gross profit	50 000
Less non-manufacturing cost	40 000
Net profit	10 000

Because only 40 percent of the produced vaccine was sold in the same accounting period, only 40 percent of the total product costs appear in the profit and loss account as an expense. The remaining 60 percent is included in the value of the closing stock which appears in the balance sheet but not in the profit and loss account. So these costs are not expenses but will become expenses in the next accounting period (assuming that the remaining 30 000 doses of vaccine will then be sold). On the other hand, all period costs (non-manufacturing) will appear as expenses in the profit and loss account because they were incurred in this period. The cost of goods sold is derived only from (part of) the product costs and not from period costs.

Another notable effect is that, because of this allocation to different periods, the unit cost of a vaccine may differ from period to period if period costs are included. For example, from the first data it appears that in order to produce 50 000 vaccines, total expenses are (in United States dollars):

Manufacturing	100 000
Non-manufacturing	40 000
Total	140 000
Number	50 000
Unit cost	2.80

But if related to year 1 the unit cost appears to be different:

Manufacturing	40 000
Non-manufacturing	40 000
Total	80 000
Number	20 000
Unit cost	4.00

It is clear that only the second version

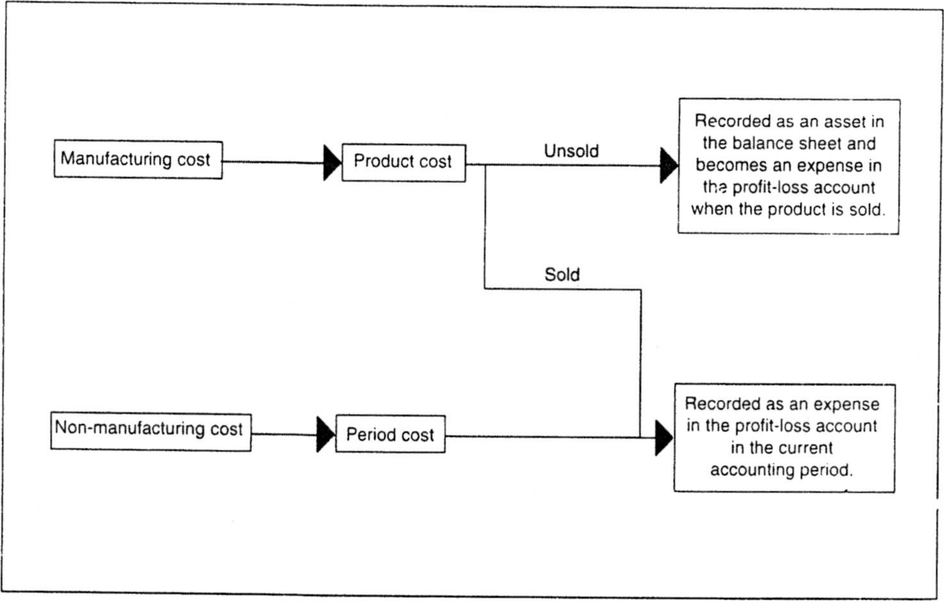

FIGURE 3
Comparison of manufacturing and non-manufacturing costs

Source: C. Drury, 1988.

(unit cost 4.00) is the correct one – if, as assumed, only 20 000 vaccines are sold in year 1. It should also be clear that the unit cost in year 2 could be different from year 1 depending on the total number of vaccines (of this particular batch) sold and the exact period costs for year 2.

Sunk costs

Sunk costs are the costs of resources that have already been acquired and that will not be affected by present and future management decisions. In a way sunk costs are by definition irrelevant costs in the planning process as the decision to incur them has been taken before. Some authors resist the use of the term sunk cost. For them, it simply applies to past expenses which may (or may not) have financial implications. These implications could be new costs such as possible interest payments on loans taken up to pay for past investments.

In the case of vaccine production in developing countries, research and development (R&D) is typically a cost item that concerns management decisions of the past. Strictly speaking there are two ways of dealing with R&D expenses in the financial statements.

In the first way, R&D expenses are considered to be investment costs and are therefore depreciated over the useful lifetime of the investment. As a result, the profit and loss account will contain an item for annual depreciation of R&D costs for the various products put on the market. In practice, however, there may be difficulties in assigning R&D costs to specific end products in a unit cost assessment.

Alternatively, R&D can be considered as period costs before the actual revenue started accruing. In this case, these costs should have appeared in the profit and loss accounts of those years in which they were incurred. This should still be reflected in the balance sheet as R&D in early years probably led to substantial negative retained earnings being carried over from the profit and loss account to the balance sheet.

In practice, however, development costs are often regarded as sunk costs and are thus not recovered through sales of final products. Often they are even disregarded in the profit and loss accounts and the balance sheet, unless they concern material assets.

Cost allocation

Veterinary laboratories that are engaged in vaccine production often also provide various other functions, such as serology services and veterinary advisory services. In order to improve the efficiency with which such laboratories carry out these functions, a manager should ideally be able to assess each function separately on a cost and revenue basis. This means that revenue and expenses need to be allocated to sub-components of the overall organization. In fact, three types of cost centres can be distinguished in a possible framework for cost control within a single manufacturing enterprise (Figure 4).

Practice shows that in the case of government-controlled veterinary laboratories, the allocation to cost centres is more of an exception than the rule even though there are tremendous differences in the kind of services offered by such laboratories, some of which belong to the public domain while others may well be commercially oriented. The establishment of cost, profit or investment centres can also be considered at the level of vaccine production when different vaccines are produced.

However, there are constraints which make the establishment of such centres more complicated in the case of animal vaccine production in developing countries.

One such constraint is the fact that the

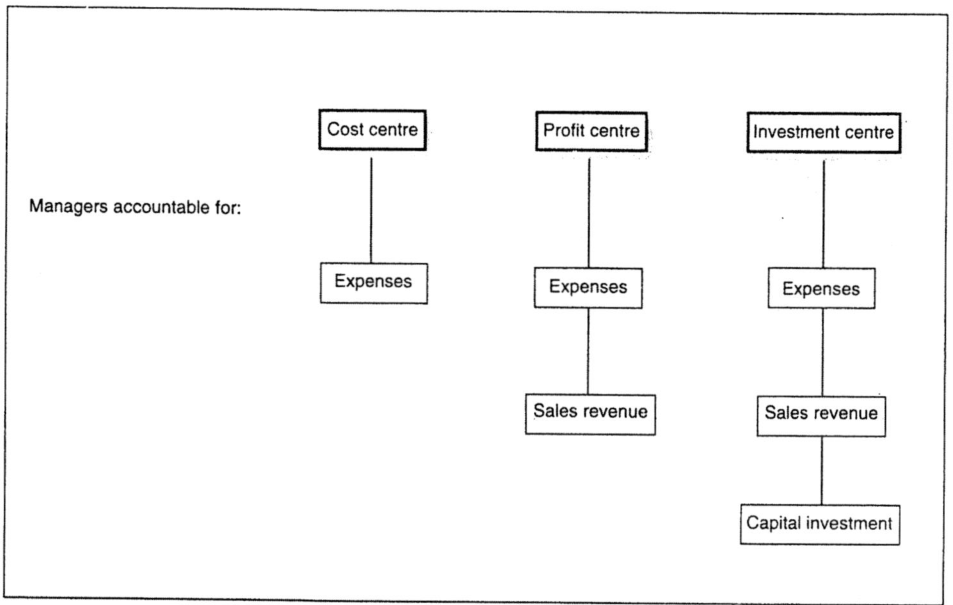

FIGURE 4
Cost control framework for single manufacturing enterprise

production of vaccines is done in batches and not continuously as for most industrial products. Nevertheless, the production process is repetitive and thus open to unit costing or cost accounting. The greater number of inputs and processing steps are very strictly defined, which in a way makes the process of unit costing easier.

Another potential constraint is that joint product costing (Drury, 1988) may complicate the financial control of the manufacturing process. Joint costs are costs of two or more kinds of outputs that are produced simultaneously by a single process and are not identifiable as individual types of products until a split-off point is reached (Horngren, 1977). This kind of joint costing can be handled by distinguishing one cost centre before and two (or more) cost centres after the split-off or, alternatively, by a cost allocation procedure based on units or value related keys.

Nevertheless, the financial management of veterinary laboratories would clearly be facilitated by establishing cost or profit centres around various core activities, one of which would be vaccine production. Others might be serological services, applied research, quality control, etc. Overall management would be easier as a number of tasks and functions could be delegated to the appropriate centre. This type of business framework is quite common in the commercial world but, unfortunately, still rare in parastatal or government institutes in developing countries.

Overhead costs

In practical terms, developing unit costings in a set-up with cost or profit centres requires the allocation of overhead costs to these centres. When, for the sake of estimating unit production cost, a veterinary laboratory differentiates expenditure according to cost centre, there are usually a number of overhead costs which can fairly easily be allocated to specific centres.

Time recording can be of help in assessing the labour inputs of employees not directly linked to a specific cost centre, for example the distribution of indirect materials such as stationery can be recorded for each cost centre. On the other hand, expenditure on general maintenance of the building, rent, heating, lighting, etc. cannot be allocated directly to specific cost centres. For this type of expense, the apportioning of cost must be based on other factors, such as the area occupied and the number of staff.

As an example, assume that in a veterinary laboratory there are two types of products – vaccine A and serological services – and that these constitute the basis of differentiation of cost centres. The unit costs of the vaccine and the serological services need to be established in order to guide management decisions on pricing, stocks and distribution. The floor area of the laboratory is 10 000 m^2, 3 500 m^2 of which is occupied by vaccine production laboratories, 2 500 m^2 by serological laboratories, 2 000 m^2 by shared production facilities and 2 000 m^2 by offices and other general facilities. If the total annual cost of rent, lighting, heating, etc. is US$50 000 then the apportioning could be done as follows: for vaccine production 35 percent of its own area plus 10 percent of the shared laboratory (50 percent of the total) plus 10 percent of the allocation for offices (50 percent of the total) which comes to 55 percent of total costs, or US$27 500. The remaining 45 percent, or US$22 500, would be the apportioned overhead cost for serological services.

Note that this method includes a second level apportioning for the expenses that are not directly linkable and that expenditure for offices could even be allocated on the basis of a specific apportioning method, for example one based on the total turnover of each cost centre.

It must be noted that there is no standard method for apportioning overhead costs; in each case a method should be found that has a causal ground for allocating costs to specific centres, such as the floor area used in relation to building-related expenses as shown above.

Similarly, labour inputs that cannot be directly allocated have to be apportioned on the basis of a key determinant, for example technicians who maintain and/or repair equipment in different departments can easily record time expenditure on job sheets for the individual cost centres. Even management staff can to some extent record time expenditure by cost centre. It is clear, however, that this cannot be done for the entire labour input of service departments or management, since part of their input is of a general nature and cannot be allocated to specific departments.

Other service departments that work for the laboratory as a whole include libraries, the stores department, accountancy and security guards. Their expenditure has to be allocated on the basis of the perceived benefits that each cost centre receives, for example the stores department's expenditure could be allocated on the basis of the number of material requisitions from each centre or on the more difficult to assess basis of the value of materials dispatched to each centre.

In advanced cost accounting systems, overhead allocation does not stop at the level of cost or profit centre, but relates to the specific tasks that pass these centres. In the context of vaccine production, this leads to cost accounting being brought down to the level of individual batches and not just to the vaccine production unit. Desirable as this may be, in government-controlled veterinary laboratories this kind of breakdown is often far too ambitious and cost allocation at the level of cost centres is usually quite adequate.

STOCK OR INVENTORY CONTROL

Inventories can be a major source of cash drain for any kind of company. This is especially so in firms that have little working capital. As vaccine producing laboratories often depend on government support for establishing a capital basis, it is clear that they very often struggle with financial constraints because of a lack of working capital. Good stock control, of both inputs and outputs, is thus an important element in the financial management of such (semicommercial) manufacturers.

Inventories must be maintained so that the customer can be served on request (Horngren, 1977). In addition, in the case of veterinary vaccines it may be necessary to maintain a certain stock of specific vaccines in case an outbreak of a specific disease requires immediate and medium- to large-scale intervention.

Inventories are cushions to absorb planning errors and unforeseen fluctuations in supply or demand and to facilitate smooth production and marketing operations. Inventories can also minimize the interdependence of different parts of the organization, so that each can work effectively (Horngren, 1977). Another reason for companies to hold stocks is for speculation whereby a firm buys in more or fewer inputs than are required from a strict managerial point of view in order to take advantage of anticipated price fluctuations. Unlike the other reasons for stockholding, this latter motive cannot be generalized in guidelines for stock control as the speculation motive is by definition a matter of uncertainty. Disregarding the speculative aspect, the problem that management faces regarding stock control is to find a good balance between the need for inventories of inputs and outputs and the desire not to tie up too much of the firm's capital in idle stocks. As far as stock control is concerned, manufacturing companies in developing countries find that the shortage of raw materials is often more of a problem than controlling excess inventories.

The question of stock valuation is important in the sense that management must decide on a policy for attaching specific values (costs or prices) to individual inputs or outputs that are released from storage for use in either manufacturing or sales. The inventory valuation methods used are usually one of the following three:

- First-in first-out (FIFO): the earliest acquired stock is assumed to be used first, so that the impact of present price effects is delayed, as the prices used reflect historical acquisition prices or unit costs.
- Last-in first-out (LIFO): the latest acquired or produced units are supposed to be used or sold first. With this method, the value of stock items released is a reflection of present (or at least recent) costings. LIFO usually leads to somewhat higher values as price levels over time generally show rather a rising tendency than a falling one.
- The obvious compromise is the use of some kind of average inventory method, which could be a moving average whereby each new addition to the stocks is lumped with the previous ones and average unit prices have to be adjusted with each change in stocks.

None of the above methods is entirely satisfactory and each has it own advantages and drawbacks.

Security stocks

The financial burden of keeping stocks of vaccines ready at hand for emergencies should, in theory, not be borne by the producing firm. In practice, however, this is usually what happens. As a result, the complex administrative channels through which reimbursement has to be channelled in case of emergency delivery constitute an additional financial bottleneck for vaccine supplying companies.

The question is whether the cost of holding such emergency stocks should and can be included in the firm's manufacturing cost and consequently be covered by the sales price of the vaccine. The answer to this question is primarily a policy issue which is related to the more general problem of differentiating between the health-related aspects of veterinary services, which are beyond the control of individual livestock owners, and those services that primarily relate to the productive activities of the livestock sector and are under the control of individual farmers.

As a general rule, cash generated from sales or the collection of receivables is an idle asset unless it is put to use internally (reinvested) or externally (invested in short-term securities). If, however, the economic situation in a country is characterized by high inflation rates, investment in short-term securities can only make sense if the real interest rate is positive, i.e. higher than inflation. If not, investments are a waste of resources. The problem in many developing countries, however, is the lack of efficiently functioning and fully developed money and capital markets (Sun, Gao and Soenen, 1993). This may mean that capital markets are not tuned to the characteristics of the economy but are centrally controlled by government.

On the other hand, manufacturing companies that are controlled and/or owned by governments may also benefit from this situation. The firm's equity is often provided by government authorities without having an explicit cost attached to it, for example enterprises have been financed in the past by state equity capital that was free of charge (Sun, Goa and Soenen, 1993). This situation came about because veterinary vaccine production was thought to belong to the government's essential tasks and was therefore monopolized under government control. The lack of competition gave companies no incentive to aim at efficiency gains and governments considered it appropriate to support these firms through the provision of equity capital, independent of the conditions in the capital markets. In recent years discussions have increasingly centred around the question of what exactly is included in the government's essential tasks. There is a tendency among donor agencies and international banking institutes to consider the support of vaccine production as non-essential for a government. Vaccinations, on the other hand, will in many cases continue to be considered as an essential task of the government and explicit government interference may therefore be deemed feasible and acceptable.

CONCLUDING REMARKS

On the basis of historical costs and with a proper accounting system it should be possible for veterinary vaccine producers to keep track of both direct and indirect costs and overheads. The principal problems that remain will be the proper allocation of overheads and the clarification of the goal of manufacturing versus other social or commercial functions. In the context of this manual it is impossible to cover the details of cost control in the different cost centres of a manufacturing firm. Nor is it possible to deal with the accounting principles behind such a cost control system in any detail. Apart from indicating some fields of special interest, reference will have to be made to the professional literature in this field.

The main purpose of this chapter has been to point out a number of problems that may arise, especially in animal vaccine manufacturing institutes or enterprises in developing countries. The role of the government, often as owner and/or controller of veterinary laboratories, is crucial in this respect. Mostly because of external pressures, this role is changing rapidly and the process of manufacturing is increasingly being left to the private and semi-private market. Whenever this is happening, businesslike approaches to the management of such manufacturing processes become increasingly important. Donor agencies may play an important role in this respect in supporting and/or organizing management training for scientific staff of such veterinary institutes.

Such actions would encourage a real incentive for improved economic performance and this in turn would lead to a better and more efficient use of scarce resources for the benefit of the community. This is the major goal of economics.

BIBILIOGRAPHY

Drury, C. 1988. *Management and cost accounting*. London, Chapman & Hall. 857 pp.

Fama, E.F. & Miller, M.H. 1972. *The theory of finance*. Hinsdale, Ill., USA, Dryden. 344 pp.

FAO. 1992. *A coordinated multi-donor programme for tick and tick-borne disease control in Eastern, Central and Southern Africa*. Report of the Formulation Mission, Rome.

Gittinger, J.P. 1982. *Economic analysis of agricultural projects*. Baltimore, USA and London, Johns Hopkins University Press. 505 pp.

Horngren, C.H. 1977. *Cost accounting – a*

managerial emphasis. London, Prentice-Hall International. 934 pp.

Naylor, T.H. & Vernon, J.M. 1969. *Microeconomics and decision models of the firm.* New York, Harcourt, Brace and World. 482 pp.

Sun, B., Gao, G. & Soenen, L. 1993. *Financial management practices in Chinese state enterprises.* RVB Research Papers, p. 1-5.

Thompson Jr., A.A. 1977. *Economics of the firm – theory and practice.* N.J., USA, Prentice-Hall. 638 pp.

van Hemert, P. 1972. *Vaccine production as a unit process.* Delft, the Netherlands, Technische Hogeschool. 175 pp.

The logistics of vaccine manufacture in developing countries

P. Hunter

Producers of veterinary vaccines in developing countries are faced with constraints not encountered by manufacturers in industrialized countries; many vaccine production centres are government-funded with limited resources, often with facilities not specifically designed for the purpose. The implementation of good manufacturing practices (GMPs) (Sharp, 1983) is difficult under these conditions. Financial constraints limit flexibility in the modification of existing plants and producers usually obtain little support from fiscal authorities owing to a general lack of insight into the requirements of vaccine manufacture.

A producer may be forced to make a particular biological product as a result of political or administrative policy, despite a lack of appropriate technology or funding. Faced with the responsibility of producing a safe and effective product under suboptimal conditions, the decision as to whether to produce or import an equivalent product must be assessed. The relatively high price of imported products needs to be weighed against the capital outlay needed to manufacture products of equivalent quality and safety. Since the role of vaccine producers is ultimately the benefit of agriculture, no advantage can be gained from insisting on producing substandard or excessively expensive vaccines locally.

While vaccine manufacturing plants should comply with certain minimal standards, the structural shortcomings of buildings should not be used as an excuse for failing to implement operational GMPs such as correct work flow procedures, hygiene and documentation. With ingenuity and dedication a safe and effective product can usually be obtained.

FORWARD PLANNING

In many developing countries animal immunization is conducted on a campaign basis and planning of vaccine production must make provision for producing large quantities of vaccines in a short period of time.

Vaccines for important diseases such as rinderpest and foot-and-mouth disease can be stored as strategic reserves; the Plowright rinderpest vaccine is stable for approximately four years in the freeze-dried state at 4°C (Doel, 1993) while foot-and-mouth disease vaccine can be stored as a frozen concentrate in liquid nitrogen indefinitely and formulated on demand. Freeze-dried lumpy skin disease vaccine stored at 4°C or -20°C will retain its original titres for two to four years (Doel, 1993).

In countries where important arthropod-transmitted diseases are endemic, there is usually a seasonal demand for vaccine in spring and early summer. Failure on the part of farmers to immunize their livestock on a sustained basis can result in massive logistical problems for producers; for example the vaccination of sheep against Rift Valley fever in southern Africa should be carried out to provide animals with adequate herd immunity during the long intra-epidemic periods which characterize the disease. Live Rift Valley fever vaccine is easily produced in large quantities and confers lifelong immunity, but at the onset of an epizootic of Rift Valley fever, farmers cannot make use of the live vaccine in pregnant animals. There is therefore a massive demand for the inactivated vaccine which requires a larger antigenic mass per dose and a longer lead time for production.

The clostridial toxoid vaccines are generally very stable and lend themselves to storage as concentrates at 4°C.

A campaign approach to production, whereby only one product is produced for a short period of time, allows the manufacture of a large amount of vaccine to supply seasonal or other demand if production capacity is restricted and prevents cross-contamination if containment facilities are suboptimal. This is also a practical approach with a vaccine such as anthrax which has a disastrous potential for the contamination of production and bottling plants.

The production of vaccines which have a very short shelf-life, such as the blood vaccines for rickettsial and protozoal diseases in Africa, need special attention with regard to planning. The procurement of susceptible animals, infection, bleeding, collection and bottling of vaccines must be carefully planned to avoid the wastage of resources. Producers may have to supply clients according to a schedule, for example weekly in the summer months but only monthly in winter.

Ordering materials

As in any production plant, ordering materials for vaccine production must be done in a timely manner, so that there is sufficient time for checking and quality control (QC). In developing countries, there is the additional problem of raw materials frequently being imported and time must be allowed for importation and release from customs. Further problems such as receiving the wrong product in a consignment of raw materials can delay production. Stockpiling crucial raw materials is advisable if sufficient storage space is available and as long as the product is stable on storage (Lambert and Birch, 1985). However, stockpiling ties up capital and adds to the unit cost of the product compared with those produced in developed countries where manufacturers can rely on a *just-in-time* approach.

Since many raw materials for vaccine production are analytical grade chemicals, most conform with the specifications of the manufacturer. Using cheap culture substrates which are available locally to reduce costs (e.g. using meat broth or corn steep for clostridial vaccines) causes complications because these substances may vary in composition from batch to batch. Additional QC tests such as protein or nitrogen content (on meat broth) and total solids (on corn steep) are necessary to eliminate poor substrates. In addition, careful growth tests must be done to ensure their suitability for use.

Since few laboratories can afford to import complete cell culture media, powdered media or individual components are usually purchased. Although buying from reputable companies may cost more it does reduce the risks of unscrupulous companies dumping poor-quality products in developing countries.

THE PRODUCTION PROCESS

Media preparation

Cell culture medium. Cell culture medium must be formulated with double-distilled water or water produced by reverse osmosis and filtered sterilely into stainless steel tanks or into bottles. If sterile room facilities are unavailable for sterile filling, small laminar flow units can be used. Careful sterility checks at 37°C and room temperature are essential if conditions are not optimal.

Bacterial culture media. Bacterial culture media are usually sterilized by heat in tanks or glass flasks – a process which is generally associated with fewer problems than sterile filling. However, the function of autoclaves and the quality of the steam used for sterilization may affect the heat-sterilization process and sterility tests must be carried out.

The preparation of agar plates or slopes should be done in laminar flow cabinets or under laminar flow units if no sterile rooms are available.

Virus vaccines

Cell lines. Cells for virus production can be obtained from culture collections or reputable laboratories, where the identity, chromosomal characteristics and freedom from extraneous agents have been established. If in-house testing is not possible intermittent checks can be done by other local laboratories that are able to check cell identity and freedom from mycoplasmal and viral contamination.

It is essential to check cell lines for extraneous viruses. As in-house facilities are seldom available for this, help should be enlisted from universities or other laboratories with experience in detecting the viruses that may affect the cells used for production. With this in mind, it is more convenient if viral vaccines produced from cell lines are manufactured on a campaign basis to eliminate the need for continual testing for extraneous viruses.

Media. The importation of complete formulated media for vaccine production is impractical owing to freight costs, despite the advantages of QC and growth checks thereby becoming unnecessary. It is more economical to buy powdered media, but cell growth checks must be done, as the quality of water used for formulation can affect the product.

Storing cell and virus seed Erratic power supplies make it essential that cell and virus stocks should be duplicated and stored at various institutes as back-up supplies.

Viral master seed stocks. The identity, purity, passage history and titres must be carefully noted. Recording the passage level of live attenuated virus vaccine strains is of major importance and failure to control this can lead to serious problems in the field.

Production

The production of live vaccines on cell culture requires less antigen and can therefore be performed in roller bottles or in Roux flasks. Inactivated virus vaccines require a large amount of antigen, which may necessitate the production of vaccine virus in suspension culture. This has been done successfully with BHK cells for rabies and foot-and-mouth disease vaccine production.

However, in developing countries it may be more practical to use a labour-intensive, scale-up monolayer system as has been used for foot-and-mouth disease vaccine production (Ubertini *et al.*, 1963) and for IBR, Aujesky's disease and PI3 vaccines (Panina, 1985).

Bacterial vaccines. The production methods of many bacterial vaccines are uncomplicated and appropriate for use in most developing countries. However, the production of vaccines for *Brucella abortus* and *B. melitensis* should not be attempted without adequate containment and biosafety facilities.

Undemanding anaerobes such as the clostridia can be produced without difficulty but strict anaerobes such as

Bacteroides nodosus require totally oxygen-free gases which are not readily available in developing countries.

Although most modern bacterial vaccines are produced in fermentation vessels, labour-intensive methods of producing vaccines on agar layers in Roux flasks are suited to the conditions in some developing countries. Clostridial toxoid vaccines such as those against botulism and tetanus are easily produced by the dialysis bag method (Sterne and Wentzel, 1950) if fermentation technology is unavailable.

Protozoal vaccines. Since the production of redwater (*Babesia* spp.) and anaplasmosis (*Anaplasma centrale*) vaccines for cattle may require the use of splenectomized cattle, the appropriate facilities must be available or the services of universities or private clinics must be elicited. Animals need to be maintained under tick-free conditions, by means of water-trenches around stables and the provision of sterilized feed.

Tick stabilate vaccines such as those prepared for *Theileria* sp. and heartwater, where the vaccine consists primarily of infected ticks ground into a suspension, must be prepared with caution because of the prevalence of tick-borne diseases which can affect humans such as tick-bite fever (*Rickettsia conori*) and the viruses which cause haemorrhagic fevers.

Serum for culture media. Foetal calf serum is rarely available in developing countries and has to be imported. Although expensive, the advantage of this is that a sterile product which has passed appropriate growth tests is received.

Normal bovine or other sera are usually more easy to obtain from abattoirs but the quality can be a problem. Collection is rarely from animals bled by trochar and inevitably the blood collected at exsanguination has high microbial contamination and resultant high endotoxin levels. However, the serum collected in this manner is cheap and, providing the laboratory has a separator for defibrination and facilities for sterile filtration, a usable product is usually obtained although the suitability of each batch for cell culture needs to be checked and stringent sterility checks are essential. Because of the risk of adventitious viruses which may be present in serum, for example BVD virus (Kriazeff, Wopschall and Hopps, 1975), bovine sera for use in live vaccines should be irradiated or heated.

The problem of the presence of antibodies in serum, which may react with the virus to be cultured, can be overcome by precipitation with polyethylene glycol (Abaracon and Giacometti, 1976; Barteling, 1974).

Downstream processing

Whether it be the removal of bacterial cells for the processing of toxoids or the concentration of virus harvests, the major concern for a vaccine producer in developing countries is the selection of methods which combine low capital outlay with low-cost maintenance. Of the variety of processes available, only ultrafiltration is suitable for large-scale processing; the equipment is simple and of relatively low cost but it has the disadvantage that purification cannot be achieved to any great extent.

Adjuvants

Adjuvants. Alum (potassium aluminium sulphate) and aluminium phosphate are relatively cheap and easy adjuvants to formulate. They are commonly used for adjuvanting toxoid vaccines. The in-house production of aluminium hydroxide gel (alhydrogel), which is the most widely used adjuvant for veterinary vaccines, is more demanding. The aluminium content, pH and conductivity need monitoring and the poor heat conduction of the gel requires careful control of sterilization. With this in mind, the cost-effectiveness of buying a commercial product which conforms to safety and efficacy requirements must be weighed against that of in-house production of the product.

Oil adjuvants. Mineral oils used for single or multiple oil formulations in veterinary vaccines are usually imported into developing countries and, because of the propensity of oil formulations for causing local reactions, attention must be paid to the quality and purity of the oils. Vaccine producers must insist on certificates of analysis and must check the containers in which the oils are delivered to ensure the absence of contamination with other products. The oils should be stored under nitrogen to prevent oxidation during storage.

Saponin. This adjuvant usually has to be imported and the producer should be aware that the quality varies with supplier. While some brands which are not highly purified have good adjuvant activities and can be used with success, for example in the anthrax spore vaccine, they can affect certain antigens such as foot-and-mouth disease virus on storage. Some initial research should therefore be undertaken to determine an appropriate supplier. Purified saponins are less likely to destroy the antigen, but are extremely expensive and some have poor adjuvant activity.

Filling and freeze-drying

The vaccine filling and freeze-drying plant is the bottleneck area in most production facilities. In developing countries the additional problem exists that equipment is imported and service back-up from the supplier becomes very important. Ampoules used for freeze-drying can be manufactured locally to keep the unit price low, but these are often not produced to specification, leading to breakages by capping machines. This is a serious problem not only because of wastage, but because it becomes a safety problem when bottling freeze-dried products such as *Brucella* sp. and live attenuated mouse-brain adapted strains of African horse sickness virus (Erasmus, personal communication).

Producers are often forced to use a filling line for both live and killed products; if this is unavoidable, live products must be bottled at the end of a week, after killed products, and the facility must then be disinfected with an appropriate disinfectant, or fumigated with formaldehyde, and allowed to stand over a weekend.

The malfunctioning of freeze-drying machines can cause a high moisture content in the product which results in poor stability of the vaccine, which is important in tropical and subtropical countries.

QUALITY CONTROL

As the number of QC tests performed increases, so does the cost of the final product, and often only essential tests are selected.

Physical and chemical tests

The manufacturer should not underestimate the value of visual inspection of the product. Numerous problems can be detected merely by looking at a formulation: the colour, consistency, presence of foreign bodies, proportion of alhydrogel and appearance of freeze-dried pellet can indicate a problem in the final product. Basic tests such as pH determination are simple to perform and give valuable information about the reagents used and in monitoring each stage of the vaccine production process. QC tests must be validated by including standards and, if necessary, by requesting other laboratories to duplicate tests.

Raw materials. The extensive QC tests performed on raw materials in developed countries are seldom performed in developing countries because of the cost. Less affluent producers must nevertheless ensure that analytical grade chemicals are used and growth tests are performed on formulated media.

In-process tests. The monitoring of inactivation is essential in order to obviate using vaccines containing non-inactivated organisms. When aziridines are used as inactivants, the inactivation process can be controlled by monitoring the pH changes during the process of cyclization of the reagent and by sampling and titration of the antigen (Bahnemann, 1990).

Moisture content of freeze dried vaccines. Since a high moisture content will affect the stability of vaccines Karl Fischer moisture determination should be performed, if possible, by the producer or an analytical laboratory. An accelerated stability test can pre-empt the issuing of vaccine with high moisture content if moisture determination tests cannot be performed.

Biological tests

Innocuity/safety testing. *Abnormal toxicity testing* is done on two guinea pigs (2 ml intraperitoneally or subcutaneously) and on five mice (0.5 ml). This test is important if the analysis of raw materials and in-process controls cannot be done.

Specific safety tests, as for the abnormal toxicity test, are essential and become all the more important if the quality of raw materials and other reagents cannot be controlled. These tests are essential for live attenuated vaccines. Susceptible target animal species are inoculated with at least one dose of the specific vaccine.

Potency testing. As with potency testing in developed countries, titrations of live organisms or serology are performed in place of challenge tests on large or small animals, where this is possible. Performing serological tests may be difficult in some countries, owing to the problem of finding seronegative animals to ensure immunological responsiveness to specific antigens. In South Africa, sheep have to be purchased from an area in the country where bluetongue does not occur and have to be maintained in insect-free stables while they are tested for their serological response to the bluetongue vaccine.

The lack of containment facilities may prevent developing countries from performing challenge tests for vaccines such as rinderpest and contagious bovine pleuropneumonia and only serology will be carried out.

PROTOZOAL AND RICKETTSIAL VACCINES

The cattle used for the production of blood vaccines, such as those for babesiosis and anaplasmosis, should be tested for infectious agents which could contaminate the blood vaccine (OIE, 1992) and sheep used for heartwater vaccine production should be free of *Anaplasma ovis, Erlichia ovis* and *Trypanosoma ovis* (Oberem and Bezuidenhout, 1987).

STORAGE

Sufficient storage capacity in cold rooms, freezers or liquid nitrogen tanks is essential for storing vaccine or antigen. A minimum requirement is a recording system for validating constant temperature control, since a loss of refrigeration or freezing in cold rooms can affect the antigen or the finished product. If temperature monitoring cannot be done electronically, manual hourly checking can be done by production staff and after hours by security staff. Ideally, alarm systems should be utilized to alert production managers to such eventualities.

DISPATCH AND DISTRIBUTION

Dispatch and distribution should preferably be undertaken by distributors with facilities for handling and dispatching the finished product. Consigning vaccines to the mercies of rail or road transport in developing countries can lead to serious losses. Vaccines are often offloaded at small railway sidings or bus depots over weekends and the recipient is only informed of the arrival of the consignment the following Monday.

Maintaining a cold chain during the dispatch of biological products is commonly believed to be an obstacle to using vaccines in developing countries. Yilma (1989) mentions a particular problem in Ethiopia with regard to hot arid conditions. Other authors (Belsham *et al.*, 1989) have stated that cold chains are often available for medical supplies and human vaccines and these can be utilized for veterinary biologicals. Effective cold packages can be devised using polystyrene containers into which frozen cool-bricks can be packed to keep vaccine within the optimum temperature range for 24 hours, provided the package is well sealed.

Cold chain monitors are available commercially. These indicate by a colour change on an indicator card whether the product has been exposed to high temperatures for any length of time. Maximum/minimum thermometers can be included in packages to monitor their ability to maintain the required temperature. In some countries, such as Lesotho, where temperatures drop below freezing in winter and vaccine is sometimes carried on horseback, inactivated vaccines such as rabies must be transported in insulated packages to prevent freezing.

POULTRY VACCINES FOR DEVELOPING COUNTRIES

Producing vaccines for intensive poultry raising systems in developing countries is uneconomic owing to the very low unit cost at which these vaccines can be supplied by large international companies. The latter also produce a wide variety of vaccines and can therefore provide the poultry producer with a complete range of products. In addition, intensive poultry farming calls for vaccines with a high safety and efficacy index. Any reactions caused by virulence of an attenuated strain, adjuvant reactions or infection with adventitious agents causing death, failure to protect, failure to gain weight or a drop in egg production will occur on a scale which affects the profit margins of the producer. *De novo* development of poultry vaccines, therefore, requires extensive efficacy and safety testing which few developing countries are able to undertake. The production of vaccines in embryonated eggs requires a source of specific pathogen-free (SPF) eggs and SPF birds are required for many of the QC tests performed for poultry vaccines.

COMPANION ANIMAL VACCINES

Developing countries vary in their demand for companion animal vaccines, other than rabies which is usually the concern of government authorities. In general, the greater the affluence of the country the more the attention given to the vaccination of pet animals. As in the case of the poultry industry, the demand for safety and efficacy of vaccines is high and, unless a producer can do sufficient research and development and safety testing, producing these vaccines is not economically viable. Producing a single component vaccine such as live attenuated distemper may be feasible, but more sophisticated consumers will demand combination vaccines which contain multiple antigens.

LICENSING OF BIOLOGICAL PRODUCTS

The situation with regard to the licensing of biologicals in developing countries varies considerably; in some South American countries government authorities have the facilities for testing vaccines and have personnel who are well informed on vaccine production facilities and processes. Other countries may have only a small government department with a few officials encumbered with the licensing of local and imported biologicals. These officials may not be well informed about vaccines and vaccine production; often minimal data on safety and efficacy is required to license a product. In the southern African region, for example, each country has its own small group of technical advisers. It may be advantageous for countries in this situation to pool resources and devise a harmonized registration and regulatory system, which will prevent duplication of registration offices and costs.

BIBLIOGRAPHY

Abaracon, D. & Giacometti, H. 1976. Vaccines against foot-and-mouth disease and virus produced in cell cultures with bovine serum treated with polyethylene glycol. *Bol. Cent. Panam. Fiebre Aftosa,* 21-22: 49-53.

Bahnemann, H.G. 1990. Inactivation of viral antigens for vaccine preparation with particular reference to the application of binary ethylenimine. *Vaccine,* 8: 299-303.

Barteling, S.J. 1974. Use of polyethylene glycol treated serum for the production of foot-and-mouth disease virus in growing BHK suspended cell cultures. *Bull. Off. int. Epiz.,* 81(11-12): 1243-1254.

Belsham, G.J., Anderson, E.C., Murray, P.K., Anderson J. & Barrett, T. 1989. Immune response and protection generated by a vaccinia virus recombinant expressing the F protein of rinderpest virus. *Vet. Rec.,* 124: 655-658.

Doel, T.R. 1993. *In* A.R. Peters, ed. *Vaccines for veterinary application.* London, Butterworth-Heinemann.

Kriazeff, A.J., Wopschall, L.J. & Hopps, H.E. 1975. Detection of bovine viruses in bovine serum used in cell culture. *In Vitro,* 11: 400-403.

Lambert, K.J. & Birch, J.R. 1985. Cell growth media. *In* R.E. Spier & J.B. Griffiths, eds. *Animal cell biotechnology,* Vol. 1, p.111. London, Academic.

Oberem, P.T. & Bezuidenhout, J.D. 1987. The production of heartwater vaccine. *Onder. J. Vet. Res.,* 54: 485-488.

OIE. 1992. *Manual of Standards for Diagnostic Tests and Vaccines for List A and B Diseases of Mammals, Birds and Bees,* 2nd edition. Paris, Office International des Epizooties.

Panina, G.F. 1985. Monolayer growth systems: multiple processes. *In* R.E. Spier & J.B. Griffiths, eds. *Animal cell biotechnology,* Vol 1. London, Academic.

Rogers, R.J., Dimmock, C.K. & de Vos, A.J. 1988. Bovine leucosis virus contamination of a vaccine produced *in vivo* against bovine babesiosis and anaplasmosis. *Austr. Vet. J.,* 65: 285-287.

Sharp, J.R. 1983. *Guide to good pharmaceutical manufacturing practice.* London, Her Majesty's Stationery Office.

Sterne, M. & Wentzel, L.M. 1950. A new method for the large-scale production of high-titre botulinum formol-toxoid types C and D. *J. Immunol.,* 65: 175-183.

Ubertini, B., Nardelli, L., Dal Prato, A., Panina, G.F. & Santero, G. 1963. Large-scale cultivation of foot-and-mouth disease virus on calf-kidney cell monolayers in rolling bottles. *Zentralbl. Veteriner. Med., (B),* 10: 93-101.

Yilma, T.D. 1989. Prospects for the total eradication of rinderpest. *Vaccine,* 7: 484-485.

PART III

Production operations

Basic laboratory services and media preparation for vaccine production

E.E. Worrall

The services to a vaccine production unit should be of the highest standard attainable and should provide a structure that is appropriate, taking into consideration the conditions and resources normally expected in a developing country. The factors that have a fundamental influence on the quality and sustainability of these services are:

- *Water supply.* Methods of water treatment should ensure high quality, and the most appropriate equipment to achieve a high standard of final water quality should be selected.
- *Electricity supply.* This service is vulnerable to supply interruption and its quality is often beyond the control of the end-user. Protective devices should be installed to ensure an uninterrupted, stabilized power supply, independent of the generating authority. Although the equipment used in the central services section is not as vulnerable to voltage fluctuation and supply interruption as the more sensitive equipment found in production units, it still requires a constant and uninterrupted supply to maintain a high standard of service.
- *Capital equipment.* Careful consideration must be given to the selection of the equipment needed to operate a central services section successfully. It should always be borne in mind that the most sophisticated is not necessarily the best and the natural desire to incorporate the latest technology should be carefully evaluated before a decision is made. At the early planning stages, scale is also a very important factor to consider.

WATER

Water is undoubtedly the most vital and fundamentally important resource required by the central services and media departments. It is therefore extremely important to ensure its uninterrupted supply and quality.

The quality of the raw water available to a laboratory depends to a great extent on the geological stucture of the catchment area and the nature and quantity of the minerals dissolved in it. In many cases the laboratory has no control over the selection of source and is obliged to rely on the supply provided by the local water authority. The source can be a well, a spring or a borehole, adjacent to and under the control of the end-user. However, the water quality is still dependent on the geological strata surrounding the aquifer.

The supply of clean drinkable water in developing countries varies considerably. In many cases the supplying authority will have carried out some form of pretreatment to give a supply fit for human consumption. Generally this means chemical flocculation followed by filtration and chlorination. These processes can introduce an increased chemical composition which must be removed before the water can be used for vaccine production. In many arid catchment areas, boreholes and wells that suffer seasonal variation are often contaminated further with particulate matter in the form of colloidal clays and laterites and may not be subjected to treatment by the local water supply authority. In such cases, the laboratory should pretreat the waters before attempting further purification.

Methods of determining the quality of the raw water

Optical clarity. This is usually obvious and can easily be determined by visual observation of a sample in a glass beaker against a transmitted light source.

Soluble mineral salts and ionic composition. A reliable measurement of the degree of dissolved solids in raw water can be made using a conductivity meter which measures its electrical conductivity in microsiemens per centimetre. This will give a good indication of the purity of raw water. Waters with a high mineral content can give readings as high as 1 500 microsiemens/cm whereas softer waters with lower mineral content can be in the region of 50 to 200 microsiemens/cm.

It should be emphasized that this measurement on its own, although a valuable indication of the general purity, cannot identify the soluble salts of calcium and magnesium which, in the main, are the cause of damaging permanent hardness. A simple colorimetric test kit is available which will determine the relative degree of hardness in the water sample and thereby indicate if the water is hard, medium or soft.

In general, soft waters, if not contaminated with particulate matter, are perfectly suitable for all washing operations and for direct feed to stills and deionizers without pretreatnent. If particulate matter is found to be a problem it can be removed effectively by coarse-clarifying unglazed porcelain candle filters which can be incorporated between the equipment and the raw water supply.

This type of filter is recommended for the small vaccine production unit because it presents a sustainable type of system, will give years of trouble-free operation and does not rely on the frequent importation of disposable cartridges which some current systems require. Furthermore, these filters can be dissassembled easily by unskilled operators, scrubbed by hand, backwashed to remove the surface film of particulate material and be back in operation within a short time.

Equipment for water purification

At this stage some consideration has to be given to scale and the volumes of media and vaccines to be produced as these have a direct bearing on the size and output of the equipment to be installed. In large units with high consumption, where raw water is pumped from a borehole or drawn directly from a river or stream and is heavily contaminated with particulate and colloidal matter, it might be advisable to treat all raw water entering the service unit by installing a sand filtration system to reduce suspended solids to less than 40 microns and give flow rates of 50 litres per minute. Such equipment is available commercially and is simple to operate and maintain, no chemical regeneration is necessary and it requires only a physical backwash service regeneration operated by a seven-day timer. For vaccine production units producing a total of approximately 15 000 litres of mixed viral and bacterial vaccines per annum, semi-industrial scale water purification equipment is the best option. It is wiser to install appropriately sized equipment which will be fully utilized rather than opting for prestigious large-scale equipment which may be grossly underutilized and involves high capital expenditure. Future increased demand should be anticipated, however, and the capacity should be able to cope with at least a doubling of demand.

Water-softening plant

Medium- to large-scale vaccine producing units in developing countries frequently opt for a central semi-industrial water-softening plant which treats all incoming raw water before reticulation to the various sections for individual uses. Although this may seem to be a good practice, such a system continues to operate effectively. Without strict monitoring and the delegation of responsibility to a responsible operator, the system breaks down and generally falls into disuse. It is also wasteful to soften all incoming water when much of it will be used for general purposes for which softened water is unnecessary and when softening large quanitites of water requires frequent regeneration of the equipment which results in operator fatigue and neglect. It is often better to install smaller individual softeners at the points where they are most required, such as the bottle cleaning department and, where necessary, to protect stills and electrically operated steam generators.

The decision to install water-softening plant is, therefore, entirely dependent on the degree of hardness of the raw water. In general, water with a degree of hardness greater than 10°dH should be softened for laboratory use, and many natural raw waters have values much greater than this (e.g. 28° hardness). A plant that delivers approximately 110 m^3 of water at 1° hardness between regeneration cycles will be adequate for most small- to medium-scale vaccine production units.

Water-softening plants are usually of the single bed resin ion exchange type, regenerated with sodium chloride. Modern units are completely automatic and have a monitoring device which actuates the regeneration cycle when the degree of hardness becomes unacceptable. The operator has only to maintain a suitable level of salt in the regeneration reservoir.

Uses for the softened water include the first wash in the bottle cleaning section, where it can greatly reduce the need for expensive detergents and soaps, and for the protection of stills, where it eliminates the build-up of damaging calcium and magnesium scale on the heating elements. Softened water should not be used to protect deionizers as the effluent contains a high concentration of sodium ions which would rapidly exhaust the ion exchange resins of the deionizer.

Water pressure

Water pressure is an important consideration and for the efficient operation of water softeners, deionizers and automatic stills the pressure on the equipment at raw water inlets should be at least 2.5 bar.

Deionizers

Deionizers are very useful for the culture media and bottle cleaning departments of the vaccine production unit where large volumes of relatively pure water are required. Most modern equipment is capable of delivering high-quality water with a purity matching glass double-distilled water of around 0.08 microsiemens/cm.

A moderately sized twin bed or mixed bed system will provide water at a flow rate of 300 litres per hour for the final rinsing of glassware and for all culture media preparation with perhaps the exception of tissue culture media which ideally should be depyrogenated.

Water purification systems based on ion exchange, reverse osmosis or a combination of both are available for the laboratory and vaccine production unit. Most systems rely on expensive factory-produced cartridge replacements when the resins are exhausted. This system is very difficult to sustain in a developing country where extreme demands on hard currency reserves lead to extended use of exhausted cartridges and a resulting fall in water quality.

A more sustainable system is one which utilizes automatic electrical flushing regeneration of the resins *in situ* whereby the resins do not require chemical regeneration nor do they become exhausted and need expensive replacement. Flow rates of 1 200 litres per hour and greater are possible with equipment only 1 m high and occupying less than 0.3 m^2 of floor space. If the equipment does not have a built-in conductivity meter, monitoring the conductivity of the effluent from the deionizer can be done by using a hand held meter.

Stills

With the exception of the most sophisticated deionizers, which contain depyrogenating cartridges, the all-glass double-distillation still is undoubtably the most reliable and sustainable system for the production of pyrogen-free water with a conductivity lower than 0.1 microsiemens/cm suitable for cell culture.

Modern automatic stills are compact and very reliable pieces of equipment which will give years of trouble-free service as long as they are protected from scale formation by the upstream installation of a suitable water softener when used in hard water areas.

Most modern equipment is provided with fail-safe and automatic cleaning devices which make it very easy to operate. Glass double-distillation units are available with outputs of up to 8.0 litres per hour and, with suitable upstream protection and a reliable power and water supply, these can be operated continuously providing ample water for cell culture vaccines.

ELECTRICITY

The central services unit must be connected to an automatic trip standby generator in order to ensure a completely uninterrupted electricity supply. Each section should be provided with sufficient power outlet sockets rated at 15 amps connected to a sub-distribution board containing automatic trip miniature circuit-breakers to protect all equipment from overloading and short-circuiting. The sockets should be located 15 cm above bench height and must be properly earthed. Sockets in the media preparation and bottle cleaning sections should ideally be of the splash-proof type.

Where three-phase 380/400v supply is required for larger equipment such as autoclaves, stills and steam generators lines should terminate via a suitable automatic trip fused switch-box.

Voltage stabilization is not normally required in the central services section as most of the equipment there is fairly robust. With the increased use of more sophisticated, microprocessor-controlled systems, however, it would be advisable, if the vaccine production laboratory is already served with a stabilized supply, to install an outlet in the media preparation room. The cold room and freezer room should be connected to a dedicated electrical supply, i.e. each piece of equipment should have its own line which is not connected to any other equipment, to avoid loss of function owing to accidental overloading with subsequent fuse trip disconnection.

Main and sub distribution boards should be equipped with an electromechanical interconnection that effectively disconnects all power when the protective cover is opened for inspection.

Electrically operated equipment handled in wet areas such as the media preparation section should be provided with residual current detection devices that switch off the supply to the equipment to protect the operator from possible electrocution in the event of serious current leakage.

THE CENTRAL SERVICE UNIT: DESIGN AND OPERATION

A central services unit is generally composed of four distinct sections:

- the decontamination section;
- the bottle cleaning section;
- the media preparation section;
- the sterilization section.

Each section has its own special function which is distinctly related and physically linked to those of the other sections in such a way as to provide the most efficient use of space and to adhere to the rules of good manufacturing practice (GMP). Ideally the central services unit should be located on the same floor as the vaccine production section and both should be accessible by a shared service corridor. In designing a new central services unit or modifying an existing one, careful attention should be given to the traffic patterns of both personnel and materials within the related sections to ensure efficient and safe operation.

The unit can be constructed from hollow concrete blocks or bricks faced with a high-quality cement screed and finished with waterproof plastic paint. All electrical wiring should preferably be surface-mounted using a ring main layout from a main distribution board through suitably fused miniature circuit-breakers to surface mounted outlet sockets located 15 cm above bench height. Where three-phase supply is required for stills, electrically heated autoclaves, steam generators and hot air ovens the outlets should be terminated with appropriately fused isolator switch-boxes. In wet areas such as the bottle cleaning and media preparation rooms all outlet sockets should be of the splash-proof type and suitable earthing should be mandatory. Great care must be taken to ensure that there are sufficient outlet sockets in each section to avoid the common and dangerous practice of overloading outlets with multiple adaptors.

The floors throughout the central services section should be of high-quality waterproof terrazzo continued 15 cm up the walls and, with the exception of those in the sterile filtration and hot and cold rooms, all floors should be provided with adequate falls to a common glazed earthenware or plastic drain running the full length of the outside walls and covered with a removable, durable, perforated grating. This last feature is essential, especially in the media preparation section, to facilitate the washing and chemical decontamination of the high-traffic working areas.

The use of factory-prepared, prefabricated benching and "flat-pack" furniture made from melamine-surfaced high-density particle board is a cheap and practical solution. This furniture can be installed by relatively inexperienced staff and is very flexible in form and function.

The decontamination section

The decontamination section is designed to deal only with hazardous contaminated materials originating from the vaccine production unit. It should be accessible from all sections of the vaccine production unit and be completely self-contained with a single access from the shared service corridor.

This section should contain a suitable reception table on which the material to be decontaminated is placed. Ideally the contaminated material should be sterilized in a double-ended autoclave, the dirty side of which is accessible from the decontamination section and the clean side from the adjacent room which houses the bottle cleaning section. All material entering the autoclave in the decontamination section should be identified with autoclave tape which will give the operator receiving it in the bottle cleaning area clear visual evidence that the load has been sterilized.

Autoclaves of this type are generally

operated by mains steam originating from either a central boiler house in relatively large vaccine production units or from smaller electrically operated steam generating units. Steam pressure of at least 15 kg per square centimetre is required to operate this type of autoclave, which should also be fitted with a water-operated vacuum system to remove trapped air and ensure efficient penetration of the load by superheated steam. The autoclave should be fitted with safety door locks to prevent the opening of either door until the pressure and temperature are within safe operational limits and present no hazard to the operator.

The cycle should be electronically controlled by solid-state circuitry. A truck and rail system for loading and unloading should be incorporated to permit complete removal of the load before handling.

Bottle cleaning

The bottle cleaning section should be situated adjacent to the decontamination section and is used for the cleaning of all glassware and equipment originating from the decontamination autoclave and of uninfected material from the vaccine unit. It houses the deionizer, still and water softener. It should have a reception bench on which all dirty but uninfected glassware, etc. can be placed. This material, together with the decontaminated contents of the double-ended autoclave, is then subjected to the washing/cleaning process.

The bottle cleaning section should have three large deep polypropylene sinks fitted with large-bore vertical overflow pipes and supplied with hot and cold water. The local construction of concrete, terrazzo or tiled sinks is not recommended since, invariably, such sinks lead to unacceptable glassware breakages and are difficult to keep clean.

It is important to consider the work flow pattern. Most operators are right-handed, so it is covenient to plan an anticlockwise flow pattern. Sterilized previously infected material originating from the double-ended autoclave and uninfected dirty material should be collected on a large table to the right of the operator. The glassware is then subjected to a hot water and detergent soak in the first sink, followed by brushing, if necessary, to remove stubborn adhesions with an electrically powered bottle brushing machine. The glassware is then transferred to the second sink on the operator's left, where it is rinsed with hot water. In the third sink the glassware receives a final rinse in deionized water and is left to drain on racks. The clean, dry glassware can then be stored in a room designated for non-sterile clean glassware in this section.

The rinsing of glassware is best carried out using pressure jet nozzles located at the base of the tap-water and deionized water rinsing sinks. These nozzles can be adapted to suit all types of bottles, test tubes, etc. and are available commercially from laboratory equipment suppliers. For larger vaccine production units it may be desirable to consider a fully automatic bottle washing machine but in most developing countries it is probably more practical to utilize human operators using the simpler equipment described previously.

Media preparation section

The media preparation section requires very careful consideration and the ultimate layout and size will depend largely on the batch sizes that are to be produced. If production batch volumes are to be greater than 50 litres per batch, it will be necessary to consider the installation of equipment capable of handling larger volumes – up to 100 to 200 litres per batch. In such cases, it is better to install steam-heated hemispherical stainless steel vessels complete with rim-mounted electric stirrers. The most convenient and practical layout would be one 50-litre capacity stainless steel hemispherical vessel fitted with a mild steel jacket and mounted on four mild steel legs and two 200-litre vessels of a similar design. The steam jacket of each vessel should also have a cold water supply to facilitate rapid cooling when required.

These three vessels constitute the preparation vessels necessary for culture media prepared from dehydrated ingredients and for the preparation of protein hydrolysates. They should be situated adjacent to one another and all steam trap and waste water outlets should be connected to a suitable floor drain along an exterior wall. All the steam pans should be covered by a suitable extraction hood venting through an adjacent exterior wall. The floor of the media preparation room should be constructed of high-quality terrazzo with a suitable fall to a glazed earthenware or plastic floor drain, covered with a removable perforated cast iron or alloy grating. The terrazzo flooring should be continued 15 cm up the walls to complete a well-drained, durable, washable surface. Culture media prepared in the vessels described above can be transferred directly by peristaltic pumps through high-capacity membrane filters housed in an adjacent sterile filtration room. The sterile filtration room should be equipped with a horizontal laminar flow cabinet and a stainless steel sink supplied with cold water and two bench-mounted gas taps connected by copper tubing to a cylinder of propane located in a well-ventilated gas store outside the building. The sterile filtrate can either be pumped directly into sterile fermenters housed in the adjacent vaccine production unit or be delivered into the appropriate final sterile glass or disposable plastic growth bottles in the filtration room prior to transfer to the production unit.

All operations within the sterile filtration room should be carried out using aseptic precautions.

Large-scale culture media which is to be sterilized *in situ* can also be pumped directly into fermenters or suitable containers using peristaltic flow inducers. This type of pump is highly recommended as the simplest means of handling liquid for both direct transfer and positive pressure filtration.

In-house processing of culture media raw materials. In vaccine production units with a suitable supporting infrastructure, where large volumes of culture media are used and where local resources such as mammalian protein in the form of waste (condemned) meat, milk by-products such as whey, vegetable protein by-products such as maize gluten and waste blood from abbatoirs are available, the processing of such raw materials can be considered as a means of increasing self-sufficiency and reducing dependency on costly imported dehydrated media.

Hydrolysates of these materials can be prepared using the three vessels already described, concentrated by vacuum evaporation to a density ot 40 percent total solids and stored at -20°C or, preferably, spray-dried to give a free flowing powder of greater stability that does not require refrigerated storage.

The media preparation section should have access to walk-in refrigerated rooms at -20°C and 4°C for the storage of perishable raw materials and finished sterile media and walk-in incubators at 37°C for the sterility testing of filtered media in bulk containers.

A complete set of formulae and standard operating procedures should be available for all culture media prepared in the section and copies distributed to all end-users. A review procedure should be adopted where new formulae can be included and existing ones upgraded when necessary. A customer request system should be instigated to help ensure the smooth operation and execution of orders and to help maintain a record of raw material consumption.

A batch numbering system should be operated for all batches of media prepared to enable identification in the event of end-user complaint and to help identify any associated procedure that may have had either a beneficial or a deleterious effect. Following sterilization by autoclaving or filtration, a representative sample of all batches of culture media should be subjected to a period of incubation at 37°C for not less than 21 days as a check on the efficacy of sterilization procedures. When large volumes of a medium are filtered without the inclusion of antibiotics, for example volumes of 20 litres in glass vessels to supply a continuous culture fermenter, it is essential to ensure the sterility of the medium by incubating the whole batch prior to use, thus avoiding costly contamination and the subsequent interruption of production schedules. The incubation period should be long enough to reveal contamination without diminishing the nutritive properties of the medium.

Sterilization section

Situated adjacent to and linked by a door into the media preparation section, this room should house the sterile autoclave and hot air oven. It is used for the final sterilization, by autoclaving or dry heat, of glassware, media and other materials from the vaccine production sections. The sterilization section should be equipped with at least two four-wheeled trolleys for the transportation of material to the vaccine production unit.

All material leaving this section should be clearly identified as sterile by the use of heat-sensitive autoclave tape secured to each item and showing unequivocally that it has been exposed to sterilizing temperatures for the necessary period.

Equipment for the central services section

Decontamination section. This section should be equipped with:

- a double-ended autoclave operated by mains steam with interior dimensions of 120 cm wide, 150 cm high and 250 cm long;
- a vacuum steam extraction facility;
- free steaming and pressure cycles that are electronically controlled;
- thermal safety locks on all doors;
- a steam-jacketed load-drying facility;
- wheeled trucks and rails for easy loading and unloading.

Bottle cleaning section. This section should be equipped with:

- a floor-mounted continuous deionizer that is electrically regenerable *in situ* and has a capacity of 1 200 litres per hour at 1.0 microsiemen/cm (e.g. Millipore DI system Model No. 9042);
- a floor-mounted water softener that is regenerable *in situ* using sodium chloride (NaCl) and has a capacity of 1 500 m^3 at 1°dH;
- a wall-mounted all glass double-distillation unit with automatic cleaning and sterilizing cycles, power and water fail-safe protection and a capacity of 8.0 litres per hour at less than 1.0 microsiemen/cm, pyrogen-free distillate (6.5 kilowatt, three-phase 380/400 V, 50 Hz);
- an electrically operated bottle brushing machine complete with assorted bottle brushes (220 V, 50 Hz);
- two heavy-duty free-standing, pressure-operated bottle/test tube rinsers for raw water and deionized water rinsing;
- a peristaltic flow inducer with variable speed control and a pumping rate from

140 ml to 33 litres per minute (220 V, 50 Hz, e.g. Watson Marlow 701U/R);

- three heavy-duty black polypropylene sinks with wide-bore vertical overflow pipes and traps, 100 cm long, 50 cm wide and 40 cm deep;
- a wall-mounted draining rack;
- a floor-mounted hot-air drying oven with fan blower, variable temperature adjustment (50° to 200°C) and timer operation, internal dimensions of 100 cm wide, 200 cm high and 150 cm deep, with adjustable shelving;
- a hand held conductivity meter with digital readout multirange of 0.1 to 2 000 microseimens/cm;
- four 100-litre polypropylene aspirators with taps, mounted on fully castoring wheeled bases.

Media preparation section. This section should be equipped with:

- two stainless steel, 200-litre capacity, steam heated, mild steel jacketed, hemispherical bottomed boiling vessels mounted on four mild steel tubular legs, fitted with steam/water vapour traps and cooling water entry and exit to the mild steel jacket and with rim-mounted 0.5 horsepower (about 375 watts) stainless steel stirrer;
- a stainless steel, 50-litre capacity, steam heated, mild steel jacketed, hemispherical bottomed boiling vessel mounted on four mild steel tubular legs, fitted with steam/water vapour traps and cooling water entry and exit to the mild steel jacket and with rim-mounted 300-watt stirrer.
- two graduated stainless steel jugs of 2-litre capacity;
- two hemispherical scoops of 2.5-litre capacity;
- a stainless steel heavy-duty dial-type centigrade thermometer;
- a stainless steel plate (40 cm by 40 cm) and frame filter press containing 20 plates with transfer plate, fitted with Saunders inlet and outlet valves with 30-mm rifled nozzles, mounted horizontally on a wheeled chassis;
- a heavy-duty peristaltic flow inducer with capacity of 140 ml to 33 litres per minute (e.g. Watson Marlow 701U/R);
- a peristaltic flow inducer/dispenser for the calibrated delivery of sterile culture media, dose range of 1.0 ml to 16 litres with positive cut-off control and with a 20:1 control ratio (e.g. Watson Marlow 501Z/R);
- a stainless steel 293-mm diameter membrane filter using 0.22-micron filtration discs (e.g. Millipore or Sartorius);
- ten heat-sterilizable polysulphone 100-mm diameter pressure-type filters using membrane 0.22-micron micropore filters;
- a multidisc cartridge filter using 0.22-micron PVDF filters with a maximum flow rate of 16 litres per hour;
- two hot plate magnetic stirrers with assorted polytetrafluoroethylene-(PTFE)-covered followers (1 000 watt, 220/240 V, 50 Hz);
- a bench model pH meter with five spare electrodes;
- two hand held battery-operated pH meters with ten spare batteries and five electrodes;
- a water bath in stainless steel, 50 cm long, 30 cm wide and 30 cm deep, with gabled lid;
- a heavy-duty bench-mounted butcher's meat mincer with feed-hopper, spare cutting blades and discs;
- six seamless stainless steel, 100-litre capacity containers with lids, mounted on fully castoring detachable bases;
- a laminar horizontal flow product protection cabinet;
- four stainless steel funnels, 50-cm diameter;

- two stainless steel powder scoops, 1-kg capacity;
- an electronic top-loading balance with 5 000 g capacity and sensitivity/ readability of 1.0 g;
- an electronic top-loading balance with weighing range of 0 to 200 g and readability of 0.0001 g;
- an electronic platform scale with weighing range of 0 to 50 kg and readability of 100 g;
- an electrically operated steam generator providing dry steam at 15 kg/cm^2, with total working capacity to provide steam for two autoclaves and three steam-heated boiling vessels in the media preparation room.

Ancillary equipment for dehydrated media production. The media prepartion section will also require the following equipment if dehydrated media are to be produced:

- a steam-operated falling film evaporator for the concentration of dehydrated media preparations and protein hydrolysates;
- an electrically heated spray-dryer for the drying of dehydrated media and hydrolysed protein concentrates;
- six polypropylene measuring cylinders of 2-litres volume;
- six polypropylene measuring cylinders of 1-litre volume;
- six polypropylene measuring cylinders of 500-ml volume;
- six pyrex glass beakers of 2-litres volume;
- six pyrex glass beakers of 1-litre volume;
- six pyrex glass beakers of 500-ml volume.

Sterilization section. This section should be equipped with:

- a single-doored mains steam-operated autoclave with water-operated steam evacuation system, steam jacketed for load-drying, free steaming and pressure cycles operated by electronic circuitry, thermal safety locks on door, operation cycle chart recorder, wheeled truck and rail loading system;
- a floor-mounted hot air oven with blower fan, temperature control of 50° to 300°C, timer-operated cycle, stainless steel lined with multiposition shelving, 100 cm wide, 200 cm high and 150 cm deep;
- two double-shelved, fully castoring four-wheeled rubber-tyred trolleys.

Laboratory furniture. Laboratories have the following requirements:

- laboratory bench tops made from 40-mm thick, high- density particle board (680 kg/m^3), with the upper surface covered in factory-fabricated melamine, heat- and chemical-resistant plastic with one long edge post formed, 3 000 mm by 600 mm by 40 mm;
- T-profile white plastic or aluminium jointing strips to conceal joints in worktops;
- silicone rubber sink sealant for the water-repellent sealing of sinks and joints in worktops.
- five under-bench floor units acting as worktop supports constructed from 18-mm high-stability melamine-faced high-density particle board, assembled by means of integral rapid assembly slotted turn catches, with cupbboards supported on black plastic adjustable legs, doors hung on 170° self-closing hinges, fitted with flush full-width aluminium finger pulls and drawers constructed from 12-mm plywood with runners of epoxy-coated steel on nylon roller carriages. The floor units should be of the following designs: i) two cupboards and two drawers; ii) four drawers; iii) single cupboard; iv) three drawers; and v) single cupboard and single drawer;

- a sink unit cupboard;
- three single-drainer stainless steel sinks;
- three black polypropylene sinks, 100 cm long, 50 cm wide and 50 cm deep, fitted with large-bore constant overflow pipes and quick-release traps.

Recommended building specifications

It is understood that buildings and services should comply completely with national building standards; however, the following specifications are offered as a guide:

Walls. Load-bearing walls should be confined to external and corridor walls. External walls should be of either double brick cavity with damp course or hollow block concrete. The external walls should be finished with mortared brick or, in the case of hollow block concrete, finished with cement rendering.

Corridor walls and the walls of hot rooms and freezer rooms should be made of hollow cement block with both surfaces cement rendered to a smooth finish.

All wall surfaces should be sealed with polyvinyl acetate (PVA) sealer before painting. Washable plastic paint should be used for all areas. In the wet areas, such as the bottle cleaning and media preparation rooms, exposed walls should be tiled from the floor to 50 cm above bench height with ceramic wall tiles using waterproof tile adhesive and waterproof grouting compound. All tile-bench junctions should be sealed with mould-resistant silicone rubber mastic.

Ceilings. Ceilings should be fitted with a false ceiling of fire-resistant fibre or cement or plasterboard. All joints and cornices should be plastered over and sealed to prevent dust entry.

Floors. Floors should be constructed of damp-proof reinforced concrete covered with terrazzo screed or tiles with terrazzo screed carried 15 cm up the walls. In high-traffic wet areas, drainage slopes of at least 1:100 should be made leading to plastic or glazed earthenware open drains situated along outside walls and covered with removable cast iron grids. All drain exits to the main waste water system should be covered with vermin-proof traps.

Doors. Doors in the filtration rooms and bottle store should be a standard 90 cm wide. All doors opening on to the service corridor and those linking the sections should be 150 cm wide to allow for easy access and to facilitate the subsequent installation of large pieces of equipment such as autoclaves and spray-dryer.

Windows. Windows should be large enough to permit adequate natural lighting and should be placed at least 120 cm from the floor. Window frames should be constructed of hot dipped galvanized steel with glass panes completely sealed with putty. Individual window openings should be of sufficient size to serve as emergency exits in the event of a fire. All opening windows should be mosquito- and fly-proofed with netting screens.

Benches. All bench tops should be factory pre-formed and melamine-surfaced, with the long edge post formed. They should be constructed from high-density particle board 40 mm thick and preferably 90 cm wide. Workbench heights should be 85 cm except in special areas where they may have a reduced height of 70 cm to serve as writing tables or for the installation of bench-top-mounted laminar flow cabinets.

Cupboards, drawers and sink units. These should preferably be factory-prefabricated, user-assembled, flat-pack units constructed from 18-mm melamine-surfaced high-density particle board and equipped with four plastic adjustable legs. These units can be used to support the bench tops giving ample kick space and allowing complete access for the cleaning of floor areas beneath and around them.

Sinks for the bottle cleaning unit should preferably be constructed from heavy-duty polypropylene, 60 cm long, 50 cm wide and 30 cm deep, with a top edge flange of 3 cm and large-bore drain fitted with a removable vertical overflow pipe to facilitate the continuous rinsing of glassware.

Shelves. Box-form shelves can be made from 18-mm melamine-surfaced high-density particle board, 30 cm wide, with supports at 50-cm centres. The walls should be drilled and plugged using plastic expandable plugs and the shelves attached using No. 8 woodscrews, through right-angled 3-mm mild steel fish-plates, firmly screwed to the back of the top inside corners of each 50-cm box-shelf partition.

Electricity supply. The unit should be surface rather than sub-surface wired using cables of appropriate cross-section to take the load with a safety margin of at least 30 percent. Surface-mounting permits easy access for electrical maintenance and also allows ready access for future modifications. All outlets, except in cases where three-phase 380/400 V, 50 Hz is required, should be 220/240 V, 50 Hz, 15 amp earthed sockets, mounted 15 cm above bench height and, in wet areas, outlets should be of the sealed, splash-proof type, fitted with residual circuit-breakers to provide full operator protection. Each section should be provided with a suitable subdistribution board equipped with miniature circuit-breakers adjusted to the correct safety amperage. The whole laboratory should be connected to an automatic start, standby generator. A large-capacity 10.5 kV voltage stabilizer should be installed to serve the whole unit and at least one outlet from this should be connected to each room to provide stabilized voltage for vital equipment where performance might be compromised by a fluctuating supply.

Dedicated lines (i.e. lines that are not shared by more than one piece of equipment) should also be installed to freezers, cold rooms and hot rooms to ensure their continuous operation.

Lighting. Laboratories should be adequately illuminated with fluorescent strip lights to give 400 lux at bench height.

Gas. Natural gas such as propane or butane should be reticulated via copper piping to the bottle cleaning and media preparation sections and should be supplied from a covered, well-ventilated central gas store, located outside the building.

Water supply. Cold water with a pressure of at least 2.5 bar should be reticulated via 1-cm galvanized steel pipes to all sections. The hot water required in the bottle cleaning section can be provided from electrically operated flash heaters or large-capacity 300-litre storage heaters.

Fire control. Fire extinguishers suitable for flammable chemicals, electrical and general fires should be located in each section.

First aid. A comprehensive first aid kit should be prominently situated in one designated room, with eyewash facilities in the media preparation room.

Modern cell culture technology for vaccine manufacture

P.J. Radlett

Since the early pioneering work on the mass cultivation of mammalian cells *in vitro,* many types of cells have been grown in a wide variety of culture systems. These have been used for the isolation and identification of viruses, the screening of antiviral and anti-cancer agents, the production of hormones, antibodies and other cellular products and, most important, the production of viruses and other organisms principally for the preparation of vaccines.

The wide range of uses for cell culture has resulted in the development of an equally wide range of cell cultivation systems, each being more or less appropriate for the required purpose. The number of cell cultivation techniques to have found broad acceptance for vaccine production is, however, much more limited, and this chapter will concentrate on these systems.

In general terms, the methods used for the production of culture media are similar, irrespective of the cell cultivation system used, but the methods appropriate to the selection and establishment of cell banks and for cell culture depend on whether the proposed cell substrate is a continuous line or derived directly from primary tissue and whether it will grow in free suspension culture or requires a suitable surface substrate for cell attachment.

An outline of the facilities required for the operation of cell culture units is given in the chapter, Basic laboratory services and media preparation for vaccine production, p.223. The scale of the vaccine manufacturing operation and the nature of the organism with which the vaccine is to be prepared will, however, have an impact on these requirements, in terms of the size and type of cell growth facility and the level of biological containment required for the associated antigen production area, of which the tissue culture unit may form a part.

SELECTION AND STORAGE OF CELL BANKS

Any cell substrate selected for vaccine production should be shown to be free from adventitious contamination. This includes bacterial, fungal and mycoplasmal contamination which would otherwise be likely to have deleterious effects on subsequent cell cultivation. Screening should also include the frequently less obvious contamination from agents, particularly viruses, which may persist in latent forms throughout the manufacturing process and cause disease or other adverse effects when injected with the vaccine into animals.

The selected substrate must also support the replication of the required organism to levels which are adequate and economic for vaccine production and should present the antigenic component in an immunogenic form and in a manner that permits its simple and cost-effective recovery for subsequent downstream manufacturing operations. Finally, the substrate and/or the components which may pass into the finished product must in themselves be intrinsically safe for the animals that will ultimately be the recipients, for the operators and for consumers of meat and meat products from the tissues of vaccinated animals.

Over the years there has been much debate on the intrinsic safety of established cell lines. In the early days of tissue culture the predominant view was that primary cells were likely to be safer because they lacked the "immortality" characteristic of continuous cell lines and, hence, the apparent risk of associated malignancy. Experience has shown that, providing the characteristics of cell lines obtained from normal tissues are carefully monitored and controlled and that the manufacturing process effectively eliminates whole cells from the product, the risks associated with their use are negligible. Furthermore, it is much more difficult to manage a cell production system in which each batch of material represents a new threat of introducing deleterious agents than it is with a cell line where a master stock can be established and thoroughly screened prior to its use for vaccine production. Petricciani (1987) has reviewed the arguments relating to the use of primary and continuous cell lines and concludes: "It is difficult to argue, however, that one is not better off with a very well tested cell system" (i.e. as offered by a continuous cell system) "and a manufacturing process which can cope with even theoretically worrisome contaminants".

In many situations the testing to which the cell substrate must be subjected will be laid down by the control authorities responsible for licensing the product. In Europe, the United States and some other countries, there are established guidelines for these requirements (EC, n.d.a and n.d.b) and, even in situations where there is not a mandatory requirement, the guidelines provide a useful and sensible basis by which the manufacturer can ensure that the products manufactured are likely to be safe to use. Against such a background, the manufacturer will identify a cell substrate which enables the production of the required antigen. In many cases this will be based on what has already been established by developments elsewhere and the manufacturer will need either to establish a new master cell bank (in the case of continuous cell lines) or to identify a suitable source of primary tissue.

Clearly, the amount of effort required to complete all the testing necessary to comply with the requirements described results in established and tested source materials with a significant commercial value. Manufacturers are unlikely either to make such materials freely available or to disclose the details of their findings. There are however, international depositories of characerized cell substrates which are unlikely to include the formally registered and tested materials but from which samples may be obtained for a nominal cost. Such organizations publish detailed information on those materials that they are able to make freely available (PHLS, n.d.) and which may often provide a source for initial culture material.

Primary cell culture

Primary tissue from an acceptable source will need to be transported to the laboratory rapidly under cool or cold conditions. Some primary tissues may be stored frozen pending culture, but in other cases there is a significant loss of susceptibility and/or viability associated with this practice.

There have been many reported techniques for handling primary tissue, but essentially all of these techniques comprise excision of the appropriate material for culture, dissociation as far as possible into a monodispersed suspension using a proteolytic enzyme (usually trypsin) either by itself or in combination with a chelating agent such as ethylenediamine tetra-acetic acid (EDTA) and dilution into a suitable growth medium. The techniques used for the dissociation and culture of a range of primary tissues are described in some detail in a number of publications, specifically in the manual edited by Kruse and Patterson (1973).

The cellular material so prepared may then require or tolerate some degree of amplification through a limited number of serial passages or transfers (usually only one or two) before evidence of senescence becomes apparent. Because of the limited life of such cultures it is not normally possible to lay down banks of substrate material and the antigen production process is usually confined to the use of simple culture flasks on a rather small scale. The amount of antigen required for a live virus vaccine is frequently much lower than that needed for an inactivated product. In consequence, this method of production may appear attractive for the preparation of live vaccines, but these are the products where the risks of live extraneous agents persisting into the final production stages are greatest. Because of the inherent risks arising from these cultures, vaccines produced in this way should be very carefully controlled prior to release. Nevertheless, where suitable continuous cell lines are not available the method still provides a satisfactory method of producing vaccines.

Continuous cell lines

When a suitable cell line for vaccine production purposes has been identified, it will be necessary to store an adequate number of ampoules of cells (as many as practicable) to establish a master bank. This bank can then be subjected to whatever testing is considered appropriate to demonstrate the suitability of the material for vaccine production purposes. From this master bank, subsidiary master and working banks can be established. An ampoule of cells can be revived from the working bank to initiate a cycle or series of cycles of production, followed by the revival of a further ampoule for additional production cycles. In this way the working banks can be made to last for a very long time before they become exhausted, when they can be replenished from the subsidiary master bank which, in turn, can be replenished from the original master bank. Such procedures make it possible to supply suitable cells on an almost indefinite basis, without the need for passaging them more than a fixed and limited number of times from the original tested material. Unlimited passaging of cells may (at least in theory) increase the risk of propagating cells with modified characteristics or of introducing adventitious contamination. A maximum of 20 passages from the master bank to the final production culture is normally considered acceptable and, in most well-managed production systems, this permits the production of several harvests without recourse to further stored material and enables production to continue for many years from the same basic cell stock.

The method of culture depends on the particular cell type and the scale and nature of the final production process. In most cases, however, either simple flat-bottomed flasks (for anchorage-dependent cell substrates) or simple stirred flasks (for cells that will grow in free suspension) are appropriate for both the production of cell banks and the preparation of seed material prior to transfer to the full-scale production system.

Cell storage

The cells held in the banks described above are almost invariably stored at low temperatures, either over or in liquid nitrogen, or at least below -65°C in a mechanical refrigerator. Doyle, Morris and Armitage (1988) have provided an excellent review of the process of cryopreservation which encompasses both the theoretical and practical aspects of the problem.

The following points are also worth noting:

- Storage over liquid nitrogen is the most satisfactory method. Storage in mechanical refigerators may, over several years, lead to some deterioration in viability. Immersion in liquid nitrogen can lead to problems with the integrity of the seal and there are risks from alternation between liquid and vapour phases if the liquid level is allowed to fluctuate.
- Some form of cryoprotectant is required. Dimethyl sulphoxide is extremely effective but is toxic and the contact time between the agent and viable cells in the liquid phase must be minimized. Glycerol is also very effective as a cryoprotectant and, because of its generally lower toxicity, may be easier to use.
- Much has been written about the freezing rate of cells and how it should be controlled. Controlled rate freezing equipment is, however, very expensive and by no means all cell substrates require this level of sophistication. Frequently, ampoules may be successfully stored directly over liquid nitrogen. Alternatively, some degree of control may be obtained by cooling ampoules in stages, through 4°C, to -20°C, -65°C and finally to the vapour phase of liquid nitrogen. In most cases, the cells in ampoules should be thawed as quickly as possible and diluted out of the preservative maintenance medium.
- Whatever the storage system adopted, the contents of the freezer will ultimately represent a considerable investment in time, resources and production potential. The importance of reliable, well-maintained facilities cannot be overemphasized and, wherever possible, dispersion of the cell stock to more than one location, or at least to more than one freezer, is recommended.
- The volume and density of the stored cells are critical factors that should be carefully optimized. Small volumes will freeze and thaw more quickly but high cell densities may rapidly modify the cultural environment, particularly the pH, during preparation and freezing. Conversely, sufficient cells are required in each ampoule to seed the revived culture adequately and at a sufficient volume to permit rapid cell amplification to full production scale.

PRODUCTION OF CULTURE MEDIUM

Much work has been directed towards the definition of culture medium for the growth of mammalian cells. The objectives of this work have varied among research workers, some concentrating on the precise definition of the nutritional requirements of cells without the inclusion of ill-defined supplements, while others have been concerned to minimize the waste of expensive raw materials. In the former case there is the obvious potential benefit of eliminating the risks of introducing adventitious agents and even of untoward vaccinal reactions when the traditional supplements such as serum and peptones are used. Defined media formulations have not, however, generally found favour for commercial vaccine manufacture, because industrial-scale yields were often lower (sometimes much lower) than could be obtained when supplements were used. Alternatively, the formulations described contained various complex additives which were too expensive for routine large-scale manufacturing operations.

Similarly, attempts to minimize the cost of culture media have not resulted in satisfactory formulations, partly because such formulations do not always provide comparable yields on serial passage over the full life of cells at the full scale of the manufacturing operation and partly because medium production costs are generally a very small proportion of the total manufacturing cost.

Water

Water is a most important constituent of the tissue culture medium and there is a requirement for good-quality water that is free from pyrogens and as free as practicable from contamination with bacteria, other organisms and impurities that may interfere with the cultivation of cells. Although impurities can be difficult or impossible to define precisely, suitable water may normally be prepared by ion exchange followed by either reverse osmosis or distillation. Assuming that a suitable primary source is available, the major problems are likely to concern the sterilization and maintenance of the purification equipment and the storage of the purified water.

The columns used for ion exchange and reverse osmosis cannot yet be simply and routinely sterilized by steam *in situ* and, in consequence, care has to be taken with the design and installation of the equipment itself and the operating and sterilization procedures. Furthermore, great care needs to be taken with the subsequent storage of water to ensure that recontamination, particularly with organisms that may produce pyrogens, does not occur. These aspects are considered in the chapter, General design and operating requirements for vaccine manufacturing establishments, p. 171.

Basic medium

The basic medium for cell culture almost always comprises a solution of sodium chloride supplemented with a range of inorganic salts to provide a balanced, isotonic medium with glucose as a carbon source. This solution is supplemented with a range of amino-acids and vitamins aimed essentially at providing all the nutritional requirements of the cells. To achieve satisfactory growth and the necessary cell densities for subsequent virus production, however, it is usually necessary to supplement the medium with an ill-defined peptone or animal serum or, most frequently, both. Although the precise formulations used for different products in different laboratories may vary extensively, most are variations of the early formulations published by pioneers in this field including Eagle (1955 and 1959).

The formulations used for cell maintainance during the virus culture phase are usually similar to those used for cell growth but for a number of systems it has proved possible to eliminate the serum from the formulation. It should not, however, be assumed that the virus replication phase takes place under serum-free conditions, since the carry over of residual medium from the cell growth phase can often be considerable.

Serum

As described above, the success of most veterinary vaccine manufacturing operations depends on the inclusion of animal serum, at least in the cell growth medium. Partly because of cost and general availability, serum of bovine origin is used almost exclusively. Many reports in the literature describe the use of newborn calf or even foetal bovine serum for cell culture. This is extremely expensive and wherever possible the use of the much less expensive and more readily available adult bovine serum is to be preferred. Whatever the type of serum used, this component is of major concern in respect to the accidental introduction of adventitious contamination. Attention has to be paid to ensure that the product is obtained only from healthy animals, is collected and processed under clean conditions and is adequately tested to give an assurance of freedom from extraneous agents. Because of the disease risks associated with this material, in many situations it is now only acceptable to use serum from countries such as New Zealand or parts of Australia in which the disease status is deemed satisfactory. Since some residual serum will very often find its way into the final vaccine, care also needs to be taken over the compatibility of the serum source and the target species for which the vaccine is intended. There have been cases of hypersensitivity associated with the use of serum from one species for the production of vaccines to be used in another.

Whatever the serum source, incorporation levels of 8 to 10 percent are frequently used for cell culture and, where care has been taken to use only selected high-quality serum, this can sometimes be reduced to 4 percent or lower without reducing cell yields. In such cases the economic benefits of using a high-quality but more expensive serum source can be justified economically. Even so, serum may well prove to be the most significant cost component of the medium, frequently exceeding all the other medium production costs combined.

Peptones

The list of peptones or similar compounds which have been used in culture medium is long and for perhaps understandable commercial reasons manufacturers are frequently reluctant to divulge the precise composition, origin and method of preparation relating to their products. In consequence, there may be significant variation between two media reported to contain a given concentration of peptone. The concentrations used in cell growth and maintenance media are frequently in the range of 1 to 5 grams per litre of medium and this alone can represent a significant proportion of the total medium production cost. The risks associated with introducing adventitious agents to this type of product are probably much lower than those associated with serum because a combination of heat treatment and enzymatic digestion is usually required in the preparation of the material. This cannot be assumed, however, and steps should be taken to gain an assurance that the risks via this route are indeed minimal.

Medium sterilization

The composition of tissue culture media generally precludes sterilization by heat and, although there were some early attempts to sterilize media by chemical means, filtration is the method used almost exclusively today. Early filtration processes relied on asbestos containing depth filters, which have been adequately demonstrated to produce a reliable sterile product – provided that the level of contamination in the unfiltered medium is controlled within reasonable limits (Telling, Stone and Maskell, 1966). Such filters have proved very effective at handling the rather difficult serum containing media. Where the nature of the medium has resulted in very low filtration volumes in relation to the filter area used or where double filtration has been used to increase confidence in the sterility of the product some reduction in cell growth potential has sometimes been experienced.

A more recent development in the manufacture of such filter media has been the introduction of asbestos free sheets, brought about by the perceived health risks associated with the manufacture of materials containing asbestos. Although such sheets are claimed to be of a sterilizing grade, this has not always been the case and caution should be exercised in using such materials for final sterilization.

More recently, cartridge-type filters have gained wide acceptance for the sterilization of tissue culture media. As with all filtration processes there is a need to control contamination in the unfiltered medium to within reasonable levels – both to reduce the number of organisms presented to the filter and to minimize the build-up of toxins and the possible degradation of the medium prior to filtration. In order to obtain economic throughputs from sterilizing cartridge filters, some form of prefiltration is generally required. This may be provided by the use of depth filters or cartridge units with a lower rating than the sterilizing filter. The presence of serum in the medium makes the use of cartridge units more difficult and the level of prefiltration required in such situations can be quite critical.

EQUIPMENT

The equipment required for cell and virus cultivation depends on the particular processes employed and is likely to be of stainless steel, glass or disposable plastic construction. Experience has shown that, where appropriate for the process, the type of equipment employed for bacterial fermentations is, with minor modifications, also applicable to mammalian cell culture and virus production. The main features of suitable static process plant are good smooth finishes and freedom from crevices and imperfections. These are particularly important in relation to stainless steel welds. Adequate valving is also essential to ensure effective sterilization and to permit the proper drainage of liquors and venting of air. Well-drained, properly arranged pipe runs are also of great importance.

The design of equipment that is to be sterilized by autoclaving should follow the same basic principles in relation to crevices, drainage and air venting, and attention must be paid to the handling of such equipment under sterile conditions including, where appropriate, its connection to static plant.

Culture equipment will require facilities for environmental control or will need to be held in a controlled environment. In some cases this can be as simple as maintaining the culture in a temperature-controlled room or cabinet, while in other cases some direct control of the culture vessel will be appropriate. It was demonstrated many years ago that temperature control could be achieved effectively in static tanks by the provision of a temperature-control loop with a heating facility directly applied to the tank (Telling and Elsworth, 1965). Despite the simplicity of this method many workers fear the effects of local overheating and still prefer an indirect system of circulating warm water – even with its attendant complexity.

Fixed culture vessels are amenable to the convenient installation of additional environmental control facilties, but these add a degree of complexity that needs to be carefully balanced against the perceived benefits. Automatic control of pH, although certainly desirable, may not be essential for many processes and, in view of the relatively slow growth rate of the cell culture, manual adjustment at intervals may be sufficient. Some form of oxygenation may be required to maximize growth yields, but it may not be necessary to resort to automatic control in order to satisfy the culture's requirements. Modern oxygen electrodes may be more reliable than their predecessors but, nevertheless, add a degree of complexity which manufacturers may prefer to avoid. The relatively low metabolic rate associated with cell culture has enabled some operators to arrange a programme of manually adjusted sparged air rates sufficient to satisfy the culture's requirements.

The more sophisticated modern manufacturing procedures may require significant downstream processing. Equipment for some of these operations, such as that for concentration by ultrafiltration, may not be amenable to sterilization by steam. In such cases a regime of chemical sterilization must be developed but this will always carry potential contamination risks. Care needs to be taken to minimize the proportion of the plant that requires chemical sterilization, and also over the interface between chemically sterilized and heat-sterilized parts of the plant.

CELL CULTURE AND ANTIGEN PRODUCTION

The basic methods employed for cell culture and antigen production depend on whether the cell source is dependent on a fixed substrate for growth and replication (anchorage dependence) or will grow in free suspension. Although the benefits of simplicity and easy scale-up associated with the operation of free suspension systems are considerable, the range of susceptible cell lines suitable for vaccine production is rather limited and many vaccine manufacturing processes are based on anchorage-dependent systems. In contrast, the use of suspension systems has permitted the bulk production of some vaccines, such as those against foot-and-mouth-disease (FMD) and rabies, which are required in particularly large quantities.

Antigens produced by culture may be used for the production of either live attenuated or inactivated vaccines. The culture methods used are likely to be similar in both cases but, because the effective dose of a live attenuated vaccine (which is subsequently amplified by replication within the tissues of the host) is generally much lower than for an inactivated vaccine (the antigen of which cannot be amplified within the recipient), the volumes required at the production stage are proportionately lower for live vaccines.

In many cases the virus is released freely into the maintenance medium following incubation of the virus culture. Where this does not take place it may be necessary to disrupt the cells by mechanical, ultrasonic or chemical means to release intracellular virus prior to proceeding with vaccine production. There are, however, situations where the whole cell containing the infectious agent is used for the production of live attenuated vaccines. In all cases except the last it will be necessary to remove the cell debris resulting from the virus replication phase prior to proceeding with vaccine manufacture, and this has been variously accomplished by sedimentation, centrifugation or filtration.

Anchorage-dependent cell systems

Conventionally, anchorage-dependent cells are grown on the flat sides of simple glass or plastic bottles. In such cases, the scale-up for bulk manufacture may require no more than the use of multiples of the largest practicable bottles that can be incubated in a conventional hot room. Many attempts have been made to increase the efficiency of such a process by increasing the surface area within each unit available for cell growth. The use of roller cultures enables almost all of the contained internal surface area to be utilized – as opposed to less than half in a conventional static culture – but introduces the additional complexity of the need for roller equipment. Nevertheless, facilities for handling large numbers of roller cultures have been developed and, for those cells that cannot be grown in free suspension, the technique probably represents the most popular approach to vaccine manufacture even today.

Additional surface area can be provided by the introduction of spirally wound plastic film within a rolling bottle or by configuring the static vessel as a series of flat plates. Such systems have been used with varying degrees of success but introduce additional problems of complexity and, as efficiency (and hence cell density) itself increases the need for some degree of environmental control within the unit, further difficulties are raised. Although the literature contains many descriptions and reports arising from the use of such systems, or their many variations, in practice none of the systems described has rivalled the simpler static flasks or roller bottles used for bulk manufacture.

Another very attractive option for the growth of anchorage-dependent cells is the so-called microcarrier culture in which the cells are grown on the surface of beads which, in turn, can be held in free suspension (van Wezel, 1967). By this method, in theory at least, the benefits of simplicity, straightforward environmental control systems and the relatively direct approach to scale-up associated with deep suspension culture, become available for the growth of anchorage-dependent cells.

In practice, however, there are a number of problems yet to be overcome, which, despite the efforts of a large number of people, have so far prevented exploitation of the full potential of the technique. The difficulties appear to be associated with the transfer of cells and beads from one scale of culture to seed the next and with the establishment of cultural conditions that provide adequate mixing to maintain the beads in suspension and permit metabolic exchange – at the same time avoiding shearing the cells from the surface of the beads.

Much work has been carried out on these systems, and many techniques have been described for overcoming the limitations but relatively few have succeeded in establishing routine large-scale production systems using this method. Despite these difficulties, however, there have been some reports of success in large industrial culture systems, although understandably few details can be found in the public domain. Of the options available, the use of specially prepared sephadex beads as the carrier substrate has been the most successful and the technique may well be worth consideration for production at the semi-industrial scale of operation, in the range of 5 to 50 litres, where the important environmental parameters required can be controlled.

A number of other systems for the growth and maintenance of mammalian cells have also been described, for example the hollow fibre and perfusion systems reviewed by Tharakan, Gallagher and Chau (1988) and Feder (1988). These techniques are applicable to the field of very high-density cell cultivation, such as that used for the production of monoclonal antibodies, where the maintenance of cells over long periods is essential and the cell growth phase is less critical. The problems of environmental control can be considerable, particularly in the former case (maintenance phase) and the equipment necessary is quite complex.

Hollow fibre systems have almost certainly not been used (and are unlikely to find favour) for vaccine manufacture. Equally, perfusion systems are unlikely to be considered appropriate for classical virus production operations in which the cell is grown and infected and the virus destroys the cell and is released. For chronically infected cell systems, where the cell is not killed but leaks virus persistently over a relatively long period of time, such techniques may well be applicable but, as yet, do not seem to have been used in routine vaccine manufacturing operations.

All of the above options are in principle amenable to use with anchorage-dependent cells from any source, including both primary cell culture and continuous cell lines. However, where more than one virus vaccine is being made from more than one cell type, precautions should be taken to segregate the manufacturing operations and operators in space and/or time to minimize the risks of cross-contamination at both the cell and the virus production stages. This aspect has been dealt with more fully in the chapter, General design and operating requirements for vaccine producing establishments, p. 171.

Whatever the cell system selected, almost invariably it will also determine the virus production system. In most cases the virus production phase comprises a change of medium, with or without a cell washing stage, and infection with an appropriate quantity of virus seed within the original culture vessel or flask followed by a suitable incubation period.

Suspension culture

Because suspension culture permits the growth of large quantities of material within a single culture vessel, in which environmental control is a relatively simple matter and which can be readily scaled to any convenient volume, it remains the method of choice for any cell or virus system capable of growth and replication in this manner. The scale-up of conventional stirred tank bioreactors has been dealt with in many reviews including Rokem (1988). The conventional stirred tank continues to be used extensively for the production of FMD (Radlett, 1987; Radlett, Pay and Garland, 1985) and rabies vaccines (Pay *et al.*, 1985), both of which have been produced in culture vessels with a capacity in excess of 1 000 litres, and its application in the veterinary field is only limited by the range of suitable susceptible cell substrates.

Care must be taken to provide a level of agitation that maintains the cells in suspension and permits efficient metabolite and oxygen transfer but avoids the damaging effects of excessive shear. The relationship between aeration, agitation and shear is a complex one and the damaging effects of aeration under some conditions have been well documented (Handa, Emery and Spier, 1987). As with the use of anchorage-dependent systems, the virus production phase is usually continued by removing the spent cell growth medium, replacing it with a maintenance medium and infecting the culture with a suitable volume of virus seed. After an appropriate incubation period the culture is harvested and processed further (Radlett *et al.*, 1972).

Another system which has been increasingly used in fermentation processes, including in some cases the production of cells in free suspension, is the airlift reactor. Essentially this is a gas/liquid contacting device, in which injected air causes liquid to circulate through an enclosed concentric tube within the reactor (Seigel, Hallaile and Merchuk, 1988). As applied to tissue culture, the main use of this method appears to have been for the growth and maintenance of hybridomas, where a requirement for relatively high cell densities results in a need for particularly efficient oxygen transfer. In principle, the technique should be appropriate for vaccine production but to date does not appear to have been widely adopted, presumably because the better-known stirred tank systems perform satisfactorily for this purpose.

CONCLUSIONS

During the last 30 years much work has been undertaken on a whole range of culture systems which have found varying degrees of application within the tissue culture field. The number of techniques that have found favour for the routine production of veterinary viral vaccines is, however, much more limited. This chapter has highlighted the various approaches that have been used to date and indicated the level of application that these techniques have found. The techniques that have found lasting favour have tended to be the simpler, less sophisticated ones and these have been amply demonstrated to be capable of routine and reliable operation, frequently at a large or very large-scale.

As with all biological processes great care needs to be taken to define the operating parameters as closely as possible and to ensure that only materials of an appropriate quality are used in the manufacturing process. In addition, all stages of production, including the manufacturing environment, must be closely monitored and controlled. When attention is paid to these issues, modern manufacturing processes can produce high-quality, effective products reliably, consistently and in the quantities required for field operations.

BIBLIOGRAPHY

Doyle, A., Morris, C. & Armitage, J. 1988. Cryopreservation of animal cells. *In* A. Mizrahi, ed. *Advances in biotechnological processes*, Vol. 7, p. 2-17.

Eagle, H. 1955. Nutrition needs of mammalian cells in tissue culture. *Science*, 122: 501-504.

Eagle, H. 1959. Amino acid metabolism in mammalian cell cultures. *Science*, 130: 432-437.

EC. (n.d.a). *General requirements for the production and control of live mammalian bacterial and viral vaccines for veterinary use.* Committee for Veterinary Medicinal Products of the EEC.

EC. (n.d.b). *General requirements for the production and control of inactivated mammalian bacterial and viral vaccines for veterinary use.* Committee for Veterinary Medicinal Products of the EEC.

Feder, J. 1988. The development of large-scale animal cell perfusion culture systems. *In* A. Mizrahi, ed. *Advances in biotechnological processes*, Vol. 7, p. 126-153.

Handa, A., Emery, A.N. & Spier, R.E. 1987. On the evolution of gas-liquid interfacial effects on hybridoma viability in bubble column bioreactors. *Dev. Biol. Stand.*, 66: 241-253.

Kruse & Patterson, eds. 1973. *Tissue culture: methods and applications.* London, Academic.

Pay, T.W.F., Boge, A., Menard, F.J.R. & Radlett, P.J. 1985. Production of rabies vaccine by an industrial-scale BHK 21 suspension cell culture process. *Dev. Biol. Stand.*, 60: 171-174.

Petricciani, J.C. 1987. Modern approaches to animal cell technology. In *Proc. 8th Meeting of the European Society for Animal Cell Technology*, p. 1-19. London, Butterworths.

PHLS. (n.d.) *Catalogue of cell lines and services, European Collection of Animal Cell Cultures.* Porton Down, UK, PHLS Centre for Applied Microbiology and Research.

Radlett, P.J. 1987. The use of BHK suspension cells for the production of foot-and-mouth disease vaccines. *Adv. Biochem. Eng./Biotech.*, 34: 130-146.

Radlett, P.J., Pay, T.W.F. & Garland, A.J.M. 1985. The use of BHK suspension cells for the commercial production of foot-and-mouth disease vaccines over a twenty-year period. *Dev. Biol. Stand.*, 60: 163-170.

Radlett, P.J., Telling, R.C., Whiteside, J.P. & Maskell, M.A. 1972. The supply of oxygen to submerged cultures of BHK 21 cells. *Biotech. Bioeng.*, 14: 437-455.

Rokem, J.S. 1988. Conventionally stirred tank bioreactors. *In* A. Mizrahi, ed. *Advances in biotechnological processes*, Vol. 7, p. 49-78.

Seigel, M.H., Hallaile, M. & Merchuk, J.C. 1988. Airlift reactors: design, operation and applications. *In* A. Mizrahi, ed. *Advances in biotechnological processes*, Vol. 7, p. 80-124.

Telling, R.C.& Elsworth, R. 1965. Submerged culture of hamster kidney cells in a stainless steel vessel. *Biotech. Bioeng.*, 7: 417-434.

Telling, R.C., Stone, C.G. & Maskell, A. 1966. Sterilisation of tissue culture medium by filtration on a large laboratory scale. *Biotech. Bioeng.*, 8: 153-165.

Tharakan, J.P., Gallagher, S.L. & Chau, P.C. 1988. Hollow-fibre bioreactors for mammalian cell culture. *In* A. Mizrahi, ed. *Advances in biotechnological processes*, Vol. 7, p. 154-185.

van Wezel, A.L. 1967. Growth of cell strains and primary cells on micro-carriers in homogenous culture. *Nature*, 216: 64-65.

Fermentation technology for the production of bacterial vaccines

F. Bover

Much has been written about fermentation technology. Elaborate equations have been developed to describe agitation kinetics, mass transfer, energy transfer, etc. but very little has been published regarding the use of fermenters in vaccine production. In this chapter the discussion is limited to the practical aspects of selecting and optimizing fermentation equipment and fermentation systems for vaccine production.

The production of a bacterial vaccine involves growing a strain of the causative organism in artificial culture under conditions that maximize the level of the protective antigen(s). Each individual aspect of the production system needs to be carefully selected but it is the manner in which the individual aspects are combined that influences the level of success attained. The way in which the bacterial strain, the culture medium, the fermentation equipment and the fermentation parameters are selected is of critical importance and each individual selection will be influenced by numerous factors.

THE ORGANISM TO BE PRODUCED

The strain of bacteria should be antigenically consistent with strains found in the target animal population. With some species of bacteria little antigenic variation has been found and so it would be appropriate to use a strain of proven production performance. With other species of bacteria there is considerable antigenic variation and careful selection of a strain or strains relevant to the target animal population is essential. For example, *Brucella abortus* Strain 19 has been successfully used in many countries as part of eradication programmes whereas with *Bacteroides nodosus* (ovine foot-rot) ten or more antigenic variants have been identified in a single country. A knowledge of the situation in the target animal population must form the basis of any strain selection.

Once the strain(s) has (have) been selected it is essential to establish a seed lot system which should then form the basis for all future development and production work for the vaccine. Seed lots should be preserved by lyophilization or stored in a suitable cryopreservative at -70°C or in liquid nitrogen.

GROWTH MEDIUM

Standard texts provide a guide to the type of media best suited for the cultivation of various species of bacteria but the medium nominated for any bacterium should be regarded as a guide only. Improved growth and the production of protective antigen may be achieved by supplementing the base medium with animal or vegetable extracts, amino-acids, peptides, nucleotides or inorganic salts. The medium formulation should be optimized for each strain of organism being produced. A large range of concentrated and dehydrated media are available from established companies such as Oxoid, Difco, BBL and Merck. The convenience of such media and their relative consistency need to be balanced against their cost – it may be appropriate to use media prepared at the vaccine production laboratory or, alternatively, a range of meat- and vegetable-based digests and infusions could be considered. Meat or organs from animals likely to be affected with bovine spongiform encephalopathy or scrapie should not be used for media preparation under any circumstances. Neural tissue from any source should not be used.

The ultimate selection should be made after careful evaluation of all such factors as the reliability and consistency of supply, cost and whether extra processing equipment and laboratory space are required. A regular review of the basis for the selection should be made but substantial changes in the medium formulation may have an impact on the efficacy of the vaccine and thus its registration status. The quantity of medium or medium ingredients held in stock should be determined after consideration of such factors as purchase lead time, projected requirements, cost, storage requirements and stability.

A clean and reliable supply of water should be available either for rehydration of dried media or for use in the preparation of digests and infusions. Where the quality or consistency of water from the local supply cannot be guaranteed it may be necessary to use distilled or deionized water. When considering the use of local water, such factors as the natural mineral content and the level of treatment with antibacterials (e.g. chlorine compounds) should be taken into account.

Media can be sterilized by heating (e.g. autoclaving) or filtration. Wherever possible, autoclaving should be used to minimize the possibility of survival of viral contaminants. This is particularly important in the production of live attenuated vaccines and the temperature and duration of autoclaving should be established after careful validation.

FERMENTATION EQUIPMENT

The selection of the actual fermentation equipment to be used will involve the careful consideration of all relevant factors: the required output will influence the size of the fermenter; the respiration requirements of the organism(s) will impact on the configuration of the vessel, the stirring system and whether or not an efficient system of aeration is required; and the level of instrumentation and control systems required also needs to be carefully evaluated. It should be clearly understood that the mere presence of sophisticated instrumentation and control will not guarantee successful fermentations. Indeed, in many laboratories efficient manufacture of vaccines is achieved with relatively simple equipment, but there are some basic parameters that should be well controlled, including sterilization, maintenance of freedom from contamination and temperature control. Where the organism being produced is zoonotic, for example *Brucella* spp. or *Leptospira* spp., extra attention should be paid to contaiment of the organisms and also to sterilization of exhaust gas.

Fermenters range in size from barely 1 litre to hundreds of thousands of litres. The selection of the appropriate size to use in vaccine production depends on anticipated yields, required vaccine volume, etc.

Fermenters can be constructed of a range of materials such as glass, glass-lined steel or stainless steel. Generally stainless steel, with the internal surfaces polished to the highest possible standard, is preferred. The most common shape for fermenter vessels is cylindrical. Although it is the normal convention to have a diameter-to-height ratio of 1:3, other configurations have been used successfully in vaccine manufacture.

It is essential to have reliable agitation and there are a large number of means of achieving this. Paddles mounted on a revolving shaft are the most common system for agitation. The difficulties in effecting reliable sealing where the stirrer shaft penetrates the top or bottom of the fermenter have led to the development of magnetically driven stirring shafts which avoid the need for direct penetration through the vessel wall. Other forms of agitation include vibrating discs, airlift and sparging systems.

TEMPERATURE AND pH CONTROL

Precise control of temperature is essential. The most common means of controlling the temperature is by circulating warm water through coils mounted inside the fermenter or through a jacket integrated into the fermenter wall. Ideally the system chosen should be capable of controlling the temperature to ± 0.5°C.

If the medium is sterilized by autoclaving in the fermenter an efficient cooling system is essential. It should be capable of cooling the volume of liquid from 121°C down to 37°C in 20 to 30 minutes to avoid exposing the medium to elevated temperatures for longer than necessary. In areas with a dry and temperate climate an evaporator cooling system will provide a cheap and efficient system for supplying the cooling needs of a fermenter laboratory. In areas with a hot and humid climate a more elaborate cooling system will be required.

Many of the fermentations associated with vaccine production are enhanced by adequate control of pH. Before pH can be controlled it must be measured and this can be accomplished quite simply by testing samples using strips of pH paper. However, more sophisticated systems, which use sterile electrodes to provide continuous measurement, are relatively common. Similarly, the actual adjustment of pH can be achieved by a simple manual system or by a complex automatic one. Only detailed knowledge of the particular fermentation system will allow a decision to be made as to how complex or precise the pH control system needs to be.

Control of the level of dissolved oxygen similarly enhances aerobic fermentations but the measurement of dissolved oxygen requires relatively sophisticated equipment. The level of dissolved oxygen can be adjusted by varying the airflow, the stirrer speed and the head space pressure.

INTEGRITY OF THE SYSTEM AND CONTROL OF CONTAMINATION

A fermenter must be capable of maintaining its integrity for the duration of a fermentation. Inoculation and sampling systems must be such that they do not compromise the fermentation by allowing the introduction of extraneous organisms. A sensible approach is to test the integrity of the fermenter and the sterilization, inoculation and sampling systems by incubating a suitable test medium (e.g. soybean case in digest medium) and simulating inoculation and sampling. The test medium should remain sterile while being incubated in such a test for at least seven, and preferably 14, days and the integrity of the air filtration should also be checked in a similar manner.

CONCLUSION

The ultimate test that any fermenter must pass is whether it provides a reliable and efficient means for the production of the required antigen. To achieve this, meticulous attention must be paid to each aspect of the chosen fermenter and fermenter system.

BIBLIOGRAPHY

Aiba, S., Humphrey A.E. & Mills, N.F. 1965. *Biochemical engineering*. Tokyo, University of Tokyo Press.

Brooks, C.H. & Russell, P.D. 1986. A unified design approach to fermenter sterility and containment. *Process Biochem.*, 21: 77-80.

Mignone, C.F. & Rossa, C.A. 1993. A simple method of designing fed-batch cultures with linear gradient feed of nutrients. *Process Biochem.*, 28: 405-410.

Norris, J.R. & Ribbons, D.W., eds. 1973. *Methods in microbiology*, Vols. 1 to 8. London, Academic.

Schügerl, K. 1985. Foam formation, foam suppression and the effect of foam on growth. *Process Biochem.*, 20: 122-123.

Scragg, A.H. 1995. *Bioreactors in biotechnology: a practical approach.* Ellis Horwood Series in Biochemistry and Biotechnology. Chichester, UK, Ellis Horwood.

The use of lyophilization in the manufacture of vaccines

J.C. Mariner

Lyophilization, or freeze-drying, is a method of preservation that greatly enhances the storage life and portability of many otherwise labile microorganisms and biological products. In regard to attenuated live vaccines, the ability to freeze-dry a viable organism is often a crucial determinant of sustainable, cost-effective application in the field. To date successful lyophilization has been confined to viruses and bacteria. No technique for freeze-drying viable eukaryotic cells has yet been developed, and this has greatly limited the impact of attenuated protozoal vaccine strains and protozoal infection and treatment schemes.

The manner in which biologicals are lyophilized influences the quality, especially the potency and stability, of the final product. Research on lyophilization has been expanding in recent years and the processes involved are now relatively well understood. This has led to an enhanced ability to control the process, greater predictability and the potential for more stabile commercial products.

Unfortunately, lyophilization remains a neglected area in the practical world of vaccine production. Biological scientists frequently view lyophilization as the realm of mechanical technicians who, in turn, confine their interests to the functioning of the machinery. Worse yet, the processes involved are best understood from the viewpoint of physical chemistry, a subject not close to the heart of most biological scientists or mechanics. As a result, lyophilization is handled as a turnkey system based on an antiquated protocol of obscure origin in which the operator follows the instructions and everybody hopes that the vaccine batch survives the ordeal.

This chapter will present some basic guidelines and concepts fundamental to successful freeze-drying. A conceptual approach will be used wherever possible. Since lyophilization of vaccines is an interdisciplinary topic involving biology, physics and chemistry, no more than a basic college introductory course level of prior training will be assumed for any field.

STORAGE METHODS AND THE ADVANTAGES OF FREEZE-DRYING

The degradation of stored biologicals occurs through chemical reactions and the fundamental task in preserving biologicals for long-term storage is to slow degradative reaction rates. Reaction rates are dependent on the effective concentration of the reactants, their mobility or activity, and temperature. Water plays an important role in degradative reactions by mobilizing reactants and facilitating structural changes in proteins (Hageman, 1988) and for effective storage, water must be removed or immobilized without disrupting the functional structure of the biological material.

Freezing is an effective method of immobilizing water and other reactants which preserves structure and function even in eukaryotic cells. However, the necessary equipment is not very portable and maintenance costs are high owing to the continuous consumption of energy. Drying at ambient temperatures is an effective means of preserving some biological materials – the product is portable and storage costs are low – but for many sensitive biologicals, the physical stresses of drying result in loss of structure and function.

Freeze-drying, drying from the frozen state, combines the advantages of both these processes. The water is first immobilized by freezing and then removed by drying under vacuum, at low temperatures and without loss of the stable frozen structure. The product retains its viability during the drying process and can then be stored at temperatures above freezing. Lyophilized materials are sealed under vacuum or with a dry inert gas, such as nitrogen, to remove the degradative reactant oxygen from the system.

OVERVIEW OF THE PROCESS

A production-scale shelf lyophilizer looks like a complicated machine but consists of three basic elements: a refrigeration system, a vacuum system for evacuating the chamber and a heating system. The dual function of the refrigeration system is to freeze the product prior to drying and to chill the condenser during lyophilization while the purpose of the heating system is to supply energy to the product. The lyophilization chamber contains a number of shelves that can be raised mechanically for stoppering the product under vacuum at the end of the run. Inside the shelves is a fluid circulation system and this fluid is either chilled by the compressor system during the freezing step or heated during lyophilization to drive the drying process.

A lyophilization run can be divided into three steps: freezing, primary drying (sublimation of ice) and secondary drying (desorption of water). In a typical run (Figure 5), the shelves are pre-chilled to the minimum possible temperature, usually in the neighbourhood of -45°C. In Figure 5 note the super-cooling phenomena in the product temperature curve (Arrow A), the initiation of primary drying after product temperatures are well stabilized at -40°C (Arrow B) and the effective end of primary drying manifested by the increase in product temperature and the drop in condensor temperature (Arrow C). In this cycle the vacuum was regulated at 100 torr (13 332 pascals) during primary drying and the transition to secondary drying. After primary and secondary drying, the vaccine harvest, combined with a stabilizing excipient, is distributed in vials, fluted butyl rubber stoppers are placed halfway in the neck of the vials and the material is loaded on to the shelves.

The product is now in direct contact with the chilled shelves and rapidly freezes. Once the product temperature reaches about -40°C, the cooling power of the compressor system is shifted to the condenser which is then chilled to a temperature of -55° or -60°C. Once the temperature of the condenser is lower than that of the product, the vacuum system is engaged and the chamber is evacuated.

At this stage primary drying has begun. During this phase the crystalline ice in the product is removed by the process of sublimation in which the product is allowed to warm slightly to a temperature just below its collapse temperature (usually about -30°C), water vapour then exits from the product and travels to the condenser where it is trapped as ice. As the water sublimes from the product, it takes thermal energy with it, thereby cooling the product. The energy of the sublimed water is released to the condenser during condensation and this tends to warm the condenser – the shelf heating system and the refrigeration compressor must work to counter these effects. After several hours all the ice has been removed from the product and the process of sublimation

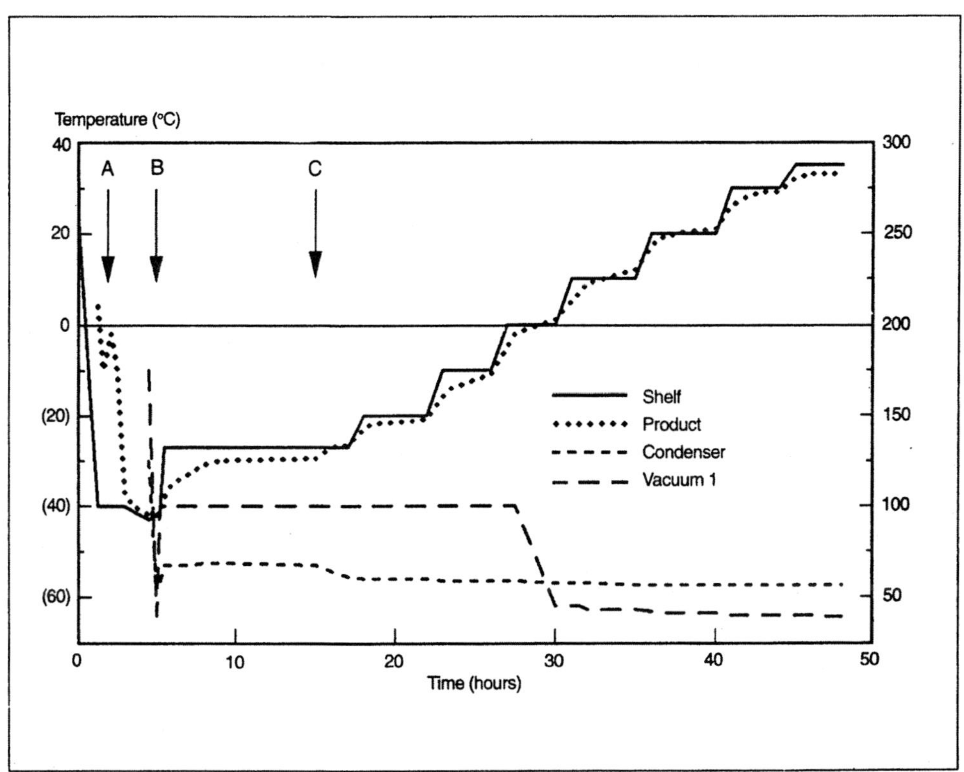

FIGURE 5
Sample lyophilization cycle

stops. The product now has a residual moisture content of 5 to 10 percent; the remaining water is not frozen but is absorbed into the solid matrix of vaccine and excipient.

Secondary drying can now begin. The function of secondary drying is to remove the majority of the absorbed water present in the amorphous solid matrix. The product is warmed slowly to temperatures above 0°C – no melting will occur because all of the bulk water, which was in the form of ice, has been removed. The condenser continues to trap water vapour as it enters the chamber atmosphere from the product and, as the end of secondary drying approaches, the product is essentially dry. High product temperatures, in the range of 25° to 35°C, can be used safely during this period to extract the small amounts of moisture that remain. For most vaccines, the goal of secondary drying is to have a product with a residual moisture level in the range of 1.0 to 1.5 percent.

The product is now sealed without opening the chamber by mechanically raising the shelves and pushing the butyl stoppers home in the neck of the vials. The product can be sealed under full vacuum or, just prior to sealing, a dry inert gas (e.g. nitrogen) can be admitted to the chamber and the product sealed under partial vacuum (0.8 atm).

BASIC PHYSICAL CONCEPTS OF LYOPHILIZATION

An understanding of the behaviour of water and solutions with water as the solvent is essential for successful freeze-drying.

Water exists in three phases: gas (vapour), liquid (water) and solid (ice). The phase of water is determined by the temperature and pressure conditions of the system. Temperature is a measure of the kinetic energy of the water molecules, i.e. their tendency to move. In the gas phase, molecules have complete freedom of movement and will distribute themselves evenly throughout a sealed container; their kinetic energy is high enough to overcome completely any intermolecular attractive forces. In the solid phase, the water molecules are tightly bound to one another in a highly ordered, crystalline structure; the molecules' kinetic energy level (tendency to move) is low and intermolecular attraction is the ruling force. Liquid is an intermediate phase where the energy level of the molecules results in some movement, but intermolecular attractive forces keep the molecules in proximity to one another.

At atmospheric pressure water is a gas at temperatures over its boiling point (100°C), a solid at temperatures below its freezing point (0°C) and a liquid at temperatures in between. As the pressure changes, the temperatures of the phase transitions, especially boiling point, change. When the pressure is reduced, liquid water has a greater tendency to become a gas, so at high altitudes water boils at a slightly lower temperature. At sufficiently low pressures, water will boil at room temperature, for example a beaker of water placed in a bell jar (or a freeze-dryer) in which a vacuum has been drawn will boil at room temperature. These relationships are best illustrated by the phase diagram Figure 6. Curves A-B and B-C are the vapour pressure curves for ice and water, respectively. Curve B-D is the vapour pressure curve for super-cooled water, a metastable state. From B-C, note that the boiling point drops with decreasing pressure. The phase diagram shows that water cannot exist as a stable liquid below a pressure of 4.58 torr (point B, the triple point). Below this point ice cannot melt, it can only sublime, as shown by the arrow.

Although most of the phase changes of water – freezing/melting, boiling/condensation and evaporation – are familiar from daily life, there is one phase change, sublimation, which may not be familiar since it occurs at very slow rates under atmospheric conditions. Sublimation is the transition of water molecules from the solid phase (ice) directly to a gas without passing through the liquid phase. Conceptually, sublimation is analogous to evaporation. Evaporation occurs from the liquid phase at temperatures below the boiling point. In the liquid phase, water molecules are continuously colliding and occasionally several molecules collide at one point and transfer all their kinetic energy to one molecule. When this happens near the surface, the molecule may break away from the body of the liquid and enter the gaseous phase. Sublimation can be viewed as the process of occasional molecules receiving enough kinetic energy to escape from the crystalline ice matrix and enter the gas phase. At low temperatures or low pressures, ice cannot melt, it can only sublime (Figure 6).

Sublimation is the critical process in freeze-drying. If the temperature is not allowed to rise and a vacuum is drawn (as in primary drying in a lyophilizer) the rate of sublimation will increase. As the water leaves the substrate, the frozen structure remains intact, the departing water molecules take their kinetic energy with them and, thus, the substrate is cooled. If the water vapour were not removed from the chamber, as the process continued water vapour would collect in the chamber atmosphere and eventually exert a pressure (the partial pressure of water vapour) which would result in condensation of water vapour on the product. This process would quickly reach an equilibrium with the amount of water subliming from the product being equal to the amount of water condensing on the product. It is the function of the chilled condenser to remove water vapour from the chamber atmosphere and, since the condenser is maintained at a lower temperature than the product, the water vapour preferentially condenses out of the chamber on to the condenser coils. Thus, an energy gradient is established from the heated shelf, to the product, to the chamber atmosphere and to the condenser.

FREEZING THE PRODUCT

The freezing of the product is a critical step. There are many methods of freezing but only one – freezing on the shelf of the lyophilizer – is practicable for large-scale vaccine production in developing countries. The rate of freezing is a major determinant in the structure of the vaccine cake owing to the fact that the freezing rate determines the size, shape and orientation of the ice crystals in the product and, after primary drying has removed the ice, the characteristics of the pores in the cake. During secondary drying these pores will act as the conduit for the desorbed water as it exits the cake.

Ice crystals form through a process of nucleation. In water solutions, the solute and impurities can act as nucleation foci and assist the process. As the product is rapidly chilled, the temperature of the solution falls significantly below zero before ice nucleation takes place; this phenomenon is called supercooling. At some point, nucleation takes place and, if the solution is sufficiently supercooled, the crystallization of ice rapidly spreads throughout the entire vial. As shown in Figure 5, the temperature of the supercooled solution returns to zero when nucleation occurs. As the crystals of pure water form, they exclude the solutes. The impurities, biological material and stabilizing excipients are concentrated in the interstices of the growing crystals and eventually these micro-environments become so concentrated that essentially no more water can be crystallized as ice.

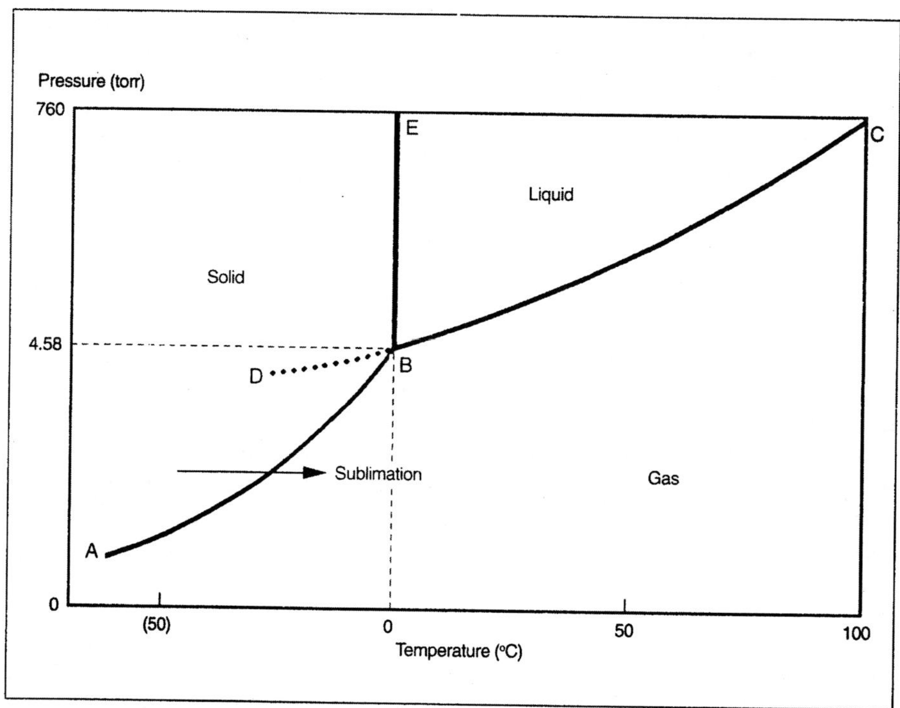

FIGURE 6
Phase diagram of water

During this process, two possible events may take place in the concentrated solute: the constituents of the excipient may form their own pure crystals; or the components may form an amorphous solid solution where the stabilizer components, biological material and unfrozen water are evenly distributed. The term amorphous means structureless and refers to a lack of regular crystalline structure. It is now commonly believed that crystallization of the excipient is undesirable, because if the stabilizer forms crystals it is not available for biological material and cannot perform the desired stabilizing interactions. A homogeneous amorphous solid is, therefore, the preferred structure.

Amorphous solids can exist in two states: rubber or glass. The glass state is an elastic solid whereas the rubber state is a deformable solid with a greater freedom of molecular motion and migration. The water present in the amorphous solid is not frozen and is said to act as a "plasticizer". The transition between the glass and rubber states is defined by an isoviscosity curve (Figure 7), the glass-to-rubber transition (T_g). As shown by the curve, the less water (plasticizer) present or the lower the temperature, the greater the tendency of the amorphous solid to be in the glassy state. Note that T_g' is the intersection of the solution freezing curve and the glass-to-rubber transition (T_g) curve. As the ice crystals form during freezing, the solute in the interstitial solution is progressively concentrated. The composition of interstitial solution can be thought of as moving from left to right across the bottom of the diagram until T_g' is reached. At this point no more water can be crystallized out of the interstitial solution and it becomes an amorphous solid. The water content of the amorphous solid is not frozen, as shown in Figure 7; it is in a metastable glassy state. The arrow indicates the portion of the T_g curve that is of interest during secondary drying and storage of the final product. As the curve shows, after the water content has been reduced to below 2 to 3 percent, the amorphous solid can support relatively high temperatures without collapsing.

The objective in freezing the product is to achieve a stable structure with the greatest immobilization of water possible and to maintain that structure through to the end of drying. Thus, the product must be chilled to a temperature below the glass-to-rubber transition temperature (T_g') of the solution.

In solutions containing one solute, T_g' is a characteristic of the solute and is independent of the initial concentration. In solutions containing multiple solutes, as with most bulk vaccines, T_g' is determined by the relative concentrations of the solutes and their respective T_g' values, i.e. the components of the immunogen harvest and stabilizing excipient. In practice, T_g' is above -30°C for most widely used veterinary vaccine formulations (Levine and Slade, 1988).

From this the following general guidelines for the freezing of vaccines can be formulated:

- Freezing should be as rapid as possible to ensure that the ice has a fine crystalline structure and the amorphous glassy material has a maximum specific surface area.
- The product must be frozen to a temperature below that of the glass-to-rubber transition of the amorphous solid component, i.e. to -40°C or the coldest temperature possible in order to insure that all vials in all locations are well below T_g'.
- In most vaccine production laboratories in developing countries, the highest freezing rate will be obtained by freezing the filled product directly on the shelf. The shelves should be chilled to the lowest possible tem-

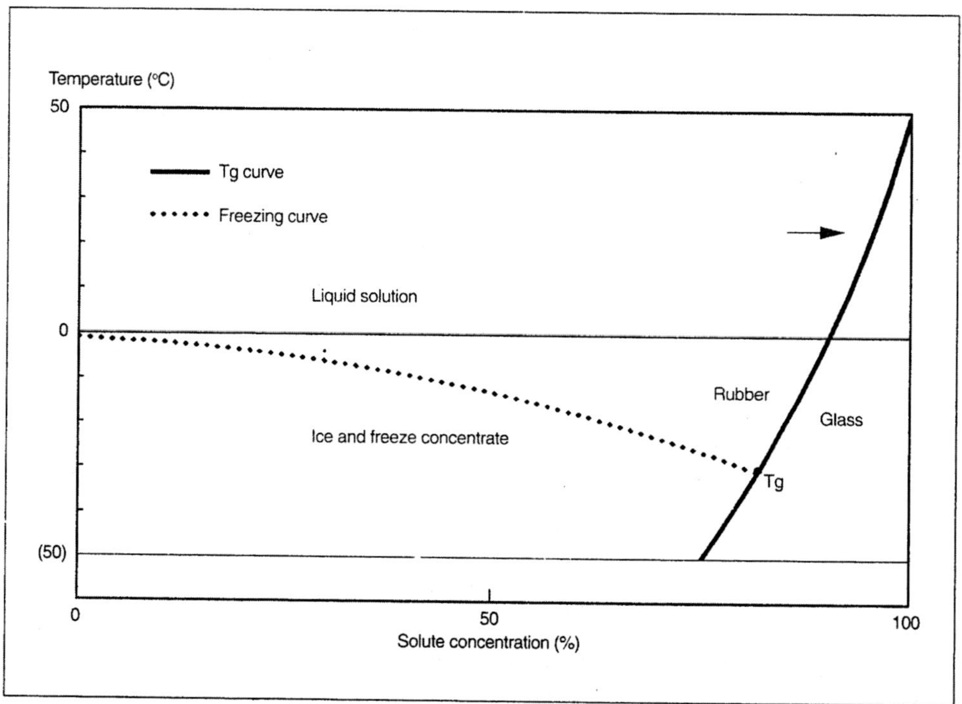

FIGURE 7
Glass/rubber transition state diagram

perature (usually -40° to -50°C) prior to loading. Pre-freezing should not be done in -20°C freezers or on inefficient pre-freezing racks. During the filling operation, filled trays can be kept cool in a +4°C walk-in refrigerator and then transferred to the chilled shelves of the lyophilizer.

PRIMARY DRYING: THE SUBLIMATION OF ICE

The product is now a mixture of ice and vitreous amorphous solid. The condenser is chilled to below the temperature of the product, a vacuum is drawn, the shelf heating system is engaged and ice begins to sublime. When the process is observed through the window a moving front of sublimation is visible descending from the top of the vaccine cake towards the bottom of the vial.

The critical concept for primary drying is collapse (melt-back). Collapse is the loss of the frozen structure, usually manifested by the destruction of the pore system left behind by the receding ice front. Once collapse occurs water is trapped within a shell of amorphous solid and effective freeze-drying is no longer possible. The resulting product will have a shrunken or foamy appearance and residual moisture levels will be higher than ideal for the stability of the final product. Collapse results when the product temperature exceeds the effective T_g' of the amorphous glass. When this happens the amorphous solid enters the rubber state and can flow while surface tension causes the fine filamentous structure of the amorphous solid to contract (Pikal and Shah, 1990). If the temperature rise above T_g' is extreme, the cake viscosity will be greatly reduced and foaming of the cake will be evident. This can be considered as being the boiling of liquid at low temperatures under a vacuum.

The fact that a frozen product can sit on a heated self and not collapse is one of the apparent paradoxes of freeze-drying and occurs for two reasons. The first reason is that sublimation during primary drying has a cooling effect caused by the fact that the water vapour exiting the substrate takes its kinetic energy with it. This is analogous to evaporative cooling and, if heat was not added through the shelf, the vaccine temperature would fall, the sublimation rate would quickly decrease to zero and drying would stop. The second reason is that the system is under vacuum and a vacuum is a good thermal insulator.

Heat can be transferred between two solid bodies by three methods: conduction; convection by an intervening gas or liquid phase; and radiation. Heat transfer between two bodies by conduction is the transfer of molecular kinetic energy (heat) through the collision of the molecules. This type of transfer can occur directly between two solids in contact but direct contact between solids is very limited – a minute intervening space is present between many of the surfaces that appear to the naked eye to be in contact. If this intervening space is filled by a gas, indirect conduction of heat can take place through the collision of the gas molecules with the two bodies and this greatly enhances heat transfer. Heat transfer by convection is the added effect of molecular flow or currents in the gas, thus, if the intervening space is a high vacuum, heat transfer by gaseous conduction and convection is severely restricted. If the lyophilization chamber is maintained under high vacuum during primary drying, appreciable heat transfer from the shelf to the product only occurs through the processes of radiation and conduction by direct contact and these are relatively inefficient methods of heat transfer.

In order for primary drying to proceed at an efficient rate, the product should be kept at the maximum safe temperature which is usually taken to be about 3°C below the collapse temperature. To maintain this temperature while sublimative cooling is occurring, significant amounts of heat must be transferred to the product and at maximum vacuum this would require high shelf temperatures. High shelf temperatures pose a number of risks to the process, especially in developing countries where power cuts are common. If the vacuum system fails, sublimation stops, the product quickly warms to the shelf temperature, collapse occurs and the batch is lost.

It has been found, however, that if a moderate vacuum level is used sublimation continues unimpeded, but heat transfer by conduction and convection is increased. Many commercial-scale lyophilizers are capable of drawing a vacuum of 40 torr (5 333 pascals) or less which, at primary drying temperatures of -30°C, is far lower than ideal (normal atmosphere at sea level is 101 325 pascals). The vacuum level should be regulated to a pressure equal to one-half of the partial pressure of water vapour over ice at the product temperature used during primary drying (Le Floc'h, 1986). In practice, this is usually in the range of 100 to 120 torr (13 333 to 16 000 pascals) when primary drying is done at -30°C. Vacuum regulation is available as a standard feature on many commercial-scale lyophilizers and as an inexpensive option on almost all modern models.

The following are guidelines for safe and efficient primary drying.

- Primary drying should be done at a product temperature 3°C below the collapse temperature (essentially T_g').
- For most veterinary vaccine preparations, primary drying can be done at temperatures of -30°C or above.
- A vacuum should be maintained at 100 to 120 torr (13 332 to 16 000 pascals) during primary drying at product temperatures of -30°C or above.
- Where good temperature control is available, shelf temperatures in the range of 3° to 4°C above the desired product temperature should be used, especially when the vacuum is regulated. This reduces the risk of product collapse and eases the transition to secondary drying.
- Primary drying can be considered to be at an end when no visible ice is present in the product, the product temperature begins to rise to the level of the shelf temperature and the condenser temperature falls (Figure 5).

SECONDARY DRYING: THE DESORPTION OF WATER

At the end of primary drying, the product cake is a porous filamentous glass with between 5 and 10 percent residual moisture. All of the crystallized water (ice) has been removed. The remaining water is absorbed within the amorphous solid and the objective in secondary drying is to remove most, but not all, of the remaining water. A certain amount of water (generally 1 to 1.5 percent residual moisture) is essential for the structural integrity and viability of live vaccines but more than this minimal level is detrimental to product stability.

At the beginning of secondary drying, the collapse temperature of the amorphous solid is still essentially equal to T_g'. As water is removed from the glass, the glass transition temperature increases (Figure 7), thus, progressively higher temperatures can be used during secondary drying without causing product collapse.

Pikal *et al.* (1990) have shown that the important determinants of secondary drying rates are the specific surface area of the amorphous glass and the shelf temperature. Their study found that products rapidly reached a plateau moisture level at a given temperature and that further drying was minimal if the product was left at that temperature for a prolonged time. Final shelf temperatures are thus a major determinant of product residual moisture content and the higher the final shelf temperature the drier the product.

In practice, many manufacturers go to high shelf temperatures (+25°C) relatively rapidly. However, exposing a humid product to high temperatures runs the risks of causing partial collapse of the product and of significant losses in potency. A more prudent procedure which also takes advantage of high final temperatures is to increase the shelf temperature step by step. At each successive temperature step, product moisture content reaches a lower level and product temperature can safely be increased to the next step. Application of this technique to rinderpest vaccine stabilized with 5 percent lactalbumin and 10 percent sucrose allows final shelf temperatures of 35° to 40°C to be used with minimal loss in product titre (> 0.3 $\log_{10}$ $TCID_{50}$). Although the stabilizer is highly hydroscopic, the residual moisture content of the final product is between 1 and 1.5 percent and product stability is sufficiently enhanced to allow use of the vaccine with a reduced cold chain (Mariner *et al.*, 1990).

It is also common practice to draw a full vacuum during secondary drying and some computer-controlled freeze-dryers have made this obligatory. Drawing a full vacuum, however, does not necessarily accelerate secondary drying (Pikal *et al.*, 1990).

The following are guidelines for safe and efficient secondary drying:

- Increase shelf temperatures in steps, allowing at least two hours at each step.
- The product temperature should rapidly equilibrate with or surpass the shelf temperature during secondary drying, otherwise significant product moisture may be present and product collapse (shrinkage) may result.
- Final shelf temperature is a major determinant of product residual moisture content and, thus, product stability.
- For most veterinary products, the final shelf temperature should be in the range of 25° to 35°C.

SELECTION AND PREPARATION OF PACKAGING

All of the effort put into freeze-drying is lost if the quality of the packaging is inadequate. Good-quality packaging assures more uniform heat transfer and drying as well as providing a robust seal capable of maintaining a vacuum over a range of temperatures. Vials and stoppers should be considered as two components of one system; the stopper must be matched to the vial. Vials should be thin and of uniform thickness to allow for rapid, uniform heat transfer. Vials manufactured from tube glass are ideal and can be obtained at prices comparable to moulded glass vials. Vials should not be recycled as complete cleaning is virtually impossible and microscopic contamination of the neck can result in microleaks during storage. New vials should be stored in a dust-free environment and rinsed with distilled water prior to use. For sterilization, the simplest and safest method is to load the vials on to the lyophilizer trays, wrap the trays in foil and sterilize in a dry oven. In this way, the sterile trays can be filled with product with a minimum of handling.

Stoppers should be coated with silicone to assist in the stoppering process at the end of lyophilization. The only function of the silicone is to reduce friction, and excess silicone may compromise the stability of the seal or contaminate the product. Properly siliconized stoppers have no visible silicone, they just feel slightly slippery. Many manufacturers provide pre-siliconized stoppers which are ideal. If silicone must be applied during preparation, spread the stoppers on a tray and either spray them lightly with an aerosol preparation or place a small amount of silicone on the hands and work the stoppers. Using either method, the stoppers should be thoroughly mixed by hand to assure a thin, even coat.

The stoppers are then autoclaved at 121°C during which they absorb a considerable quantity of moisture. This moisture will not be removed during lyophilization but will equilibrate with the product cake during storage resulting in a significant rise in residual moisture and loss of stability (Held and Landi, 1977; Le Meste *et al.*, 1985). Thus, a well-dried final product with 1 percent residual moisture at the time of exit from the apparatus can have residual moisture of 5 percent or more after six months storage at 4°C if the stoppers are used directly from the autoclave without drying.

It is recommended that stoppers be subjected to four hours of drying at 135° to 142°C in a drying oven just prior to use. These drying conditions will not damage the stoppers but temperatures and times in excess of these may cause them to harden and lose their "rubber" sealing properties. Stoppers should be packed in cotton sacks or in another porous material in moderate quantities to ensure adequate drying throughout. Vacuum-drying in the autoclave cannot be recommended as a general procedure as the efficiency of this treatment varies greatly between machines (Mariner and Sassu, 1993). There is also limited data to suggest that stoppers made from chlorbutyl are superior to those made from isobutyl in terms of reduced moisture absorption and desorption.

The following are guidelines for the selection and preparation of packaging:

- The use of new, tube glass vials with matching stoppers is highly recommended.
- The integrity of the vacuum seal should be evaluated under conditions of temperature stress. A simple test is to submerge a sample of the final product in a water bath at 45°C for 24 hours and observe the cake for evidence of contamination with aspirated water.
- Stoppers should be dried at 135°C for four hours following autoclaving.

PRODUCT FORMULATION

The content of the product profoundly affects the physical processes of lyophilization. In veterinary vaccines, excipients tend to be composed of a protein, a sugar and a buffer system. An ideal excipient would have the following properties:

- immunological and pharmacological inertia;
- it stabilizes the biological during freezing, drying and storage;
- it dries readily at moderate primary drying temperatures without collapse;
- low cost and ready availability;
- it is easily sterilized;
- it rehydrates rapidly;
- it has an elegant appearance.

Unfortunately, the ideal stabilizer has yet to be found. As an example, skim milk powder used in the production of contagious bovine pleuropneumonia vaccines does well in all categories except that it is difficult to sterilize. Disaccharides such as sucrose, lactose and trehalose work well in viral vaccines but require longer drying times at optimum concentrations for stability and, in addition, trehalose tends to add to the cost of the product.

Freezing and drying have been shown to be different stresses and the mechanisms of stabilization are becoming clear. During the freezing of proteins, any solute that is preferentially excluded from the surface of the protein results in a protective shell of hydration and, owing to the non-specificity of the interaction, a wide range of additives exhibit cryostabilizing effects. During drying more direct interaction between the stabilizing additive and proteins is required. Disaccharides perform well as stabilizers of proteins during freezing and drying (Crowe *et al.*, 1990) and have also been shown to stabilize phospholipid membranes during drying (Crowe *et al.*, 1987). Disaccharides are able to stabilize proteins during drying by replacing water at hydrogen binding sites. They are also believed to stabilize membranes by forming favourable interactions with the polar head groups of the phospholipids, thus conserving the proper intermolecular spacing between the phospholipids after the removal of water. Monosaccharides such as glucose are able to stabilize proteins during freezing by the preferential exclusion mechanism, but are unable to take on the hydrogen binding role required of a good drying stabilizer. For freeze-drying, stabilizers that protect against both freezing and drying stresses are necessary and disaccharides are the biological stabilizer of choice.

The role of the protein component is to increase the structural stability of the cake, protecting it against collapse. Live vaccine preparations would have low protein contents if additional protein were not added. On average disaccharides have low T_g' values (about -30°C) whereas proteins tend to have moderate T_g' values (about -10°C). Excipients that combine a protein with a stabilizing disaccharide result in a solution with a T_g' value in the range of -15° to -25°C, a more practical drying temperature in commercial-scale freeze-dryers. For extensive tables of T_g' values, see Franks (1990) or Levine and Slade (1988).

The following are guidelines for the selection and use of excipients:

- For live veterinary vaccines, excipients should contain a protein, a disaccharide and a buffer system.
- The collapse temperature of the cake is determined by the relative concentration of the excipient components. In less efficient lyophilizers the risk of collapse can be reduced through the selection of components with high T_g' values or through changes in the relative concentration of components.
- Whenever possible excipients should be added at the time of harvest, prior to freezing, to take advantage of their cryoprotective effect.

QUALITY CONTROL OF LYOPHILIZATION

The objective of freeze-drying is to increase the shelf-life of the product while maintaining the purity and potency of the bulk harvest. The quality control tests which relate directly to the efficiency of the lyophilization are the titration of the vial filling pool and the final product, the measurement of residual moisture content in the final product, vacuum testing and accelerated stability testing.

Titration procedures for the major veterinary vaccines are already well described (PANVAC, 1993). The important parameter for assessing freeze-drying efficiency is the loss during lyophilization or the difference in titre between the filling pool and the final product. In rinderpest vaccine production these losses are typically in the order of 1 $\log_{10}$ $TCID_{50}$ per millilitre, however a more appropriate freeze-drying cycle can reduce these losses to less than 0.3 $\log_{10}$ $TCID_{50}$ per millilitre (Mariner *et al.*, 1990).

A number of techniques are available for the measurement of residual moisture (May *et al.*, 1982). These techniques measure different forms of residual moisture and, in practice, no technique measures absolute water content. It is difficult to compare residual moisture measurements made using different testing procedures, but in-house standards can and should be developed based on one reproducible technique. In the past, a quantitative chemical method of measuring residual moisture, the Karl Fischer test, was introduced into several laboratories in developing countries. Unfortunately, the Karl Fisher test is not very objective, is highly sensitive to moisture contamination and involves the use of absolute alcohol which is difficult to ship. Gravimetric and thermogravimetric tests are simple, accurate techniques applicable to laboratories in developing countries.

In the gravimetric test, vaccine is weighed, placed in a vacuum desiccator for a period of two weeks and then reweighed. The residual moisture is calculated as the weight loss divided by the initial weight of the vaccine expressed in percent. This technique has the advantage of requiring simple apparatus normally available in vaccine production laboratories: a sensitive balance (0.1 mg), a vacuum pump and a desiccator. The thermogravimetric method was originally developed for residual moisture measurement using a vacuum oven. However, a wide range of thermogravimetric balances are now available for measuring residual moisture. These devices combine a balance with a heating element and allow the residual moisture test to be completed within two hours. Their cost is comparable to a good balance and most can be used as a balance when not measuring residual moisture. Many of these devices are designed for measuring the moisture in foodstuffs, etc. where large sample sizes are affordable (10 g). Institutes purchasing a moisture measurement balance for vaccines should select one capable of working with 1 g samples (a 1-mg or 0.1-mg balance) and good temperature regulation in the range of 60° to 70°C.

The recommended temperature for measuring residual moisture in vaccines without charring the sample is 60°C. The moisture analyser can be set to this temperature and left until the sample weight (moisture content) becomes constant. This can take several hours and protocols for measuring moisture at higher temperatures (70°C) have been developed which greatly reduce the test time. High temperature protocols must be validated by testing samples in parallel at 60°C.

The recommended method for determining product stability is accelerated stability testing. In this test, the product is placed at elevated temperatures, usually 37° or 45°C, and samples are taken over time. The data is then plotted with titre on the Y-axis and time on the X-axis – if the data is linear or can be segregated into linear components the slope of the line can be determined using linear regression. This slope is termed the degradation constant (k) which is the best measure of vaccine stability and is independent of many non-stability parameters such as initial titre. By comparing k values for a specific temperature for vaccine batches produced under differing lyophilization protocols, the relative effect of the protocol on vaccine stability can be determined. This is an essential step in product development.

There are also more advanced applications of k values and accelerated stability testing. If measurements of k are made at three temperatures (e.g. 37°, 45° and 56°C) the three k constants can be related using the Arrhenius equation and the slope of the Arrhenius equation can be used to predict the value of k at lower temperatures. The advantage of this procedure is that vaccine stability can be predicted at moderate temperatures such as 4° and 10°C where tests would have to be prolonged over several years to observe an effect. Mariner *et al.* (1990) provide an example of the application of this technique to rinderpest vaccines.

The following are minimum guidelines for quality control of the lyophilization process:

- Determine the loss of potency during lyophilization.

- Where vials are sealed under vacuum, spark-test a random sample of the final product.
- Measure the residual moisture using a recognized method.
- Determine the degradation constant (k) at 37° or 45°C on representative lots of vaccine for each product formulation and / or freeze-drying protocol.

STORAGE OF LYOPHILIZED PRODUCTS

As a general recommendation, live lyophilized veterinary vaccines in stoppered vials should be stored at temperatures between +4° and -20°C. Lyophilized products in stoppered vials should never, under any circumstances, be stored at temperatures below -20°C. The glass-to-rubber transition temperature for butyl stoppers is about -70°C which means that at these very low temperatures the stopper will be in the glassy state and lose all of its desirable sealing properties. Furthermore, if the stoppers are not adequately dried, the water content may cause them to lose their elasticity at more moderate temperatures such as -30° and -40°C. Thus, at temperatures below -20°C, the stoppers will begin to harden and loss of vacuum is a very real risk.

Butyl stoppers are relatively impermeable to water and gas at low temperatures, but diffusion can take place over a period of years. Vaccines should be stored in a dry environment to reduce the risk of moisture contamination. Light can also cause significant degradation of the product, particularly in the case of rinderpest vaccines, and all vaccines should be stored in the dark.

CONCLUSION: A NOTE ON VACCINATION ECONOMICS

Freeze-drying is a critical step in the vaccine manufacturing process. Product formulation as well as the time, temperature and vacuum settings used during lyophilization affect product potency, stability and portability.

With the current emphasis on privatization and cost-recovery, minimizing production costs is an important concern. Eliminating unnecessary expense will be a prerequisite for survival in a competitive private market, but maintaining or improving the quality and presentation of the product will be equally important. Many producers in developing countries are obsessed with shortening lyophilization cycles and skimping on the cost of vials, but this is a false economy.

The estimated cost of vaccinating an animal against rinderpest in Africa ranges between US$0.30 to $0.75. However, it is important to remember that vaccine costs represent less than 10 percent of the cost of vaccinating an animal and that vaccine quality is the single most important determinant of vaccination success or failure. A poorly packaged and lyophilized product may be a cent cheaper per dose, but is much more prone to cold chain failures. Veterinarians and paying consumers will insist on products that work and are cost-effective in the field. The optimal efficacy and portability of a well lyophilized product is essential for success in the market.

BIBLIOGRAPHY

Crowe, J.H., Carpenter, J.F., Crowe, L.M. & Anchordoguy, T.J. 1990. Are freezing and dehydration similar stress vectors? A comparison of modes of interaction of stabilizing solutes and biomolecules. *Cryobiology*, 27: 219-231.

Crowe, J.H., Crowe, L.M., Carpenter, J.F. & Aurell Wistrom, C. 1987. Stabilization of dry phospholipid bilayers and proteins by sugars. *J. Biochem.*, 242: 1-10.

Franks, F. 1990. Freeze-drying: from empiricism to predictability. *Cryo-Letters*, 11: 93-110.

Hageman, M.J. 1988. The role of moisture in protein stability. *Drug Dev. Ind. Pharm.*, 14: 2047-2070.

Held, H.R. & Landi, S. 1977. Water permeability of elastomers. *J. Biol. Stand.*, 5: 111-119.

Le Floc'h, L. 1986. Principles of freeze-drying. Maurepas, France, Société Usifroid.

Le Meste, M., Simatos, D., Preaud, J.M. & Precausta, P.M. 1985. Factors influencing changes in moisture content during storage of freeze-dried vaccines in vials. *J. Biol. Stand.*, 13: 177-184.

Levine, H. & Slade, L. 1988. Principles of "cryostabilization" technology from structure/property relationships of carbohydrate/water systems: a review. *Cryo-Letters*, 9: 21-63.

Mariner, J.C. & Sassu, K. 1993. *Residual moisture of chlorobutyl vaccine vial stoppers.* PANVAC Vaccine Bulletin No. 3, addendum. Addis Ababa, Pan African Veterinary Vaccine Centre.

Mariner, J.C., House, J.A., Sollod, A.E., Stem, E., van den Ende, M.C. & Mebus, C.A. 1990. Comparison of the effect of various chemical stabilizers and lyophilization cycles on the thermostability of a Vero cell-adapted rinderpest vaccine. *J. Vet. Microbiol.*, 21: 195-209.

May, J.C., Grim, G., Wheeler, R.M. & West, J. 1982. Determination of residual moisture in freeze-dried vaccines: Karl Fischer, gravimetric and thermogravimetric methodologies. *J. Biol. Stand.*, 10: 249-259.

PANVAC. 1993. *Standard operating procedures.* Addis Ababa, FAO/Pan-African Rinderpest Campaign/Pan African Veterinary Vaccine Centre.

Pikal, M.J. & Shah, S. 1990. The collapse temperature in freeze-drying: dependence on measurement methodology and rate of water removal from the glassy phase. *Int. J. Pharm.*, 62: 165-186.

Pikal, M.J., Shah, S., Roy, M.L. & Putman, R. 1990. The secondary drying stage of freeze-drying: drying kinetics as a function of temperature and chamber pressure. *Int. J. Pharm.*, 60: 203-217.

Inactivation of antigens for veterinary vaccines (1)

Viral vaccines

H.G. Bahnemann

For many years antigens for viral vaccines were inactivated by treatment with formalin (an aqueous formaldehyde solution) but, as early as the 1950s, suspicions were being voiced that formalin-inactivated foot-and-mouth disease (FMD) vaccines had, in some cases, caused the disease after application, although the same vaccines had passed official innocuity tests (Lucam, Mackowiak and Magot, 1958)

In studies of the inactivation of poliovirus with formalin in the years 1955 to 1958 it was shown that the inactivation process is complex and not a first-order or linear reaction (Gard and Lycke, 1957). Formalin reacts with many chemical groupings of proteins, which leads to the phenomenon of the "membrane effect" in which the reactions "close" the outer protein shell of the virus before the nucleic acid of the infectious genome has been destroyed. Even after prolonged incubation of the inactivated antigen, infectious nucleic acid can emerge and lead to a replication of the virulent virus. This can cause a subclinical infection or even lead to disease in the vaccinated animal.

The membrane effect alters the surface proteins of the virus and modifies and reduces the antigenicity of the antigen. It also stabilizes the antigen.

In the late 1950s and early 1960s a new inactivant for FMD virus was reported in the literature (Brown and Crick,1959) and used later by a leading FMD vaccine manufacturer. This inactivant was N-acetylethyleneimine, or AEI, which belongs to the group of alkylating substances.

It was shown that the inactivation curve produced with this substance was linear (Graves and Arlinghaus, 1967) which meant that the inactivation reaction was more specific for the nucleic acid. The inactivation rate and end point could be calculated, and this was a great improvement in the control of the inactivation process. It was also demonstrated that the inactivating agent produced an antigenically superior vaccine (Girard *et al.*, 1977) owing to the fact that alkylating substances react very little with proteins and therefore do not alter the antigenic components of the virus.

Nevertheless, AEI was patented, which prevented a more widespread application of this inactivant. Other alkylating substances were therefore investigated, such as ethyl-ethyleneimine (EEI) (Bauer, 1970) and ethyleneimine (EI) (Bahnemann, 1973). They also inactivate in a linear mode but were not readily available for large-scale application and had the disadvantage of requiring the handling of a highly toxic liquid.

A preparation of ethyleneimine – binary ethyleneimine (BEI) – was described slightly later (Bahnemann, 1975). It was produced by cyclization of bromo-ethylamine HBr (BEA) under alkaline conditions (NaOH solution). The cyclization process proceeds with a considerable pH drop from about 13.5 to 8.5 which can be followed and visualized by use of the pH indicator β-naphthol violet (BNV). BEA is used at a low concentration and this results in a concentration of 0.5 percent of EI and means that BEI is much less dangerous to handle although reasonable caution must still be used in its preparation and application.

The three substances required for the preparation of BEI – BEA, NaOH and BNV – can readily be obtained from several chemical supply companies and are not expensive.

For all these reasons the application of BEI in the preparation of veterinary viral vaccines has become widespread. The largest application is in the preparation of FMD vaccines but many other viral vaccines for animals have also been produced with BEI as the inactivant (Bahnemann, 1990).

THE PREPARATION OF BEI AND ITS USE AS AN INACTIVANT

The preparation of BEI is fairly simple and straightforward. The first step is to prepare a 0.175 N solution of NaOH. It is strongly advised that this solution be prepared from NaOH pellets and with distilled water, always on the same day that the BEI preparation is to be made. In order to indicate the pH drop and control the cyclization of the BEA, a solution of 1 percent BNV in distilled water is prepared. From this stock solution 0.5 ml is added per litre of the 0.175 N NaOH solution. The resulting colour is a pale violet.

The BEA salt is then dissolved in the prewarmed (37°C) NaOH solution to a concentration of 0.1 molar (M) (20.5 g BEA per litre of 0.175 N NaOH). The cyclization to BEI is allowed to proceed for at least 30 minutes. After about 15 minutes the colour of the solution should have changed to a pale orange and if there is no colour change after about 30 minutes the solution should not be used for inactivation and should be discarded.

The 0.1 M BEI solution is then added to the virus suspension at a concentration 1 to 3 percent. This gives a final concentration of 1 to 3 millimolar BEI. Care must be taken that the virus suspension is already at the selected inactivation temperature (whether 26°C, 37°C or another) before the BEI is added under slow stirring.

The inactivation should proceed in two phases. The first phase, occupying perhaps a third or even half of the total inactivation time, occurs in the first vessel where the BEI was added and the inactivation began. For the second phase, the virus suspension should be transferred through a valve in the bottom of this vessel to a second vessel. This procedure is important to avoid any accidental recontamination of the inactivated virus suspension with infectious virus remaining on the vessel wall above the liquid level, or in dead spaces (dead-end tubes, valves etc.) of the inactivation vessel, after neutralization of the BEI.

Residual BEI has to be hydrolysed after inactivation. This can be done immediately after inactivation or after storage of the inactivated antigen and before vaccine formulation. The hydrolysation is carried out with a sterile 1 M Na-thiosulphate solution, which is added at equimolar concentration (to BEI), i.e. at 10 percent of the volume of the BEI solution used. The thiosulphate solution can be sterilized by autoclaving.

INACTIVATION CONTROLS

For each batch of virus supension, the inactivation rate (decrease of viral infectivity) should be calculated to allow the determination of the actual end point of the inactivation process. In the industrial production of viral vaccines, the inactivation rate can be expressed in log units of virus infectivity inactivated per hour.

The inactivation rate is calculated from infectivity titrations of samples taken after different intervals from the beginning of the inactivation process, for example, after one, two, three and four hours. From the values of the infectivity titres, the slope of

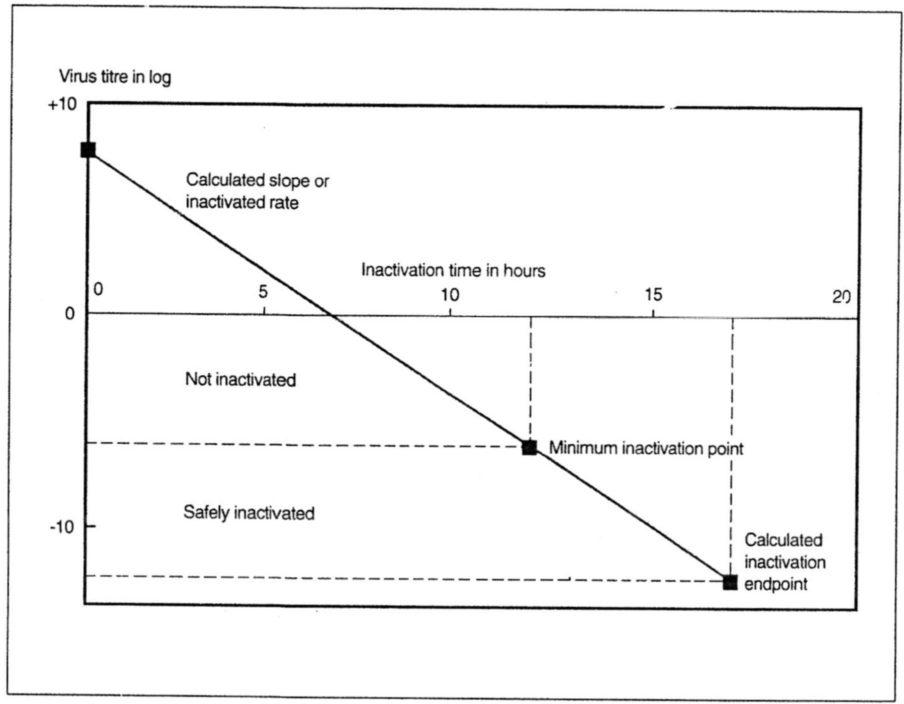

FIGURE 8
Control of inactivation of viruses with BEI

the inactivation curve, or the inactivation rate, is calculated by determination of the least squares regression line. With the known inactivation rate it is possible to calculate the minimum inactivation point and the minimum inactivation time required to reach that point.

The minimum inactivation point is defined as one log unit of virus infectivity below the point where one infectious particle is present in the total volume to be inactivated. For example, a virus titre of 10^{-3} means that there is one infectious particle in 1 000 ml or 1 litre. The minimum inactivation titre would therefore be 10^{-4}. From the known inactivation rate it can then be calculated at what time this titre is reached.

For a proper calculation of a safe inactivation time, the initial virus titre, the volume of the virus suspension and the inactivation rate have to be considered. A virus suspension can only be considered to be safely inactivated if the calculated inactivation end point is below the minimum inactivation end point (Figure 8).

In addition to the inactivation end point calculation the successful inactivation has to be controlled by innocuity tests in cultures of susceptible animal cells. Cell culture innocuity tests should be done with at least two serial subcultures of the maintenance medium at appropriate time intervals. The inactivated virus suspension can only be used for vaccine preparation after the inactivation end point calculation and the cell culture innocuity tests indicate complete inactivation.

OPERATIONAL CONSIDERATIONS

The inactivation of viral antigens should be carried out in an intermediate area that has a limited connection to the virus production area and no direct connection to the vaccine preparation area. The virulent antigen should only be inactivated in this area and can only be considered as inactivated on successful completion of the innocuity tests.

This means that the inactivation area has to be large enough to accommodate a laboratory for innocuity testing and storage facilities (cold rooms, tanks) for the antigen being tested. Only after the innocuity tests have shown that the antigen is properly inactivated can it be passed to the vaccine preparation area.

BIBLIOGRAPHY

Bahnemann, H.G. 1973. The inactivation of foot-and-mouth disease virus by ethylenimine and propylenimine. *Zentralb. Veterinaermed. B,* 20: 356-360.

Bahnemann, H.G. 1975. Binary ethylenimine as an inactivant for foot-and-mouth disease virus and its application for vaccine production. *Arch. Virol.,* 47: 47-56.

Bahnemann, H.G. 1990. Inactivation of viral antigens for vaccine preparation with particular reference to the application of binary ethylenimine. *Vaccine,* 8: 299-303.

Bauer, K. 1970. Die Inaktivierung des Maul- und-Klauenseuche (MKS) Virus durch Aethylaethylenimine und die Eignung des inaktivierten Virus zur Impfstoffherstellung. *Zentralb. Bakterial. Parasitenkd. Infektionskr. Hyg. Abt. I. Orig.,* 213: 285-297.

Brown, F. & Crick, J. 1959. Application of agar-gel diffusion analysis to a study of the antigenic structure of inactivated vaccines prepared from the virus of foot-and-mouth disease. *J. Immunol.,* 82: 444-447.

Gard, S. & Lycke, E. 1957. Inactivation of polio virus by formaldehyde: analysis of inactivation curves. *Arch. ges. Virusforsch.,* 7: 471-493.

Girard, H.C., Bayramoglu, O., Erol, N. & Burgut, A. 1977. Inactivation of O_1 FMD virus by binary ethyleneimine (BEI). *Bull. Off. int. Epizoot.,* 87: 201-217.

Graves, J.H. & Arlinghaus, R.B. 1967. Acetylethlyeneimine in the preparation of inactivated foot-and-mouth disease vaccines. *Proc. 71st. Ann. Meeting US Lvstk San. Assoc.*, p. 396-403.

Lucam, F., Mackowiak, C. & Magot, A. 1958. La vaccination anti-aphteuse en France: étude statistique de ses résultats. *Bull. Off. int. Epizoot.*, 49: 230-256.

Inactivation of antigens for veterinary vaccines (2)

Bacterial vaccines

H. de Ree

Vaccines for veterinary use are preparations containing antigenic substances which are applied for the purpose of inducing a specific and active immunity in animals against infectious diseases caused by bacteria and the toxins produced by bacteria.

In most cases veterinary bacterial vaccines are prepared with inactivated whole bacteria but in some vaccines the antigen is an immunogenic part of the bacterium, for example fimbriae or toxins. Toxins and whole bacteria have to be inactivated, otherwise the antigens will induce disease, and the inactivation of bacteria or toxins has to be examined carefully before the antigen can be included in a vaccine.

REQUIREMENTS FOR INACTIVATION

Requirements for the registration of veterinary vaccines are described in a European Pharmacopoeia Monograph (European Pharmacopoeia Commission, in press).

Inactivation kinetics

The inactivating agent and the inactivation procedure should be shown, under the conditions of vaccine manufacture, to inactivate the bacterium or the toxin. Adequate data on inactivation kinetics should be provided and normally the period of inactivation used in production should exceed the time shown to be adequate by the inactivation kinetics by at least 33 percent. The testing of the inactivation kinetics should carried out at least once.

Conditions for inactivation

Prior to inactivation, care must be taken to ensure a homogeneous suspension, free from particles that may not be penetrated by the inactivating agent.

Control of the inactivating agent

Appropriate tests must be carried out to demonstrate that the inactivant has been removed or depleted, or that any residues are safe, once the inactivation process has been completed. For example if formaldehyde is used as the inactivating agent then a test for free formaldehyde must be carried out.

Innocuity testing

A test for complete inactivation should be performed on the harvest immediately after termination of the inactivation procedure and, if applicable, the neutralization or removal of the inactivating agent. The test selected must be appropriate for the growth of the bacteria being used for vaccine production and must consist of at least two passages in production media or in media prescribed in the monograph specific to the vaccine being produced. No evidence of any live microorganism must be observed.

Bacterial toxoids are prepared from toxins by diminishing their toxicity to a very low level or by completely eliminating the toxic activity.

INACTIVATING AGENTS

Inactivation of bacterial suspensions is carried out with chemical agents such as formaldehyde or thiomersal. Sometimes inactivation can also be performed with heat. Concentration of the inactivating agent and the temperature during the inactivation process must be determined and the presence of the inactivating agent in the ultimate vaccine (i.e. the final product) has also to be determined. The test for the determination of free formaldehyde can be made by an analytical method but also with a dipstick method, which is an easy and fast method. Not more than 0.05 percent m/V of free formaldehyde can be present in vaccines unless the higher concentration has been shown to be safe.

INACTIVATION OF BACTERIAL SUSPENSIONS

The method for inactivating bacterial suspensions can best be described by means of an example in which bacterium X is used as an antigen in an inactivated whole bacteria vaccine and the chemical inactivation is carried out with the inactivating substance Y.

For a general determination of the inactivation kinetics an inactivation curve can be established at the laboratory scale but this has to be confirmed later with a batch at the production scale.

After the bacterial fermentation has been completed the inactivant Y is added directly to the culture. Some substances also react with media components and it is therefore better to wash the bacteria first and to resuspend them in saline buffer before the agent Y is added.

After careful mixing to a homogenous suspension the bacterial culture is transferred to another vessel. This step is performed to circumvent the possibility that droplets of bacterial suspension on the inner part of the vessel, which do not come in contact with the inactivating agent, will reinfect the inactivated suspension.

The inactivation process is always carried out at a fixed temperature and the bacterial suspension has to be at that temperature before the start of inactivation. This is particularly necessary for very large volumes of production material since large volumes need a long time to reach the inactivation temperature.

Laboratory-scale inactivations will give an indication of the inactivation kinetics. Before and during the inactivation, samples are taken from the inactivation vessel and the live bacteria are counted by a validated method. The inactivation curve can be predicted for larger-scale productions by using the information from the laboratory batches. Reliable inactivation curves also have to be determined on large batches.

Differences between the kinetics for laboratory-scale batches and production batches are shown in Figure 9. At the laboratory scale it was demonstrated that inactivation of *Actinobacillus pleuropneumoniae* with a 0.1 percent thiomersal solution was complete within within days at 37°C. At the production scale (300 times larger than the laboratory scale), the inactivation was not complete after two days at 37°C and the inactivation time had to be prolonged by five more days.

With this inactivation curve the real inactivation time, including the 33 percent excess time, can be determined. Therefore, in the example shown in Figure 9, the total inactivation time has to be ten days.

The innocuity test to demonstrate complete inactivation has to allow optimal growth conditions for the agent X. For example, the inactivation of leptospira can be carried out with thiomersal but leptospira will not grow in the presence of small traces of thiomersal. Therefore, it is impossible to demonstrate that a sample taken directly from the inactivated suspension still contains live leptospira. The thiomersal has to be removed by a washing step or by diluting the sample so that the thiomersal is below the inhibiting concentration. Another method is to

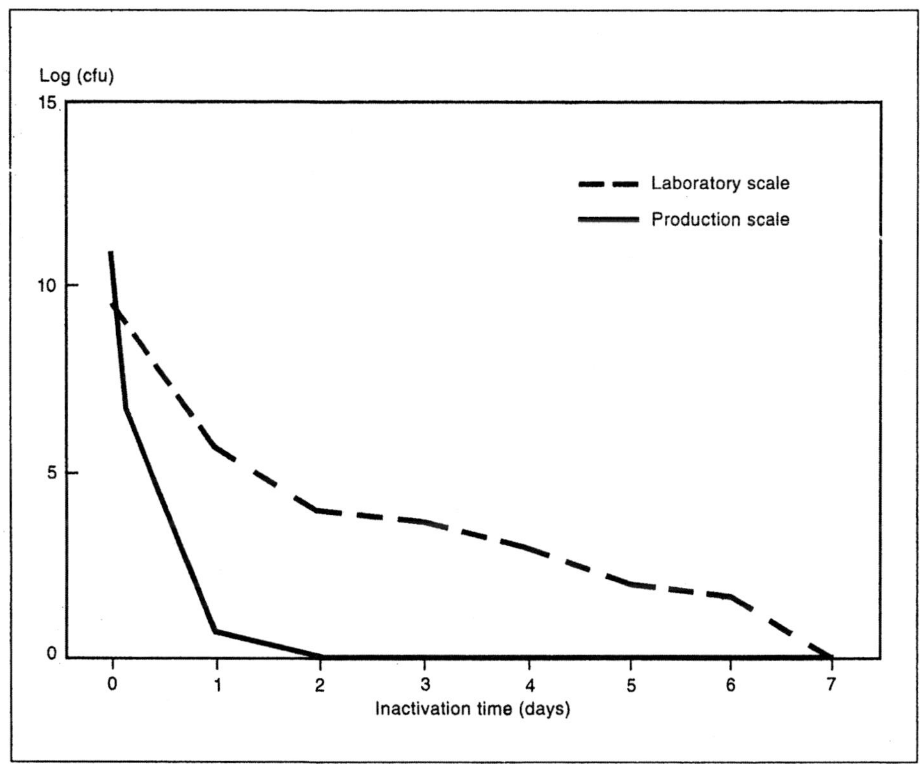

FIGURE 9

Inactivation curve of Actinobacillus pleuropneumoniae

neutralize the inactivating agent, for instance thiomersal can be inactivated with thioglycolate, but some bacteria are also sensitive to thioglycolate. This method cannot be used, for example, with leptospira. It is very important that the sensitivity of the test used is carefully determined.

The innocuity test has to be performed immediately after the prescribed inactivation process. Batches of inactivated antigen are often stored before being mixed with another antigen batch or with an adjuvant prior to the final vaccine formulation.

Sometimes several inactivated antigen batches are mixed before the formulation of the final vaccine, in which case the final vaccine formulation has to be tested for innocuity once again. This is necessary because of the possibility that in the production process inactivated batches are mixed accidentally with live bacterial suspensions.

It can be difficult to carry out inactivation tests on a final vaccine because the presence of the adjuvant can cause problems. If this is the case, the test should be performed on a sample of the inactivated batch, taken immediately before the addition of the adjuvant. Antigen batches that have been sampled according to this method should only be stored in the vessel from which the sample was taken.

INACTIVATION OF TOXINS

The requirements for bacterial toxins are the same as those described for the inactivation of bacterial suspensions. Absence of toxin activity in toxoid preparations has to be demonstrated in an animal model or in a cell test. The activity of the dermo-necrotic toxin of *Pasteurella multocida* can, for instance, be measured with the aid of Vero cells.

The irreversibility of the toxoiding process has to be determined by using the buffer for the final vaccine, without the adsorbent, and making a batch of purified toxin containing the same toxoid concentration as in the final vaccine. This batch is divided into two equal parts. One is kept at 5° ± 3°C and the other at 37°C for six weeks. Thereafter, both preparations are tested with a suitably sensitive assay for active toxin. Both must be free from any toxic activity.

BIBLIOGRAPHY

European Pharmacopoeia Commission. *Vaccina ad usum veterinarum.* European Phamacopoeia Monograph. Sainte-Ruffine, France, Maisonneuve. (in press)

Adjuvants in veterinary vaccines

R. Bomford

Adjuvants are materials that are added to the antigens in a vaccine to stimulate an immune response. They can improve the performance of vaccines in various ways:

- They can increase the immune response induced by a given quantity of antigen. In general, live attenuated vaccines work well without an adjuvant, but inactivated or subunit vaccines, particularly highly purified recombinant antigens, usually require one.
- They can reduce the quantity of antigen needed to generate a protective immune response and may enable the vaccine to be made more cheaply. Fortunately some of the most widely used adjuvants, such as aluminium hydroxide gel ($Al(OH)_3$) or saponin, are not expensive and are easy to incorporate in vaccines. Whenever a decision is taken to include an adjuvant in a vaccine, it is worth titrating the antigen to see if a saving can be made.
- They can prolong the immune response so that only one administration of vaccine is required to protect the animal over its life span or season of exposure to the pathogen. This results in a saving of husbandry costs.
- They can be used to stimulate specific components of the immune response, such as particular antibody isotypes or cell-mediated immunity, which may be important for protection against the pathogen in question. In the majority of adjuvanted vaccines against bacterial and viral diseases that are currently used it is probably the circulating antibody that is important, but future vaccines against protozoal or multicellular parasites may need to induce mucosal or cell-mediated immunity to be effective and, as discussed in this chapter, there are adjuvant formulations that will achieve this.

The purpose of this chapter is to describe the procedures for using the adjuvants most widely included in veterinary vaccines and to provide a brief overview of new adjuvants that may find their way into future vaccines. For a more thorough review of the usage of adjuvants in particular veterinary vaccines, and of their mechanism of action, see Dalsgaard, Hilgers and Trouve (1990).

MINERAL GELS

Salts of aluminium, calcium, zinc, beryllium and other elements have been used as immunological adjuvants, but those most commonly found in human and veterinary vaccines are $Al(OH)_3$) and aluminium phosphate ($AlPO_4$) (Bunn, Nervig and Pemberton, 1986; Bomford, 1989a). $Al(OH)_3$ is used as an adjuvant for veterinary vaccines containing purified bacterial toxins, whole bacteria or inactivated viruses (Bunn, Nervig and Pemberton, 1986; Dalsgaard, Hilgers and Trouve, 1990) principally in large animals and also in some bacterial vaccines for poultry. However, the use of oil adjuvants for viral vaccines in poultry is increasing (Zanella and Marchi, 1982; McKercher, 1986). In some cases $Al(OH)_3$ may be used together with other adjuvants, for instance with saponin in foot-and-mouth disease (FMD) vaccines (Dalsgaard, 1978) or with an oil emulsion in sheep foot-rot vaccine (Thorley and Egerton, 1981).

There are two methods of preparing vaccines adjuvanted with $Al(OH)_3$. The first consists of mixing the antigen with a solution of alum, $KAl(SO_4)_2$, followed by the addition of NaOH, which will cause a precipitate of $Al(OH)_3$ to form according to the equation:

$$2KAl(SO_4)_2 + 6NaOH = \\ 2Al(OH)_3 + 3Na_2SO4 + K_2SO_4$$

Vaccines prepared in this manner are referred to as alum-precipitated.This method can lead to somewhat variable results (Joo, 1973) and it is now more usual to add the antigen to pre-formed $AL(OH)_3$ gel, which can be prepared by adding 1 N NaOH to a 10 percent solution of alum, the precipitated gel being washed with saline or phosphate-buffered saline. Alternatively, ready-prepared $Al(OH)_3$ gels such as Alhydrogel (Superfos, Denmark) or AluGel-S (Serva, Germany) which have been tested for properties such as purity, stability and adsorptive capacity can be purchased.

The formulation of the vaccine is a simple process of ensuring a uniform mixing of the antigen and gel although care needs to be taken to ensure that the pH and electrolyte content of the mixing solution are suitable for optimal adsorption. Vaccines made by mixing the antigen with $Al(OH)_3$ are referred to as aluminium-adsorbed antigens.

$Al(OH)_3$ should be stored in containers made of aluminium, pyrex glass or inert plastic at 4°C. It should not be frozen, as this can be detrimental to the gel structure and adsorptive potential. It can be repeatedly sterilized by autoclaving (120°C for one hour), checking that the gel phase is always submerged beneath the aqueous phase to avoid dehydration changes. Because of the poor heat conductivity of suspensions of $Al(OH)_3$ gel, it is desirable to carry out sterilization in a stirred vessel.

The effectiveness of $Al(OH)_3$ as an adjuvant depends crucially on obtaining a good adsorption of the antigen to the gel (Lei, 1985; Seeber, White and Hem, 1991). Adsorption takes place by ionic interaction, under conditions in which the gel and the antigen carry opposite charges. At neutral, physiological pH $Al(OH)_3$ is positively charged and the majority of proteins are negatively charged, so adsorption is not usually a problem.

It is, however, essential to check that adsorption has occurred and this can be achieved by incubating a constant amount of antigen with varying amounts of gel overnight followed by centrifugation and measurement of the concentration of antigen remaining in the supernatant by an appropriate assay. If the majority of the antigen is not adsorbed by the quantity of gel it is intended to use in the vaccine, the following steps may be taken:

- First, check the electrolytes that are present in the antigen solution. Monovalent ions have no effect on adsorption at normal concentrations, but multivalent anions such as phosphates, sulphates or borates can interfere with adsorption.
- Second, test the adsorption of the antigen to $Al(OH)_3$ under different conditions of pH. The antigen and gel can be adjusted to different pH values prior to mixing, at pH intervals of 0.5 over a range compatible with the stability of the antigen and the pH requirements of the vaccine.
- Third, consider replacing $Al(OH)_3$ with $AlPO_4$, the latter being negatively charged at physiological pH and, hence, suitable for the adsorption of proteins which have a high isoelectric point and are positively charged at physiological pH (Seeber, White and Hem, 1991).

The quantity of $Al(OH)_3$ to be used in a vaccine is best determined by titration in the target species. As a general guideline, the most important veterinary vaccines for cattle and pigs contain approximately 2 to 10 mg Al as the total aluminium content of a dose of vaccine. The dose-response curve of the adjuvant effect of $Al(OH)_3$ is bell-shaped (Hennessen, 1965), so that including too much adjuvant could reduce the stimulation of the response. It could also increase the risk of local reactions, although aluminium-adsorbed vaccines are generally well tolerated. The optimum dose of $Al(OH)_3$ does not change with the dose of antigen (Hennessen, 1965), so that once an optimum dose of $Al(OH)_3$ has been determined for one dose of antigen, it is possible to titrate the antigen keeping the dose of $Al(OH)_3$ constant.

SAPONIN

Saponins are natural products very widely distributed in the plant kingdom. Chemically they consist of a sterol or triterne ring structure, to which is attached one or more sugar chains. Since the ring structures are hydrophobic and the sugars are hydrophilic, saponins often possess a detergent-like activity and will lyse red blood cells.

In relation to vaccines the major application of saponin has been its use in the formulation and potentiation of FMD vaccines and some bacterial vaccines (Dalsgaard, 1978; Dalsgaard, Hilgers and Trouve, 1990). Saponin is a particularly good adjuvant for experimental vaccines against protozoal parasites (Bomford, 1989b).

The complex chemical structure of saponins gives great scope for heterogeneity, through changes in either the ring structures or the sugars. Not only are there differences among the saponins extracted from different plants, but even a single species of plant may produce a considerable variety (Price, Johnson and Fenwick, 1987).

It cannot be stressed too strongly that not all saponins are adjuvants and that a saponin intended for vaccine use should have a defined botanical origin and should be extracted in a reproducible manner. Saponins are produced in large amounts for the photographic industry or as foaming agents for soft drinks, and many preparations are sold as "saponin" without any indication of their origin, chemical nature or degree of purity.

The choice of a saponin is simplified by the fact that the saponins currently in use in veterinary vaccines are all extracted from one species, the bark of the South American tree *Quillaia saponaria.* Preparations of *Quillaia* saponin may differ in adjuvant activity according to the source or method of extraction, and the activity of new batches should be checked. A purified preparation containing a mixture of *Quillaia* saponins, named Quil A (Dalsgaard, 1978), is produced commercially as a standardized adjuvant for veterinary vaccines (Superfos, Denmark). Recently a defined component of *Quillaia* saponin (QS-21) which is adjuvant-active but lacks toxicity has been isolated (Kensil *et al.*, 1991). This is also produced commercially under the trade name Stimulon (Cambridge Biotech, United States) and is beginning to be used in veterinary vaccines.

Although it is preferable to use *Quillaia* saponin when available because of its proven efficacy in veterinary vaccines, saponins from other plants, *Gypsophila* and *Saponaria,* have shown adjuvant activity in experimental systems (Bomford *et al.*, 1992). These saponins are similar in structure to those of *Quillaia,* being hydrophilic with two sugar chains. Therefore, saponins other than those derived from *Quillaia,* might be considered for veterinary vaccines, provided their adjuvant activity is confirmed, their source is well defined and they are produced in a manner that yields a consistent product.

Saponins are supplied as lyophilized powders and are very stable at room temperature under dry conditions. They are water-soluble and may be sterilized by filtration.

The dose of saponin to be used in a vaccine is best titrated in the target species. The recommended dose of Quil A for cattle vaccines is 250 to 750 micrograms per dose of vaccine (Superfos, 1994), but possibly four to five times this amount of the less purified food-grade preparations of *Quillaia* saponins will be required.

Saponins are potentially toxic, causing both local and systemic side-effects, and new batches should be checked in the target species for effects such as lameness or loss of appetite. However, with a good-quality saponin preparation it is usually possible to find a dose that is adjuvant-active and non-toxic.

IMMUNOSTIMULATING COMPLEXES

The original idea behind immunostimulating complexes (ISCOMs) was to form a mixed micelle of surface antigen from enveloped viruses and saponin. This was achieved by splitting the virus particles with a detergent and centrifuging them into a solution of saponin which yielded cage-like structures around 35 nanometres in diameter (Morein *et al.*, 1987). However, it subsequently proved difficult to prepare ISCOMs from recombinant viral antigens, and it was realized that cholesterol and phospholipid, which are present in virus envelopes, are essential parts of the structure. Experimental protocols for preparing ISCOMs from lipid-free antigens now include these two lipids (Morein *et al.*, 1987; Dalsgaard, Hilgers and Trouve, 1990) and empty ISCOMs containing saponin and lipids but no antigen can also be made. Antigens require a lipophilic region in order to be incorporated into ISCOMs. This is available naturally in the surface proteins of enveloped viruses with their transmembrane region, and other antigens such as synthetic peptides can be adapted to associate with ISCOMs by conjugation to fatty acids.

The procedure for preparing ISCOMs from whole enveloped virus particles involves the purification of the virus on a lectin column, its solubilization with the detergent N-decanoyl-N-methyl-glycoside (MEGA-10) at a final concentration of 5 percent for two hours, the addition of Quil A to a final concentration of 0.1 percent and dialysis against 0.05 molar ammonium acetate buffer (Carlsson, Alenius and Sundquist, 1991). The ISCOMs should form spontaneously after the dialysis, but this needs to be checked by electron microscopy.

A great many ISCOM-based experimental veterinary vaccines have been prepared from enveloped viruses (Morein *et al.*, 1987; Dalsgaard, Hilgers and Trouve, 1990; Carlsson, Alenius and Sundquist, 1991), and two commercial ISCOM vaccines against equine influenza have been launched (Iscotec, Sweden; Equip, Pitman-More, United Kingdom). ISCOMs appear to be very effective for inducing mucosal immunity after oral immunization (Mowat and Donachie, 1991).

OIL EMULSIONS

The prototype oil-emulsion adjuvants are the so-called Freund's adjuvants, named after their inventor Julius Freund. The Freund's incomplete adjuvant (FIA) is a water-in-oil emulsion of mineral oil stabilized with the emulsifier mannitol mono-oleate. Freund's complete adjuvant (FCA) is the same emulsion with the addition of killed cells of mycobacteria in the oil phase. FCA is an extremely powerful adjuvant, but much too inflammatory for vaccine use. The adjuvant active component of mycobacteria has been identified and synthetic analogues of this, the muramyl dipeptides, are being used in new adjuvant formulations.

A variety of veterinary vaccines against bacterial and viral diseases of cattle, pigs, sheep and poultry are adjuvanted with oil emulsions (McKercher, 1986; Dalsgaard, Hilgers and Trouve, 1990). These vaccines find a particular application in FMD vaccines for pigs (Anderson, Masters and Mowat, 1971; McKercher and Graves, 1977) and inactivated viral vaccines for poultry (Zanella and Marchi, 1982). Oil-emulsion adjuvants are particularly suitable for vaccines that will be required to give long-term protection. The antigen, being enclosed in the water droplets in the continuous phase of the oil is released slowly and provides a long-term stimulation of the immune system.

The technical factors that need to be taken into account for oil emulsions are the choices of oil and emulsifying agent, the proportions in which they are mixed together and with the antigen, the conditions of emulsification and the quality control of the finished emulsion.

The oil should be a light mineral oil of low viscosity containing hydrocarbons with a chain length of 12 to 30 atoms. Hydrocarbons of a lower chain length are more inflammatory (Gupta *et al.*, 1993). The following oils have all been found to be satisfactory in veterinary vaccines: Drakeol 6VR (Penrecco, United States), Marcol 52 and Marcol 82 (EXXON), Sontex 55 (Marathon Marco, United States), Vestan A50B (Fina) and Whitrex 307 (Mobil).

The usual emulsifying agent is a mannitol mono-oleate and it is preferable to use a product specially refined to be of injectable quality such as Arlacel A special (ICI, United States) or one of the range of Montanides (SEPPIC, France), rather than material intended for industrial use, which may contain impurities. These emulsifiers can be sterilized by autoclaving (120°C for 90 minutes) or filtration.

The ratio of oil to emulsifier is usually 9:1 by weight, although this can vary a little with different Montanides, and sterile ready-made mixtures of oil and emulsifying agent are available – the Montanide ISA adjuvants (SEPPIC, 1994). The proportion of the aqueous phase may be between 25 and 50 percent by weight, but the viscosity of the final emulsion increases with the water content.

A water-in-oil emulsion prepared with the emulsifying agents Span 85 (sorbitan triolate) and Tween 85 (polyoxyethylene 20 sorbitan triolate) has been described (Bokhout, van Gaalen and van der Heijden, 1981). The ratio of aqueous phase to mineral oil (Marcol 52) to emulsifying agents is 8:9:1 (by volume) and the Span 85 and Tween 85 are mixed in a ratio of 54:46 (by volume).

Industrial-scale emulsification can be carried out on a batch-to-batch basis in tanks of up to 300-litre capacity or by using two tanks of 300- to 1 000-litre capacity with an in-line homogenizer. Suitable homogenizers are sulplied by Silverson (Chesam, United Kingdom). The oil and the emulsifier are mixed in the tank at low speed and then the aqueous phase is added over about five minutes while the speed of homogenization is increased to around 4 000 rpm.

Homogenization is continued for about four minutes and the temptation to overhomogenize should be resisted because too much agitation may increase the viscosity of the emulsion, reduce its stability because of coalescence of water droplets and lead to overheating which could damage the antigen.

The following properties of the finished emulsion require to be checked:

- *The nature of the emulsion.* Is the emulsion water-in-oil, or oil-in-water? The simplest way of checking this is to place a small drop of the emulsion gently on the surface of cold water. If the emulsion is water-in-oil the droplet should not spread out over the surface and should only break up, with difficulty, into large pieces when agitated. If, however, the emulsion is oil-in-water, the droplet will disperse immediately and mixing will produce a uniform milky suspension. The two types of emulsion can also be distinguished by their electrical conductivity, measured with a conductivimeter. The conductivity of water-in-oil emulsions is <5 microsiemens, whereas that of oil-in-water emulsions is >5 millisiemens.

- *The viscosity of the emulsion.* This can be measured by a rotating viscometer. The viscosity of the emulsion will vary according to the emulsifying agent and the proportion of the aqueous phase, but it should preferably not be higher than 400 centipoises from the point of view of ease of injection.
- *Stability of the emulsion.* The preparation should be stored at 4°C and checked regularly for changes in appearance or conductivity over a period of six months.

There is a tendency for oil-emulsion adjuvants to cause granulomatous reactions at the site of injection, the possible causes of which are reviewed in Gupta *et al.* (1993). The most important points relating to these reactions can be summarized as follows:

- The intensity of adverse reactions is to some extent dependent on the antigen that is used, crude bacterial antigens being worse than well-purified viral antigens.
- Different species show different susceptibilities to the adverse effects, poultry being particularly resistant.
- The probability of causing adverse reactions can be reduced by optimizing the emulsion constituents as described above.

NEW ADJUVANT SYSTEMS

The new adjuvant systems which are being developed for human recombinant vaccines against viruses are reviewed in Bomford (1992). Some of these are now undergoing clinical trials in humans in vaccines against AIDS (Bomford, 1994). It is worth mentioning a selection of these formulations here, because they often show a more powerful adjuvant activity than $Al(OH)_3$ with model antigens and, hence, might find their way into veterinary vaccines in the future.

Monophosphoryl lipid A (MPL)

The lipid A fraction of bacterial endotoxin is a powerful adjuvant but too toxic to include in vaccines. MPL is a less toxic derivative produced by removing one of the phosphate groups of lipid A isolated from remutants of *S. typhimurium* and *S. minnesota.* It works best as an adjuvant when incorporated into oil-in-water emulsion of squalene (a constituent of shark oil) together with trehalose dimycolate, a surface-active molecule of bacterial origin. This formulation is available commercially as the Ribi Adjuvant System (Ribi Immunochem, United States).

Pluronic polymers

Pluronics are block copolymers of polyoxyethylene and polyoxypropylene, and their adjuvant effect is also best expressed in oil-in-water emulsions of mineral oil or squalene stabilized with Tween. This adjuvant system is sold under the trade name Titermax (CyTRx, United States).

Muramyl dipeptide (MDP)

MDP, a synthetic molecule, is an analogue of the minimal structure of the peptidoglycan of the mycobacterial cell wall that mediates the adjuvant activity of mycobacteria in FCA. The original MDP was too pyrogenic for vaccines, but less toxic analogues have been discovered. One of them, threonyl MDP, is formulated with a pluronic oil-in-water emulsion of squalene as the Syntex Adjuvant Formulation-1, SAF-1 (Syntex, United States). Another that is commercially available is glucosaminylmuramyldipeptide, GMDP, (GERBU, Germany).

ADJUVANTS FOR ANTIPARASITE VACCINES

Vaccines against protozoal and multicellular parasites would be of great value for animal husbandry in developing countries but have proved very difficult to develop, partly because of the need to identify the protective antigens and also because it is likely that immune mechanisms other than circulating antibody may play a role in protection. Adjuvants may help to solve the latter problem, and the special adjuvant requirements of parasite vaccines are reviewed in Bomford (1989b). As regards vaccines against protozoa, it is striking that saponin is a highly effective adjuvant, not only for experimental infections of mice but also for the protection of cattle against babesiosis. The situation with helminth vaccines is more complicated, in that there is evidence that the IgE antibody may be one component of immunity, the best adjuvant being $Al(OH)_3$ which preferentially stimulates IgE, at least in mice; although there is also evidence for the importance of cell-mediated immunity in other experimental systems, in which the best adjuvants are saponin or *Bacille Calmette Guerin* (BCG).

CONCLUSIONS

It is likely that the adjuvant requirements of the standard bacterial and inactivated viral veterinary vaccines will continue to be met with mineral gels, saponin and oil emulsions or combinations of these adjuvants. However, these do not solve all the problems of long-lasting immunity after a single vaccination and induction of mucosal and cell-mediated immunity. This may demand the introduction of new adjuvants or, alternatively, the problem may be solved with live recombinant vaccines which are expensive to develop but cheap to produce. An anti-rabies vaccine based on a vaccinia virus vector is already being used to protect foxes in Europe, and oral veterinary vaccines against enteric diseases with salmonella vectors are under development.

BIBLIOGRAPHY

Anderson, E.C., Masters, R.C. & Mowat, G.N. 1971. Immune response of pigs to inactivated FMD vaccines: response to emulsion vaccines. *Res. Vet. Sci.*, 12: 342-350.

Bokhout, B.A., van Gaalen, C. & van der Heijden, P.J. 1981. A selected water-in-oil emulsion: composition and usefulness as an immunological adjuvant. *Vet. Immunul. Immunopathol.*, 2: 491-500.

Bomford, R. 1989a. Aluminium salts: perspectives in their use as adjuvants. *In* G. Gregoriadis, A.C. Allison and G. Poste, eds. *Immunological adjuvants and vaccines*, p. 35-42. New York and London, Plenum.

Bomford, R. 1989b. Adjuvants for anti-parasite vaccines. *Parasitol. Today*, 5: 41-46.

Bomford, R. 1992. Adjuvants for viral vaccines. *Rev. Med. Virol.*, 2: 169-174.

Bomford, R. 1994. Adjuvants in AIDS vaccines. *In* D.E.S. Stewart-Tull, ed. *Adjuvants: theory and practical applications.* New York, John Wiley and Sons.

Bomford, R., Stapleton, M., Winsor, S., Beesley, J.E., Jessup, E.A., Price, K.R. & Fenwick, G.R. 1992. Adjuvanticity and ISCOM-formation by structurally diverse saponins. *Vaccine*, 10: 572-577.

Bunn, T.O., Nervig, R.M. & Pemberton, J.R. 1986. Metallic salts as adjuvants for veterinary biologics. *In* R.M. Nervig *et al.*, eds. *Advances in carriers and adjuvants for veterinary biologics,* p. 105-113. Ia., USA, Iowa University Press.

Carlsson, V., Alenius, S. & Sundquist, B. 1991. Protective effect of an ISCOM bovine virus diarrhoea (BVDV) vaccine against an experimental BVDV infection in vaccinated and non-vaccinated pregnant ewes. *Vaccine,* 9: 577-580.

Dalsgaard, K. 1978. A study of the isolation and characterisation of the saponin Quil A. Evaluation of its adjuvant activity with special reference to the application in the vaccination of cattle against foot-and-mouth disease. *Acta Vet. Scand.,* Suppl., 69: 7-40.

Dalsgaard, K., Hilgers, L. & Trouve, G. 1990. Classical and new approaches to adjuvant use in domestic food animals. *Adv. Vet. Sci. Comp. Med.,* 35: 121-159.

Gupta, R.K., Relyveld, E.H., Lidblad, E.B., Bizzini, B., Ben-Efraim, S. & Gupta, C.K. 1993. Adjuvants – a balance between toxicity and adjuvanticity. *Vaccine,* 11: 293-306.

Hennessen, W. 1965. The mode of action of mineral adjuvants. *Prog. Immunobiol. Stand.,* 2: 71-79.

Joo, I. 1973. Mineral carriers as adjuvants. *Symp. Series Immunobiol. Stand.,* 22: 123-130.

Kensil, C.R., Patel, U., Lennick, M. & Marciani, D. 1991. Separation and characterization of saponins with adjuvant activity from *Quillaja saponaria* Molina cortex. *J. Immunol.,* 146: 431-437.

Lei, J.C. 1985. Aluminium hydroxide gel – guidelines for adsorption. *Vaccine,* 3: 54-55.

McKercher, P.D. 1986. Oil adjuvants: their use in veterinary biologics. *In* R.M. Nervig *et al.,* eds. *Advances in carriers and adjuvants for veterinary biologics,* p. 115-119. Ia., USA, Iowa University Press.

McKercher, P.D. & Graves, J.H. 1977. A review of the current status of oil adjuvants in foot-and-mouth disease vaccines. *Dev. Biol. Standard.,* 35: 107-112.

Morein, B., Lovgren, K., Hogland, S. & Sundquist, B. 1987. The ISCOM: an immune stimulating complex. *Immunol. Today,* 8: 333-338.

Mowat, A.M. & Donachie, A.M. 1991. ISCOMS – a novel strategy for mucosal immunization? *Immunol. Today,* 2: 383-385.

Price, K.R., Johnson, I.T. & Fenwick, G.R. 1987. The chemistry and biological significance of saponins in foods and feedingstuffs. *CRC Crit. Rev. Food Sci. Nutr.,* 26: 27-135.

Seeber, S.J., White, J.L. & Hem, S.L. 1991. Predicting the adsorption of proteins by aluminium-containing adjuvants. *Vaccine,* 9: 201-203.

SEPPIC. 1994. *Montanide and Montanide ISA. Adjuvants for vaccines.* SEPPIC Technical Bulletin. Paris.

Superfos. 1994. *Guidelines for use of lyophilized Quil-A.* Technical Bulletin. Vedbaek, Denmark, Superfos Biosector.

Thorley, C.M. & Egerton, J.R. 1981. Comparison of alum-absorbed or non-alum-absorbed oil-emulsion vaccines containing either pilate or non-pilate *Bacteroides nodosus* cells in inducing and maintaining resistance of sheep to experimental foot rot. *Res. Vet. Sci.,* 30: 32-37.

Zanella, A. & Marchi, R. 1982. Inactivated vaccines in oil emulsions in the control of the infectious disease of poultry. *Dev. Biol. Stand.,* 55: 19-32.

Bottling, labelling and packaging of vaccines

V.A. Srinivasan, A.P. Kariath and P.B.V.P. Bangar Raju

Product presentation to attract customers has been receiving great attention in recent years and manufacturers of biological products all over the world are being forced to adopt new methods of packaging to make their products more competitive and attractive. However, bottling, labelling and packaging is a comprehensive subject which requires to be described from the point of view of mandatory requirements as well as customer satisfaction.

CONTAINERS

Containers are vital components in the drug and biological product dispensing system. An ideal container is chemically and physically inert and in no way affects the contents it holds. The dosage and presentation of products may vary and hence containers are required to be chosen according to the colour, quality and composition of the product, the storage conditions and the final state of the preparation, i.e. liquid, freeze-dried, etc. Vaccines are presented in either glass or plastic containers as single-dose or multi-dose packs depending on the requirements of the user.

Glass containers

Glass is principally silicon dioxide with varying amounts of metal oxides. The glass containers used for vaccine preparations should be tested for chemical inertness. Quality control tests can determine the amount of alkali released from a particular grade of glass under specified conditions to ensure there is no hydrolysis or leaching.

Glass containers suitable for packaging pharmaceutical preparations are classified as types 1, 2 and 3. They have the following properties:

- *Type 1* is borosilicate glass and is principally silicon dioxide and boric oxide. It has the least leachability and a low thermal coefficient of expansion. Type 1 glass is suitable for all products and should be the first choice whenever the use of glass is inevitable.
- *Type 2 and 3* glasses contain relatively high proportions of oxides of sodium and calcium which make them chemically less resistant.

Glass vials are convenient for the visual inspection of the contents but their main disadvantages are undue weight, larger space requirements and fragility.

Plastic containers

Various polymers of thermoplastics are used in the pharmaceutical industry. Polypropylene is the most common polymer used in the veterinary vaccine manufacturing industry. Owing to their thinner walls, plastics are not easily breakable and are less heavy than glass, making them economical to transport and preventing loss through breakages.

Controls

On receipt of containers from the manufacturer, an adequate number of samples should be taken and tested to confirm that they match the required specifications. To check vaccine containers for freedom from manufacturing defects, quality control tests should be conducted for the determination of the dimensions of bottles, for example bottle and neck sizes, usable volume, wall thickness and general configuration compared to the manufacturer's specification. There should also be tests caried out to confirm the absence of leakage.

In addition to the above, long-term vaccine storage tests should be carried out to assess the ability of the containers to hold the contents in a safe and sterile condition over a defined period of time.

Every manufacturing plant should decide on the type of containers to be used for filling various products and should insist on the usage of only approved materials tested against specification. Proper care must be taken with regard to the storage of containers prior to use to avoid mix-ups, contamination and damage.

Closures

Containers are usually sealed with bungs which enable the withdrawal of contents by means of a hypodermic needle without loss of integrity. Bungs are made principally from either natural rubber (latex) or a synthetic polymer such as butyl or neoprene.

The ideal rubber closure should be chemically inert and no component of the vaccine should be absorbed or adsorbed. Butyl rubber bungs are most commonly used in the vaccine industry and are siliconized to make them non-reactive. Epoxy-coated butyl bungs are less prone to leaching and shedding of particulate material.

Rubber closures should be tested for elasticity, puncture resistance, hardness, porosity and inertness. Rubber bungs that exhibit the property of a low water vapour transmission rate are preferred for sealing freeze-dried products. Rubber bungs for freeze-dried products must have the appropriate slotting to ensure the effective removal of moisture during freeze-drying operations.

Aluminium seals

Aluminium is used to hold the rubber closure in place and provide a tamper-proof seal. As most vaccines have to be stored at low temperatures, the selection of aluminium seals is critical since they tend to corrode at low temperatures. Caps made of 0.2- or 0.3-mm thick aluminium sheet are preferable. It is possible to obtain single caps with a "tear-off" system at the centre of the cap or double caps with additional tamper-proof arrangements.

Seals should be subjected to thorough checking, especially of physical parameters such as thickness, diameter and height, so as to facilitate easy handling on automatic sealing machines. Where a variety of vaccines are manufactured, it is advantageous to have coloured seals to differentiate the various products. Such coloured seals must be tested for non-leaching of colour. Seals can be embossed with the name or logo of the manufacturer. As the seals are delicate, adequate care has to be taken to avoid damage while transporting from the supplier to the vaccine manufacturing unit.

BOTTLING REQUIREMENTS

The environment in which the product is processed has a direct effect on its quality. If the work area is contaminated or dusty, even products containing the best-quality ingredients can become unacceptable so the environment must meet the standards required for the operation. The work of the filling section consists of bottle preparation, filling and labelling. The ideal flow plan for these activities and the work areas needed follows:

- bottle washing area;
- preparation area;
- sterilization area;
- sterile bottle holding area;

- filling area;
- inspection area;
- quarantine area;
- labelling and packing area;
- storage area.

Bottle cleaning area

The operations in the bottle cleaning area comprise: bottle washing, bottle preparation, bung and seal washing and sterilization.

In the pharmaceutical industry, cleanliness of the final containers is of extreme importance to ensure safety of the product. Irrespective of whether they are plastic or glass, all containers should be washed free from dust particles and inert materials. The size of the work area depends on the type of bottle washing machine used and the number of containers to be handled. An area of 10 by 8 m is adequate for washing approximately 20 000 vials of 100-ml capacity per day.

Adjacent to the bottle cleaning area there should be a zone dedicated to the unpacking of cartons of new containers. Such an arrangement helps in keeping the other areas free of dust, which is often brought in with the cartons.

Washing of bottles. The washing of containers involves cleaning with powerful jets of detergent, hot water, distilled water and compressed air. Bottles are washed by means of a rotary washing machine or a tunnel washing machine.

The sequence used by a rotary washing machine is as follows: freshwater wash with detergent; first compressed air flush; hot water wash; second compressed air flush; distilled water wash; and third compressed air flush.

Tunnel washing machines work essentially in the same sequence as the rotary washing machine except that the movement is linear.

Bottles are cleaned on the outside by spraying hot water and distilled water through nozzles.

The loading and unloading of bottles are normally carried out manually by the operator. Automatic loading and unloading facilities are available for some machines, but these inevitably increase the initial purchase price.

The washed bottles are subsequently sent to the preparation area.

The washing area requires good exhaust systems, as heat and humidity are likely to be high.

Bung and seal washing area. Bungs come in direct contact with the final product and should therefore be subjected to thorough cleaning. The bungs are initially boiled with a mild detergent and then washed with hot water. To avoid particle shredding, agitation is carried out using compressed air. This is followed by rinsing with distilled water. The bungs are siliconized before being packed into stainless steel boxes for sterilization. The siliconization of rubber closures is carried out using commercially available silicone-release agents. Silicone, being an inert substance, does not react with the vaccine but forms a thin film that reduces the reaction of the vaccine with the rubber closures. Silicone also helps in the insertion of bungs into the necks of bottles either manually or with the use of an automatic bunging machine.

The aluminium seals are initially washed with tap water followed by filtered distilled water and dried. After inspection any defective seals are removed before the remainder are processed for sterilization.

Preparation area

In the preparation area washed bottles, bungs and seals are packed into suitable stainless steel containers for sterilization and are visually checked for cleanliness before packing. A sterilization indicator strip is placed on the lid of the container and marked with details of the type of material, the date of sterilization, etc.

Sterilization area

The sterilization section should adjoin the aseptic filling area and be provided with facilities for sterilization. The sterilizers should have double doors and be installed across the wall so that sterilized containers can be unloaded directly into the aseptic area. Both dry-heat sterilizers and autoclaves are normally installed to cater for the sterilization requirements of glass and plastic containers, respectively. Materials sterilized by dry heat include glass containers and aluminium seals.

Polypropylene containers, bungs and also the garments used by operatives are sterilized by autoclaving. The autoclave cycle should include three vacuum pulsings before sterilization and vacuum drying after sterilization.

The sequence of autoclaving should be as follows: three consecutive cycles of vacuum pulsing and steam injection; sterilization at 134°C for five minutes; vacuum drying for 20 minutes; and sterile air injection.

The sequence of dry-heat sterilization should be as follows: drying for one hour at 80°C; sterilization for three hours at 160°C; and cooling with high-efficiency particulate adsorption- (HEPA-)filtered air for 30 minutes.

Sterile bottle holding area

The sterile bottle holding area is part of the sterile filling area. The size of this area depends on the filling rate and the number of containers filled per day. The doors on the sterile side of the autoclave and the dry-heat sterilizer open into this area where the sterilized materials are unloaded and allowed to cool and the area is supplied with HEPA-filtered air to ensure that the containers, bungs and aluminium seals remain sterile.

Filling area

The area at the centre of the filling operations is held under positive pressure with HEPA-filtered air to minimize the risk of contamination. Bottling machines are arranged sequentially under laminar airflow units to enable continuous flushing with HEPA-filtered air. The speed of the air should be maintained at 100 +/- 20 feet (approximately 6 m) per minute.

The construction of the filling area requires special attention. The walls, ceilings and floor should be smooth, impervious and constructed with waterproof material to enable regular cleaning. All light fixtures, utility service lines, etc. must be shrouded or recessed to reduce dust accumulation. Mechanical equipment and table tops should be covered with stainless steel. There should be no sinks inside the filling area. The passage of the product from the sterile filling area to the outside non-sterile area should be such that the conveyor belt stops at the perimeter of the sterile area and the passage of filled containers should be across a stationary surface.

The HEPA filters for the filling area should have an efficiency of 99.97 percent in removing particles of 0.3 microns or larger. Filters should be regularly validated for efficiency using appropriate tests. The room should be air-conditioned and humidity controlled (temperature of 22°C and relative humidity of 40 percent) to ensure the comfort of personnel and the avoidance of sweating while they work. The filling area should be monitored at regular intervals by the use of "settle" plates to assess microbial counts and any deviation from those normally observed should be properly dealt with. Entry to the filling area should be restricted to authorized persons only.

Personnel working in the filling area must be adequately trained, neat, orderly and reliable in order to ensure the safety of operations. Facilities created to ensure product safety can be rendered virtually useless if personnel do not take sufficient care to observe aseptic precautions. Sterile, dirt-free garments and gloves must be worn before entry into the sterile areas. Garments should be such that operators feel comfortable when wearing them and the material should shed no fibres or particles.

Entry into the sterile filling area should be through a three-room entrance. In the first room, outside footwear should be removed. The hands should be thoroughly scrubbed with germicidal soap and dried. The second room should be the changing room where sterile garments and gloves are put on and the third room is for the disinfection of gloves before entering the filling area.

Filling may be carried out in the sterile filling area using one of the following devices:

- a semi-automatic filling machine with manual stoppering;
- an automatic filling machine with manual stoppering;
- an automatic filling machine with automatic stoppering.

The appropriate method can be chosen on the basis of the turnover of bottles required. Automatic stoppering machines are expensive.

Devices used for bottling. The filling of vaccines into containers is best done by using aseptic filling machines. Vaccines do not undergo terminal sterilization, so the product must be transferred from the bulk container or blending vessel into the final container with the utmost care during filling operations.

The delivery of vaccine into the final containers is achieved using a syringe that delivers a pre-set volume of liquid. The syringe is made of either glass or stainless steel. The delivery of liquid into the container is through a nozzle, the size of which varies according to the neck of the vial and the volume to be delivered.

The syringe is mounted on a motor-driven shaft and the piston slides backwards and forwards with the rotation of the shaft. The syringe assembly consists of two ball valves which control the inflow and outflow of the liquid. While retracting, the sliding piston causes a negative pressure which opens the inlet valve to allow the liquid to flow into the syringe the forward motion of the piston shuts the inlet valve and opens the outlet valve to deliver the liquid. Filling machines can have syringe assemblies delivering product into a fixed number of vials at one time. They have arrangements for holding vials at a point immediately below the nozzles. The nozzle slides down into the vial and during its upward motion delivers the liquid into the vial – by the time the nozzle has moved up to the vial neck delivery is complete. The bottles then move away on the conveyor belt as the transport-stopping mechanism is released, a fresh set of vials move into place and the filling process is repeated.

The movement of vials, nozzles and syringes and the delivery of the product are all synchronized by controls provided with the equipment. The tubing and syringes used for filling are easily dismountable for cleaning and sterilization. They are made of non-corrosive metals such as stainless steel (grade 316) and siliconized rubber. Some of the vaccines contain certain additives, such as aluminium hydroxide, and to prevent these from settling in the bulk container prior to filling, a magnetically coupled stirrer mechanism has to be provided.

Personnel. The key personnel involved in the various filling operations should have adequate qualifications recognized by the pharmaceutical and biologicals control authority of the country concerned. All other personnel employed in the filling process should be adequately trained in aseptic operations and handling sterile products and should be familiar with all the various operations that are being carried out.

Inspection area

The containers filled with vaccine leave the filling area and are brought to the inspection area. Each container should be checked thoroughly for underfilling, improper sealing and the presence of extraneous material. Containers that do not meet requirements should be discarded.

Quarantine area

Vaccine containers should be stored separately in a designated area until all the mandatory tests are completed. After a batch has been cleared following quality control tests, the vaccine bottles are labelled and transferred to the commercial cold store prior to despatch.

Labelling and packing area

The term "labelling" describes all labels and other written or printed material placed on a container or on any package or wrapper in which it is enclosed. The labelling of vaccines (both bacterial and viral) must provide the user with all the information needed to ensure the safe and proper use of the product. Incorrect labelling is one of the most frequent causes of product misuse and product recall. Consequently, most government regulations insist that labels should carry the following information:

- The name of the preparation;
- the composition of the vaccine and the quantities of its individual ingredients;
- the name and percentage of bacteriostatic agent contained in the vaccine;
- the route of administration;
- storage conditions;
- the batch or lot number;
- the date of manufacture;
- the expiry date;
- the name and address of the manufacturer;
- the manufacturing licence number that has been given by an appropriate government authority.

The label should also indicate that the product is meant for veterinary use only, in accordance with the pharmaceutical and biological regulations of the appropriate authority of the country concerned.

Types of labels. Different types of labels are used in the pharmaceutical industry:

- paper labels of 70, 83 or 90 grams per square meter (gsm) on chromo-art paper;
- pre-gummed paper labels of 70, 83 or 90 gsm;
- pre-gummed polyvinyl chloride (PVC) labels.

Selection of appropriate labels is important to ensure their retention on containers during storage and transport at low temperature. Labels for each individual product should be stored separately to avoid their misapplication.

Controls. Each batch of labels should be checked and cleared for use on receipt according to the set procedures. The printing of labels in mass should be avoided. Excess labels bearing a particular batch number should be destroyed after completion of labelling of that batch and before commencement of labelling of subsequent batches.

Rejected labels should be counted and destroyed to avoid confusion. The area and equipment for the labelling operation should be thoroughly checked for any leftover labels from previous batches. The area where labels are stored should be accessible to authorized personnel only. Checks should be made on the number of labels used against the number issued and proper reconciliation of the figures must be achieved. Any discrepancies should be investigated before the batch is released.

Packaging and distribution. The term "packaging" refers to all the materials and methods that help to make the product available to the customer in a suitable, convenient and safe manner.

The distribution of vaccine should essentially be carried out in such a way that vaccine is maintained at temperatures appropriate to avoiding the deterioration of its components. The transport of vaccine in tropical countries where atmospheric temperatures in summer may reach 45°C needs special attention. Packaging materials require careful selection and rigorous testing and will, in general, include such items as polystyrene boxes, corrugated boxes and cool packs.

Some of the important attributes of efficient packaging follow:

- The particular package used should ensure that the quality of the product is maintained until it reaches the customer.
- It should be pilfer- and tamper-proof.
- It should have adequate information about the product in addition to instructions regarding storage and transportation.

Vaccines are thermolabile and so require to be transported under conditions in which the temperature is maintained at between 2 and 8°C. The mode of transport should ensure there is no break in the cold chain. Transportation under cold chain conditions from supplier to point of application involves the use of insulated boxes with adequate cooling material to ensure the maintenance of required temperatures. Alternatively, refrigerated vans may be used to transport vaccines, but this method is very expensive and somewhat cumbersome.

The insulated boxes used for transport should be cheap and efficient. Expanded polystyrene (EPS) boxes, popularly called "thermocole boxes", are used for transporting vaccines and these are designed to meet the above requirements. The size and wall thickness of the box chosen depends on the number of vaccine containers to be transported in each box and on the anticipated transit time.

Figure 10 gives the specifications of an EPS box used for transporting ten bottles of vaccine packed in 300-ml containers for a period of 18 hours and maintained within the temperature range of 2 to 8°C.

EPS boxes should be manufactured with a density of polystyrene granules of 30 kilograms per cubic meter. The external dimensions of the box should be 424 mm by 355 mm by 233 mm. The box should be provided with two grooves on the lid to carry two cool packs as in Figure 10. The weight of each box should be 560 g +/- 5 g.

Cool packs. To maintain the required low temperature within the box for extended periods, cool packs are used. These contain brine frozen at -20°C or a gel containing a mixture of guar gum, gelatin, carboxy methyl cellulose and distilled water similarly frozen. These preparations act as a "heat sink" to maintain the temperature of the vaccine between 2 and 8°C. For transporting 20 bottles of vaccine, each of 300-ml capacity, two cool packs of the dimensions given in Figure 10 are required.

The containers that form the cool packs are made from high-density polyethylene as shown in Figure 11. They are designed to fit into the lids of EPS boxes and are embossed with the logo and name of the manufacturer. Cool packs should be able to withstand temperatures in the range of -20° to +40°C and a suitable cap should be provided to fit tightly on to the filling port of the cool pack body.

The heat absorbance capacity of cool

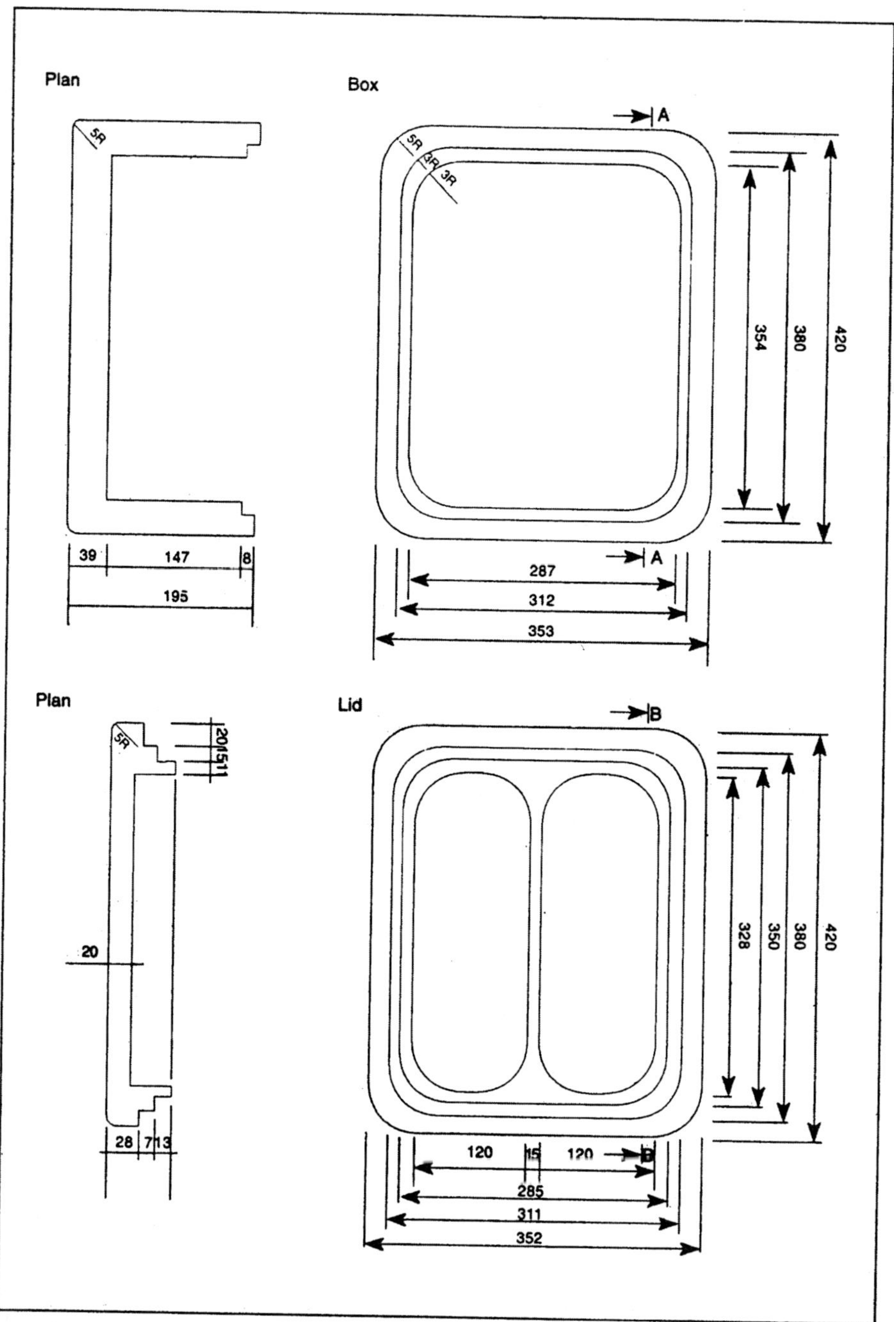

FIGURE 10

Dimensions of a polystyrene box and lid suitable for transporting 20 300-ml vaccine bottles. (Dimensions in mm)

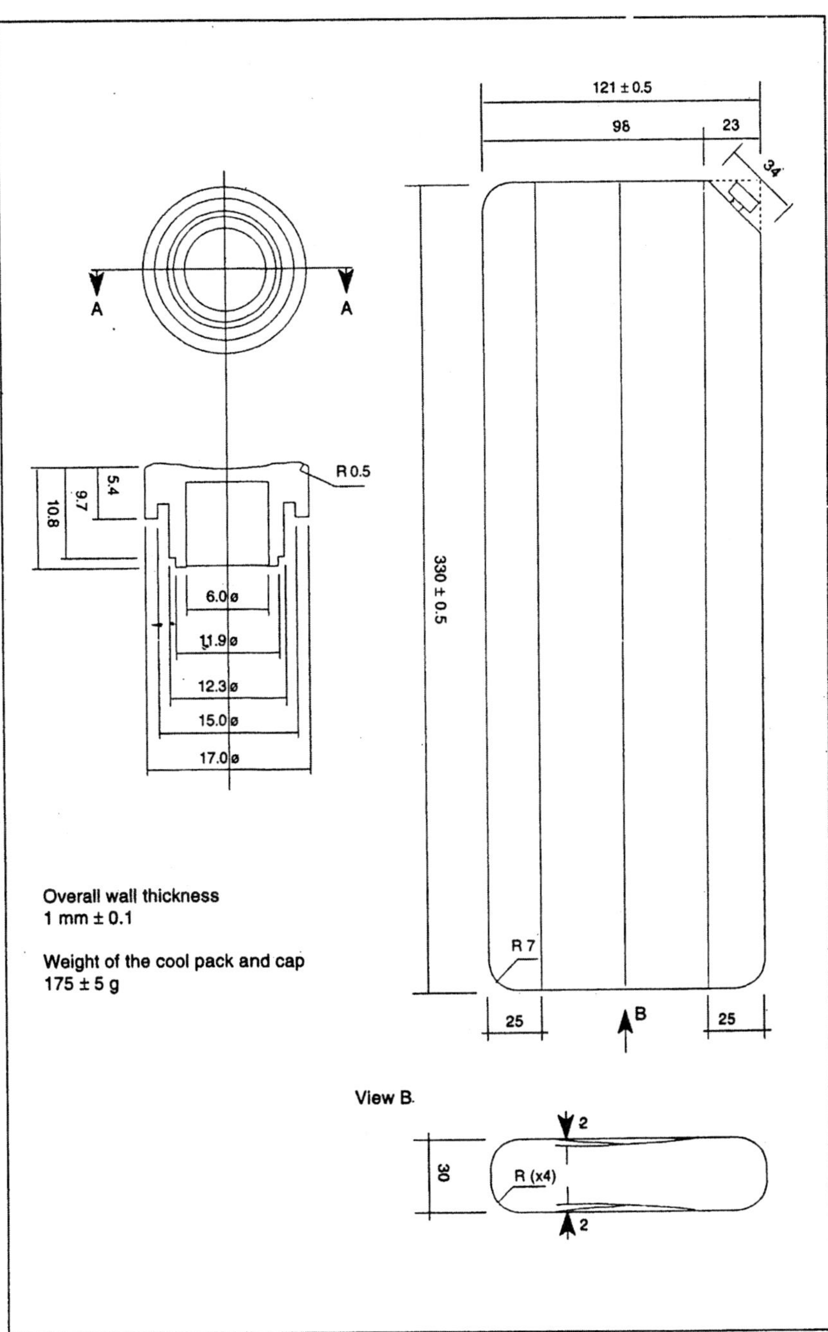

FIGURE 11

Dimensions of a cool pack

packs depends on their effective volume and the temperature at which they are frozen, for example a 2-kg cool pack frozen at -20°C has a capacity to absorb approximately 208 000 Calories of heat.

The number of cool packs used depends on the type of product to be transported. For the transport of some vaccines, for example foot-and-mouth disease (FMD) vaccine, where freezing is contraindicated, the utmost care should be taken to provide the optimum number of cool packs to ensure maintenance of the cold chain without actual freezing. Cool packs should ideally be fixed in the lid of EPS boxes. EPS boxes and cool packs can be used several times if necessary – provided they are not damaged in transit.

Corrugated boxes. Vaccine packed in EPS boxes with cool packs is protected further by transportation of the EPS box in an external corrugated box. An obvious advantage of the use of such a box is that, in addition to protecting the fragile contents, it also permits the attachment of instructions related to handling of the box during transportation and the address of the customer/consignee. Corrugated boxes should be made from three- or five-ply virgin kraft paper of 100 to 120 gsm depending on the particular requirement.

The strength of such boxes is directly related to the specifications of the material (its gsm) and the number of layers (plys) used in its construction. The following is an indication of the bursting strength of this type of material:

- paper of 100 gsm bursts at strains of 2 kg/cm^2;
- paper of 120 gsm bursts at strains of 2.5 kg/cm^2;
- paper of 150 gsm bursts at strains of 3.0 kg/cm^2.

BIBLIOGRAPHY

HMSO. 1985. *British Pharmacopoeia (Veterinary).* Medicines Commission, pursuant to the Medicines Act 1968. London.

Remington. 1990. *Remington's Pharmaceutical Sciences,* 18th edition. Easton, Pa., USA, Mack Publishing Company.

United States Pharmacopoeial Convention. [year]. *The United States Pharmacopoeia,* 21st revision. Rockville, Md., USA.

PART IV

Quality assurance and quality control

Quality assurance and good manufacturing practice

J.P. Soulebot, V.J. Palya, M. Rweyemamu and D. Sylla

In recent years, quality assurance (QA) and good manufacturing practice (GMP) have become increasingly important in the pharmaceutical industry. They are of particular importance in the manufacture of veterinary vaccines since such products have the following specific characteristics:

- The active ingredients are almost always produced by the manufacturer (and not as is generally the case by another industry, as for example with chemicals).
- Vaccine production usually requires cultivation steps, including growth of the appropriate organism and the use of substances of animal origin, which makes it easy to introduce a contaminant and to amplify low levels of contamination.
- As the end product is not usually subjected to a final sterilization step, prior to final formulation its constituents should be particularly well protected against contamination and cross-contamination.

Manufacture requires the handling of live organisms which are sometimes pathogenic for humans and/or animals. The release of these agents, with the possibility of contamination/cross-contamination, has to be regarded as a serious danger and, depending on the organism involved, the workers and the environment, together with all the materials, should be well protected. Moreover, the level of risk is further exacerbated by the large number of animal species and potential pathogenic agents. The variety of products manufactured is very great but the volume of manufacture is sometimes quite low, so manufacturing operations based on the sharing of equipment and facilities is common. In addition, other activities such as diagnosis and research are frequently linked to manufacture and this may result in opportunities for cross-contamination.

Vaccine manufacture is a complex activity, with risks, which is carried out in a complicated environment. Particular aspects of the work are important in relation to potential problems of contamination, for example contamination of the product, cross-contamination, possible amplification of contamination organisms and contamination of workers and the environment.

These factors, together with the inherent variability of biological agents and materials and the relative inefficiency of quality control tests in providing adequate reassurance for final products, means that the roles of the QA system and GMP are of the utmost importance. Not only should the requirements of general current GMP for medicinal products be applied, but also the specific requirements of particular products.

The need to maintain control over all aspects of GMP cannot be overemphasized.

In this chapter an overview of QA and GMP, with special attention to some of the particular requirements of vaccine manufacture, will be given. It has to be emphasized that responsible persons in vaccine manufacturing must have a good knowledge of the requirements of QA and GMP, and those responsible for research and development have to appreciate the significance of QA.

The European Union's (EU) guidelines on GMPs for medicinal products (EC, 1992a) dedicates an entire annex to immunological veterinary medicinal products (IVMPs).

QUALITY ASSURANCE

Quality

The International Organization for Standardization (ISO) defines quality as: "the totality of features and characteristics of a product or service that bears on its ability to satisfy stated or implied needs" (ISO, 1994).

For medicinal products, the main components of quality, as defined by ISO, are:

- *safety;*
- *efficacy* to produce the expected effect;
- *quality,* in the narrow sense of analytical and manufacturing quality.

These are particularly important but, among others, the following should be added:

- simplicity of use (administration, storage, etc.);
- compatibility with immunoprophylaxis, if required;
- the overall cost of the product, which should be reasonable.

A medicinal product (as well as any other type of product) can only meet the required standard of quality if it has been properly designed and manufactured. This is ensured through the application of a QA system.

ISO gives the following definition of QA: "All those planned actions and systemifications necessary to provide adequate confidence that a product or service will satisfy given requirements for quality" (ISO, 1994) and the EU guidelines add the following:

> Quality assurance is a wide-ranging concept which covers all matters which individually or collectively influence the quality of a product. It is the total sum of the organized arrangements made with the object of ensuring that medicinal products are of the quality required for their intended use. (EC, 1992a.)

QA is a comprehensive system, designed, documented, implemented and furnished with personnel, equipment and other resources so as to provide assurance that products will be consistently of the required quality. The system therefore involves obtaining high quality at every level, from design to manufacture, product servicing and follow-up.

Figure 12 shows the relations between the different parts of QA.

Quality assurance for design

QA should ensure the avoidance of any design defect. The possibility of defects should always be borne in mind because they may affect all batches and their occurrence is virtually inescapable. Defects can be particularly costly, for example incomplete inactivation conditions as a result of a design defect in the manufacturing process may lead to disease in vaccinated animals.

New methods and rules enable the implementation of QA procedures into the design of manufacturing processes related to the production of vaccines.

Design reviews. These are defined by ISO as: "a formal documented, comprehensive and systematic examination of a design to meet these requirements and to identify problems and propose solutions" (ISO, 1994).

Good laboratory practice. Good laboratory practice (GLP) refers to laboratory organization and the conditions under which trials are planned, carried out and reported (OECD, 1981; EC, 1987, 1990b and 1992b).

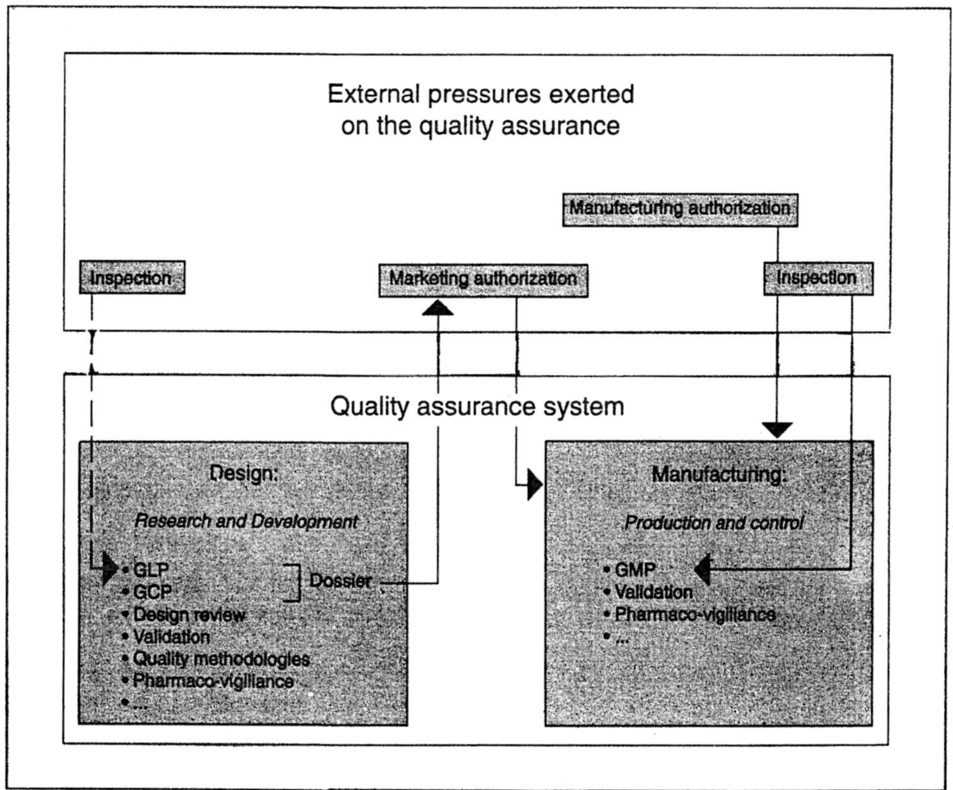

FIGURE 12
The quality assurance system

GLP also applies to the non-clinical trials designed to assess the properties and safety of veterinary medicinal products so that the quality and integrity of future trial results can be guaranteed.

The EU guidelines (EC, 1992b) indicate that the system of QA appropriate for the manufacture of medicinal products should ensure that such products are designed and developed in a way that takes account of GLP.

Good clinical practice. Good clinical practice (GCP) is defined as a series of measures that must be implemented to ensure the quality and authenticity of the scientific data obtained through trials (EC, 1992c). For GCP purposes, clinical trials mean systematic studies made in the field on target species.

Quality assurance for design and manufacture

Important aspects of QA concern both product design and manufacture.

Validation. Validation is the action of proving in accordance with GMP principles that any procedure, process, equipment, material, activity or system leads to the results expected.

There should be complete validation of manufacturing processes to ensure the continuous conformity of vaccine batches to required standards (EC, 1990a).

Production methods. Methods that ensure product quality and standards for the management of QA work (ISO, 1987a and 1987b) should be in operation.

Pharmaco-vigilance. Procedures to monitor the use of products in accordance with good standards of pharmaco-vigilance should be established. This will allow data on rare and unexpected effects to be recorded and analysed.

It must be emphasized that in both the design and manufacture of products, the prevention of defects is a better policy than relying on the results of certain in-process tests or tests of the final product (Soulebot, 1992).

With regard to control tests, it is best that they be carried out as far upstream in the process as possible. If a purity test has to be performed, it is easier to test the starting materials thoroughly than to test the dozens of batches of final product derived from those starting materials. Similarly, the results of inactivation tests will be of greater significance if carried out on the unformulated antigen suspension – whereas the results of similar tests on the final product may be significantly affected by the presence of adjuvants, excipients, etc. It will always be better to take measures to avoid the contamination of starting materials, and to make sure that the inactivated biological agent really is inactivated, by the thorough application of duly validated processes.

QUALITY ASSURANCE FOR MANUFACTURE: GOOD MANUFACTURING PRACTICES

QA applied to manufacture is represented mainly by GMPs, defined in EC (1992a) as: "GMP deals with that part of QA which ensures that products are produced consistently and controlled to the quality standards appropriate to their intended use".

Principles

QA (and GMP) should ensure the avoidance of any manufacturing or product defect. In order to achieve this purpose, the following general principles and aims should be adhered to:

- The holder of a manufacturing licence must manufacture medicinal products so as to ensure that they are fit for their intended use, comply with the requirements of the marketing authorization and do not place animals at risk owing to inadequate safety, quality or efficacy.

- The attainment of these objectives is the responsibility of senior management and requires the participation and commitment of staff in many different departments and at all levels within the company. This also applies to the company's suppliers and distributors.
- To achieve these quality objectives consistently, there must be a comprehensively designed and properly implemented QA system that incorporates GMP and quality control. The system should be fully documented and its effectiveness monitored.
- All parts of the QA system should be adequately resourced with competent personnel and suitable and sufficient premises, equipment and facilities.

The purposes of QA

The QA system intended for the control of the manufacture of medicinal products should ensure the following:

- Medicinal products are designed and developed in a way that takes account of the requirements of GMP and GLP.
- Production and control operations are clearly specified and GMPs adopted.
- Managerial responsibilities are clearly defined.
- Arrangements are made for the manufacture, supply and use of the appropriate raw materials and packaging materials.
- All necessary controls on intermediate products, and any other in-process controls and validations, are carried out.
- The final product is correctly processed and checked, according to the necessary defined procedures.
- Medicinal products are not sold or supplied before an appropriately qualified person has certified that each production batch has been produced and controlled in accordance with the requirements of the marketing authorization and any other regulations relevant to the production, control and release of medicinal products.
- Satisfactory arrangements are made to ensure, as far as possible, that the medicinal products are stored, distributed and handled in such as way as to maintain their quality throughout their shelf-life.
- There is a procedure for in-house inspection and quality audit which regularly appraises the effectiveness and applicability of the QA system.

GMP for medicinal products

GMP is that part of QA that ensures that products are consistently produced and controlled to the quality standards appropriate to their intended use and as required by the marketing authorization or product specification.

GMP is concerned with both production and quality control. The following are the basic requirements of GMP:

- All manufacturing processes are clearly defined, systematically reviewed and shown to be capable of consistently manufacturing medicinal products of the required quality and complying with their specifications.
- Critical steps in the manufacturing process and significant changes to that process are validated.
- All the necessary facilities for GMP are provided, including: appropriately qualified and trained personnel; adequate premises and space; suitable equipment and services; correct materials, containers and labels; approved procedures and instructions; and suitable storage and transport.
- Instructions and procedures are written in clear and unambiguous language, specifically applicable to the facilities provided.

- Operators are trained to carry out procedures correctly.
- Records are made (manually and/or by recording instruments) during manufacture to demonstrate that all the steps required by the defined procedures and instructions are taken and that the quantity and quality of the product was as expected. Any significant deviations should be fully recorded and investigated.
- Records of manufacture and distribution, which enable the complete history of a batch to be traced, are retained in a comprehensible and accessible form.
- The method of distribution of products minimizes any risk to their quality.
- A system is available to recall any batch of product from sale or supply.
- Complaints about marketed products are examined, the causes of quality defects investigated and appropriate measures taken in respect of defective products so as to prevent reoccurrence.
- Rigorous standards of hygiene and cleanliness are applied.

Quality control

Quality control (QC) is that part of GMP that is concerned with the taking of samples during production, the specifications related to the product and the tests to be applied. It is also concerned with the organization, documentation and release procedures to ensure that the necessary and relevant tests are actually carried out and that materials are not released for use, or products released for sale or supply, until their quality has been judged to be satisfactory.

The following are the basic requirements of QC:

- Adequate facilities, trained personnel and approved procedures are available for sampling. Raw materials, packaging materials, intermediate, bulk and final products should be inspected and tested and, where appropriate, environmental conditions should be monitored for GMP purposes.
- Samples of starting materials, packaging materials, intermediate products, bulk products and final products are taken by qualified personnel and by methods approved by the requirements of QC.
- Test methods are validated.
- Records are made (manually and/or by recording instruments) that demonstrate that all the required sampling, inspection and testing procedures have been carried out. Any deviations should be fully recorded and investigated.
- The final products contain only active ingredients that comply with the qualitative and quantitative composition specified in the marketing authorization, are of the purity required and are enclosed within their proper containers and correctly labelled.
- Records are made of the results of inspection and the testing of materials, intermediate, bulk and final products is correctly assessed against specifications. Production assessment includes a review and evaluation of the relevant production documentation and an assessment of any deviations from specified procedures.
- No batch of product is released for sale or supply prior to certification by an appropriately qualified person in accordance with the requirement of the marketing authorization.
- Sufficient samples of starting materials and products are retained to permit future examination of the product if necessary. Products should be retained in their final packs unless exceptionally large packs are produced.

GOOD MANUFACTURING PRACTICES

GMPs are concerned with such issues as:

- personnel training, organization, safety and hygiene;
- premises and equipment;
- documentation;
- production;
- quality control;
- contract manufacture and analysis;
- complaints and products recall;
- in-house inspections.

Personnel training, organization, safety and hygiene

The establishment and maintenance of a satisfactory QA system and the correct manufacture of medicinal products rely on people. There must be sufficient qualified personnel to carry out all the tasks that are the responsibility of the manufacturer. Individual responsibilites should be clearly understood by the individuals and recorded. All personnel should be aware of the GMP principles that affect them and should receive initial and continuing training, including hygiene instructions, relevant to their needs. Staff should be well motivated.

The following are some of the important aspects relating to personnel in vaccine manufacturing establishments:

- Key personnel are the head of production, the head of quality control (who must be independent from each other) and the qualified person(s) who must ensure that each batch has been produced and checked in accordance with regulations and the marketing authorization.
- Basic and appropriate training should be given, according to training programmes.
- Personnel should be protected against possible infection, particularly in the case of microorganisms known to cause disease in humans that are either handled directly or used in work with experimental animals. Where appropriate, personnel should be immunized.
- Adequate measures should be taken to prevent microorganisms being carried outside the plant by personnel.
- The risk of contamination or cross-contamination of vaccines by personnel is particularly important. Prevention should be achieved by a set of measures and procedures (the use of protective clothing, etc.).
- Detailed hygiene programmes should be established.

Premises and equipment

Premises and equipment must be located, designed, constructed, adapted and maintained to suit the operations to be carried out. Their layout and design must aim to minimize the risk of errors and permit effective cleaning and maintenance in order to avoid cross-contamination, the build-up of dust or dirt and any other adverse effect on the quality of products.

Premises. Premises should be designed in such a way as to control the risk to both the product and the environment. This can be achieved by the use of containment, clean, clean/contained, contained and controlled areas.

Live biological agents should be handled in *contained areas*. The level of containment will depend on the pathogenicity of the microorganism.

Inactivated microorganisms and non-infected cells isolated from multicellular organisms should be handled in *clean areas*.

Open-circuit operations involving products or components that are not subsequently sterilized, should be carried out within a laminar airflow workstation (grade A) in a grade B area (see Table 14).

Other operations where live biological agents are handled (quality control, research, diagnosis) should be appropriately contained and separated if production operations are carried out in the same building or in buildings in close proximity to those used for production.

Containment premises should be easily disinfected and have the following characteristics:

- an absence of direct venting to the outside;
- ventilation with air held at negative pressure – air should be extracted through high-efficiency particle absorption (HEPA) filters;
- a system for the collection and disinfection of liquid effluents – solid waste should be disinfected, sterilized or incinerated as appropriate;
- a changing room designed and used as an airlock, equipped with appropriate showering facilities;
- an airlock system for use when equipment is being transferred;
- in many instances, a barrier-type double-door autoclave.

With the exception of blending and subsequent filling operations, only one biological agent should be handled at a time within each area and production areas should be designed to permit disinfection between production runs with different organisms, using validated methods.

The characteristics of *clean areas* are well known and described in the GMP literature. Clean areas have a ventilation system with air under positive pressure (see Table 14).

Clean/contained areas have the characteristics of both clean and contained areas, but have a ventilation system with air at negative pressure. The outside section of the changing room is under positive pressure, the inside section is under a negative pressure that is higher than that of the work area. There is therefore an air pressure barrier. This type of area is used when it is necessary to protect the product and the environment against the handling of live organisms during certain production processes, for example the inoculation or harvest of roller bottle cultures during virus multiplication steps.

TABLE 14

Air classification system for the manufacture of sterile products

Grade	Maximum permitted number of particles per m³ equal to or above:		Maximum permitted number of viable microorganism per m³	Possible final filter efficiency[1] (%)
	0.5/µm	5/µm		
A laminar airflow workstation	3 500	None	Less than 1[2]	99.997
B	3 500	None	5[2]	99.995
C	350 000	2 000	100	99.950
D	3 500 000	20 000	500	95.000

Notes:

Laminar airflow systems should provide a homogeneous air speed of 0.30 m per second for vertical flow and 0.45 m per second for horizontal flow.

In order to reach air grades B, C and D, the number of air changes should generally be higher than 20 per hour in a room with a good airflow pattern and appropriate HEPA filters.

The guidance given for the maximum permitted number of particles corresponds approximately to the United States Federal Standard 209 C as follows: Class 100 (grades A and B), Class 10 000 (grade C) and Class 100 000 (grade D).

It is accepted that it may not always be possible to demonstrate conformity with particulate standards at the point of fill when filling is in progress owing to the generation of particles or droplets from the product itself.

The air pressure differentials between rooms of successively lower risk should be at least 1.5 mm water gauge.

[1] Given as an indication, percentage determined by BS 3928.

[2] The low values involved here are only reliable when a large number of air samples are taken.

Box 1
Definitions

Clean area
An area with defined environmental control of particulate and microbial contamination, constructed and used in such a way as to reduce the introduction, generation and retention of contaminants within the area.

Clean/contained area
An area constructed and operated in such a manner that will achieve the aims of both a clean area and a contained area at the same time.

Contained area
An area constructed and operated in such a manner (and equipped with appropriate air handling and filtration) so as to prevent contamination of the external environment by biological agents from within the area.

Containment
The action of confining a biological agent or other entity within a defined space.

Controlled area
An area constructed and operated in such a manner that some attempt is made to control the introduction of potential contamination (an air supply approximating to grade D [Table 13] may be appropriate) and the consequences of accidental release of living organisms. The level of control exercised should reflect the nature of the organism employed in the process. At a minimum, the area should be maintained at a pressure negative to the immediate external environment and should allow for the efficient removal of small quantities of airborne contaminants.

Primary containment
A system of containment that prevents the escape of a biological agent into the immediate working environment. It involves the use of closed containers and biological safety procedures along with secure operating procedures.

Secondary containment
A system of containment that prevents the escape of a biological agent into the external environment or into other working areas. It involves the use of rooms with specially designed air handling, airlocks and / or sterilizers for the exit of materials and secure operating procedures. In many cases it may add to the effectiveness of primary containment.

Animal houses should be separated from other production premises.

Documentation relating to the premises should be readily available.

Equipment. The equipment used should be designed and constructed to meet the particular requirements for the manufacture of each product.

Before being put into operation it should be assessed and validated as suitable for the process. Subsequently every piece of equipment should be regularly maintained and validated.

Where appropriate the equipment should ensure the satisfactory primary containment of the microorganism involved in the process and should be designed and constructed to allow easy and effective decontamination and / or sterilization.

Separate incubators should be used for infected and non-infected containers, and also for different organisms or cells in general.

Careful consideration should be given to the procedures and equipment aimed at avoiding environmental contamination (wastes, effluents, etc.).

Documentation

Good documentation constitutes an essential part of the QA system. Clearly written documentation prevents errors arising from spoken communication and permits the tracing of a batch's history. Specifications, manufacturing formulae and instructions, procedures and records must be free from errors and available in writing. The legibility of documents is of paramount importance.

Important aspects of documentation include:

- Specifications, manufacturing formulae, processing and packaging instructions, procedures and records are of paramount importance.
- It is particularly important that the data generated by the monitoring of various aspects of GMP (equipment, product, premises, etc.) are rigorously assessed and that informed decisions are made and recorded.

Production

Production operations must follow clearly defined and validated procedures in accordance with the relevant manufacturing and marketing licences. Careful attention must be paid to the constant monitoring of production and to in-process controls.

Starting materials. The properties required of starting materials should be clearly defined in written specifications. This is particularly important for substances of animal origin when the geographical origin and the animal species from which the materials are derived should be included. Special attention should be paid to the supplier's QA system.

Where possible, heat is the preferred method for sterilizing starting materials.

Media. Media should preferably be sterilized *in situ* or in line. Heat is the preferred method.

Seed lot and cell bank systems. In order to prevent the undesirable drift of properties that can ensue from multiple generations (i.e. many serial growth passages), a seed lot or cell bank system should be used. Seeds and / or cells should all be adequately characterized, tested, stored, etc.

Operating principles. Accidental spillages, especially of live organisms, must be dealt with quickly and safely.

The formation of droplets and the production of aerosols or foams should be avoided. Centrifugation and blending should be carried out in appropriate contained or clean / contained areas or in a closed system when it is necessary to prevent the transfer of organisms.

A closed system or laminar airflow cabinet should be used for operations such as the transfer of sterile media.

Equipment, the external surfaces of containers, etc. must be disinfected before transfer from a contained area and liquid and solid waste must be sterilized or disinfected.

Quality control

QC is concerned with sampling, specifications and testing, as well as with the organizational, documentation and release procedures that ensure the necessary and relevant tests have been carried out and that materials are not released for use, or products released for sale or supply, until their quality has been judged satisfactory. QC is not confined to laboratory operations, but must be involved in all decisions that may affect the quality of the product. The independence of the QC section from the production group is considered fundamental to the satisfactory operation of QC.

Important aspects of QC include:

- Control laboratories should apply good quality-control laboratory practice.
- In-process controls play an especially important role. Important controls that cannot be carried out on the final product should be performed at an appropriate stage of production.

Contract manufacture and analysis

Manufacture under contract and analysis must be properly defined, agreed and controlled to avoid the misunderstandings that could result in a product or service of unsatisfactory quality. There must be a written contract between the contractor and the customer which clearly establishes the duties and liabilities of each party. The contract must clearly state the procedures used by the qualified person when releasing each batch of product for sale.

Complaints and product recall

All complaints and other information concerning potentially defective products must be reviewed carefully according to written procedures. A system should be in place to recall from the market, in a prompt and effective manner, all products known to be, or suspected of being, defective.

In-house inspections

In-house inspections should be conducted for the purpose of monitoring the implementation of and compliance with GMP principles and to propose corrective measures where necessary.

They should be conducted in an impartial and independent manner, following a pre-arranged programme, and should be recorded. Statements of the actions subsequently taken should also be recorded.

Most countries have their own GMP guidelines or regulations which are compulsory. Other countries are covered by the World Health Organization guidelines (WHO, 1992) which should be followed. The United States Code of Federal Regulations (CFR) (USDA, 1994), as well as EU requirements (EC, 1991a and 1991b), will also be very helpful.

There is now a move to apply the same regulations across a group of different countries, as for example in the Member States of the EU.

MAINTENANCE OF THE QUALITY ASSURANCE SYSTEM: INSPECTIONS

The integrity of the QA system, after its implementation, can only be maintained (and the introduction of undesirable small changes in the operation resisted) by the application of both internal and external pressures or checks.

Internal pressure is represented by verification and validation from in-house inspections, design reviews and the continuous attention of top management. External pressures are those exerted by competition and customers. The latter exercise direct pressure by placing orders or not. Indirect pressure is exerted by legal authorities, through official licensing (manufacturing and marketing licences) and official inspections (see Figure 12, p. 299). Such inspections are very important. Their degree of implementation differs considerably from one country to another and between GMP and GLP and an appropriate and uniform system of inspection is highly desirable.

CONCLUSIONS

When applied to vaccines, the QA system assures users that the necessary standards of quality in relation to products have been maintained (i.e. products have been suitably designed and produced and properly inspected at a reasonable cost). The QA system should also allow the manufacturer and the national control authorities to reduce costly and time-consuming control tests that offer only a relative degree of reliability.

Such developments are to some extent new in regard to the concepts and practice of vaccine manufacture. Confidence in the product and the manufacturing process is best achieved when standards and methods of working are properly challenged by an appropriate and efficient system of QC.

The requirements of an efficient QA system should facilitate batch release and permit easy, free and fair trading and/or the exchange of vaccines for use in different regions.

BIBLIOGRAPHY

EC. 1987. Council Directive 87/18/EEC of 18 December 1986. *Off. J. Eur. Comm.*, No. 15/29 of 13.1.87.

EC. 1990a. Council Directive 90/677/EEC of 13 December 1990. *Off. J. Eur. Comm.*, No. L373/26-28 of 31.12.90.

EC. 1990b. Commission Directive 90/18/EEC of 18 December 1990. *Off. J. Eur. Comm.*, No. L11/37-50 of 13.1.90.

EC. 1991a. *General requirements for the production and control of inactivated mammalian bacterial and viral vaccines for veterinary use.* Commission of the European Communities, III/3181/91-EN.

EC. 1991b. *General requirements for the production and control of live mammalian bacterial and viral vaccines for veterinary use.* Commission of the European Communities, III/3182/91-EN.

EC. 1992a. *EEC guide to good manufacturing practices for medicinal products.* Rules Governing Medicinal Products in the European Community, Volume IV, January 1992, p. 1-165.

EC. 1992b. Commission Directive 92/18/EEC of 20 March 1992. *Off. J. Eur. Comm.* No. L97/1-23 of 10.04.92.

EC. 1992c. *Good clinical practice for the conduct of clinical trials for veterinary medicinal products.* III/3767/92, CVMP, EC.

ISO. 1987a. ISO, 9000, Geneva, Switzerland, International Organization for Standardization.

ISO. 1987b. ISO, 9004. Geneva, Switzerland, International Organization for Standardization.

ISO. 1994. *Quality management and quality assurance – Vocabulary.* ISO 8402:1994 Geneva, Switzerland, International Organization for Standardization.

OECD. 1981. *Good laboratory practice in the testing of chemicals.* Good Laboratory Practice Principles, Organisation for Economic Co-operation and Development. Annex II to Council Decision of 12.5.1981, C81.30 final.

Soulebot, J.P. 1992. FEDESA's point of view: quality, application to IVMPs (immunological veterinary medicinal products). *Dev. Biol. Stand.*, 79: 201-211.

USDA. 1994. *Animals and animal products,* CFR title 9. Animal and Plant Health Inspection Service, United States Department of Agriculture.

WHO. 1992. WHO Technical Report Series 823 No. 32. WHO Expert Committee for Medicinal Products Specifications, Geneva, Switzerland, World Health Organization.

The principles of good laboratory practices, including safety in vaccine production and quality control

C.A. Mebus

The general principles of good laboratory practice (GLP) and quality control (QC) in veterinary vaccine production apply to both live and inactivated viral and bacterial vaccines. The first part of this chapter will address the general principles of good laboratory practices associated with the production of a biological product and the second part will be more specific on requirements for quality assurance.

GENERAL PRINCIPLES OF GOOD LABORATORY PRACTICE

A biological product must be pure, safe, potent and efficacious. To produce such a product there must be a proper facility that has been inspected and approved as appropriate for the manufacture of safe biological products. Close attention must be given to all the parameters associated with production of biological products, i.e. to ensure a good-quality product production must be carried out in accordance with good laboratory practices (GLPs). GLPs are a set of rules, operating procedures and practices that describe how laboratory procedures, tests and studies are planned, performed, monitored, recorded and reported, to ensure the quality and integrity of the data generated by a laboratory. These procedures and practices should be detailed and written in a clear manner, so that someone unfamiliar with them could perform the work, for example the operation and/or calibration of an instrument should be described, the speed at which to run the centrifuge should be given and the way in which to handle record charts should be described. These procedures and practices are generally written by the manufacturer and approved by the regulatory authority.

MANAGEMENT

Laboratory management is responsible for providing appropriate facilities, qualified personnel and good equipment, reagents and materials and for maintaining personnel records and ensuring that written and approved standard operating procedures, protocols and schedules are established and documented for all aspects of production.

There should be a document that specifies the authority, responsibility and interrelation of all laboratory personnel (management and staff) involved in the production of biological products. The laboratory organization should include a person responsible for ensuring that GLPs are in place, a technical manager who has the overall responsibility for production and a quality control manager who is responsible for all aspects affecting product quality, including maintenance, calibration, validation, monitoring of equipment and instruments and testing of the final product. The quality control manager should report directly to senior management.

THE FACILITY

Plans of the property showing the location of all buildings and blueprints on which are listed all the activities carried out in these buildings should be developed and made available. To minimize opportunistic cross-contamination, specific buildings should be dedicated to the production of particular biologicals and there should be no diagnostic and/or research activities in such buildings.

Buildings should be designed and constructed to prevent cross-contamination during the process of production. Halls, rooms and production areas should be arranged to provide maximum biological security and minimal contamination of the production areas. Thus, the areas with the greatest potential for contamination of the product should be the furthest removed from the production area. Offices, eating areas, dressing rooms, toilet facilities and warehouse areas should be located so that they are accessible without passage through the production areas. Personnel and materials moving to a biological production area should not pass through the production area designated for another product.

The air supply to a production area should preferably be high-efficency particle absorption- (HEPA-) filtered and come directly from outside the building. Air pressure gradients within the building should be designed to minimize the potential for cross-contamination and exhaust air from a production area should not be recirculated to another production or building area.

In production areas, the floors, walls, ceilings and doors should be made of materials that will prevent cross-contamination and that can be easily cleaned and disinfected.

Water should be free of pollution and impurities and there must be an adequate supply and distribution of hot and cold water.

The sanitary system must have the necessary traps and vents and a disposal method that minimizes pollution. All maintenance and repairs should be documented.

The area around the building should be well-drained, clean and free of clutter. Animal facilities should be located away from production buildings and should be properly drained and ventilated and kept in a sanitary condition. An effort should be made to minimize the fly and rodent populations in the surrounding area and to keep the production areas free of these pests.

PERSONNEL

Each person working in biological production should have a personal file that includes a curriculum vitae, documentation of education and training and a detailed job description including to whom the person reports and details of those whom the person supervises.

Before working with a particular organism or agent, management must evaluate the potential for human infection and, if needed, implement immunization and/or other necessary precautions. Each area of the facility should have defined and documented operating procedures.

Production personnel must be competent in microbiological and good laboratory techniques through education and/or training. Before entering a biological production area, personnel should either change their clothes for clean laboratory clothing or cover their street clothes with appropriate laboratory garments. Hair covering, face masks, gowns and shoe covers should be used in production areas. Eating, smoking or any unsanitary practice should be prohibited in a production area.

To maintain a high level of competence, staff should receive periodic training in laboratory techniques and quality control procedures. Staff should be given opportunities for training in specific practices or of observing them in other institutions.

STERILIZATION

There should be written standard operating procedures for the washing and sterilization of all containers, instruments and equipment parts that will be in contact with the product. A recording device should be used with each sterilization cycle to ensure that the proper time, temperature and/or concentration of the sterilizing agent have been achieved. Items subjected to sterilization procedures should be labelled and dated.

Sterilization can be accomplished using live steam at a temperature of at least 120°C for not less than 30 minutes or dry heat at a temperature of at least 160°C for not less than one hour. If an instrument risks damage from either of these treatments, it can, instead, be boiled for not less than 15 minutes or subjected to chemical sterilization, for example ethylene oxide or formaldehyde would be acceptable if found to be effective.

LABELLING

Labels for identification should be placed on all ingredients, components of a biological product, biologicals in any stage of preparation and completed biological products. The label should include the date of preparation and the initials of the preparer.

SEED ORGANISMS

Responsibility for the storage of organisms to be used as master seeds should be assigned to a particular individual. All vials of seed material should be labelled and stored in a secure location and the record for all seeds should contain a documented history, test results and an accurate inventory. Protocols for the testing procedures used should also be on file.

The microorganism seeds used to produce biological products should be free of extraneous agents including viral, bacterial, mycotic and chalymydial organisms. This is best accomplished using a master seed principle. The master seed is a microbiological agent at a specific passage level from which all other seed passages are then made. When developing a vaccine, the master seed and the passage level (i.e. the number of seed passages, which is usually five) that will be used for production must have been shown to be pure, safe, potent and efficacious. The production seed is the specific passage level used to produce the antigen in the product and the working seed is a passage level that lies between the levels of the master seed and the production seed. Working and production seeds have to be shown to be free of any extraneous agent.

In viral vaccine production, the same benefits can be obtained by using a master cell principle for those cell lines used to produce viral antigen. A master cell is a supply of cells at a specific passage level from which working cells and production cells originate for the production of a biological. Master cells will have been shown to be free of extraneous agents and to be non-oncogenic, while working and production cells must be shown to be free of any extraneous agent.

STERILITY

To maximize the probability of the final product being free of extraneous agents, only certified (tested) working and production seeds and cells should be used. Media, if they cannot be heat-sterilized, should be filtered and tested for freedom from any extraneous agent before use. There should be protocols for filtration and for the testing of material for sterility.

The following are examples of ways to maintain sterility:

- Materials that need to be kept free of contamination should only be worked with in biological cabinets or in isolation rooms by people who are properly dressed, to minimize the possibility of contamination.

- Work in cabinets or isolation rooms should be properly planned.
- Work with non-infected material should be done first, followed by work with infected material.
- After working with infected material, the area should be decontaminated and allowed to remain idle for sufficient time to allow dilution by air changes to minimize cross-contamination.
- The potential for bacterial contamination in a production area can be evaluated by incubating bacteriological media that have been exposed to the air in the area for 10 to 20 minutes.

OUTLINE OF PRODUCTION

Each biological product should have a detailed outline of production containing a protocol and guidelines. Where applicable, the outline of production should be in such detail that production could be carried out without prior experience.

An outline of production is made up of several sections.

Composition of the product

This section includes the source and passage history of the organism(s) and, if applicable, the relative proportions of organisms in the product.

Cultures

This section comprises:

- protocols and schedules (or frequencies) for identifying the organism(s) and frequency of identification;
- a protocol for determining the purity of culture(s) and, if applicable, the virulence of the organism(s) as well as the range of passage levels or subcultures to be used in production;
- the composition of the media to be used for seed and production cultures; sources of media ingredients, eggs, cell culture or tissues used; protocols for production of the media; and the methods used to determine the growth-promoting qualities of the media and their freedom from contaminants.

The protocols for production of media should include the formula, source and quality of ingredients; instructions on the storage and handling of ingredients; the quality of water required; equipment; the quality of glassware; procedures for product formulation and testing; the conditions for storage and handling of formulated media; and the product expiry date.

The protocol for testing the sterility and growth-promoting qualities of media should include preparation and testing of QC media, the source and care of QC cultures and media performance testing. Records must be made concurrently with the performance of successive steps in the production and testing of each lot of medium.

The record for each lot of medium should contain the name of the supplier, the lot number, the date of purchase, the date the seal was broken for each medium ingredient; the pH and osmolarity of the medium; the date the medium was prepared; and the initials of the preparer.

The outline of production should also include:

- a description of the containers used to grow organism(s) and instructions on how they are to be sterilized;
- storage conditions for seed cultures;
- the protocol for preparing inoculum;
- the technique for inoculation together with protocols for the preparation of production media and the titre and volume of the inoculum for each size and type of culture container;
- the duration and conditions of incubation;
- a description of the characteristics of growth and the characteristics of contamination;

- a description of the method of attenuation, if any, before the organism is used for production.

Harvest

This section comprises:

- the minimum and maximum time allowed between inoculation and harvesting and the characteristics of the culture at harvest;
- the protocol for the preparation and handling of cultures for harvesting;
- the protocol for harvesting;
- criteria for acceptable harvested material and the procedure for determining acceptability;
- instructions for the handling of discarded material not used in production;
- any additional pertinent information.

Preparation of the product

A detailed description should be given of every step from the harvest of the antigenic material to the completion of the product in the final container, emphasizing the following:

- the method of inactivation, attenuation or detoxification, if applicable;
- the composition of the preservative, adjuvant or stabilizer, the stage of production and the method of addition. (The proportions used should be stated in such a manner that the final concentration of the added component can be calculated.);
- the protocol for the method and the degree of concentration;
- if the product is standardized to a specific concentration of antigen, the procedures used to achieve this concentration and the calculations made in doing so should be given;
- serials: i) the method of assembly of units to make a serial (illustrate by example); ii) the volume of an average serial; iii) the volume of a maximum serial; and iv) other pertinent information;
- the volume of fill for each size of vial;
- a description of the method and technique for filling and sealing the final container;
- the protocol for lyophilization including procedures for determining the moisture content;
- the amount of antigenic material per dose or doses in the final container and how this is determined;
- conditions for storage of the finished product.

Permitted antibiotics and amounts per millilitre of biological product in the United States are:

• Amphotericin B	2.4 micrograms
• Nystatin (Mycostatin)	30.0 units
• Tetracyclines	30.0 units
• Penicillin	30.0 units
• Streptomycin	30.0 micrograms
• Polymyxin B	30.0 micrograms
• Neomycin	30.0 micrograms
• Gentamicin	30.0 micrograms

Permitted combinations of the above include:

- penicillin and streptomycin;
- either amphotericin B or nystatin with any of the other antibiotics alone or with a combination of penicillin and streptomycin or polymyxin B and neomycin.

Testing

A description should be given of how samples of the final product are collected, stored and tested. Protocols should be provided for the determination of purity, safety, potency, moisture content and any other test performed on the product. Each test protocol should include the minimum requirement for a satisfactory test.

Post-preparatory steps

This section should include:

- the form and size of the final container in which the product is to be distributed;

- a description of the conditions for storage.

Finally, the outline of production should include bibliographical references and any relevant appendixes.

LABELLING

All biological products should be properly labelled and packaged before leaving the production establishment. The final container label should include the following information: the name of the product; the name and address of the producer; the recommended storage temperature; the number of doses in the vial; the use, dosage and route of administration for each animal species for which the biological product is recommended; the expiry date; the serial number; and warnings or cautions, if applicable.

The expiry date is based on the earliest date of harvest and the date of the last satisfactory potency test. If applicable, the date of lyophilization should be given. A stability record should be established by testing each serial for potency at release and at the approximate expiry date.

The following are examples of warnings or cautions for products containing live or dangerous organisms: "Burn this container and all unused contents"; (for multidose vials) "Use entire contents when first opened"; "Do not vaccinate within [state number] days of slaughter"; and "Do not vaccinate pregnant animals".

The following information should be provided on the label, carton label or an enclosed leaflet: full instructions on the use of the product; if applicable, schedules of use; names of preservatives; and any restrictions on use of the product.

Containers of diluents to be used for reconstituting biological products should include on the label: the words "sterile diluent"; the name of the biological product with which it is packaged; its recoverable quantity in cubic centimetres or millilitres; the serial number; and the name and address of the producer. All necessary warnings as covered by the label for biological products should be placed on the diluent vial to cover its use and handling after reconstitution.

STORAGE

Completed biological products should be stored at 2° to 7°C, unless a different temperature has been shown to give better stability.

RECORDS

Each biological production facility should keep detailed records of all the activities carried out within the establishment. These should include a daily log of production area use. Records should be made concurrently with the performance of successive steps in the production of each lot and should contain the date and time of all critical steps, the identity and quantity of all ingredients added or removed and sufficient detail to give a clear understanding of each step in the preparation of the product. The charts and temperature records made during preparation of ingredients, sterilization of equipment or manufacture of a product are part of the record for the lot being produced. For each lot there should also be detailed records of the tests performed on ingredients, seeds, the product during manufacture and the completed serials or subserials of the product.

The facility should have a record of the location of all biologicals being prepared and the quantities held in storage and distribution channels.

QUALITY ASSURANCE

The protocols and testing procedures that were mentioned earlier can be regarded as contributing to the QC and quality assurance (QA) of biological products in the process of manufacture. These procedures are of considerable value to the manufacturer in indicating the efficiency of the process, thus, it is of major importance that the performance of these critical factors should be documented in appropriate records. The QA monitoring of production and testing of a product should be performed by personnel not associated with the production process. The personnel responsible for QC and QA should report directly to senior management.

The requirements and procedures for testing the quality of a product should conform to the standard requirements established by the country or region in which the product will be used. In addition to tests performed by the manufacturer, product quality should be verified by a national or regional control authority's reference laboratory. Examples of standard requirements can be found in the United States Code of Federal Regulations (CFR) (USDA, 1994) and the European Pharmacopoeia (European Pharmacopoeia Commission, 1985). New test methods developed by the manufacturer should be approved by the national or regional control authority's laboratory before being used to evaluate a product.

When possible, test procedures should include a standard reference reagent, such as a virus, bacterial culture or antigen, for direct comparison with the product. Similarly a standard test reagent, sucha as a serum, antitoxin, fluorescent antibody conjugate, toxin, virus, bacterial culture or antigen, should be used to assure the correct sensitivity of the test. These reference preparations and reagents should be made available by a national or regional reference laboratory. Protocols for calibration, validation, monitoring and maintenance schedules for instruments and equipment should be based on published recommendations such as those contained in the College of American Pathologists. Instruments should be monitored frequently enough to ensure that they operate within tolerance limits 95 percent of the time.

CONCLUSIONS

The quality of a biological product is dependent on close attention to all factors directly or indirectly involved in production. These start with the design and operation of the facility, include the performance of the process and lead eventually to the testing and use of the product. The producer of a biological product must always remember that it is the manufacturer, not the user, who is responsible for ensuring that the product is pure, safe, potent and efficacious.

BIBLIOGRAPHY

College of American Pathologists. *Laboratory instrument evaluation, verification and maintenance manual.* Northfield, Il., USA.

European Pharmacopoeia Commission. 1985. *European Pharmacopoeia,* 2nd edition. Sainte-Ruffine, France, Maisonneuve.

USDA. 1994. Viruses, serums, toxins and analogous products; organisms and vectors). In *Animals and animal products,*. CFR, title 9. United States Department of Agriculture.

USDA. *Good laboratory practices for non-clinical laboratory studies.* Washington, DC, USA, Food and Drug Administration, United States Government Printing Office.

The role of reference and regional laboratories

A.I. Donaldson and V. Astudillo

International organizations such as the Food and Agriculture Organization of the United Nations (FAO), the Pan American Health Organization of the World Health Organization (PAHO/WHO), the Office internationale des Epizooties (OIE) and the Commission of the European Community (CEC) have designated a series of laboratories worldwide as reference laboratories, collaborating centres and regional laboratories. These laboratories are viewed as an essential part of the organizations' respective missions to promote animal health and prevent the spread of disease through international trade in animals and animal products. The lists of FAO and OIE reference laboratories and FAO Collaborating Centres are given in the FAO/OIE/WHO (1995).

The largest network of reference laboratories (RLs) is for foot-and-mouth disease (FMD) – reflecting the international importance of the disease and the requirement for technical support so that its control and eradication can be on a regional basis. Under the aegis of FAO, OIE and CEC, different networks link a world reference laboratory, RLs, a community coordination institute and national laboratories and serve as a model for the role of reference and regional laboratories. In this chapter the background to these designated RLs and descriptions of their activities are provided.

WORLD REFERENCE LABORATORY FOR FMD

The Institute for Animal Health, Pirbright, United Kingdom (formerly the Animal Virus Research Institute) was designated by FAO in 1958 as the World Reference Laboratory (WRL) for FMD. The terms under which the WRL agreed to operate are:

- to perform tests for the presence of FMD virus on specimens sent by Member Governments of FAO and the European Commission for the Control of FMD;
- to identify the virus if present and/or the strain and antigenic properties of the isolated virus(es) if deemed necessary;
- to send all relevant information regarding the results of such tests to the government(s) requesting the test(s), with duplicate copies sent to the Animal Production and Health Division of FAO in Rome.

At the 1959 Session of the European Commission for the Control of FMD it was agreed that the WRL would be responsible for examining strains of virus found in Europe that were suspected of being types other than O, A and C, i.e. exotic strains. Additional responsibilities for the WRL were the subtyping of strains of the virus, maintenance of a reference collection of all confirmed subtypes and corresponding antisera and the supply of such antisera to other laboratories on request.

The 28th General Session of OIE in May 1960 recognized the Institute for Animal Health, Pirbright, as the WRL for FMD and authorized it to handle all seven serotypes of FMD virus. Thus the WRL became uniquely sanctioned by both OIE and FAO to manipulate all seven serotypes of FMD virus.

Between 1958 and 1993 the WRL processed 18 200 samples from more than 110 different countries. It has also played a leading role in developing and standardizing methods for improved FMD diagnosis and virus strain characterization (Ferris and Donaldson, 1992).

REGIONAL REFERENCE LABORATORIES FOR FMD

Five regional RLs for FMD are recognized. These are:

- the Pan American Foot and Mouth Disease Center (PAHO/WHO), Rio de Janeiro, Brazil, which is designated by FAO and OIE as the regional RL for South and Central America;
- the Botswana Vaccine Institute (BVI), Gaborone, Botswana, is the OIE-designated regional RL for Southern Africa;
- the FMD Centre, Pakchong, Thailand is the FAO- and OIE-designated regional RL for FMD for Southeast Asia and Oceania;
- the Institute for Animal Health, Pirbright, United Kingdom, is the community RL for Member States of the European Union;
- the Central Veterinary Institute (CDI-DLO), Lelystad, the Netherlands, is the community coordinating institute for FMD vaccine for the European Union.

The expected functions and activities of OIE-designated RLs for FMD were reviewed by the OIE FMD and other Epizootics Commission in 1989 and adopted by the International Committee of OIE at the General Session in May 1989. They are as follows:

- The RL should act as the reference laboratory for the countries in the region and should collect and compile epidemiological data from the region with the collaboration of the national veterinary services.
- All RLs must operate under high disease-security conditions as recommended in the FAO guidelines on minimum standards (FAO, 1993). The high security systems should be regularly inspected by the relevant authorities (national and regional).
- Samples for FMD diagnosis should be received from the national veterinary services in the region.
- If a country wishes the WRL to perform the diagnosis then samples should be sent simultaneously to both the RL and the WRL.
- If a virus isolate is suspected of belonging to a serotype previously exotic to the region, samples should be sent to the WRL for confirmation and storage.
- The RL should be equipped and skilled to provide an initial diagnosis (serotyping) rapidly.
- The RL should be equipped and skilled for the determination of the serological responses of animals in terms of the serotypes of FMD virus in the region.
- The RL should use a sensitive and specific test. For this purpose it should maintain a stock of regional serotypes of FMD virus, inactivated antigens of exotic types and the appropriate immune sera.
- The RL should be equipped to propagate any FMD isolates in animal hosts and cell culture systems.
- In the case of an uncertain diagnosis, the RL should send a sample of the virus from the primary case to the WRL for confirmation and further characterization. Ideally, an aliquot of field material should be sent but, if this is not possible, animal passage material obtained from the original host species, or low cell culture passage material is acceptable. The history of animal or cell culture passage material should be provided.

- Further virus characterization should be carried out by the most up-to-date techniques, but only as a second priority.
- The RL should participate in collaborative studies with the WRL and other RLs.
- The RL should provide regular training courses in FMD diagnosis, epidemiology and disease control and should organize collaborative studies with national laboratories for the standardization of tests.
- On request, the RL should assist national laboratories by supplying reagents as required.
- The RL should perform tests and provide advice about vaccines for prophylaxis and emergency control. The definitive test is the cattle challenge test. Advice can be given, based on the results of indirect tests provided a correlation has been established between the indirect test and the cattle challenge test.
- Results and epidemiological data should be compiled and presented regularly to OIE, FAO and the WRL.
- All requests for the supply of FMD virus from any other laboratory, including the WRL, should be made through official channels, i.e. the central veterinary authority of a country must make an official approach in writing to the proposed supplier of the virus on behalf of the requesting laboratory.
- The supply of an FMD virus which is exotic to the country of the requesting laboratory should only be undertaken according to OIE and FAO procedures.

FAO expects its regional reference centres to operate along very similar lines.

The Pan American Foot-and-Mouth Disease Center

The Pan American Foot-and-Mouth Disease Center (PAFMDC) was established in 1951 as part of a technical cooperation project of the Organization of American States. Planning of the centre, which offers an international service, was done by the Pan American Sanitary Bureau, in collaboration with the InterAmerican Institute of Agricultural Sciences. Operation of the centre is the responsibility of the bureau.

The centre was built on a site and in buildings donated, together with utilities and a proportion of the labour costs, by the Brazilian Government. Major financial support was provided by the Organization of American States, and additional collaboration in specific parts of the technical and training phases of the centre's programme was received from FAO and the United States Department of Agriculture (USDA). During its formative years the work of the centre was devoted to: the training of national laboratory and field staff responsible for the control of FMD in the Americas; diagnostic services, including identification of the virus; field consultations in control and prevention techniques; and research on the nature of FMD virus and allied viruses.

National FMD control and eradication programmes were first established in South America in the early 1960s and consisted of a network of vesicular disease diagnostic laboratories, vaccine control units and field offices, the latter being responsible for disease monitoring and surveillance and the implementation of disease control procedures. PAFMDC was pivotal to these activities through the technical and advisory services it provided, particularly in the characterization of vesicular virus diseases, the production, standardization and supply of reagents to other diagnostic laboratories in the region and the training of personnel.

A continental vesicular diseases surveillance system (CVDSS), developed by PAFMDC, began operating in 1977. This linked the centre with field offices and laboratories throughout the region. Information on vesicular disease outbreaks in individual countries is sent to the centre where it is collated and analysed to create continental disease status information which is then passed on to participating countries weekly, monthly and/or annually. The WRL, FAO and OIE also regularly receive these data.

Through this system the development of emergency disease situations, such as outbreaks in normally disease-free areas or a sudden increase in outbreaks in endemic areas, can be identified at an early stage and neighbouring countries alerted. PAFMDC's regular monitoring and characterization of virus strains circulating in the field is an important part of the CVDSS since it can identify antigenic changes and the need to alter the spectrum of strains included in vaccines. The possibility of emerging epizootics is particularly likely where there is a decrease in vaccination coverage or increased animal movement owing to trade. The links in this network are shown in Figure 13.

Significant antigenic and immunogenic differences are identified between field isolates and vaccine strains. If there are also epidemiological data indicating an increased disease incidence among vaccinated animals, PAFMDC will recommend to the relevant national authority or authorities that the strains of virus in commercially produced vaccines be changed. This may be effected by adding the new strain to the existing formulation, by substituting one of the strains or by producing a monovalent vaccine to be used together with the commercial vaccine.

Experience has demonstrated, however, that it is not advisable to substitute any strain in a vaccine when the field isolates can be covered with existing vaccine strains following intensified vaccination and revaccination. An example of this was the prediction of a type A epidemic in the Rio Plata basin region three months before its occurrence which allowed the forewarning of national authorities. The alert began in 1987 when PAFMDC established that a strain of virus, later identified as A-81 Argentina/87, present in the Rio Plata region was immunogenically different from the strain being used at that time in vaccines. PAFMDC wrote to the head of the national diagnostic laboratory in Argentina, giving details of the antigenic and immunogenic properties of the field isolate and pointing out the fact that revaccination would be necessary to achieve an acceptable level of protection and that if such measures were not immediately adopted an epidemic could be expected.

The Botswana Vaccine Institute

In 1977, Botswana suffered three outbreaks of FMD, almost simultaneously, caused by SAT 1 and SAT 2 viruses. In the Makgadikgadi area, where an outbreak of SAT 2 occurred, cattle were vaccinated with an imported vaccine but protection was poor. As imports were the only source of vaccine, the Botswana Government decided to build its own vaccine institute (in association with the company IFFA-Mérieux) but, since it was estimated that it would take at least three years to design and construct a permanent vaccine production plant and the need for vaccine was urgent, it was decided to tackle the problem in two phases as follows (Falconer, Mannathoko and Cuinet, 1982).

- *Phase 1*, an emergency phase, designed to produce limited amounts of vaccine while maintaining maximum disease security;
- *Phase 2*, establishment of the permanent institute, designed initially to produce 21 million monovalent doses of vaccine per year.

It was decided to use a mobile virus laboratory in order to enable work on FMD

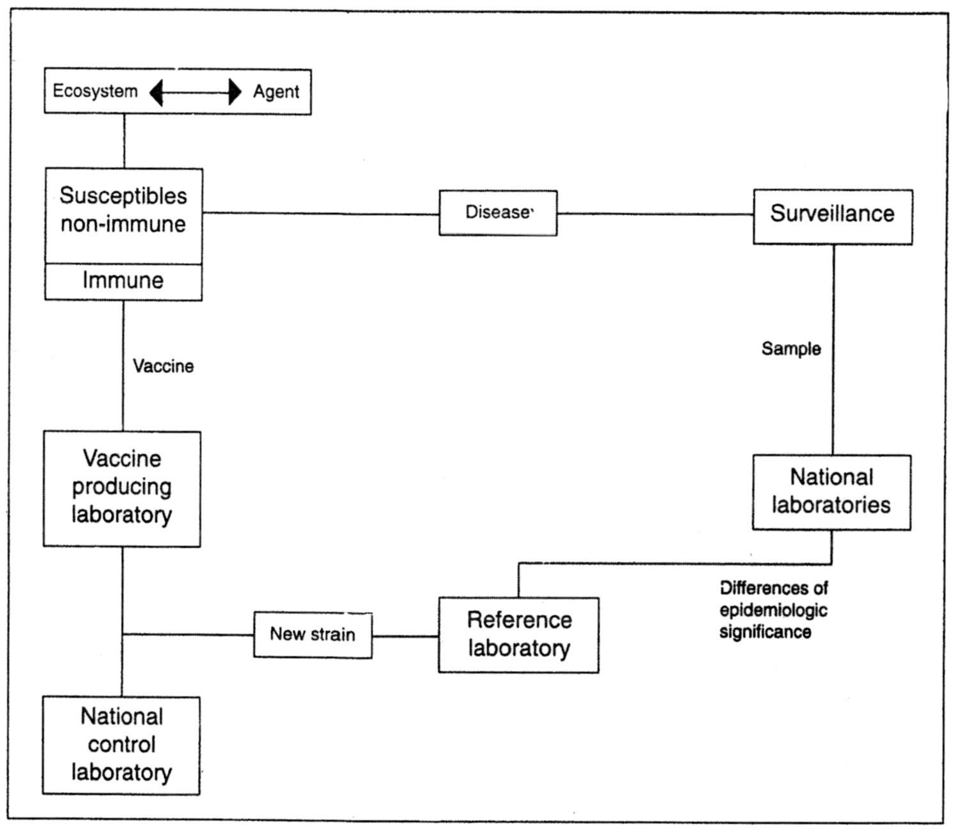

FIGURE 13
Reference system activation flow

viruses to be undertaken as quickly as possible. In August 1978, the laboratory was flown from France to Botswana in a Hercules aircraft and installed on a site in Gaborone. To provide facilities enabling work to be done outside the module's viral zone area, a large prefabricated building was erected, encompassing all the activities of Phase 1.

Financing to build, equip and run the Phase I facilities was provided by the European Community. Seven weeks after the arrival of the mobile laboratory the first batch of vaccine was produced. Phase 2, the construction of a permanent vaccine institute, started at the end of March 1980 and was completed in August 1981. The permanent, commercial vaccine institute started production in September 1981 and was soon producing on an industrial scale that allowed the exportation of vaccine to other African countries. The Frenkel method of production was used initially, utilizing bovine tongue epithelial tissues harvested at the Botswana Meat Commission abattoir at Lobatse. Additional tongue tissues were obtained from the Zimbabwe Cold Storage Commission abattoir in Bulawayo, Zimbabwe. Later BHK-21 suspension cells were introduced for vaccine production and currently the two methods are used according to need.

Initially, owing to the lack of secure facilities, it was not possible to test the vaccines produced at BVI on cattle in Gaborone and a small field laboratory at Motopi, northwestern Botswana, was used instead. Since the end of 1979, one batch out of every four produced has been subjected to a potency test in cattle and these tests are now carried out in high containment facilities at BVI, Gaborone.

One of the main responsibilities of BVI, in addition to the production of FMD vaccines specifically suited to the epidemiological situation of the countries in the region, is to study the different strains of FMD virus present in southern Africa and other parts of Africa. At the practical level, this has resulted in an increasing demand from neighbouring countries for the rapid diagnosis of suspected disease (Guinet *et al.*, 1982).

In 1985, during the 53rd General Session of OIE, BVI was designated as an RL for FMD in Africa.

Foot-and-Mouth Disease Centre, Pakchong, Thailand

The FMD centre at Nong Sarai, near Pakchong, in Nakhon Ratchasima Province, about 150 km northwest of Bangkok was established in 1958. It belongs to the Division of Veterinary Biologics of the Department of Livestock Development within the Ministry of Agriculture and Cooperatives. Early work, which was assisted by FAO and provided equipment and experts, concentrated on the isolation and identification of field strains of FMD virus. The laboratory developed the capability of producing vaccines in 1960 and this heralded the start of the FMD vaccination campaign in Thailand. Over the following three decades, and with technical and financial assistance provided by the Japanese and Australian governments, the facilities at Pakchong were considerably expanded.

REFERENCE LABORATORIES IN THE EUROPEAN COMMUNITY

As part of its policy for harmonizing the control of FMD in the European Community, as provided for in Directive 85/511/EEC, CEC decided that it would designate a community RL for FMD and a community coordinating institute for FMD vaccine.

Community Reference Laboratory for FMD

The Institute for Animal Health, Pirbright, was designated as the community RL for FMD by CEC in September 1989. Under

Articles 1 and 2 of a five-year contractual agreement, which came into effect on 1 April 1990, the agreed functions and duties are:

- To ensure liaison among the laboratories of the Member States with regard to the standards and methods of diagnosis of FMD and differential diagnosis, where necessary, in each Member State specifically by: i) receiving field samples from Member States and certain third countries with a view to determining their identity; ii) typing and full-strain characterization of FMD virus from the samples referred to in i) and communicating the results of such investigations without delay to the Commission and the Member State concerned; iii) building up and maintaining an up-to-date collection of FMD virus strains; iv) building up and maintaining a collection of specific sera against FMD virus strains;
- to support the functions of national laboratories, in particular by: i) storing and supplying to national laboratories cell lines for use in diagnosis, together with virus and / or inactivated antigens, standardized sera and other reference agents; ii) organizing and operating periodic comparative trials on FMD diagnosis at Community level and the transmission of the results of such trials to the Commission and the Member States;
- to provide information and carry out further training, in particular by: i) gathering data and information on the methods of diagnosis and differential diagnosis used and distributing such information to the Commission and the Member States; ii) making and implementing the necessary arrangements for the further training of experts in laboratory diagnosis with a view to harmonizing diagnostic techniques; iii) organizing an annual meeting where representatives of the national laboratories may review diagnostic techniques and the progress of coordination.

Under Article 3 of the contract it was agreed that:

- The RL shall operate according to recognized conditions of strict disease security as indicated in FAO, 1985.
- The RL shall formulate and recommend the disease security measures to be taken by the national laboratories in matters of FMD diagnosis, in accordance with the minimum standards referred to in the previous paragraph.

The community coordinating institute for FMD vaccine

The Central Veterinary Institute (CDI-DLO) at Lelystad, the Netherlands, was appointed as the community coordinating institute (CCI) for FMD vaccine by CEC in December 1992 and commenced its activities as a department within the CDI-DLO on 1 January 1993 under a renewable annual contract.

The functions and duties of the CCI are:

- to standardize the methods of control of FMD vaccines by national laboratories prior to authorization of vaccines by the competent authority of the Member State.
- to coordinate the control of FMD vaccine by national laboratories in each Member State specifically by: i) occasionally, or on request, receiving representative samples of batches of FMD vaccine intended for use in the Community including that produced in third countries (for use in the Community, in Community-supported vaccination campaigns or in animals intended for importation into the Community) and testing such vaccines for innocuity and potency; ii) carrying out comparative studies to ensure that innocuity and potency testing in each

Member State is of uniform methodology; iii) testing, by means of cross-immunity assays in live cattle, the efficacy of existing vaccines against important new field strains of FMD virus and communicating the results of such assays without delay to the Commission and the Member States; iv) gathering data and information on control procedures and vaccine tests and periodically transmitting such information to the Commission and Member States;

- to coordinate training and research among the various national laboratories by: i) making and implementing the necessary arrangements for the further training of experts in vaccine verification and testing with a view to harmonizing such techniques; ii) organizing an annual meeting where representatives of the national laboratories may review vaccine control and testing techniques and the progress of coordination;
- to operate according to recognized conditions of strict disease security as indicated in FAO, 1985;
- to formulate and recommend the disease security measures to be taken by the national laboratories in accordance with the standards already defined.

REFERENCE LABORATORIES AND THE QUALITY OF FMD VACCINES

The following activities of RLs have a bearing on the quality of FMD vaccines:

- *Antigenic suitability:* the antigenic characteristics of contemporary field strains of geographical relevance to the region must be constantly monitored by the RL so that advice can be given about the suitability and selection of strains already present or to be incorporated in vaccines. Suitable tests for this purpose include: virus neutralization; plaque reduction; mouse protection tests; and the liquid phase blocking enzyme-linked immunosorbent assay (ELISA) using bovine sera from a serum bank of vaccinated and revaccinated cattle. These procedures provide results from which an indirect prediction can be made of the protection likely to be conferred by selected vaccine strains against a field strain or strains and are especially appropriate in emergency situations. In the case of routine prophylactic vaccination campaigns, where speed is not so critical, the ultimate test is that of the cattle challenge. However, this has the disadvantages of high cost, greater disease security risk and the fact that it raises animal welfare considerations.
- *Independent testing of vaccines:* the RL should carry out independent and impartial quality testing of vaccines for use in different countries of the region, taking into consideration the prevailing epidemiological situations, to ensure that vaccines are suitable, potent and safe. To achieve these aims the RL should define the decision-making rules for the approval of vaccines and be capable of undertaking control assays including: vaccine production process control (antigen characterization and titration); antigenic payload (146S content) measurement (Barteling and Meloen, 1974); establishing the stability of the final emulsion; toxicity testing to ensure there are no adverse reactions in animals; and potency control tests in cattle. However, the latter are likely to be progressively replaced in the future by serological tests that demonstrate a good correlation between *in vitro* and *in vivo* results.
- *Innocuity testing:* these are essential to ensure that vaccines have been fully inactivated and are safe and sterile.

Recommended tests of innocuity include the inoculation of BHK-21 monolayer cultures (Anderson, Capstick and Mowat, 1970) and / or susceptible cattle.

- RLs should maintain stocks of reference virus strains and their antisera for supply to vaccine producers in the region.

MONITORING AND FINANCIAL SUPPORT OF REGIONAL LABORATORIES

The designation of a regional laboratory as an RL carries with it the obligation to undertake the duties and activities listed at the start of the chapter. This should be fully explained by international organizations and appreciated by candidate laboratories before they accept the designation. Furthermore, there must be a regular monitoring procedure to ensure that designated RLs are fulfilling their duties and satisfying the demands and expectations of the countries in the region.

Monitoring should be done on an annual basis through meetings of the relevant authorities of the countries of the region, by the provision of reports from the laboratories of their activities and through visits by groups of experts from international organizations (i.e. OIE, FAO, EU, PAHO / WHO).

Generally, the financial support of RLs is provided mainly by the host government and in part through specific programmes and projects. It is advisable that laboratories seeking to become designated or already performing reference work should accurately estimate the cost of these activities and request complementary funding from their usual sources or search for other sources to fulfil their needs. These other sources may include research contracts with central or local governmental agencies, international organizations and livestock associations.

Alternatively, a candidate RL may be able to persuade an international organization to meet the majority of its costs under a contractual arrangement. The advantage of the latter is that both parties should be fully aware in advance of their commitments and so both financial and technical programmes can be more effectively planned.

Note. While this chapter has been primarily concerned with describing the functions and activities of the five regional RLs involved in the control of FMD, it should be noted that, in support of FAO's Global Rinderpest Eradication Programme (GREP), there are now three regional laboratories that promote the control of the disease. Two of these are located in Africa (Senegal and Kenya) and the Pirbright Laboratory of the United Kingdom's Institute of Animal Health has recently been appointed as the FAO WRL for rinderpest. In addition, the Pan African Veterinary Vaccine Centre (PANVAC), Debre Zeit, Addis Ababa, Ethiopia, supports GREP by providing laboratory services to ensure that only vaccines of the appropriate quality and standard are used in the control campaigns currently under way in African countries.

BIBLIOGRAPHY

Anderson, E.C., Capstick, P.B. & Mowat, G.N. 1970. *In vitro* method for safety testing of foot-and-mouth disease vaccines. *J. Hyg., (Camb.)*, 68: 159-172.

Barteling, S.J. & Meloen, R.H. 1974. A simple method for the quantification of 140S particles of foot-and-mouth disease virus (FMDV). *Arch. gesamte Virusforsch.*, 45: 362-364.

Falconer, J., Mannathoko, M. & Guinet, J.J. 1982. Methods of control of foot-and-mouth disease in Botswana. *Ann. Virol. (Inst. Pasteur)*, 133: 151-155.

FAO. 1985. Minimum standards for laboratories working with foot-and-mouth disease virus *in vitro* and *in vivo*. *Report of the 26th Session of the European Commission for the Control of Foot-and-Mouth Disease,* Rome.

FAO. 1993. Security standards for FMD laboratories. *Report of the 30th Session of the European Commission for the Control of Foot-and-Mouth Disease,* p. 67-78. 27-30 April 1993, Rome.

FAO/OIE/WHO. 1995. *Animal Health Yearbook 1994.* Rome.

Ferris, N.P. & Donaldson, A.I. 1992. The World Reference Laboratory for Foot and Mouth Disease: a review of thirty-three years of activity (1958-1991). *Rev. sci. tech. Off. int. Epiz.,* 11: 657-684.

Guinet, J.J., Piroird, R., Falconer, J. & Fargeaud, D. 1982. Present results of serological and immunological studies of foot-and-mouth disease virus at the Botswana Vaccine Institute. *Rev. sci. tech. Off. int. Epiz.,* 1: 369-386.

Description and documentation of production and quality control of veterinary vaccines

S. Ullah and G. Blocks

The products produced by veterinary biological or pharmaceutical manufacturers ultimately affect human lives, so it is necessary that companies not only produce a good-quality product that is safe, pure and efficacious but prove adherence to the regulations and guidelines that ensure every step within the manufacturing process has been carefully planned, monitored, traced and accounted for. By ensuring compliance to regulations and guidelines through these methods, companies demonstrate their ability to control the manufacturing process.

Adherence to all requirements concerning the product and processes is evidenced through documentation, so it is apparent that the documentation system is one of the most critical and complex areas of compliance with current good manufacturing practices (GMPs).

Note: It may seem as though the information in this chapter is relevant only to the functioning of large, highly developed, multinational companies. It should be noted, however, that the emphasis on the stringent control of processes, the need for testing and the development of accurate and reliable documentation, demonstrates admirably the important principles involved in establishing effective systems for quality control and quality assurance in any biological production organization – no matter how small. The lessons of this chapter are therefore strongly recommended to all those involved in vaccine production including those in small production organizations such as government veterinary laboratories in developing countries.

The initial focus of this chapter will be the general principles and premises behind GMP and the establishment of baseline criteria for developing effective documentation systems within production and quality control.

Owing to the brevity of this chapter relative to the subject matter, methodologies should not be considered comprehensive but, rather, should provide key information that producers can utilize to initiate a successful documentation system.

GENERAL PRINCIPLES

In establishing manufacturing operations, many companies equate regulations with current good manufacturing practices – indeed, it is common within the pharmaceuticals and biologicals industry to use the terms interchangeably. While GMPs are incorporated into the regulations – and in some countries are regarded as the law – clarification of what is meant by GMP should be made.

Regulations are written parameters and methodologies established by a country's government that ensure (when adhered to) that the consumer will receive a safe, pure and efficacious product of high quality. Regulations are essentially the law and non-compliance can result in censure, fines or closure of businesses. Deliberate and wilful disregard for the law can in some instances result in fines or criminal charges being levied. (Countries may use titles incorporating the word regulations, guidelines, rules, etc. when describing regulations, for example the European

Union's (EU) GMP guideline is called a guideline but is enforced as regulations throughout the EU.)

Governments must oversee all aspects of industry, including such diverse companies as meat processing facilities, medicated feed plants, biotechnology, pharmaceutical and biological manufacturing, so regulations tend to be broad and parameters vague. This is deliberate on the part of governments to allow for latitude in the way companies can produce products while still adhering to the spirit of the law.

It is the interpretation of the regulations that is difficult for many companies to decipher, institute and apply. Indeed, incorrect interpretation is the most common cause for a company to be prosecuted for non-compliance. By stating what companies must do, yet not specifying exactly how they must do it, governments have allowed for the industrial growth of manufacturing while ingeniously providing a barometer against which to measure a company's true understanding of the pharmaceutical business and all applicable laws.

GMPs are the current guidelines practised by companies that have successfully interpreted, assimilated and applied the regulations and any additional addenda to these regulations. Because regulations from countries may vary in stringency, acceptable process methodologies and requirements, it should be noted that there is more than one method of achieving successful compliance and numerous options and methods for practising GMP exist.

The common barometer for measuring a company's regulatory success is contingent on one principle: the establishment, through documentation, of accountability, traceability, standardization, reliability and control of all operational elements that have an impact on the product. Successful application of this concept should ensure a comprehensive controlled manufacturing operation and accelerate a company's global marketability by requiring minimal adjustments to another country's compliance criteria.

Traceability tracks every item and every step in a process from its source (i.e. from an individual or a substance) as a raw material, to the provider of the source substance/equipment (the vendor or supplier), through manipulations at the manufacturing facility (the processes) and as it is sent to market (distribution). This information, in conjunction with appropriate assessment measures, provides the assurance that every aspect of the process has been evaluated, monitored and controlled.

Reliability (as evidenced through validation and other documentation) assures that equipment, processes and systems will consistently perform at high standard levels that ensure a safe, pure and efficacious product.

Standardization and reliability of procedures, testing methodologies and results are achieved when companies employ one set of standards and procedures to perform specific functions. By establishing uniform guidelines and providing written instructions that allow for the consistent performance of procedures there is a significant decrease in the number of variables that could adversely affect the product.

By tracking and accounting for every component and variable in the process, a documented history of a given batch or serial on a given day is provided and corroborated through batch records, bench records, logbooks and other supporting information.

Processes and corresponding documentation that can account for every phase of manufacturing that requires testing (and can anticipate and plan the establishment of contingency procedures for undesired variables such as manufacturing discrepancies, unplanned deviations, investigations and rejected batches) are indicative of controlled systems.

It is necessary that regulatory agencies, customers, the public at large and the manufacturing company be assured that every action has been taken to guarantee that the best possible product is manufactured. Without documentation to prove that the above measures were consistently met, the best possible product is vulnerable to negative conjecture, claims, lawsuits and postulation owing to a lack of proof to the contrary.

It can therefore be surmised that every company that enters into the highly regulated arena of industrial veterinary biological or pharmaceutical production has the responsibility for:

- adherence to all applicable government regulations;
- application of current GMPs on a daily basis;
- meeting the contractual and possible regulatory requirements of customers;
- producing every product under controlled conditions designed to ensure that the safety, purity, quality and efficacy of the product are consistently optimal;
- continually monitoring every process to ensure standardization and reliability of procedures, testing methodologies and results;
- providing evidence of compliance to the above through concurrent and thorough documentation.

In order to establish and maintain a documentation system that will address these concerns adequately, management must have a thorough understanding of the integrative aspect of the processes and systems within the industry.

DEFINITIONS

Accessibility. As it applies to documentation accessibility means the use of a location that allows for the retrievability of controlled documentation within a reasonable amount of time (usually 48 hours), yet restricts and controls the access of unauthorized persons to the area.

Accountability. Accountability allows for each process and every component or individual involved in the processes to be evaluated, analysed and continually gauged for negative or positive effects on the system and the resultant product. Once analysed this information can be used to improve the control of a given process or system.

Auxiliary documents. Forms, diagrams, charts, logs, schematics and attachments which help to document, track and facilitate the steps in a process may be included in the batch record or referenced and kept elsewhere.

Batch record. A working copy of a master batch record, the batch record is essentially the written diary of a specific batch. Batch records trace the documented manipulations of the components and raw materials once the production process begins. For guidelines concerning batch records see Developing the infrastructure for a documentation control system (p. 349).

Bench record. This term refers to laboratory records and can apply to the raw data or the documentation that has been transcribed from the raw data. The difference between batch records and bench records is that batch records give a history of a specific product or process on a given day while bench records document the results of laboratory testing. Because bench records are essentially a compilation of testing data, the information may not be in chronological order and the data presented must be correlated to protocols or pharmacopoeias to get the complete story. Well-written batch records tell a comprehensive story that incorporates the integration of many manufacturing processes. The production of biologicals involves numerous laboratory manipulations, so considerable skill must be used to convert the resulting bench record data into a batch record.

Cleaning feasibility studies. Tests are carried out to determine the effect of various cleansers (and methods of cleaning) on surfaces of different porosity, location and environmental conditions (e.g. the effects of heat, cold and light). Studies also help to determine the virucidal or bactericidal and fungicidal qualities of various disinfectants and the effectiveness of various solutions.

Control documents. Control documents are regulated documents that contain proprietary or confidential information concerning a company's processes, policies, ideas and methods. These documents are assigned unique identifying numbers which provide traceability and accountability for the records by allowing companies to establish and monitor who gets them and what version or revision of the document is the most current.

Controlled systems. The corresponding documentation of the integration of systems, processes and procedures, which can account for every phase of manufacturing and testing, becomes the control system. Controlled systems are challenged and validated prior to use to determine weaknesses. This allows potential problems to be anticipated and planned for in advance by providing for deviations, discrepancies, investigations and revisions.

Critical control point. A significant point in a process at which a pivotal decision is made, a critical control point affects (either directly or indirectly) the safety, purity and efficacy of the product.

Deviations. A planned or unplanned variation in a process that departs from the established steps of that process is a deviation. Planned deviations are tested and justified prior to implementation and should not affect the safety, purity, potency and efficacy of the product. Unplanned deviations are departures from the norm and should not affect the safety, purity and efficacy of the product. Companies often use the term "unplanned deviations" to describe manufacturing discrepancies.

Discrepancies. Unplanned variations in the process or procedure that could adversely affect the safety, purity, potency and efficacy of the product are referred to as discrepancies. It should be noted that, while deviations may or may not require investigation, discrepancies should always be investigated and the investigation should extend to other batches where the problem may have occurred. If it is decided after investigation to release a product affected by either unplanned deviations or discrepancies, a written scientific justification for that decision should be supplied with the product.

HEPA filters. High-efficiency particle adsorption (HEPA) filters are used to filter the air and to reduce the number of particles sized greater than 0.5 microns that enter a controlled environment. HEPA filters are used in conjunction with a manufacturing facility's air-conditioning system.

Investigation. A comprehensive and in-depth examination of the evidence elicited from reviewing the steps in a process, the investigation should be an objective, controlled exercise that focuses on root causes and provides information that can effectively resolve discrepancies within a process or system.

Justification. An objective, scientific rationale (based on the data and situation) that supports the proposed decision is referred to as a justification.

Logbooks. Collation of data which effectively track certain activities in a process, logbooks are essentially the diary of a process and should present information in chronological order.

Material transfer forms. A form that accompanies raw material, equipment, components or product from one location to another, the material transfer form identifies the item(s), the origin and destination of those item(s) and who is responsible for the movement. Completed material transfer forms are usually retained in a readily accessible, centralized area.

Procedures. Step-by-step instructions that delineate how to perform a specific function in a process, procedures should be concise, to the point and written at a level that the persons with the requisite educational/experience background can understand. Procedures do not have to include every step in the process but significant steps must be a part of the procedure.

Process. A combination of a series of procedures that, when performed in a specified sequence, accomplishes a significant result within a system is referred to as a process.

Regulated functions. Operations that have written parameters and methodologies specified by the government or other regulatory entity, regulated functions have a direct or indirect impact on the product to the extent that non-compliance could adversely affect its safety, purity and efficacy. The requirements of regulated functions are inferred and outlined by laws (regulations).

Stability programme. The stability programme is a programme designed to monitor and determine the effects of environmental or physical factors on a finished product over a period of time.

PRODUCTION PROCESSES

The manufacturing operation is the engine that drives a company. Essentially, all other departments exist as support systems to augment, support and justify the results generated by the production department.

It is a common fallacy that production's main function is simply to produce, while concerns for quality are the responsibility of support systems such as quality assurance, regulatory affairs and quality control. In reality, the largest burden of proof of regulatory compliance falls on the shoulders of production owing to the impact of integrative functions and processes between production and other departments.

To understand the concept of integration, the direct processes of production need to be defined and a description of the processes from other systems that impact on production needs to be given.

Direct processes of production

In order to address effectively the application of processes to production documentation systems it is important to focus on system components and the importance of systems integration.

All operations are composed of systems which can be broken down into a series of related processes. These processes require interaction between departments at various stages of their implementation and, because it is important to demonstrate control of an operation by documentation that shows the history and control of each process, it is necessary to decide on the key places where integration may occur – and to have records that demonstrate and support that decision.

The following production processes integrate with processes in other departments or systems although their key functions are the responsibility of production.

Receipt of raw material and components. Production receives raw material, such as the ingredients for the formulation of media, reagents and starting materials, and components, such as vials, ampoules and stoppers. These materials are received from another department (material management) through the generation of a bill of materials document.

The bill of materials lists the ingredients and components to be used in a certain process. This document is a part of the batch record and identifies items by stock or equipment identification control numbers.

Every movement of starter materials should be traceable, so documentation such as material transfer forms which identify the department transferring the material, the destination of material, the date of transfer, the reason for transfer and the person documenting this information, should be maintained.

Formulation or manipulation of starter materials. Materials used in production must usually be manipulated in some way prior to their use in the making of product. Manipulations can be divided into several functions.

Equipment such as fill line tubing, needle heads, fluid pumps, filter housings, surgical instrumentation (forceps, scissors, etc.), laboratory glassware, starter and final containers, must be cleaned and sterilized prior to use. The log records, sterilization charts and oven charts can be part of the initial batch record if the equipment will only be used in the production of one batch but, if the equipment is to be used for several products, such records should be stored separately and filed by "run" number and date of processing. In this instance, it will be important to reference which run date or number and which equipment was used on each batch record. This will help to facilitate finding the information during batch record review, investigations or an audit.

(Alternatively, when using the same equipment for several products, copies of the charts and other records can be incorporated into each product's batch record, as long as this is acceptable to government or contract regulations. When this method is used, the information describing where the original documentation is located should be referenced on every copy.)

Media must be prepared, filled and, whenever possible, sterilized.

Starter materials must be calculated and weighed and the amounts used and returned to storage should be documented (usually on the bill of materials).

The designation and identification of all components must be facilitated (e.g. the designation of fill tubing should be sent to the tissue culture production section and documentation for specific pathogen-free [SPF] eggs should go to the egg culturing section). This information is usually a part of the sterilization equipment run records and is supported by the page(s) of the batch record that require documentation of the specific equipment, components and ingredients used.

Information should be augmented by departmental logbooks which identify when material was manipulated (e.g. autoclaved, weighed and formulated) and on what piece of equipment and who performed the manipulations.

(Because of the correlation of batch

record information with logbooks and equipment, cleaning and media preparation records, it is critical that the correct information, such as equipment identification numbers, actual dates of preparation and dates transferred, be checked and verified for accuracy.

Examples of the types of discrepancy that can arise are given in The application of quality assurance to production and quality control systems (p. 354).

Preparation of the operation environment. Production is responsible for the cleaning, disinfecting and, when necessary, the fumigation of rooms used in production. In addition, the monitoring of air differentials, laminar airflow cabinets, clean rooms and HVAC systems is the responsibility of production. These activities will require the retention of logbooks and the logging of dates of cleaning and types of cleansers/ disinfectants used.

If cleansers require mixing or dilution prior to use this is usually described in a type of batch record or logsheet. Schedules that demonstrate the adequate rotation of cleansers (to decrease the likelihood of microbiological resistivity) as well as cleaning feasibility studies for various cleansers must be available.

Monitoring of operation environments. Using various plating techniques and air sampling equipment, the production department continually monitors the microbial flora and air particulate concentration for every room where production takes place. The results may be documented in the batch record or the information and where to find it can be referenced in the batch record while the actual data are stored separately.

Initial operations (production run). The preparation of cell systems (i.e. the opening of eggs, grinding of tissue, etc.), inoculation, media changes, harvesting, filtering, the addition of antimicrobial agents and incubations are all examples of initial production processes. The documentation required for these processes will consist of an initial batch record, a bulk product batch record or a defined section of a comprehensive batch record (when the material is to be used to make a single final product).

Intermediate operations. Intermediate operations include storage and corresponding environmental monitoring (i.e. monitoring of freezer temperatures), sampling (archive or reserve samples for bulk solution traceability) and thawing.

When the preferred method of producing batches involves the formulation of serials (the use of initial batch solutions to make more than one type of product) the initial batch record (bulk solution batch record) is linked to the target product final batch record and the intermediate or bulk solution is referenced in the final batch record.

The batch record for the bulk solution is kept as a separate record and references every product that the bulk solution was used in. The batch record system a company decides to use should be defined in the product licence and must be well thought out and coordinated, see Developing the infrastructure for a documentation system (p. 349).

Final operations (formulation and filling). The final stages of processing involve such processes as blending, the addition of other formulating ingredients such as stabilizers, adjuvant, preservatives, etc., filling, volume checks, lyophilization (if applicable), sealing, inspection, packaging and labelling. The records generated at these stages are the final batch record and should include the records for packaging and labelling.

Packaging and labelling. This stage involves the retrieval of product from an environmentally controlled storage area, the manipulation of that product in order to package and label it and the return of the product to quarantine storage pending release.

The movement of controlled product that by virtue of its composition needs a certain temperature environment requires the documented monitoring of temperature and of the time that the product is outside the controlled environment. The documented monitoring of the controlled environment (e.g. freezer or refrigerator) requires an established procedure and frequency.

In addition, parameters of the temperature at which the product can be stored should be specified and the temperature at which immediate action must be taken (the critical action level, which is based on a critical control point) should also be recorded.

At least three types of logs are indicated by the above information:

- the log or printout used to demonstrate periodic monitoring of the temperature of the controlled environment;
- the log that documents the movement of product into and out of the controlled environment;
- the documentation within the batch record of the times of the actual packaging and labelling operations. (This information is correlated to the log information that documents the time the product was taken out of and returned to the controlled environment.)

In addition, the time out of storage is correlated to the product outline and labelling information to ensure that the time it took to process the batch did not exceed that stipulated and therefore that the safety, purity, or efficacy of the product are not jeopardized.

THE INTEGRATION OF SYSTEMS AND DEPARTMENTS WITH PRODUCTION

The complex process of documenting production processes requires that companies be aware of the relationship of other departments to the actual manufacturing operations. In order to facilitate this awareness, background information is required concerning each system that has to be included in the process. Because each system is usually the purview of a specific department, the information has to be structured to indicate the department, provide some background information concerning the department's primary focus and describe briefly how production integrates with that particular department or system.

It should be noted that the information provided here is cursory and does not include the systems integration between every department but outlines the foci of documentation on the systems of manufacturing (production) and quality control and the impact of those systems that should integrate with them.

Regulatory affairs

In order to market a biological or drug product, specific information must be submitted to the regulatory agencies that govern the industry within the country concerned.

The information submitted should outline the specifics of the manufacturing process and will usually include:

- building location and design (blueprints and legends);
- equipment and services (utilities) specifications (validation data);
- a list of the types of products a facility expects to produce;
- the procedures by which the product will be produced (including manufacturing, testing and monitoring methodologies);
- research and development data

(including master seed origin, raw materials, etc.).

The regulatory affairs department works closely with the government on a continual basis and serves as a liaison between the company and the regulatory agencies. Functions usually associated with regulatory affairs are: submission of new drug information; interpretation of licences and regulatory contracts; submission of revised product data; interpretation and application of company policies versus government regulations; the writing and facilitating official responses to government audits and the review and determination of information to put on product inserts, master labels and packaging information.

The establishment of criteria for all areas of the business that have to do with administrative aspects of regulatory compliance is also the responsibility of regulatory affairs.

The regulatory affairs department is also responsible for determining the adequacy of processes, procedures, master batch records and testing criteria as they pertain to changes in submissions or government expectations, as well as for facilitation and expedition of market withdrawals, recalls, etc. (In some companies, some or all of these duties may be under the purview of the quality assurance unit.)

Integration of production with regulatory affairs. The documentation generated and submitted by regulatory affairs is utilized to create master batch records, standard operating procedures, quality control protocols and other documents. These documents must be reviewed and compared whenever there are revisions or amendments to ensure that any changes to processes, procedures, raw materials, building or equipment specifications, etc. do not contradict the original submitted documents.

It should be recognized that all regulatory documents are in a state of flux. This means that as regulations, procedures, raw materials or equipment change or are clarified, the documentation within each system will need to be reviewed, evaluated and possibly revised to reflect and support the change.

Production should establish a mechanism for continually notifying regulatory affairs of any changes to processes, procedures, equipment or raw materials. New submissions should be made and government approval obtained prior to the initiation of new processes.

In addition, before writing or revising procedures, changing significant steps in the master batch record, approving manufacturing deviations or otherwise altering existing techniques, the procedures and proposed changes should be compared with the actual product outline or product licence submission. Changes that go outside the parameters established in the product outline may require an amendment to the licence (and scientific justification) prior to the change.

Regulatory affairs should apprise production of all changes and amendments and of new interpretations of procedures. It is also recommended that prior to submissions of research and development data, production is apprised and actively participates in the development of the procedures and processes that are to be a part of the product licence.

Documentation generated by regulatory affairs and continually utilized by production includes: the product outline, information concerning labelling operations, changes to the outline and facility blueprints and legends.

Research and development

Research and development (R&D) has considerable impact on the everyday operations of production. It is important to recognize the function of R&D and to incorporate that function with the actual production process.

R&D is responsible for developing ideas into products, for example, beginning with an isolated viral strain, R&D works to develop seed that is potent, yet has minimal adverse reactive characteristics. Using feasibility studies in conjunction with seed manipulations (passages) an optimum seed preparation is developed (the master seed) and R&D must then work to build up a master seed bank that will sustain production of the product for a specified period.

The integration of R&D with production. R&D is responsible for testing and ensuring the feasibility of product use and must develop the processes used to manufacture the product. Consideration must therefore be given to the following factors:

- feasibility of the potential product as a viable vaccine that will incorporate sufficient viral activity with minimal adverse reactivity;
- reproducibility of experimental bench activity in the "real world" (i.e. in the manufacturing process);
- testing and evaluation of excipient and other raw material in conjunction with the biological component (i.e. testing for compatibility and stability);
- testing and evaluation of the packaging (composition of vials and stoppers, labelling requirements, etc.) to establish baseline criteria for compatibility and stability testing data;
- evaluation of the effects of heat, cold, light, agitation and other environmental variables on the stability of the biological component;
- development of the manufacturing and test methodologies that will be used in the actual processes.

It should be recognized that, although R&D is responsible for developing the methods of producing and testing products, the real proving ground for the success and feasibility of R&D manipulations takes place in production.

Many ideas work well in R&D laboratories where creativity, quick adjustments and manipulations using state-of-the-art equipment may be the norm and can occur throughout the evaluation process. Current GMP requirements are applied rather loosely (if at all) during the initial stages of research to allow for all avenues to be explored and such latitude is not usually allowed during actual manufacturing. Owing to the complex, stringent control mechanisms and to the recognition that production equipment is often idiosyncratic after years of use and wear, such variables as process or ingredient adjustments can only be made after serious consideration and must undergo thorough, prescribed and controlled testing. Production using methods that still need adjustments to the actual process is usually restricted or totally prohibited.

The testing methodologies developed in R&D must be reproducible on a large scale and should incorporate and reflect the methodologies that the quality control unit will actually utilize. New methodologies that cannot be referenced to manuals or pharmacopoeias usually require the approval of government testing agencies prior to use in actual production.

For successful conversion of a production process from a laboratory to a manufacturing environment the following guidelines should be utilized:

- Apprise production of the progress of products that have been approved. Visit the production site and find out the actual methodologies and equipment that are being used.
- It is far easier to assimilate a new product that uses existing methodologies than it is to create or revise a process, every effort should therefore be made to simulate the conditions,

equipment, processes and procedures that production uses. This should minimize the number of alterations a production process requires when it is transferred to the manufacturing environment.

- The validation of processes must be performed on the actual equipment that will be producing the product. This is especially critical for formulation and lyophilization processes where idiosyncrasies of equipment, utility requirements and even the availability of specific raw ingredients could compromise all of the hard work of regulatory affairs and R&D.
- It is important to recognize the importance of validation and to ensure that process validation is complete before writing final versions of the standard operating procedures (SOPs) for that process. The information gathered during the testing and challenging of the process will help to determine the critical control points and the types of SOPs that will need to be written. In addition, SOPs that compensate for the weaknesses of a process can be developed after those weaknesses have been determined during validation.
- Idiosyncrasies of equipment and processes are not only the characteristics of different manufacturers; the wear and tear from normal production use can change such diverse critical aspects as door seal integrity (and therefore the vacuum), sensor or thermocouple capabilities (for lyophilizers) or fill lines or needles for filling machines. Companies should be aware that reproducing the results with similar equipment from the same manufacturer using the same ingredients may not be acceptable for validation or product submissions – only the actual equipment used, with the actual procedures followed, can be used for such purposes.
- R&D should be aware of the manufacturing and regulatory restrictions of production. It is important to incorporate the GMP requirements of manufacturing operations in the training of the staff of support systems that are integrated with the production department.
- R&D should be apprised of the process validation requirements in enough detail to enable informed decisions to be made about developing processes or manipulations.
- The performance of pilot batches should be facilitated by R&D but production personnel should perform all the manufacturing manipulations.

Incorporating these guidelines should help to ensure that the success of the R&D department's efforts is not delayed during actual production.

The documentation that is generated by the R&D programme includes the results and evaluation data of feasibility studies, initial stability data, bench records and pilot batch data.

Quality control

In many companies, the functions of quality control (QC) and quality assurance (QA) are combined and the unit that provides testing is also the unit that determines the appropriateness of a batch for release. In addition, regulatory guidelines do not always provide an accurate distinction between the two quality units; however, owing to the types of responsibilities given to each unit, a distinction is inferred and, whenever possible, should be defined.

QC is essentially the support system for production which performs the sampling and testing of raw materials, bulk, intermediate and final product. QC also helps to facilitate or augment any analytical laboratory testing such as sterility testing of formulation vessels, validation of tests (as required for the production processes) and monitoring of the stability programme. Because most guidelines specify that the evaluation and analysis of all manufacturing processes must take place prior to the release of the product and that such an evaluation must be performed by an independent unit not directly answerable to or influenced by production, it will be readily apparent that the QC unit (which is used to augment and test elements of the production process) should not be responsible for reviewing data performed and generated within its own department. It could not, therefore, fulfil the requirements of an independent unit.

QC utilizes controlled, standardized methodologies to test ingredients at various stages of the production process. Information, such as formulas for calculations and test procedures, is usually defined in pharmacopoeias.

If possible, the QA unit should be considered a separate department from QC.

Integration of production with QC. Most QC interactions with production involve testing at various stages of the production process and it is very important that there is continuing communication between production and QC. Changes in production caused by scale up or changes of equipment, mixing methods, ingredients, etc. can affect the application of antibiotics, pH requirements etc. during the production process and therefore have an impact on the success of QC testing. Production should apprise QC of any changes in the manufacturing process that could have ramifications on the testing of the product.

The documentation generated by QC consists of the testing records (also referred to as bench records, QC protocols, etc.); for additional information concerning QC see The role of quality control (p. 347).

Materials management

The initial integration of records which signifies the beginning of a production run involves the scheduling, receipt, storage and transfer of materials. The documentation of these actions has a significant impact on the records generated by production.

Materials management may also be referred to as distribution, logistics or production management and is responsible for the receipt, storage, inventory and distribution of raw materials as well as the scheduling of production runs and the distribution of the final product. Owing to GMP requirements, materials management is also responsible for the traceability and accountability of all raw material and components as well as for the maintenance of adequate inventory levels.

These responsibilities require the tracking and reconciliation of all materials used in the production process, together with a continual monitoring of the inventory to ensure the rotation of stock and that the oldest product in stock is utilized first. Materials management should also work in conjunction with QC to ensure that incoming shipments of raw material are adequately sampled and tested prior to their release to production.

The records maintained by materials management include: inventory cards; manufacturer, vendor and supplier lists; production schedules and logistical data; environmental monitoring logbooks for the recording of storage temperatures; material transfer forms; customer return documentation; and distribution records.

Integration of materials management with production. Production should work closely with the materials management team to ensure that production deadlines, back order issues and other logistical information is adequately recorded and passed on. Providing accurate information concerning raw material usage, the amount of material scrapped (rejected) and reprocessed, the tracking of material and the manipulations performed with material, is vital to establishing an efficient and controlled materials management process.

Production should establish processes that allow for the traceability and accountability of product usage and manipulations. This generally entails having records of when material was used, the process and/or equipment it was used with, the amount of material used, the amount (if any) returned to inventory, the lot numbers used, the date and the signature of the person performing the task(s).

Material transfer forms should be filled out accurately and should accompany any material that is to be handled in several departments.

Allowances should be made in production schedules for maintenance, environmental monitoring, R&D and validation test runs. In planning production runs, production must also consider the requirements of in-process testing and sampling of raw materials and any assays or tests that may be required prior to use of the raw material. Failure to comply with these considerations may lead to failure of the product at the final QC stage.

Examples of the documentation generated by materials management and utilized by production are: material transfer forms, bill of material data, vendor/supplier information and schedules.

Quality assurance

A successful QA programme involves the routine interaction of the QA unit with production (and with all other regulated departments) which allows the QA department to appraise operations continually and to ensure that there is communication and implementation among all integrating departments. Owing to the dynamics of manufacturing products, the timely communication of changes and amendments is extremely important to the production process.

The QA function involves the interpretation of government regulations as they apply to everyday operations and should encompass the monitoring of all regulated departments. The data generated from monitoring is collated and evaluated to determine whether patterns or trends exist. Trends are usually key indicators that a system or process may need revalidation, adjustment or possible SOP revisions.

The functions that may be incorporated under the title of QA are:

- *document control* which involves the creation of the master batch record and coordination and issuance of the production batch record and SOPs;
- *line inspection teams* which inspect line clearances and examples of the product while it is being produced (e.g. check the fill volumes and labels);
- *labelling control* which controls and tracks the dispensing of labels, inserts and cartons that contain prescriptive information;
- an *investigatory and auditing unit* which facilitates investigations of manufacturing deviations and discrepancies, monitors all regulated processes, advises on projects that require a knowledgeable view of integration of systems, performs pharmaco-vigilance and evaluates trends of adverse reactions and their subsequent impact on processes and products;
- a *GMP trainer* who facilitates the training of personnel in regulations and the practical applications of GMP – the GMP trainer may also fulfil another function within QA;
- a *validation team* which facilitates the testing and challenging of equipment and processes to ensure reliability and determine the contingencies or support

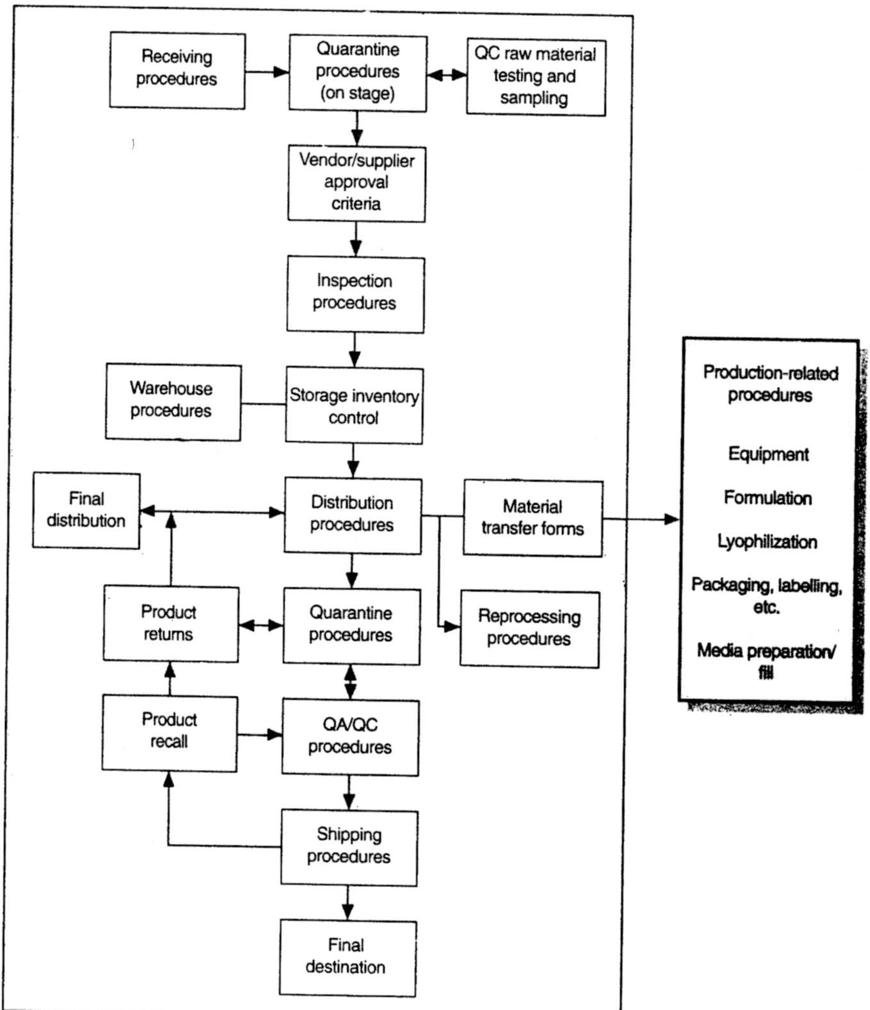

FIGURE 14

Flowchart showing production method, procedures and processes involved in material management

processes that are needed to augment a system – this includes data that will be incorporated into SOPs, tolerance parameters and maintenance programmes.

The types of documentation generated by QA include: audit reports,trend analysis data, annual product reviews, validations, evaluation and feasibility studies and release data.

The primary role of QA is to monitor continually and evaluate the application of GMP to processes and systems by utilizing audits, trend analysis, studies, etc. All regulated departments and departments that support regulated functions integrate with the QA unit and, in addition, QA performs self-assessments and evaluations.

Integration of production with QA. Companies that are proactive are discovering the advantages to having a supportive QA unit. When implemented correctly, QA works in conjunction with production to troubleshoot, investigate and solve manufacturing problems and issues. Realistic goals and empathetic attitudes are required of both departments to ensure that evaluations and corrective actions address the control of processes and systems. The following are guidelines for successful interactions between QA and production:

- Production should consult QA before implementating any revisions to processes, equipment or procedures. Owing to the comprehensive vantage point of QA, the impact of production decisions on all departments can be considered and anticipated. This will help to minimize the corrections, reworkings and other discrepancies that occur when all the ramifications have not been considered.
- QA should ensure that the present working conditions, standards and practices are considered when addressing corrective action criteria. The implementation of quality need not be expensive or time-consuming. The onus is on QA to learn the variables and factors within production and to tailor a solution that incorporates the present operation conditions with a feasible interpretation of the regulations.
- The key to successful interaction is open communication. It is beneficial for both departments to participate in departmental GMP training that provides insights into the function, responsibilities, purpose and limitations of the respective departments.

Engineering and maintenance

Together with QC, engineering and maintenance works daily with the installed processes to ensure the reliability, functionality and control of all equipment, services and processes.

The engineering and maintenance department serves as the technical support system for the facility, all equipment and services (utilities) and production. Changes or modifications of the building, services, equipment or engineering programmes should require the involvement of engineering, production, QA and regulatory affairs prior to implementation. Significant changes could affect the integrity of the manufacturing process so it is important to justify and validate all changes.

Integration of engineering and maintenance with production. Production should work closely with the engineering department to establish preventive maintenance and calibration schedules, discuss forthcoming upgrades of the facility and/or equipment and establish guidelines for the facilitation of validation protocols.

The types of documentation generated by production in conjunction with engi-

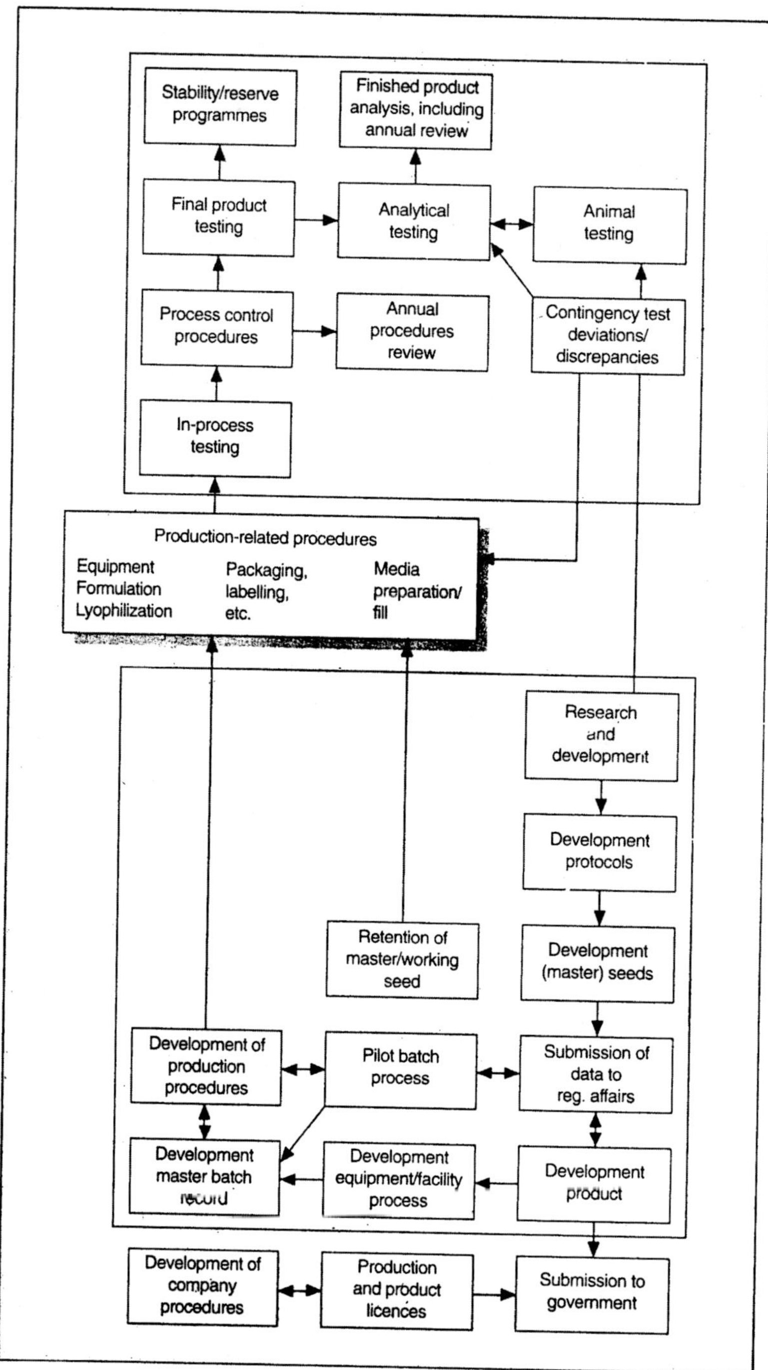

FIGURE 15
Flowchart showing production method, procedures and processes for product development and quality control

neering and maintenance are: equipment history files, maintenance and calibration schedules, manufacturer or supplier information, validation records (if not retained by a separate validation team), filter change records and equipment repair work orders.

Documentation control

Owing to the complexity of pharmaceutical and biological processes, companies have a tendency to departmentalize tasks when designing the documentation system, which results in a fragmented system that must be continually monitored, amended, revised and augmented. To remedy this situation, it is necessary to understand the flow of operations prior to establishing or revising a documentation system. Documentation exists and is mandatory for every regulated system within the manufacturing facility; therefore consideration of the facility, product, processes and systems should be paramount.

Documentation control essentially involves the dissemination of master batch records, SOPs and other forms that serve to corroborate production processes. Charts delineating regulated systems, the flow of operations and the key components of documentation are given in Figures 14, 15 and 16.

Integration of production with the documentation control system. The master batch record and SOPs are often perceived as the main components of the production documentation system, leading to the emphasis usually being placed on developing these formats instead of developing a comprehensive system.

A common error which occurs within the industry (and which creates considerable confusion and discrepancies) is to allow different departments to develop their own SOPs, including procedure formats, control numbering systems and methodologies, independently of an overall company plan. This often results in a myriad of formats, numbering systems, logs and procedural steps being developed even when all departments are performing the same or similar tasks. Because streamlining procedures reduces the amount of paperwork, contributes to the standardization of operations and increases manufacturing productivity, production should write multifunctional SOPs wherever possible (see Developing the infrastructure for a documentation control system on p. 349).

Another key area in documentation control is the process for revising existing documents. Revision of existing documents generally requires a review of the product outlines to ensure that new information or proposed procedures are not in conflict with the original submissions. Product outlines are regulated documents containing proprietary information. This means that they should be managed under a controlled system that designates specific numbers for each document and tracks the whereabouts of all copies of the product outlines including the current version.

Steps should be taken to ensure that the revising and amending of existing documents occur in a controlled manner and that the personnel in all integrative systems are aware of the impending changes and are prepared to modify their records accordingly. This is generally performed through a change control procedure. Production should also ensure that all changes that occur are reflected in the SOPs and that new copies are distributed to each department and obsolete copies are retrieved and destroyed. It is largely through the coordination efforts of the documentation control department that records are adequately maintained.

Companies that do not have the resources for a separate documentation

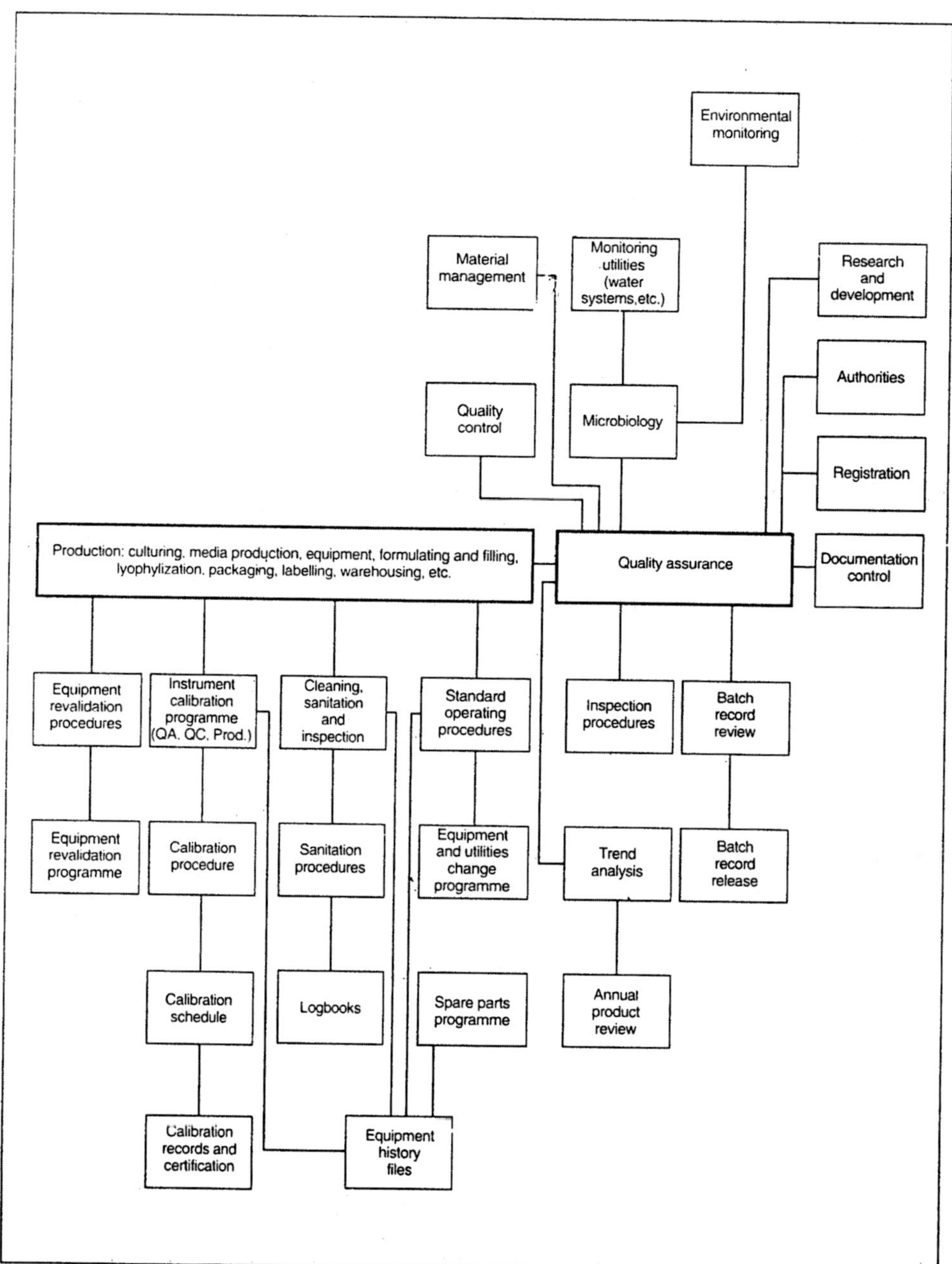

FIGURE 16
Flowchart showing quality assurance-related procedures

control unit (which is usually a component of the QA department) may integrate these functions with another department.

Although it is beneficial to assimilate the documentation control concept throughout the company, dividing document control responsibilities among various departments is not recommended. A centralized, secure area for the retention of batch records, production outlines, protocols, etc. should be utilized. Access should be limited to authorized personnel only and careful monitoring and logging of the batch records removed from the area should be performed.

The types of documentation generated and maintained by the documentation control department include: the master batch record log, the master SOP tracking log, the batch record issuance log, the form tracking log, the master company signature list and the master control records (batch records, SOPs).

Purchasing

Although purchasing is usually not considered a regulated department, the purchasing department does make decisions that can have a critical impact on production and ramifications on regulation.

Specific ingredients and processes are defined in the product outline, so it is very important that the company's purchasing department is aware of the production criteria prior to contracting with vendors. Owing to the technical nature of this information, it is recommended that the personnel involved be experienced in the processes, ingredients and component composition and that an evaluation of vendors' manufacturing and QC processes, as well as pricing factors, be considered before selecting a supplier. Purchasing personnel should also be made aware of all pertinent regulatory requirements that could affect the criteria for ordering certain products, services or equipment.

Integration of purchasing with production. In procuring equipment, products and services for a regulated industry, purchasing personnel need to be aware of the regulatory impact of their decisions. All too often, purchasing departments obtain deals for the company, only to have the money and effort saved nullified by the costs of regulatory redress.

Staff from purchasing, QA, production and engineering and maintenance should confer whenever major equipment purchases or changes in existing services need to be made. It is often required that company personnel audit the site and evaluate the suitability of a specific supplier. Purchasing personnel should undergo auditor's training or be accompanied by the company's in-house auditor whenever a new vendor is to be assessed.

Ideally, the persons responsible for procuring goods and services for production should undergo GMP and advanced technical training. Personnel should have an understanding of the ramifications of choosing certain kinds of flooring, duct work, irradiation services, etc.

The types of documentation that are generated by purchasing and that have an impact on production are: purchase orders, evaluation of vendors (vendor/supplier approval programmes), documentation of the continual monitoring of vendors and the establishment (if feasible) of a vendor/supplier certification programme.

Packaging and labelling

Information is constantly being revised, updated and clarified, so it is critical that there is an open dialogue among regulatory affairs, production and labelling control. The instructions provided on labels, inserts and cartons must reflect the same instructions submitted to the government and procedures for the facilitation of this dialogue should be written and followed.

Packaging and labelling are the production processes that are usually initiated after product testing is complete and the results of all tests have been found acceptable. The operations involved are: removal of the final product from quarantine storage, clearing away evidence of other labelling operations from the production lines, visual inspection of the vials, continual monitoring of the packaging and labelling lines and the actual process of packaging and labelling.

Key aspects of this process are the receipt, sampling, inspection, storage and dispensing of labels, inserts and cartons (these are usually functions of a division of the QA unit in conjunction with regulatory affairs).

Integration of production with packaging and labelling. On receipt of labels from labelling control, it is imperative that the production department, and all support systems, participate in the control and monitoring of the labelling operation. The procedures to be defined and followed should include: proofing or review of labels; disposal of obsolete old labels; and effective retrieval, reconciliation and destruction of defective labels. The personnel in packaging are in the position of inspecting the product and labels for extended periods of time, so it is beneficial for them to be aware of information concerning specific product parameters (such as temperature or light exposure restrictions, label and cap coloration).

In addition, each department that integrates with another assumes some of the responsibility for evaluation and criticism at the point of integration. This includes not only the labelling, but also the review of line status signage (identification of the type of product and batch number to be labelled and the phase in the process that is being performed – start-up line clearance, tear-down or changing of the line information), the expiry date, reconciliation records, etc.

It is important that key activities (such as line clearances to ensure that all labels from previous runs are removed and that no evidence of the previous run exists) are performed, verified and documented.

It is also of key importance that labels be accounted for and that a limit for label reconciliation discrepancies (how many can be unaccounted for without requiring an investigation) be established and followed. There should be investigations of all discrepancies that surpass the discrepancy threshold.

Microbiology

When a company can afford the implementation of a separate unit to perform environmental monitoring (in this instance, environmental monitoring refers to particulate and environmental flora sampling), the testing and plating of personnel and production areas and the testing for pyrogenicity, cleaning validation studies, etc., it is beneficial to have a separate microbiology department.

A testing department separate from QC allows routine production tests to be performed by one department (QC) while the other department monitors auxiliary factors that have an impact on the production process.

The microbiology department is usually concerned with the monitoring and culturing of production process components such as water systems, the evaluation of gown sterilization techniques, the testing of sterility and pyrogenicity, the manufacture and testing of various culture media (used to culture bacteria, mycological and parasitic organisms) and the evaluation of microbiological testing results.

Integration of production with the microbiology department. The microbiology department provides periodic monitoring of all production environments (including the environmental hoods used in QC), establishes criteria for the periodic testing and culturing of clean room and laboratory environments, tests filters (including HEPA filters), undertakes tests of personnel gowning techniques and subsequently cultures all samples taken. The department must schedule the testing and evaluation of test data in such a way that a minimal time elapses between materials/environments being sampled, cultured and evaluated and materials being used. This reduces the likelihood that sampled material could be used in other products or processes prior to the results of the initial culturing being available.

Where the resources of a company do not provide for a separate microbiology department, these responsibilities may be divided between QC and production.

The types of documentation generated within this microbiology include: culturing protocols, bench record information, data and evaluation of personnel gowning and room environmental results. These types of data are considered auxiliary and are usually retained within the microbiology department. Specific information, such as the results of settling plates used during a production run, can be referenced in the batch record.

THE ROLE OF QUALITY CONTROL

The QC unit is generally responsible for all of the sampling and testing of ingredients, components, reagents and raw or starting materials. The test phases include initial sampling and testing of raw materials, in-process testing, the testing of intermediate bulk materials, animal testing and final product testing.

QC must also test for anomalies, perform periodic reassays of reagents and participate in testing involved in investigations and manufacturing discrepancies. The general instructions for tests are outlined either in a country's regulatory guidelines or in pharmacopoeias; but, in cases where more than one test methodology is listed, QC must ensure that the procedures used are the same as the procedures written in the product outline.

QC should also ensure that all raw materials and components are identical to the list provided to the government in the outline. When changes in either procedures or ingredients are indicated, regulatory affairs should be notified prior to implementation.

QC data are usually presented in the form of bench records which provide the results from tests and should include the formulae used and the type of test performed, as well as referencing the established test methodology. The procedures utilized should also be referenced along with all other pertinent data (the age of the animals being tested, product outline parameters, etc.).

Other types of documentation generated by QC are: raw material assays, QC sampling logs, stability programme data, certificates of analysis, equipment QC, laboratory instrumentation calibration programme, logbooks and scheduling of the animal-handling facility and the supporting documentation.

As with production, the QC unit involves specific interactions and communications with other departments. The departments that integrate with QC are: R&D, regulatory affairs, materials management, engineering and maintenance and QA.

R&D and regulatory affairs

The test methodologies invented or designed by R&D must be incorporated into a format that can be utilized by a controlled laboratory. The latitude allowed within R&D is usually not permissible within QC. Most countries have established specific methodologies for the testing, assaying and evaluation of test manipulations. In addition, companies that export must also incorporate or augment their country's testing requirements with the explicit methodologies mandated by their customer.

The stability programme (which may be initiated by R&D but is maintained by QC) is a mechanism that monitors the effects of such elements as time, preservatives, heat, light, vial/stopper composition and temperature on the product.

Initially, R&D may perform an abbreviated version of this programme to determine the selection of vials, stoppers, raw materials, etc. on the viability of the product. This information is critical in creating an expiry date, storage temperatures and product ingredients. The QC unit utilizes this information to establish the parameters for monitoring the product.

The ongoing product/component interaction should be monitored constantly to determine if certain factors such as container or stopper composition, preservatives, heat and light react adversely with the product over time. This is the main premise for establishing a stability programme. Since the data produced could affect the product's expiry date, ingredients or components, QC should continually update the regulatory affairs department and alert it to any data that arise on the questionable stability status of a product.

Materials management

One of the responsibilities of the QC unit is to ensure the quality of all components used to make a product, so QC must perform in-process sampling and testing of raw materials and components. This involves establishing sampling programmes that specify the amount of each product to be sampled and the acceptable quality level (AQL) that must be achieved on inspection.

The AQL for vials, for example, would require establishing the type of glass, the colour, size and shape of each vial. Another element could be whether the imperfections identified are classified as critical, major or minor, and how many of each kind of imperfection could be allowed within the vial and within each sample size.

QC personnel usually have a designated space within the materials management area to sample each shipment. Using good lighting and such tools as callipers, tape measures and spatulas various items are sampled and the results are documented.

Suppliers often furnish certificates of analysis which may describe the tests done by the supplier and the results. It is suggested that certificates from other companies be augmented with parallel sampling and testing until a degree of confidence can be developed. This includes the periodic assay or testing of various raw materials (including reagents) to determine testing characteristics and to provide baseline data from which to establish supplier approval criteria.

Companies should remember to establish a programme for the reassay of reagents and ingredients that are retained for a period of one year or more.

Engineering and maintenance

One of the responsibilities of QC is to monitor the water systems of the company (if this is not performed by a separate microbiology unit), so it is important that QC be apprised of any impending changes to service systems or existing drains and of any remodelling of the facility. In addition, engineering and maintenance must perform or assist in the calibration and validation of the various instruments in the QC laboratory.

The majority of instruments in the laboratory will require a schedule of monthly, quarterly, biannual or annual calibration. Reagents and controls generally have built-in QC measures that require the testing or challenging of the control prior to use.

Quality assurance

The QA unit is responsible for the review of all QC data prior to release of the final product. QA monitors QC to ensure adherence to all applicable standards and test methodologies.

DEVELOPING THE INFRASTRUCTURE FOR A DOCUMENTATION CONTROL SYSTEM

Storage

Documents should be stored in a secure location with limited access. In order to facilitate documentation reviews such as annual product reviews, trend analyses, SOP revisions, evaluations of master batch records, lyophilization cycles, etc., it is essential to maintain various types of documentation in centralized locations.

The centralization of processes and documents allows the number of system variables and personnel involved to be more effectively controlled. A system that is accessible to several departments is vulnerable to the vagaries of departmental interpretation.

The following are recommendations for the storage of records and other documents:

- Provision should be made to ensure the storage of controlled records for a specified period of time.
- Records should be stored in a safe, secure area and efforts should be made to minimize the damage that could be caused by environmental factors such as humidity and water.
- Records should be stored in an area where they are easily retrievable and should either be located at the site where the activities described took place or should be readily accessible to authorized inspecting personnel.
- Procedures should be established for the storage and retention of records and should include the methods of storage used and the steps necessary to retrieve information.
- Procedures should exist for the revising, correcting, tracking and destruction of all controlled documentation.
- In order to facilitate storage requirements, a log should be retained delineating the numbers of controlled documents, who has copies of these documents, when they were distributed and when obsolete copies were returned.
- A procedure should exist for the archiving of records. Consideration should be given to storage periods, the types of records that should be retained, how records should be packaged for storage and who has authorization to store and retrieve archived information.

Development of master documents

Master documents are the original permanent copies of documents from which authorized working copies are made. The purpose of master documents is to have an official copy that contains the original information of the process and, when combined with copies of all of the retired (obsolete) master documents, they chronicle the information necessary for the formulation of a specific product, procedure or process.

There should be only one set of master documents. Appropriate identification of this set can be made by virtue of the original signatures, by its being printed on controlled, specially designed or coloured paper (possibly paper with a watermark or of a special restricted colour or company letterhead paper) or by its being stamped with an authorized red stamp. The key is to have some identifying characteristic that makes it possible to distinguish a master from a copy. Accessibility to the identifying characteristic (coloured or letterhead paper, for example) should be restricted.

Among the master documents are the SOPs, which are step-by-step instructions used to perform a specific function in a process. Procedures should be clear, concise and to the point. Text should be written in language that persons with the requisite education and experience can understand.

For a procedure to be effectively described there are key elements that must be present in the document format. The following information may be written as a cover sheet or in the form of a header/footer on the first page of the document:

- *SOP title:* a descriptive title of the function to be performed;
- *procedure number:* a sequential control number assigned to the procedure;
- *departmental category:* the department to which the procedure applies;
- *page number:* each page must be numbered;
- *effective date:* the date the procedure is to be officially used is typed in here. This date must be after the date of the final signature;
- *approval signatures:* appear in the blocked section and should be handwritten;
- *written by:* the signature of the person who wrote the SOP.

Packaging/labelling. Because information is constantly being revised, updated and clarified, it is critical that an open dialogue exists among regulatory affairs, production and labelling control. The instructions provided on labels, inserts and cartons must reflect the same instructions submitted to the government. Procedures for the facilitation of this dialogue should be written and followed.

The persons responsible for reviewing and approving an SOP should have a background commensurate with the subject matter they are reviewing. It is the responsibility of all signees to have a working knowledge of the subject matter and to evaluate the document in the light of their area of expertise.

The approval of production SOPs usually involves the departmental supervisor or head, the production manager, regulatory affairs and QA. (In companies where QA functions as the regulatory liaison, it may not be necessary to have the signature of the head of regulatory affairs.)

The following information should also be contained in the SOP:

- *objective:* explaining the main purpose of the procedure and defining whether the purpose is to outline the method of operation, maintenance, etc.;
- *scope:* the exact limitations of the procedure, which define the targeted elements. The procedure may be directed towards a function, a piece of equipment, a certain process, etc.;
- *responsibility:* direct responsibility should be assigned to an individual title or group, to ensure that the procedure is enforced;
- *procedure:* step-by-step directions written in wording that the person performing the task can understand;
- *review and retention:* a statement regarding the date for regular review (review of procedures should take place at least once a year) – the process for revising documents and making them obsolete may be written on each cover sheet if desired.

SOPs should pertain to specific equipment or processes. When SOPs describe the functions of a larger process, it is suggested that the last step or a reference section direct readers to the next SOP. (If a company does not have an SOP coordinator or a documentation control unit, leading references to the next SOP should be avoided.)

Any numerical values written in the SOP should have tolerance parameters whenever possible. Parameters should be realistic and, wherever possible, be broad enough to allow moderate process fluctuations. Numerical values that indicate the specific actions to be performed must be linked to documents that allow the verification of that action.

It is important to remember that the master batch record will contain abbreviated information from SOPs that specifies the significant steps. For example, a record specifying that a certain step must be verified must provide a logbook, a batch record or some other document that, when filled out, indicates that the verification took place. Information that has incorporated numerical fluctuation (i.e. tolerance) is represented as in the following example: the temperature 37°C ± 5°C means the allowable temperature range for that product is 32°C to 42°C. This means that a product found within that range is acceptable for use.

In devising tolerance ranges for processes, the data to justify ranges should be provided within the product outline.

Documents that specify time parameters must be linked to documents that allow verification of that information, for example: "Agitate the liquid for five minutes ± one minute".

There should be a logsheet or batch record providing the following information: the times the agitation began and ended; who it was performed by, with the date; and who it was verified by, with the date.

All SOPs should follow the parameters and specifications of the product outline.

All reviews of revised SOPs should incorporate a correlation of the current version of the document (if it is a revision) and the product outline.

The routing of SOPs and SOP revisions should be documented on an SOP master log.

Development of historical records

Historical records are the working batch records. The master batch record is a blank format that has been designed with specific instructions to produce a specific product of a specific size, potency, etc. The batch record is essentially the diary of all of the processes and procedures performed on a given day to produce a specific product. In a manual system, this will be the document that actual performance information is recorded on.

Batch record. A batch record is basically an abbreviated form of a process SOP that, when filled out, becomes the diary for a specific lot of a product made on a particular day.

Batch records are derived from master batch records and are authorized copies of the master document.

The following information pertains to master batch and working batch records:

- The formulation information and the equations used for scale up should be written under the guidance of regulatory affairs, R&D and the department(s) involved in scale up.
- All equations and significant steps pertaining to the production of a batch should be described.
- Master documents are always printed on official company paper. (Working batch records are copies of the master.)
- The standard type of documentation to be found in a batch record includes: the name of the product; the product registration or drug code number and the lot number of the initial product (or the raw material lot numbers)
- A bill of materials page should describe the materials and ingredients to be used and the quantity requested, with space provided in which the quantities used and returned to inventory (i.e. stores) can be documented. An example of a bill of materials record is as follows:

Product code	Material	Raw material (No.)	Expiry date	Quantity required	Quantity used	Quantity returned	Operator's initials	Date
6215400	6mm West 4880 grey stoppers, siliconized	540STPRS	6 July 1998	7 500				
7348221	20-cc type II clear flint glass vials	321GLSCC	6 July 1998	7 500				

- Original auxiliary records or copies, with a note of where the originals can be referenced, should be included in the batch record.
- All documentation that reflects the significant steps in a process such as inoculation, incubation, harvesting, centrifuging, mixing, filling, packaging and labelling should be included in the batch record.
- References and documentation should be made describing what containers and pieces of equipment were used, when the equipment was sterilized and who performed the critical steps.
- Data such as inoculation and candling results should be included in the batch record.
- Lyophilization steps should be described step by step.
- The formulae used to perform calculations for specific gravity, multiplicity of infection and fill volume criteria should be an integral part of the batch record.
- Monitoring fill volume, line clearances and other processes that are exclusive to the operation of a specific batch should be included in the batch record.
- The specific logs used to monitor filling, sealing and labelling phases of the process should be included in the batch record.
- A monitoring record should supply the following information: product name, code number, issue date, potency, etc.; any specific instructions on the monitoring procedure (e.g. "A representative vial for each nozzle should be checked at 30-minute intervals as per SOP 001.11.111"); the filling machine name; the equipment identification number; the fill room number; the manometer reading; who performed the operation, with date; the number of fill needles used; the acceptable fill range (e.g. 5.0 ml to 5.3 ml); the target range (e.g. 5.2 ml); the time started; and the time ended. A specimen monitoring record is shown in the box on the next page.

The record would then indicate an immediate readjustment of the fill volume and would probably have start and finish times of 8:40 am and 3:10 pm, respectively.

Records such as refrigeration monitoring records and the making of media or cleaning solutions are usually indicative and apply to processes that will be used for several products. These preparation records are usually written as process batch records and are retained in specific areas of the department that performed the work. The product batch record may reference the media preparation or disinfection preparation batch records but

Vial number	Time	Amount (*ml*)	Vial number	Time	Amount (*ml*)
1	8:00 am	5.25 ml	1	2:30 pm	5.13ml
2		5:20 ml	2		5.22ml
3		5.12 ml	3		5.21 ml
4		5.20 ml	4		5.18 ml
1	8:30 am	5:12 ml	1	3:00 pm	5:11ml
2		5:20 ml	2		5:26 ml
3		5:32 ml[1]	3		5:23 ml
4		5:29 ml	4		5:08 ml[2]

[1] Fill volume out of range, fill operator called and instructed to adjust needle number 3.
[2] Low fill, fill operator called and instructed to adjust needle number 4.

copies of these types of documents need not be included with the batch record.

- Batch records should contain a documentation list stating the documents that are to be found in the batch record, the results of the batch record review and whether the record is acceptable for release based on the review.
- A completed batch record usually has copies of the QC records including the certificate of analysis and the results of the testing that was performed for final product testing.

Maintenance and retention of auxiliary records

Records that support the production processes or provide documented proof of certain activities, such as lyophilization and autoclave charts, validation data, feasibility studies and stability data must be regularly maintained, monitored, updated and retained. Lyophilization, autoclave and oven charts should be maintained in the batch record when the load includes only those items that are traceable to a specific product. For example, autoclave records for stoppers or lyophilization records should be maintained in the batch record but autoclave records for media or tubing, which could be traceable to other products, may be copied with the original referenced document or the records may be kept separate and the batch number of the autoclave run referenced in the batch records.

Examples of other records that are auxiliary and may be stored separately (and referenced by a control number in the batch record) are: the results of microbiological monitoring; validation information; QC records that provide data for more than one product; preventive maintenance records for equipment; calibration records; sanitation and disinfection records; and inventory records.

Whether this practice is acceptable is contingent upon the regulations of each country's government and the requirements of importing customers (when applicable).

Control and tracking documentation

Control documents are regulated documents that contain proprietary or confidential information concerning a company's processes, policies, procedures or ideas. These types of documents are assigned unique identifying numbers which provide traceability and accountability by allowing the company to establish and monitor who gets the documents and what version or revision of the document is most current, as well as by coordinating the replacement of obsolete documents. Examples of controlled documents are product outlines, SOPs, batch records and labels.

Assigning control numbers involves the systematic application of a sequence of numbers to documents in order to track information and the corresponding recipients. Examples of tracking documents are logbooks, routing forms, perpetual inventory control cards and material transfer forms.

The information written in the batch record is correlated to the documentation in logbooks. Logbook documentation should complement the data in the batch record, so the following points should be considered:

- Documentation should be made as soon as work has been completed whenever possible. For instance, verifications should be signed by a witness immediately after the worker completes the procedure. When information is signed a day or two later, the accuracy of the information can no longer be assured, especially as it is already apparent that the personnel involved have a questionable memory demonstrated by their inability to sign the record on time.
- The same personnel who sign the "Performed by" and "Verified by" sections of the batch record should also sign the appropriate sections of the logbooks.
- Information in logbooks should be in chronological order and, wherever possible, books should be bound as opposed to loose-leaf binders.
- Significant information in either logbooks or batch records should be handwritten and not typed, stamped or computer printed.
- Master logs should describe the master documents on file and what revision number or version number is current.

Change control procedure

This procedure provides a mechanism whereby the revision or amendment of regulated documents is effectively monitored, evaluated and controlled. It involves establishing the critical control points, the authorization personnel and the criteria for making a decision for approval or rejection of a proposed change.

The change control procedure should require that several departments review proposed revisions to any procedure, equipment or processes. These include changes in temperature ranges, incubation times, ingredients, filling and manipulation of the product, testing and storage.

The procedure should be designed to eliminate the possibility of a process conflicting with the product outline and should provide for the justification of clerical as well as scientifically sound changes.

Change control procedures are considered critical and should take into account information provided by the evaluation of pertinent documents, the expertise of persons reviewing the change and the justification written to support the change. Discrepancies in any of these criteria could result in the invalidation of the change (which could jeopardize all the products made subsequently to the change).

An example of a change control procedure form is given in Figure 17.

THE APPLICATION OF QUALITY ASSURANCE TO PRODUCTION AND QUALITY CONTROL SYSTEMS

The success of a company's implementation of GMP can generally be evaluated by a review of the documentation within or surrounding the production process. From the focal point of a batch record, which is a diary of a particular batch of product, an auditor can evaluate SOPs, the product outline, QC data, distribution, purchasing and inventory records. In addition, the proficiency of regulatory affairs, labelling, engineering and mainte-

Company name ______________________
Form control ______________________
Address ______________________

Attachment I of SOP ______________________
Effective date ______________________
Supersedes ______________________

Section 1 – Responsibility: author/initiator of change
Document title ______________________
Proposed document revision number __________
Document number ______________________
Date initiated ______________________
Draft initiated by ______________________

Indicate change(s) (x):
() Revise SOP
() Convert policy to procedure
() Revise production batch record
() Convert procedure to policy
() Change validation parameters
() ______________________

Indicate type of change(s) (x):
() Clerical corrections
() Make amendment to SOP*
() Addition of step(s)
() Make attachment to production batch record
() Deletion of step(s)
() Revalidation
() Clarification of existing information
() Other (explain)

* Must be justified by department head

Section 2 – Responsibility: department supervisor or designate
Evaluate the information in Section 1 in conjunction with the document submitted.
Determine if change is feasible and warranted.

() Approve as is
() Approve as corrected
() Revised draft required prior to approval (If checked return to author)

Reviewed/approved by ______________________
Department supervisor or designate
Date ___ / ___ / ___
☛ Route approved document to education trainer

Section 3 – Responsibility: Education training
Education training review the revised document and determine if training is necessary.

() Training indicated
() Original training is sufficient

Reviewed/approved by ______________________
Education trainer or designate
Date ___ / ___ / ___
☛ Route to quality assurance

Section 4 – Responsibility: QA manager or designate
QA review proposed change(s). Indicate below justification(s) (x):

() Directed by regulation
() Provides clarification to document
() Directed by in-house requirements
() Reflect to actual practice
() Not a significant step
() Does not affect safety, purity, potency of product
() Correction action
() New process/equipment
() Other (document) ______________________

() Approved as is
() Revised draft required prior to approval
() Approved as corrected

Reviewed/approved by ______________________
Quality system manager or designate
Date ___ / ___ / ___
☛ Route to QA

Section 5 – Responsibility: QA
() Revalidation of process required
() Validation not applicable
() Validation of step required

Document ______________________
() Approved as is
() Approved as corrected
() Revised draft

Reviewed/approved by ______________________ Date ___ / ___ / ___
QA director or regulatory affairs

FIGURE 17

Sample documentation change control form

nance, documentation control and QA can be evaluated by using the batch record.

If a company fails to understand the need for integration of systems (and the corresponding documentation), an audit such as this wil be damaging for the company and revealing for the auditor.

It is important to remember that one of the primary reasons for the proliferation of documentation is to provide information to regulatory agencies and other auditing bodies. Since the lack of appropriate documentation is a key indicator of inadequacies within a system, and poor or incorrect documentation may be indicative of questionable or inappropriate operations, documentation review is the key focus of any audit.

By reviewing the batch record in conjunction with supporting documentation, auditors are able to make a relatively accurate evaluation of the manufacturing processes and systems.

The methodology for performing a systems audit via the batch record is as follows (the name of the department usually responsible is indicated in brackets):

- The auditor asks to review specific batch records and, because the information must be in accordance with the product submissions and licences, also asks for the product outline.
- If a specific licence has stipulations to meet contractual agreements (for countries that export), licence amendments, addenda and contracts may also be requested.
- If the batch record does not provide step-by-step documentation of the process but instead resembles a bench record, SOPs specific to that product and supporting functions will be requested.
- Beginning with the bill of materials, the auditor will ensure that the materials used reflect the specifications submitted to the government or agreed to in the contract. This encompasses the dilutions of ingredients and reagents, special treatments of media, the type of packaging containers, stipulations that specific manufacturers or vendors must be used, the amounts dispensed of each ingredient, lot numbers used, etc.
- If there are discrepancies in the information listed above, auditors will usually ask to see the change control procedures (regulatory affairs and/or documentation control), the annual review of procedures documentation (regulatory affairs and/or QA), certificates of analysis, which evaluate incoming raw materials (QC), documentation of the process of scale up or converting R&D batches into production batches (regulatory affairs and R&D), the supplier approval process (QA and purchasing) and the procedure for developing a master batch record (documentation control). If lot numbers are not used in a controlled, sequential manner, or if it appears that more of a lot number was documented as having been used than was received by the company, inventory records as well as procedures will be scrutinized (inventory control or materials management).
- Any ingredient that indicates the involvement of outside vendors or suppliers (such as the need for irradiation, HVAC filter changing and cleaning services, suppliers of media, eggs and tissue) will involve the evaluation of the purchasing department and should include the QA unit. Whether a company implements audits of outside contractors and includes the participation of the QA unit prior to the purchase of major equipment or supplies is a direct reflection of the company's understanding of GMP requirements. Lack of QA involvement

in the decisions of building a facility or purchasing equipment and supplies inevitably leads to GMP infractions which must be remedied or justified later.

- Both the ingredients and the formulation steps of the batch record are reviewed against the product outline and appropriate procedures (regulatory affairs, production, QC).
- The parameters for inoculation, harvesting and incubation will be compared with the product outline and contract requirements. Auditors will request logbooks to ensure adequate maintenance and disinfection of equipment and compare the dates, names, locations and equipment in the batch record with the dates, names, locations and equipment in the logbooks' lists of equipment (production, QA).
- The actual usage of ingredients will be compared with the amounts dispensed and remaining, as well as with the chronological order of lot numbers. Key points will be whether there is a system in place to ensure that the oldest ingredients are used first; a tracking system to ensure that all raw materials are reconciled; traceability of where and when ingredients were used; and an established action level threshold beyond which the company will investigate inventory discrepancies (materials management, production).
- Testing methodologies will be compared with pertinent pharmacopoeias, licence submissions and sampling plans. Evaluation methods and data will be reviewed (QC, microbiology).
- All numerical values of temperatures, incubation periods, mixing times, etc. will be reviewed and correlated to the equipment-use logs which indicate the dates of operation, the cleaning and disinfection of the various areas, environmental monitoring data (e.g. manometer readings, settling plate or air particulate sampling) and the personnel who have performed significant steps.
- The methods companies use to handle returned product, complaints and product recalls, as well as the review of equipment specifications, history and validation records, utility systems and building design are also common areas of assessment.
- Autoclave and Lyophilization charts and logs give definitive information concerning the functions of a system that encompasses equipment maintenance, biological indicator monitoring, product management, calibration, disinfection and cleaning, validation, product outlines, manufacturing discrepancy and deviation processes, quarantine/holding and rejection/disposal information. The documentation commonly reviewed at this juncture includes: equipment history files; preventive maintenance and calibration programmes; validation and revalidation data; cleanser feasibility studies (for effectiveness of disinfectants and cleansers); utility system data, especially water systems; lubrication programmes; and load configurations (production, engineering and maintenance, microbiology, regulatory affairs, QA).

The information given here is by no means comprehensive, but it should convey the relevancy and importance of documentation. As this information is reviewed, it becomes apparent why an adequate and comprehensive documentation system is necessary.

The complexity of the documentation and integration of the production processes require the use of resources that can provide an overview of the systems inherent in the manufacturing of veterinary vaccines. It is recommended that in the development of systems for a new facility, the requirements of documentation should be given paramount importance. Companies that have an interest in retroactively addressing documentation issues or that wish to improve an existing system are encouraged to assess their manufacturing systems. A successful systems review will reveal the documentation inadequacies in existing processes while providing the initial springboard for addressing and developing new documentation requirements.

BIBLIOGRAPHY

EC. 1992. *Guide to good manufacturing practices for medicinal products in the European Community.* Rules Governing Medicinal Products in the European Community. Vol. IV.

FAO. 1994. *Quality control testing of rinderpest cell culture vaccine, standard operating procedures.* FAO Animal Production and Health Paper. Rome.

USDA. 1994. The 21 Code of Federal Regulations (CFR) 211s and 600 series, FDA, Washington, DC, United States Government Printing Office.

Assessment of potency in bacterial vaccines

P.A. Knight

Regular performance of potency tests on every production lot is essential for the maintenance of efficacy in most bacterial vaccines. Failure to perform such tests has often resulted in a gradual decline in potency and vaccines from previously untested sources rarely perform satisfactorily when tested. Potency tests are prescribed in most bacterial vaccine monographs and where these have been consistently applied the incidence of failure in the field has been very low. It is, however, important to recognize that mere conformity to the requirements of a pharmacopoeia does not guarantee that a new formulation will necessarily prove efficacious in the field. It is always essential to demonstrate that a representative batch of any new formulation elicits the required level of protection or of protective antibody in the target species.

This chapter is concerned with the principles on which valid potency tests should be based, in cases where pharmacopoeial requirements are inapplicable or unavailable and considers the potency tests laid down in three major compendia, viz. the European Pharmacopoeia, which is mandatory throughout the European Union (EU), Chapter Nine of the United States Code of Federal Regulations (USDA, 1994), which is mandatory in North America, and the British Pharmacopoeia (British Pharmacopoeia Commission, 1985), which is harmonized with the European Pharmacopoeia but contains some unique monographs and is widely available in many developing countries. In the British Pharmacopoeia all the veterinary monographs are contained in a single volume, so it may be more convenient to use than the European Pharmacopoeia where they are scattered through several volumes.

Although the requirements contained in these documents are not binding to veterinary vaccine producers outside the EU, the United States or the United Kingdom, they are based on extensive experience of the production and control of effective bacterial vaccines and the methods that they prescribe have been well tried. Their adoption in other countries can, therefore, avoid the lengthy and expensive process of test development and validation. In the case of new vaccines, for which no pharmacopoeia requirement is relevant, validation of a potency test method and, where appropriate, a reference preparation should be integrated into the process of vaccine development.

KILLED VACCINES

The majority of bacterial vaccines are killed. They may contain whole inactivated cultures, suspensions of killed organisms, exoantigens from culture supernatants or extracted somatic antigens. The need for potency tests of killed vaccines has sometimes been questioned, particularly for those in which the protective antigens can be identified and measured, on the grounds that if the right quantity of antigen is present, the potency will always be satisfactory. This is not so. Potency tests are essential to the consistent production of efficacious killed vaccines because the potency of the final product is affected by a wide range of variables which cannot be completely controlled. Although the impact of these variables can be defined in a few instances, in most cases it is impossible to predict from the density of a culture, the concentration of a toxoid or its antigenic profile, the potency of an adjuvanted final vaccine prepared from it. This is because the expression of protective antigens is affected by the quality of the growth medium and the time and conditions of culture growth. The immunogenic quality and quantity of protective antigens are also affected by small differences in conditions of detoxification. The immunogenicity of the protective antigens in the final vaccine is affected to varying extents by adjuvants and other antigens which are either deliberately added to form multivalent products or are present as impurities in the final formulation.

Although a few monovalent, unadjuvanted vaccines prepared from highly purified antigens that do not require inactivation are issued for human use without any potency test, none are as yet available for veterinary applications. For all inactivated veterinary vaccines it remains impossible to predict the potency of a batch of vaccine on the basis of antigen content, culture density or previous experience.

The foregoing points emphasize the importance of maintaining rigorous standardization of every aspect of the manufacturing process and the need to control accurately the quantity of protective antigen in a dose of vaccine whenever it can be measured.

An ideal potency test should meet two requirements. It should: measure a response that is relevant to the efficacy of the vaccine; and provide assurance that the size of that response is sufficient to guarantee efficacy.

Measurement of the immune response

The method of measurement or titration of the response is critical to the relevance of the test that assesses the efficacy of the vaccine. Most potency tests on veterinary bacterial vaccines rely on the use of a challenge with live organisms to measure immunity in the test animals.

Challenge methods have the advantage that they are perceived to demonstrate efficacy directly. This is undoubtably true when the route of administration is analogous to the route of infection in the field or when the pathology of the laboratory infection is similar to that of the natural disease. However, it is a far less reliable guide if, for example, an intraperitoneal challenge is used to determine the potency of a vaccine directed against an enteric or respiratory disease. Thus, vaccines based on adhesin antigens of *Escherichia coli*, which are highly effective against colibacillosis in piglets, completely fail to protect mice against intraperitoneal challenge with live *E. coli* in the laboratory. Similarly, the relevance of intraperitoneal challenge of laboratory animals to the efficacy of vaccines directed against swine erysipelas or the pneumonic forms of *Pasteurella haemolytica* is questionable. Nevertheless, live challenges are the most relevant indicator of potency for the majority of inactivated bacterial vaccines.

Challenge tests, however, do have considerable disadvantages. They are inefficient, using large numbers of animals to obtain limited information. The procedures to which the animals are submitted are so severe that in the EU such tests can only be tolerated in the absence of a satisfactory alternative and many laboratories are active in the development of methods to replace them. In addition, the use of challenge methods precludes the determination of potency for more than one component in a multicomponent vaccine with a single group of animals. For these reasons there are considerable attractions in the use of non-challenge methods of evaluating the immune response, provided that such methods can be shown to reflect the efficacy of the vaccines concerned with sufficient accuracy.

The best-established examples of non-challenge methods are found among the clostridia, where the substantial role played by lethal toxins in the pathogenesis of the relevant diseases allows the potency of many vaccines to be determined in terms of the antitoxic response elicited by the vaccine in rabbits and titrated *in vivo* or *in vitro*. For many years such tests have been instrumental in maintaining high levels of efficacy in a range of clostridial vaccines used in Europe, Australasia and North America, despite the fact that in almost every case antitoxic immunity provides only a part of the total protection offered by the vaccine.

As the antigens responsible for protection against bacterial diseases have been identified, vaccines based on these antigens have been developed. The routine potency tests of such vaccines have been based on levels of antibody directed against the protective antigens. Although some authorities might describe such tests as immunogenicity rather than potency tests, they may furnish as good an index of efficacy as a challenge test, provided that the antibodies measured are specific to the molecular species responsible for protection. Ideally the antibodies measured should be shown to neutralize the biological action of the protective antigen. Thus, for example, antibodies directed against adhesins should be shown to block adhesion of bacteria to target cells, and those directed against toxins should be shown to prevent their toxic effects.

Unfortunately, apart from the clostridia, serological techniques such as enzyme-linked immunosorbent assay (ELISA), immunoprecipitation or agglutination have measured antibodies directed against preparations of the protective antigen(s) (which are often only partially purified) without making reference to their biological activity.

The value of such techniques as indicators of potency depends on their specificity for the protective antigen(s). Use of monoclonal antibodies (MAbs) directed against the protective antigen in capture or competition ELISAs provides a useful means of attaining specificity when such MAbs are available. Alternatively, specificity may be attained by exhaustive purification of the protective antigen(s).

Purification of large protein antigens is not always easy, even from the native state, and may be impossible for preparations derived from formalin-inactivated cultures. The choice of serological technique is not critical but ELISA offers a wider range of strategies for the attainment of specificity and many methods based on the use of MAbs are only practicable with ELISA. Detailed descriptions of a variety of methods for the serological evaluation of antitoxins are included in the World Health Organization (WHO) manual for potency testing of diphtheria, tetanus and pertussis vaccines (WHO). However, for those laboratories that lack facilities for reading ELISA tests, a more limited range of strategies for the attainment of specificity is still possible. Although tests based on the agglutination of bacterial cells have been widely used in the past, they are often dominated by immunoglobulin M (IgM) responses to O antigens and the number of antigens presented by whole organisms is so large as to make the attainment of high specificity for protective ones extremely difficult. Some of these difficulties may be overcome by the use of agglutination inhibition and single radial diffusion techniques.

Whatever method of response evaluation is chosen, it is important to establish that the selected method, when applied to sera from vaccinated animals, reflects their resistance to challenge and that results from the complete test reflect the relative efficacy of different vaccines in the target species. It is also important that all serological data are related to a laboratory reference preparation which should preferably consist of a pool of typical test sera. This is essential in order to ensure that the results obtained on different occasions or even different plates are validly comparable.

Potency test formats

The other element of the test is the elicitation of an immune response in animals. This may be observed in laboratory animals or in animals of the target species. While the latter possess obvious advantages in terms of the ease with which test results can be translated into evidence of field efficacy, the greater ease of standardization, management and containment of challenge infections, together with the better prospects of using statistically adequate numbers, have favoured the use of laboratory animals for most tests.

An ideal potency test should provide a quantitative estimate of the potency of the vaccine, which would be the same if the test were performed at any laboratory and which would exactly reflect the efficacy of the vaccine in the target species. As well as estimating the potency of the vaccine an ideal potency test would also indicate a level of confidence that the true potency exceeded minimum requirements. Because tests that rely on an absolute level of response are affected by the varying levels of sensitivity of the animals used, the potency of a vaccine in an ideal test should be determined in comparison with a standard or reference preparation.

The classical six-point assay is designed to provide that comparison. In such a test the responses of groups of animals receiving three dose levels of the vaccine under test are compared by challenge, titration or serological methods with the responses of similar groups given dilutions of a standard vaccine.

Standard and reference preparations. Standard vaccines may be supplied by national control authorities such as the United States Department of Agriculture (USDA) or international bodies such as the European Pharmacopoeia Commission or WHO. If no appropriate national or international standard is available, and particularly if the vaccine to be tested is a new formulation, a batch of vaccine of proven efficacy should be adopted as a local reference preparation.

A standard or reference vaccine should be qualitatively identical to the test vaccine. Strong interactions frequently occur between the components of multivalent vaccines. When these occur it is often better to adopt a separate multivalent reference preparation than attempt comparison with a single component reference. Use of such reference preparations may facilitate potency testing of several vaccine components in a single group of animals, resulting in considerable cost savings. If a reference preparation is intended for use over a period of more than three years it should be lyophilized and then, preferably, tested for efficacy in the target species. If this is impracticable, the lyophilized material should be shown to be identical in potency to the liquid vaccine that has been proved to be efficacious. Particular care needs to be taken when lyophilizing vaccines that contain aluminium adjuvants as these often suffer recrystallization, resulting in a substantial loss of potency when the vaccine consists entirely of adsorbed soluble antigens. The effect is largely mitigated when whole bacterial cells are present.

Challenge tests. When the immune response of animals is evaluated by challenge, the proportion of animals surviving in each treatment group is used to estimate the 50 percent protective or effective dose (ED_{50}) values for test and standard vaccines. The method of calculation of ED_{50} values is not specified but, if access to a computer is available, the preferred method is probit analysis which makes the most efficient use of the available data. The quantitative estimation of potency by six-point assays assumes that the dose-response curves of the test and standard vaccines are linear and parallel and it is usual to verify that estimates of potency are valid in this respect. (A computer program for probit analysis is available from WHO, Biologicals Division, Geneva 27, Switzerland. This estimates the relative potency of the test vaccine, together with its confidence limits, and verifies the statistical validity of the estimate.)

In the absence of a computer, ED_{50} values can be calculated by the methods of Reed and Muench (1938), provided that the available data satisfy the requirements of that method (i.e. test groups show 100 percent and 0 percent effects), or by use of tables of precalculated data such as those of Toothill, Robinson and Adams (1969). An estimate of the potency of the vaccine under test relative to a standard - the relative potency (RP) – can then be calculated as the quotient of the ED_{50} value estimated for a standard preparation divided by the ED_{50} estimated for the vaccine under test. These methods, however, are less effective than probit analysis and do not test the statistical validity of the data or estimate confidence limits.

Quantitative response tests. The six-point assay described above is applied to quantal data (i.e. proportions of survivors). The same principle can also be applied to quantitative (continuous) data such as scores or titres. The scores or titres are used to estimate the potency of the test vaccine relative to the standard by parallel-line analysis. It is usual to transform both the dose levels and the response data to logarithms at the beginning of the analysis unless they are already in a logarithmic form such as serial dilution numbers. Assays based on quantitative data usually require smaller numbers of animals than quantal assays and are therefore preferable. A computer program for parallel line analysis, similar to the one referred to above for probit analysis, is also available from WHO.

Although six-point assays provide the best estimate of the potency of a vaccine, they are rarely used in veterinary applications because of the large numbers of animals that they require. The tests for *Pasteurella multocida* and swine erysipelas vaccines in the North American and European requirements need 120 and 96 mice per test, respectively.

Absolute response level tests. The majority of the tests prescribed by pharmacopoeias do not make use of a reference preparation but base the criterion of acceptance on the elicitation of a defined level of response by a fixed dose of vaccine. This approach requires a high degree of standardization of the laboratory animals which may vary from strain to strain depending on their diet and other conditions of husbandry. The effects of these variables (which can be very large) are difficult to isolate and may influence the observed potency value of the vaccine under test. This can lead to the rejection of good vaccine or the acceptance of bad. A partial solution to this problem can be found in the occasional use of a reference vaccine to verify that it elicits a typical response in the hands of the testing laboratory. A suitable reference vaccine with target ranges for six clostridial vaccines is available from the Central Veterinary Laboratory, Weybridge, Surrey, United Kingdom. For other types of vaccine, the only means of establishing that the animals in a laboratory are producing typical results is to re-test material previously tested by a reputable laboratory, elsewhere.

Single point comparative tests. A third approach has been adopted by WHO to overcome the cost problem of six-point assays for human vaccines against diphtheria and tetanus while retaining the use of a standard vaccine (WHO). These tests are designed to provide assurance that a dose of the vaccine under test is significantly superior to a defined dose of a reference vaccine. The advantage of this method is that it offers a direct comparison of the vaccine under test with an established reference preparation but requires only one-third of the number of animals needed to determine the RP.

In the form prescribed by WHO the test offers statistical confidence that the potency of the vaccine is superior to that of the reference dose. The difficulty with this approach is that it predicates that routine batches of vaccine will be substantially better than the minimum required to protect the target species and this may not always be so. Such superiority should be sought whenever possible since definitive challenge tests in the target species are almost invariably performed shortly after vaccination is complete and make no allowance for declining immunity in the period preceding a recall vaccination.

If a comparative test is to be set up, the following procedure is recommended:

i) Establish the dose of reference vaccine (D) that is just enough to achieve minimal protection in the target species after one or two doses. If a minimum requirement has already been defined, D is the dose of reference material that exactly meets that requirement.

ii) Establish the dose of reference vaccine that, using a one- or two-dose schedule, elicits a minimal measurable response in the chosen laboratory species (d). For a challenge test the response should be approximately 10 percent protection; for an antibody response test, at least 80 percent of the animals should respond, but the titres should be low.

iii) Calculate the laboratory animal test dose (t) as the dose recommended for the target species (T): $t = T.d/D$.

iv) Inoculate groups of laboratory animals with doses d and t of the reference and test vaccines respectively. The number of animals required is discretionary; if D is much lower than T few animals will be needed; if D is only slightly greater than T very large numbers will be required. There is therefore a strong incentive to produce highly potent vaccine.

v) For both groups, follow the same vaccination and challenge or serum sampling schedule as was used for ii) above.

vi) If responses were evaluated by challenge, determine whether the response to the test vaccine (P) was significantly greater ($P < 0.5$) than those to the reference preparation by Chi-square test (Fisher's contingency tables are the most convenient way of doing this). If responses were evaluated as titres or numerical scores, they should be transformed to logarithms unless they are already in logarithmic form (end-point tube numbers from titrations involving serial dilutions and some scores are already log transformed). Using the transformed data, determine whether the responses to the test vaccine are significantly greater than those to the reference using Student's "t" test or Welch's variation if the group variances are unequal.

vii) The test vaccine is satisfactory if it

elicits a significantly greater response than the reference preparation. Alternative criteria adopted for some veterinary vaccines have included requirements that the response to the test vaccine should be simply greater or even not significantly inferior to the reference preparation. Such reduced criteria do not automatically provide assurance of adequate potency but rely on the use of minimum numbers of animals to provide confidence.

WHO does not permit the use of single-dose tests until data from six-point assays have confirmed that the assumptions of linearity and parallelism of dose-response curves, which underlie all biological tests and assays, are justified. Since evidence of linearity and parallelism is not required, even from the six-point assays prescribed for veterinary vaccines, it appears inappropriate to require it for veterinary applications of the single-point comparison described above.

Pharmacopoeial tests. The tests prescribed in the European and British pharmacopoeias and in the United States Code of Federal Regulations are summarized in Table 15.

Clostridial vaccines

Clostridial vaccines may be prepared from toxoids, whole anacultures (bacterin-toxoids) and, very occasionally, bacterins alone. With the exceptions of *Clostridium haemolyticum* and *Cl. chauvoei*, which are tested by challenge of guinea pigs with live bacteria, both the European Pharmacopoeia and the United States CFR prescribe antitoxin response tests for all the major clostridial vaccines, whether bacterial cells are included or not. The form that the tests take and the criteria of acceptance imposed by the two compendia are summarized in Table 16.

Live challenge tests for clostridia. Potency tests involving challenge of guinea pigs with live organisms are prescribed for *Cl. chauvoei* vaccines by the United States CFR

TABLE 15

Potency tests applied to inactivated bacterial vaccines

Causative organism	European and British pharmacopoeias	United States CFR	Reference used?
Clostridium novyi	Antitoxin titre	Antitoxin titre	No
Cl. perfringens A	Not included	Not included	No
Cl. perfringens B, C, D	Antitoxin titre	Antitoxin titre	No
Cl. septicum	Antitoxin titre	Not included	No
Cl. tetani	Antitoxin titre	Antibody titre	No
		or toxin challenge	Yes
Cl. haemolyticum	Not included	Challenge	No
Cl. botulinum C, D	Toxin challenge	Toxin challenge	No
Cl. chauvoei	Live challenge	Live challenge	No
Cl. sordellii	Not included	Antitoxin titre	No
Leptospira interrogans hardjo	Not included	Not specified	No
L. i. pomona	Not included	Live challenge	No
L. i. canicola	Live challenge	Live challenge	No
L. i. grippotyphosa	Not included	Live Challenge	No
L. i. icterohaemorrhagiae	Live challenge	Live challenge	No
Escherichia coli	Absolute response	Not included	Yes
Pasteurella multocida	Not included	Live challenge	Yes
Pasteurella haemolytica	Not included	Not included	No
Erysipelothrix rhusiopathiae	Live challenge	Live challenge	Yes
Brucella abortus	Live challenge	Not included	No
Mycoplasma	Not included	Not included	No

TABLE 16
Compendium requirements for clostridial vaccines

Species	European requirements			United States requirements		
	Test animal	Test type	Criterion	Test animal	Test type	Criterion
Cl. perfringens C	10 rabbits	AT resp.	10 Bu/ml	8 rabbits	AT resp.	10 Bu/ml
Cl. perfringens D	10 rabbits	AT resp.	5 Eu/ml	8 rabbits	AT resp.	2 Eu/ml
Cl. perfringens B	10 rabbits	AT resp.	10 B+5E u/ml	No United States requirement		
Cl. botulinum C, D	20 mice	Tox. chall.	> 80% live			
Cl. botulinum C	5 mink	Tox. chall.	> 80% live			
Cl. novyi B	10 rabbits	AT resp.	3.5 u/ml	8 rabbits	AT resp.	0.5 u/ml
Cl. septicum	10 rabbits	AT resp.	2.5 u/ml	No United States requirement		
Cl. sordellii	No European requirement			8 rabbits	AT resp.	1 u/ml
Cl. tetani poly	10 rabbits	AT resp.	2.5 u/ml			
Cl. tetani mono	10 guinea pigs	AT resp.	7.5 u/ml	10 guinea pigs	Ab resp. (ELISA)	2 Au/ml
Cl. tetani horse	10 guinea pigs	AT resp.	30 u/ml			
Cl. chauvoei	10 guinea pigs	Live chall.	10/10 live	8 guinea pigs	Live chall.	> 80% live
Cl. haemolyticum	No European requirement			8 guinea pigs	Live chall.	> 80% live

Notes: AT resp. = antitoxin response; Tox. chall. = toxin challenge; Live chall. = live challenge

and the European Pharmacopoeia and for *Cl. haemolyticum* vaccines by the United States CFR alone. The United States method for both involves a lower vaccine dose but permits a proportion of deaths among the vaccinates in a two-stage test in which vaccines that protect seven-eighths of the animals are accepted, those protecting less than five-eighths are rejected while intermediate results invoke a second test.

Spore preparations are available from the United States Plant and Animal Protection Service for both *Cl. chauvoei* and *Cl. haemolyticum* but their routine use is unlikely to be practicable for laboratories outside the United States. Challenge preparations can be prepared by culture of *Cl. chauvoei* in Buddle's medium containing 0.5 percent glucose until the first signs of gas appear. A satisfactory culture should contain at least 1 000 50 percent lethal doses (LD_{50}) per millilitre when injected intramuscularly in broth containing 2.5 percent calcium chloride. Should it prove impossible to achieve this level of virulence, a more virulent culture may be obtained by inoculating Buddle's medium with blood from a guinea pig at the point of death from *Cl. chauvoei* infection. If -70°C refrigeration, solid carbon dioxide (CO_2) or, better, liquid nitrogen is available, it is preferable to divide the culture into 2-ml aliquots and freeze at -70°C or lower. The lethality of the culture can then be determined before it is used. Culture stored at -70°C or in solid CO_2 will retain its full lethality for several weeks. If stored under liquid nitrogen it is stable for up to a year. It is advisable to dilute the fresh or stored culture to contain 100 LD_{50} doses in each challenge dose.

The United States type of test, by setting the final pass criterion at close to 75 percent protection, makes the outcome less susceptible to distortion by the death of a single non-responsive guinea pig. Despite this relaxation the overall stringency of the United States and European tests are very similar.

Challenge with *Cl. chauvoei* subjects guinea pigs to gangrenous lesions in the leg followed by invasion of the ventral body wall. The need for a less traumatic alternative has been widely recognized. An alternative test, based on the measurement of antibody responses in vaccinated animals by an ELISA method (based on surface antigens) has been approved in Australia. Such tests do not reflect all of the protective antigens present in the bacteria and the supernatant components of anaculture vaccines, but they have been shown to correlate well with the performance of similarly formulated vaccines in challenge tests.

It has been found that relatively crude sonicates and sodium dodecyl sulphate (SDS) extracts of bacterial cells can be used as antigens to sensitize polyvinyl chloride (PVC) or polystyrene plates. Before an ELISA method can be accepted for any particular vaccine, it is essential that a correlation be established between the serum titre corresponding to a marginal pass and the results of the associated challenge test.

No challenge test is prescribed for *Cl. haemolyticum* in Europe but some manufacturers have adopted tests based on the anti-beta-haemolysin response of rabbits which are performed in parallel with the tests for *Cl. perfringens, Cl. novyi, Cl. septicum* and *Cl. tetani*. This permits the potency of *Cl. haemolyticum* components in multivalent vaccines to be assessed in the same group of rabbits as the other components. Beta-haemolysin is the most prominent toxin produced by *Cl. haemolyticum*. Although there is no direct proof of its importance as a protective antigen there is evidence that most of the protection provided by *Cl. haemolyticum* vaccines is derived from the supernatant, and vaccines controlled and formulated on the basis of beta-haemolysin content have proved consistently effective in the field. Beta-haemolysin toxins, toxoids and antitoxins can be titrated according to the principles discussed below for the lethal toxins of other clostridia but with the use of *in vitro* indicators such as haemolysis of sheep erythrocytes or coagulation of ovolecithin.

Antitoxin response tests for clostridia. The great majority of clostridial vaccines are tested for potency by inoculation into rabbits and subsequent measurement of their antitoxin titres. This allows the costly immune response phase of the potency test to be shared among all the components of a multivalent formulation. European and United States requirements are broadly parallel – where they exist – the main differences being that larger vaccinating doses, higher response criteria and larger numbers of animals are used in Europe than in the United States.

The vaccination doses used by both authorities are large and are far beyond the upper asymptote of the dose-response relationship for most of the components. It is therefore dangerous to rely on potency test results for the adjustment of the antigen content of vaccines. With the exception of the USDA test for tetanus, the titres of pooled rabbit sera are determined by toxin neutralization (TN) tests. In TN tests the volume of a test toxin solution required to neutralize a defined quantity (e.g. 1 unit) of standard antitoxin is first determined. This is the L+ dose. The volume of each test antiserum required to neutralize the lethal effects of an L+ dose of the same toxin is the reciprocal of the serum titre expressed in units per millilitre.

In principle, the serum titre is equal to the number of units of standard antitoxin required to neutralize the test dose of toxin, divided by the volume of test serum required to produce the same effect on the same occasion. Although the toxin neutralization tests prescribed by the European and United States requirements are described in different terms both are based on the same principles – the United States method determines only the minimum acceptable titre, while the European method provides a quantitative estimate of titre. It is recommended that manufacturers should determine titres quantitatively so that adverse trends in potency can be recognized and remedied before the point of batch failure is reached.

Before testing an unknown serum it is necessary to select a suitable test dose of toxin. This is the smallest quantity of toxin which, when mixed with a defined dose of standard antitoxin (e.g. 1 unit or 0.1 units) produces an end-point effect when injected into an animal or exposed to an *in vitro* indicator. This quantity is described as L+ for 1 unit or L+/10 for 0.1 units, if the indicator is death.

Similarly, it is possible to define test doses for paralytic end points (Lp and Lp/10), for intradermal reactions (Lr and Lr/10) and for haemolytic end points (Lh and Lh/10). It is preferable to select an end point as close to neutrality as possible, such as 50 percent effect for an L+, an Lp or an Lr in the animal tests and 30 percent haemolysis in haemolytic tests.

Although toxin neutralization tests may be performed at either high or low concentrations it is important that the concentration of toxin in the test mixture and the dose of toxin administered to the indicator (the test dose) should be kept constant. This is because the test antisera (produced by two-dose immunization of rabbits) are far less avid than standard preparations which are prepared from hyperimmunized horses. In consequence, the apparent titres of test antisera are reduced when the concentration of reactants in the test mixture is low. In practice, the test dose needs to be large enough to contain at least ten indicating doses of toxin and small enough to be neutralized by 0.1 ml of a serum of the lowest acceptable titre, for example the minimum requirement for *Cl. septicum* in the European Pharmacopoeia is 2.5 units per millilitre. The highest possible test dose would therefore be 0.25 units equivalent (L+/4). In order to test down to 2.0 units per millilitre a level of L+/5 has been chosen which is the lowest level that can be supported by a good toxin which should contain ten lethal doses in one L+/5 dose.

Outline of test method. (The following description assumes that mixture volumes containing four test doses will be appropriate but other volumes are equally valid.) Having determined the test dose of toxin, select, on the basis of previous assays, an estimate of the titre of the test serum and calculate the volume required (v) to neutralize four doses of toxin and the volume of serum (m) that would be required if the true potency of the serum was of the lowest acceptable titre. Prepare a series of mixtures containing four times the test dose of toxin and one of a logarithmically graded series of volumes of the test antiserum, centred on n and including m at its upper end.

Prepare a parallel series of five mixtures, each containing the same amount of toxin and 120, 110, 100, 90 and 80 percent of the standard antitoxin dose against which the toxin test dose was determined. Make up the total volume of each mixture to four times the volume to be administered to the animal or other indicator system. Allow the mixtures to react for 30 to 60 minutes at 20° to 25°C before inoculating them into the animal or *in vitro* indicator. Volumes of 0.2 or 0.5 ml of mixtures containing *Cl. perfringens*, *Cl. septicum* and *Cl. sordellii* toxins are injected intravenously into mice, whereas mixtures containing *Cl. novyi* toxin are injected subcutaneously over the base of the tail and mixtures containing *Cl. tetani* are inoculated subcutaneously over the lumbar region of the spine.

The inoculated animals are observed for 48 or 72 hours and deaths are recorded, except for animals injected with *Cl. tetani*, which are observed for four days. An end point of minimal tetanic paralysis is used in many countries. In mice injected as described above, the end point is manifested as failure to retract either hind leg. The test is valid if a coherent end point is obtained in the standard range but, if the end point for the standard is found to be more than 10 percent above or below the expected value, the estimate of titre for the test serum should be adjusted proportionately.

Alternative indicators. Although the standard pharmacopoeial tests for clostridial antitoxins use death or paralysis of mice as indicators of excess toxicity, many of the toxins have other biological activities that are also suitable indicator effects for toxin neutralization tests. Table 16 shows some of the alternative indicators that have been shown to be valid indicators for clostridial toxins.

The use of alternative end points retains the toxin neutralization principle and represents a minimal change from the official lethal test method. It can result in considerable savings without prejudice to the reliability of the test provided that the alternative activity is a property of the same molecular species as the lethal toxin. There is evidence that the cytopathic activity of *Cl. perfringens* C filtrates for EBTR cells is not caused by the beta toxin and this gives cause to question the identity of the dermo-necrotic moiety of *Cl. septicum* and the cytopathic moiety of *Cl. novyi* B with the corresponding alpha toxins. In all other cases there are no reasons to doubt this assumption.

Serological tests based on assays of antibodies without reference to the toxin neutralization (TN) principle have been proposed for many of the clostridia. Most of the methods proposed have used ELISA methodology, but tests based on passive haemagglutination (PHA) and single radial diffusion (SRD) have also been proposed. ELISA methods offer the best prospects of consistent correlation with the titres obtained from TN tests. PHA and SRD require less-sophisticated equipment and reagents than ELISA but PHA at least is excessively sensitive to IgM antibodies which do not generally neutralize toxins.

In at least one instance (the United States test for tetanus) an ELISA method has been adopted as definitive. The value of such tests is primarily dependent on the purity of the antigen used and, for tetanus at least, there is evidence that simple ELISAs based on highly purified antigen can produce results that are almost identical to those

TABLE 17

Non-lethal indicators of clostridial toxins

	Indicating activities	Comments
Cl. perfringens alpha	Dermo-necrotic	Not used for test
	Haemolysin	Reflects lethal test
	Phospholipase C	Reflects lethal test
Cl. perfringens beta	Dermo-necrotic	Reflects lethal test[1]
	Cytopathic	Not identical to lethal toxin
Cl. perfringens epsilon	Dermo-necrotic	Reflects lethal test[1]
	Cytopathic	Reflects lethal test[1]
Cl. novyi alpha	Dermo-necrotic	Not used for test
	Cytopathic	Reflects lethal test[2]
Cl. septicum alpha	Dermo-necrotic	Reflects lethal test[2]
	Cytopathic	Reflects lethal test

[1] Lethal and alternative activity neutralized by the same monoclonal antibody.
[2] Correlation between lethal test and alternative incomplete.

obtained by TN over the range of titres expected from potency tests.

More elaborate strategies such as toxin binding immunoassay (TOBI), developed for the accurate measurement of low titres, and ELISAs based on antigen capture by non-neutralizing monoclonal antibodies, developed to overcome the poor correlation problems between TN and serological tests for diphtheria antitoxin, offer only small gains in tetanus potency tests.

The accuracy with which the results of serological tests reflect those of TN tests for other clostridial toxins has not been critically evaluated.

Clostridial potency tests based on toxin challenge. Toxin challenge tests are performed on *Cl. botulinum* vaccines only and their use for other clostridia is not recommended. The tests prescribed by the United States and European authorities both require the animals to be challenged intraperitoneally 21 days after a single dose of vaccine but differ in certain respects. In the United States, five mink receive a full recommended dose. These, with three controls, are challenged with 10 000 LD_{50} of toxin and all controls must die while 80 percent of vaccinates survive for seven days. In Europe, 20 mice receive 0.2 ml of one in eight dilution of vaccine. These, with ten controls, are challenged with 25 paralytic doses of toxin. All controls must show specific botulinum paralysis and 80 percent of vaccinates must show no signs of botulinum paralysis for seven days.

(In some countries special permission is required before undertaking tests in which animals are subjected to intoxication with *Cl. botulinum.*)

Test reagents. Although some authorities provide standard toxin materials, it is important to recognize that the definitive standard for the test is always the standard antitoxin. Standard antitoxins may be laboratory or national preparations that have been calibrated directly or indirectly against the relevant international standard. International standards are provided by WHO through the Statens Seruminstitut, 80 Armager Boulevard, Copenhagen, Denmark, for *Cl. botulinum, Cl. novyi, Cl. septicum, Cl. perfringens alpha, Cl. sordellii* and *Cl. tetani* antitoxins. *Cl perfringens beta* and *epsilon* antitoxin standards are distributed by the WHO/FAO Laboratory for Biological Standards at the Central Veterinary Laboratory, United Kingdom.

These preparations are not intended for use as working laboratory standards but should be used to calibrate national standard preparations or, in countries where these have not been produced, laboratory working standards.

Laboratory working standards are best prepared from a large pool of sera typical of the samples intended for test. The pool is carefully calibrated against the relevant national or international standard by the exact method laid down in an authoritative compendium such as the European Pharmacopoeia, preferably with the collaboration of the national control laboratory. The use of a laboratory reference preparation of the same species as the test sera is, of course, unavoidable for ELISA tests but is also highly desirable for other serological tests and TN tests using alternative indicators, where differences in avidity between standard and test preparations can lead to misleading results.

Although neither European nor United States requirements invoke a standard vaccine, it is useful to verify that the animals in a testing laboratory are of similar sensitivity to those used when the requirements were formulated. For this purpose a reference preparation, for which "normal" responses have been established by collaborative assay, has been prepared by the Central Veterinary Laboratory.

In many cases it will be necessary for laboratories to prepare their own test toxins. Test toxins can be prepared from production cultures by harvesting them a few hours earlier than for vaccine production. The toxic supernatant may be separated from the cells by centrifugation or filtration. (*Cl. perfringens epsilon* toxin is present as a prototoxin and the filtrate should be incubated for one hour with 2 percent pancreatic homogenate before stopping the reaction with soybean trypsin inhibitor.) The filtrate is concentrated and partially purified by precipitation with ammonium sulphate. Further purification is not recommended since it is likely to result in reduction of the crucial ratio of toxicity to L+. The resulting precipitate may be dried in a vacuum over phosphorous pentoxide and ground to a homogeneous powder from which weighed quantities can be dissolved to prepare the test toxin solution. When weighing dried toxin it is important that the whole contents of the bulk container are thoroughly mixed on each occasion since the surface layer often deteriorates. It is advisable to prepare sufficient toxin solution to last for several weeks and to stabilize it with 40 percent glycerol. The concentration of toxin should be high enough to ensure that not more than 5 mg of glycerol is injected in the test mixture.

If equipment for freeze-drying is available it is preferable to redissolve the toxin and dialyse it against buffered saline, then add an excipient such as 5 percent hydrolised gelatine to stabilize it before dispensing the resulting solution as accurately as possible into ampoules and then freeze-drying.

The minimum lethal dose, L+ and protein nitrogen content of the solution should be measured before freeze-drying and only solutions that contain a sufficient number of lethal doses per L+ dose should be dried. The number of L+ and indicating doses per container should be determined as accurately as possible before using the toxin.

The number of LD_{50} or minimum lethal dose (MLD) per L+ dose or the equivalent ratio of non-lethal indicating doses is critical to the suitability of a toxin. Each test dose (the quantity of toxin contained in the volume of toxin-antitoxin mixture injected into an animal or exposed to an *in vitro* indicator) should contain at least ten indicating doses. Suggested minimum levels for specific toxicity are included in each assay method in the British Pharmacopoeia. Limits for purity of test toxins are similarly included but these are less critical.

Leptospira vaccines

Little is known of the identity of the antigens responsible for the protective effects of *Leptospira* vaccines. There is therefore no rational basis for serological potency tests and the only methods recommended depend on challenge. All but one of the five serovars of *L. interrogans* used in vaccine production are lethal for hamsters (the single exception is *L. interrogans hardjo,* which infects but does not kill). Some serovars can also be tested in guinea pigs but, since hamsters are more robust and suitable for all serovars, it is convenient to use them in every case.

Both European and United States requirements specify inoculation of hamsters with a small fraction of the dose intended for the target species, followed at an interval of about 16 days by a challenge of between 10 and 10 000 LD_{50} of a virulent strain, which should preferably be a local isolate. The animals are observed for 14 days post challenge. European and United States requirements for four serovars are summarized in Table 18.

Leptospira cultures do not easily survive freeze-drying and most laboratories therefore maintain them in liquid culture. It is frequently necessary to passage the strain through hamsters to regain virulence before growing the challenge culture on Korthof's medium. (*L. interrogans* serovars are dangerous to humans. All manipulations should be carried out in safety cabinets and protective clothing – gloves, goggles and masks – should be worn during inoculation of animals. Infected animals and their excreta should be decontaminated before disposal.)

The European and United States requirements differ in the vaccination dose as a proportion of the target species dose, the number of animals used and the pass criteria which make provision for a repeat test. In these respects the United States requirement is slightly more stringent but less likely to fail to produce good vaccine than the European.

No potency test is prescribed for serovar *hardjo* but a renal infection end point can be substituted for the lethal challenge in a test based on comparison with a reference vaccine. Renal infection is determined 14 days post challenge by aseptically removing hamster kidneys and crushing them in a syringe. The crushed tissue is then inoculated into Korthof's medium and incubated for 14 days before examination for viable leptospires.

The crushing of kidneys is likely to generate spurts of infected fluid. This procedure should therefore be performed in a glove box. An alternative potency test based on the elicitation of agglutinins in guinea pigs has also been proposed for *hardjo*. Although production of agglutinins has been shown to correlate with efficacy in calves it is unlikely that the IgM antibodies measured in the test are important to the protection of calves.

Escherichia coli vaccines

Vaccines against bovine, ovine and porcine colibacillosis may depend on at least three distinct protective mechanisms; somatic antigens, adhesin antigens and enterotoxin. It is unlikely that somatic antigens alone will furnish adequate protection. No requirements for *E. coli* vaccines have been issued by USDA and no international standards or reference preparations exist, but monographs covering porcine and bovine vaccines recently completed for the European Pharmacopoeia provide a suitable basis for a review of potency tests for these vaccines.

Both monographs describe a test under potency which is not intended to be routinely performed for batch release but is prescribed in order to establish that one or more lots of the vaccine are effective against each of the strains or immunotypes against which protection is claimed. A vaccine lot shown to be satisfactory in this test may then be adopted as a reference preparation in the batch potency test (see Standard and reference preparations, p. 362). In the potency test, pregnant females of the target species are vaccinated and the resistance of their progeny to oral

TABLE 18

Comparison of European and United States requirements for leptospiral vaccines

Serovar	Vaccinating dose		Number of doses		Survivors required for pass		
	US	Europe	US	Europe	US test 1	US test 1 + repeat	Europe
Icterohaemorrhagiae	1/80	1/40	14-18	15-20	> 7/10	> 14/20	> 7/10
Canicola	1/80	1/40	14-18	15-20	> 7/10	> 14/20	> 7/10
Pomona	1/800	NI	14-18	NI	> 7/10	> 14/20	NI

challenge with heterologous strains bearing each of the claimed antigen types is compared with those of unvaccinated controls. The monograph requires 15 controls and 15 piglets from vaccinated gilts or sows, or five controls and ten calves or lambs from vaccinated dams, to be challenged.

The criteria governing the outcome of the test are too complex to be summarized in detail here but they correspond to protection indices ranging from 0.55 to 0.67 for pig vaccines and 0.875 for vaccines intended for ruminants. For manufacturers operating in countries not bound by the European Pharmacopoeia a protective index of 0.7 might be taken to represent an adequate level of protection. (The protective index is calculated by subtracting the percentage mortality of vaccinated animals from that of control animals and dividing the result by the percentage mortality of the control animals.)

The prescribed batch potency test may be performed in rabbits, guinea pigs or mice. Rats can also be considered for some of the adhesin antigens. The test depends on serological determination of the response to protective antigens after one or two doses of vaccine and requires that the mean response shall not be significantly ($P < 0.05$) inferior to the response elicited by a reference vaccine of proven efficacy under the same conditions.

Good assay practice dictates that the reference vaccine is tested in parallel with the test vaccine on every occasion. If the mean titre from the test vaccine is less than the reference the difference should be tested for significance by Student's "t" test. To satisfy the European Pharmacopoeia, the mean of the log titres elicited by the test vaccine must be shown to be not significantly inferior to those elicited by the reference vaccine.

Although this criterion avoids the release of grossly inferior vaccine it offers no assurance that the vaccine is as good as the reference and a requirement that the test vaccine is significantly superior to the reference would be preferable if such a standard could be consistently maintained. A test based on serological responses in the target species is also permitted for pig vaccines but, since no acceptance criterion is included, it is difficult to see how this could be applied.

Any valid serological method may be used in the batch potency test but ELISA methods are favoured by the European Pharmacopoeia. Although methods based on bacterial agglutination or PHA have been used, the achievement of consistent results of appropriate specificity has often proved difficult. However, the use of ELISA methodology does not, in itself, guarantee specificity or reproducibility and test antigens need to be purified with great care. The use of monoclonal antibodies in competition ELISAs offers a short cut to specificity for some antigens. Monoclonal antibodies directed at many of the protective antigens are available from the Central Veterinary Laboratory, United Kingdom. Although these recognize only one of several epitopes expressed by the test antigen, this deficiency is less serious than the intrusion of accessory antigens in partially purified preparations.

Use of the batch control test prescribed by the European Pharmacopoeia is dependent on the establishment of a statistically significant correlation between results of the batch control test and the full potency test described in the previous paragraph. While it would theoretically be possible to establish a relationship between the outcomes of full and batch control tests over a range of batches of vaccine, such a study would be prohibitively expensive. It is therefore more practicable to establish a correlation between the proportion of progeny protected against challenge and the colostrum titre of their dams as measured by the serological method developed for the batch control test. If a direct ELISA is used, a change of conjugate and laboratory reference preparation will be required before it can be applied to the target species.

Pasteurella vaccines

Vaccines against mammalian and avian strains of *Pasteurella multocida* and mammalian strains of *P. haemolytica* are considered here. No European requirements for any *Pasteurella* vaccines exist but the United States CFRs contain requirements for vaccines against both avian and mammalian strains of *P. multocida.*

The mammalian vaccine requirements are applicable to each of the immunotypes present in the vaccine. Three fivefold dilutions of the test vaccine and three identical dilutions of a standard vaccine are inoculated intraperitoneally into groups of 20 mice. The dose volume prescribed is one-twentieth of the lowest dose volume prescribed for the target species but, for laboratories not constrained by the requirements, a fixed dose of 0.5 ml may be more convenient. The standard may be provided by USDA or may be an in-house reference preparation. The initial dose is repeated after 14 days, the animals challenged intraperitoneally with 100 to 10 000 LD_{50} of a virulent culture ten to 12 days later and the proportion dying in each of the treatment groups is recorded for ten days after challenge.

The test is valid if the proportion of survivors in at least two of the groups that received standard vaccine lies between 0 and 100 percent and if the 50 percent end-point dilution for the standard lies between the highest and lowest dilution. There are no requirements for the dose response regressions to be linear or parallel. Instead the relative potency (RP) is determined as the reciprocal of the 50 percent end-point dilution of the test vaccine, divided by the equivalent figure for the reference. The method of calculation of 50 percent end-point dilution is not specified but it would be appropriate to determine the 50 percent effective dose (ED_{50}) by a standard LD_{50} calculation such as probit analysis or Reed and Muench (1938). If the protection afforded by the test preparation is so complete (>80 percent survivors at the lowest dose) that a 50 percent end point cannot be determined, while a valid end point is obtained for the reference preparation, the vaccine is satisfactory.

The acceptance criterion requires that the RP is 0.5 or more. If this criterion is not met, two further tests may be performed and a (geometric) mean value for the RP determined. There are complex provisions for the exclusion of very low initial estimates if repeat tests are satisfactory.

Although the form of the data produced in this test is suitable for full statistical evaluation by a method such as parallel line probit analysis, the actual data may not satisfy the strict validity requirements of such assays very often and the less rigorous approach is therefore justified. Although simplified, single-dose level tests have never been used for *Pasteurella* vaccines, it is probable that their use could offer assurance of potency with smaller numbers of animals than the prescribed six-point assay.

Most strains of *P. haemolytica* are far less virulent for mice than *P. multocida* but the virulence of most strains of *P. haemolytica* can be enhanced sufficiently to allow a challenge of 100 LD_{50} by inclusion of either 5 percent yeast or 5 percent hog gastric mucin in the challenge suspension. The choice of enhancing agent can only be determined by trial and error – some strains respond to yeast and others to mucin, in an apparently random fashion, and a few strains respond to neither.

No requirements for killed *P. haemolytica* vaccines exist in either the United States

CFR or the European Pharmacopoeia, but the USDA test for *P. multocida* bacterins could be applied to *P. haemolytica* with the use of virulence enhancement. However, the relevance of the mouse test to protection is questionable, particularly for the pneumonic forms and, in view of the large number of strains included in many vaccines, it may be more realistic to accept a serological test of consistency without any particular claims to the measurement of efficacy.

Serological tests currently being developed by some manufacturers to detect antibodies directed against leukotoxins and other virulence factors offer a prospect of replacing the challenge tests with serological alternatives that are in fact relevant to protection, in the near future.

The United States CFR includes requirements for avian vaccines prepared from strains of *P. multocida* types 1, 3 and 4. In each case 21 birds of the target species are vaccinated with the recommended dose and revaccinated three weeks later. After 14 days of observation, 20 of the vaccinated birds and ten unvaccinated controls are challenged with a virulent culture of an appropriate specified strain: X-73 for type 1, P-105 for type 3 and P-1662 for type 4. The numbers of birds dying during the 14 days following challenge are recorded. At least eight of the ten control birds must die for a test to be valid. If six or fewer of the 20 vaccinates die, the vaccine passes. If nine or more die the vaccine fails. If seven, eight or nine die the test is repeated and if the total number of vaccinates dying in both tests is 15 or fewer out of 40, the vaccine passes.

Erysipelas vaccines

Both United States and European requirements include potency tests in which the responses of three groups of mice receiving graded doses of the vaccine under test are compared with those of mice receiving three similar doses of a standard preparation. However, the European test has several advantages. The standard used is the WHO International Standard for swine erysipelas vaccine or a laboratory preparation that has been calibrated against it. This allows vaccines to be standardized on an international basis. The United States test is similar in structure to that for mammalian strains of *P. multocida* described above and does not yield a truly quantitative estimate of potency. The European test, from similar numbers of animals but using statistical methods such as parallel line probit analysis, can provide relatively precise estimates of potency.

Three groups of 16 mice are vaccinated subcutaneously with 0.5 ml of three graded dilutions of the test vaccine on a fivefold range (dilutions of 1/5, 1/25 and 1/125 are suggested). Similarly, three further groups of mice, which have been randomly allocated from the same population, are vaccinated with three similarly graded doses of the standard preparation (0.2, 1 and 5 units are suggested). Ten mice from the same population are retained as unvaccinated controls. After 21 days all the mice are challenged intraperitoneally with enough of a virulent culture to kill the unvaccinated controls in three days. The proportion of mice surviving challenge by eight days in each treatment group is counted and the proportions used to calculate the potency of the test vaccine relative to the standard by a suitable statistical method such as parallel line probit analysis. No formal requirements of parallelism or linearity are required, but normal statistical requirements of validity are usually easy to satisfy. The vaccine passes if the estimate of potency exceeds 50 units per dose for swine.

Although the above test is statistically more satisfactory than many potency assays there is some evidence that it does not reflect the ability of vaccines to protect swine against percutaneous challenge very accurately. The United States version of the test is very similar in principle and therefore unlikely to be more reflective of efficacy in swine.

Brucella vaccines

No requirements for inactivated *Brucella abortus* vaccines are included in the United States CFR, but a monograph in the British Pharmacopoeia specifies a challenge potency test in guinea pigs.

Inject 12 or more guinea pigs intramuscularly with one-tenth of the cattle dose. (If the vaccine is formulated as a water-in-oil emulsion do not attempt to dilute it.) Set aside six or more unvaccinated controls from the same population. After 40 days, inoculate the vaccinated guinea pigs and six unvaccinated controls intramuscularly with a suspension containing 5 000 organisms of a suitable CO_2-dependent strain of *B. abortus* (strain 544 grown in trypticase soy broth containing 5 percent equine serum may be suitable). The virulence of the suspension should be sufficient to produce a 50 percent infective dose (ID_{50}) in guinea pigs with fewer than 100 organisms. Thirty-five days after challenge weigh and kill the vaccinated and control guinea pigs and aseptically remove the spleen from each animal. Weigh each spleen and homogenize the tissue in casamino acids solution. Inoculate a volume of homogenized suspension corresponding to 0.05 g of spleen into a suitable medium and incubate at 37°C for four days.

The vaccine is satisfactory if the following criteria are satisfied:

- viable *B. abortus* organisms of the challenge strain are present in all the spleen suspensions from control animals but in not more than 25 percent of those from vaccinates;
- The mean weight of spleens in the vaccinated animals expressed as a percentage of total body weight is not more than 0.3 percent;
- the geometric mean serum agglutination titre of the vaccinated animals 35 days after challenge is not more than 600.

Care should be taken to avoid accidental self-inoculation with oil-emulsion vaccines. The process of extraction and homogenization of spleens infected with the virulent challenge culture is potentially hazardous and these manipulations should be performed in safety cabinets with barriers to contain sudden spurts of infectious material, as well as the aerosols generated during homogenization.

Although the above test is lengthy and costly to perform, it is the best available index of potency for a vaccine against which serological responses are notoriously unreliable.

Parallel test methods may be applied to other inactivated *Brucella* vaccines.

LIVE VACCINES

A minority of bacterial vaccines consist of suspensions of live organisms whose virulence has been reduced to permit their safe administration to the target species.

Routine potency tests in laboratory animals are not generally appropriate for such preparations. Potency is better guaranteed by the careful evaluation of the protective efficacy of vaccine prepared from a master seed strain in the target species and careful control of the numbers of bacteria in serials produced from it. The United States CFR uses a set formula in the majority of its requirements for the control of potency of live bacterial vaccines. This entails the adoption of a strict seed lot system in which no more than five subcultures are permitted between the final product and the master seed lot. This is supported by the performance of a challenge test in the target species every three years to show that a pilot batch, containing a carefully determined number of organisms derived from the master seed, is able to protect the target species.

If the number of organisms in the pilot batch is insufficient to attain the required level of protection a further pilot batch containing more organisms may be prepared and tested. If a master seed continues in use for more than three years, new pilot batches must be prepared and tested at three-year intervals. Further batches prepared from the same master seed can then be released on evidence that the viable count is high enough to ensure that twice the number of organisms shown to be protective in the original potency test will be present until the expiry date.

Bacterial counts on the pilot batch should be performed in five replicates using dilutions that ensure that between 30 and 300 colonies appear on each plate. Counts for the release of serials should be performed in duplicate. The test methods prescribed for five vaccine classes in the United States CFR are summarized in Table 19.

Some living bacterial vaccines, however, do not multiply in the host but consist rather of a mass of preformed antigens, which may incorporate adjuvants and are more similar to killed preparations.

Live *Pasteurella* vaccines

There are no European or British requirements for live *Pasteurella* vaccines. The tests in the United States CFR are based on the formula described above. The main test parameters and criteria of acceptance for the three vaccine classes specified in the requirements are summarized in Table 18. In contrast to tests on killed vaccines, vaccinates and controls must be housed separately.

Pilot batches prepared from new seed lots of *P. multocida* for bovines are used to vaccinate calves that are challenged by a

Table 19

Potency tests for live bacterial vaccines in the United States

	Pasteurella multocida		*P. haemolytica*	Anthrax	Erysipelas
	Bovine	Avian	Bovine		
Animals used Vaccinated Control	 10 calves 5 calves	 20 birds 10 birds	 10 calves 5 calves	 30 guinea pigs 12 guinea pigs	 20 swine 10 swine
Days to challenge	14 to 21	14 or more	14 to 21	14 to 15	14 to 21
Challenge strain	Virulent pneumonic	Virulent *P. multocida*	Virulent pneumonic	Virulent for guinea pig	Virulent strain
Route of challenge	Respiratory	Intramuscular	Respiratory	Subcutaneous	Not stated
Evaluation	Symptom scores 4 to 10 days post challenge	Survival for 14 days post challenge	Symptom scores 4 to 7 days post challenge	Survival for 10 days post challenge	Symptoms and pyrexia over 7 days post challenge
Acceptance criteria	Vaccinate score significantly better than control ($P < 0.05$)	> 7 controls die, > 13 vaccinates survive	Vaccinate score significantly better than control	> 9 controls die, > 26 vaccinates survive	> 79% controls affected > 89% vaccinates clear

respiratory route, such as aerosol or tracheal instillation, with a virulent culture preferably of a local isolate of *P. multocida*. Resistance to challenge is evaluated by a numerical scoring system. The score should take account of the extent and severity of lung lesions and whether the animal dies. It may also take account of post challenge symptoms, but the importance assigned to these observations should be much less than that assigned to mortality and lung pathology. Surviving calves are killed painlessly after a fixed interval within the range of four to ten days post challenge. The extent and severity of lung lesions are assessed in these animals and in any animals that may have died and a numeric score is assigned to each animal. The mean scores for the vaccinate and control groups should be compared statistically using Student's "t" test. For the pilot vaccine to satisfy the requirements of the test, the mean score for the controls must be significantly greater than for the vaccinates.

New seed lots of *P. haemolytica* type 1 for bovines are tested by a similar procedure. The interval from vaccination to challenge by the respiratory route with a pneumonic strain of *P. haemolytica* is the same but the symptoms among the control animals are not expected to include pyrexia and surviving calves should be killed earlier – between four and seven days after challenge.

Live *P. multocida* vaccines for birds are tested by similar methods. If more than one species of bird is indicated on the label, the efficacy of a pilot batch prepared from each new master seed lot must be demonstrated in each of them. The potency test conforms to the formula described above and the main test characteristics and criteria are summarized in Table 19. The challenge culture should be of a virulent avian strain, preferably of local origin. If the pilot batch fails to meet this requirement, another batch containing more bacteria may be prepared and tested for potency (and safety).

Bacillus anthracis vaccine

Potency tests for living anthrax vaccines based on challenge are included in both United States and European requirements. However, the United States CFR relies on a spore count for the release of final vaccine and only requires a potency test when new master seed lots are introduced, whereas the European Pharmacopoeia requires a potency test on every lot of final vaccine. The difference may perhaps be explained by the inclusion of adjuvants in some European vaccines. It follows that the United States test is suitable for the control of monovalent vaccines that contain no adjuvant whereas the European method is more suitable for vaccines containing other antigens, adjuvants or other components capable of modifying the immune response elicited by a given number of spores.

The United States CFR requires that new master seed lots are tested for potency by a method based on the formula that has already been discussed. The test differs from other formula-based tests in that large guinea pigs each weighing 400 to 500 g are used instead of animals of the target species. Since the test is carried out in this species the challenge strain does not have to be virulent for sheep. The Pasteur vaccine strain is therefore recommended. Although the requirement specifies that the challenge dose should contain 4 500 LD_{50} doses, it allows two out of 12 survivors among the controls and is therefore less severe than the European requirement.

Although the number of spores in each batch of vaccine prepared from the master seed is determined from the number present in the pilot batch there is an overriding requirement that the number of spores should not in any case be less than 2 million per dose. The number of spores is verified by direct count on every batch of final vaccine.

The European requirements make provision for vaccine strains of three levels of virulence. Mild strains, such as the Sterne strain, which are harmless to guinea pigs and mice are tested for potency in guinea pigs. Intermediate strains which are lethal for guinea pigs but harmless for rabbits are tested in rabbits and less attenuated strains which kill a proportion of rabbits must be tested in the target species. The following method relates to vaccines prepared from the Sterne strain, but the numbers prescribed are the same for each test species. The potency test is performed on every lot of final bulk vaccine or on each filling lot.

Ten guinea pigs are inoculated subcutaneously with the minimum dose prescribed on the label for sheep and observed for 21 days. If more than two of the guinea pigs die from non-specific causes, the test is repeated. After 21 days, the vaccinates are challenged with 100 LD_{50} of a strain of *Bacillus anthracis* that is virulent for the test species used and three unvaccinated controls are challenged with 10 LD_{50} of the same preparation. For guinea pigs the Pasteur vaccine strain is sufficiently virulent and less hazardous to operators and the environment than fully virulent strains.

The test is valid if all the control animals die within ten days. The vaccine passes the test if all of the vaccinates survive for ten days. If one vaccinate dies the test may be repeated but all the vaccinates must survive in the repeat test.

A bacterial count is performed on every batch to confirm that the count stated on the label is valid.

Live swine erysipelas vaccine

Potency requirements for live swine erysipelas vaccines are included in the United States CFR. The outline of the requirements conforms to the formula already applied to anthrax and live *Pasteurella* vaccines.

Potency test variables are summarized in Table 19. Since body temperature is an important index of protection, the body temperature of the vaccinates and of ten unvaccinated controls are measured daily for 14 to 21 days to establish a baseline. All 30 swine are then challenged with a virulent culture of *Erysipelothrix rhusiopathiae*. A suitable culture is available from the United States Animal and Plant Inspection Service. The animals are observed for seven days post challenge during which time at least 80 percent of the controls must register a temperature greater than 105.6°F (40.9°C) on two consecutive days and also show typical signs of infection such as hyperaemia of ears and abdomen, moribundness, skin lesions, depression, arthritis or death, in a valid test. If at least 90 percent of the vaccinates remain free of the above signs, with body temperatures remaining below 104.6°F (40.2°C), the master seed lot is satisfactory.

Live *Brucella abortus* (strain 19) vaccine

No test of efficacy is required for strain 19 vaccine released in the United States where potency is assured by viable count determinations alone with minimum requirements of 3×10^9 and 3×10^{10} live organisms per dose for reduced and standard dose formulations, respectively. These are supported by requirements that no more than 5 percent of the colonies obtained when the vaccine is plated on potato agar should be frankly rough and no more than 15 percent, in total, deviant from typical smooth colony morphology.

It is suggested that any laboratory producing strain 19 vaccine outside the United States should verify the efficacy of its product by the European Pharmacopoeia method described below whenever a new master seed is adopted and in any case at intervals of not less than three years.

The requirements for strain 19 vaccine in the European Pharmacopoeia include a potency test in which 12 guinea pigs are vaccinated intramuscularly with one-fifteenth of the calf dose of the test vaccine in 1 ml. After an interval of not less than 40 days, the vaccinates, together with six unvaccinated controls, are challenged with a virulent CO_2-dependent strain of *B. abortus*, such as strain 544. (1 LD_{50} of the challenge suspension should contain no more than 100 organisms.) After a further 35 days, the animals are weighed and killed. The spleen of each animal is weighed and then emulsified and a volume of suspension equivalent to 0.05 g of spleen is inoculated into a suitable medium such as trypticase-soy, containing 2 to 5 percent equine serum. The inoculated medium is incubated for four days at 37°C. The test is valid if the spleens of all the control animals are infected. The potency of the vaccine is satisfactory if 75 percent or more of the spleens from the vaccinated animals remain uninfected.

This potency test is supported by a viable count requirement of 4×10^{10} viable organisms per calf dose. The European requirement is thus far more stringent than the United States one in this case.

Live *Salmonella dublin* and *Salmonella cholerae suis* vaccines

Monographs for live vaccines against both *Salmonella dublin* and *S. cholerae suis* in the British Pharmacopoeia do not include any potency test and rely entirely on viable count. These monographs have been written for a single specific strain in each case and the required viable count of 2.5×10^9 organisms per dose would not necessarily be appropriate for other strains. Laboratories preparing vaccines from other strains would be advised to adopt the formula used by the United States CFR and maintain a strict seed lot system supported by efficacy tests on pilot batches produced from each new master seed to validate release on the basis of bacterial count alone.

Other live bacterial vaccines

It is recommended that the formula applied by the United States CFR should be adopted as a guiding principle in the evaluation of potency in live vaccines for which no compendial requirement exists.

BIBLIOGRAPHY

British Pharmacopoeia Commission. 1985. *British Pharmacopoeia (veterinary).* London, Her Majesty's Stationery Office.

European Pharmacopoeia Commission. 1985. *European Pharmacopoeia.* 2nd edition. Sainte-Ruffine, France, Maisonneuve.

Reed, L.J. & Muench, H. 1938. A simple method of estimating the 50 percent end point. *Amer. J. Hyg.*, 27: 493-496.

Toothill, J.P.R., Robinson, W.D. & Adams, A.G. 1969. *Precalculated ED_{50}, PD_{50} and LD_{50} statistics.* Symposium Series in Immunobiological Standardisation, Vol. 10, p. 183-220. Basel, Switzerland, Karger.

USDA. 1994. *Animals and animal products.* CFR title 9. Animal and Plant Health Inspection Service, United States Department of Agriculture.

WHO. *Manual of test methods for diphtheria, tetanus and pertussis vaccines.* World Health Organization (Biologicals Division), Geneva, Switzerland.

WHO. *Requirements for diphtheria, tetanus, pertussis and combined vaccines.* Technical report series 800, World Health Organization, Geneva, Switzerland.

Potency control of modified live viral vaccines

C. Terpstra[1]

Since Pasteur's pioneering work on the attenuation of rabies virus by the serial passaging of "street" virus in rabbit brains and use of the "fixed" virus in animals and humans (1885), modified live viral (MLV) vaccines have been developed against a vast number of viral diseases of humans and animals.

The development of most viral vaccines, however, did not begin until the introduction and large-scale use of tissue culture techniques at the end of the 1940s when antibiotics became available. Until recently, MLV vaccines were obtained in much the same way as in Pasteur's time, i.e. by multiple passages in cell cultures, embryonated eggs or in another animal species to which the virus is not naturally adapted. After a certain number of passages the virus is tested for vaccine efficacy and safety. Using this rather empirical approach, a number of highly efficacious vaccines have been developed. For example the cell culture-adapted Kabete O strain against rinderpest received over 90 passages in bovine kidney cells (Plowright and Ferris, 1962) and the so-called Chinese strain (C strain) of swine fever virus over 800 passages in rabbits (Lin and Lee, 1981). Both vaccines are highly immunogenic and safe. A single vaccination with the Plowright vaccine protects for over ten years against a lethal challenge with virulent rinderpest virus (Plowright, 1984) and pigs vaccinated once with the C strain were fully protected against challenge with the virulent Brescia strain of swine fever virus five to six years later (Terpstra, unpublished results).

Attenuation usually reflects the selection of certain variants already present in a heterogenous population of wild-type virus, a single-step mutation or a multistep mutation. This process of alteration can hardly be influenced and its results are largely unpredictable. A more accelerated approach, although with an equally unpredictable outcome, is physical or chemical mutagenesis. Examples of the first category are the temperature-sensitive mutants used in some vaccines against virus-associated respiratory disease. A promising example of chemical mutagenesis is the serially mutagenized MV P12 variant of Rift Valley fever virus (Morill *et al.*, 1987; Hubbard, Baskerville and Stephenson, 1991).

Conventional vaccines are to a certain extent developed by "trial and error" procedures, although modern biotechnology has created tools for the well-defined engineering of vaccines. The design of such vaccines, however, requires knowledge of the nature of immunogens, the mechanisms underlying virulence and immunity and the mapping of non-essential virulence genes. Examples of MLV "biotech" vaccines are deletion mutant vaccines and vector vaccines. The latter category uses vaccinia or other poxviruses, herpesviruses and perhaps in the future also adeno- or other viruses as carriers and expression

[1] The author would like to thank A. Dekker and A.H. Kroese for statistical assistance and T.G. Kimman for critical reading of the manuscript.

systems of genes from heterologous microorganisms that code for immunizing proteins.

Without the systematic use of vaccines against, for example, foot-and-mouth disease (FMD), rinderpest and swine fever it would have been impossible to control these diseases, let alone eradicate some of them from certain regions of the world. Indeed, vaccination has become one of the most cost-effective forms of veterinary health care.

Vaccines, whether developed conventionally or constructed by biotechnological means, must be evaluated for efficacy and safety before being released to the field.

The production of MLV vaccines should be based on a seed lot system. A stock of master seed virus is produced and all batches of vaccine are prepared from this within a limited number of passages. The master seed virus is subjected to extensive testing to ensure that it is immunogenic, sterile and free from extraneous viruses, as well as from pathogenic and, where applicable, oncogenic effects. A seed lot system offers the advantage that efficacy tests and, if necessary, safety tests on each batch of vaccine can be limited. In general, the minimum requirements for safety seem to be better defined and more severe than those for efficacy. The primary and ultimate goal of a vaccine, however, is to be efficacious.

This chapter describes various aspects of efficacy, *in vivo* and *in vitro* assays for determining the potency of vaccines and criteria for assessing the endurance of immunity and the value of field trials.

ASPECTS OF EFFICACY

Vaccine efficacy can be defined as the degree to which a vaccine induces a protective immunity in the target host. In most viral diseases a natural infection induces a strong and long-lasting protective immunity against reinfection and, particularly, stimulates immunological memory. Ideally an MLV vaccine simulates the natural infection without causing disease. However, there is no such thing as a perfect vaccine. A vaccine that is completely safe cannot usually induce as strong an immunity as the natural infection.

In descending order of value, the following levels of protection can be distinguished in vaccinated animals:

i) prevention of the initiation of a primary infection;
ii) reduction of virus replication at the site of entry;
iii) prevention or reduction of virus spread to other critical tissues such as blood;
iv) prevention of the virus shedding into the environment;
v) prevention or reduction of transmission of the virus to contact animals;
vi) prevention of the development of clinical disease;
vii) prevention or reduction of economic losses.

In addition: the offspring of vaccinated animals should be protected against intrauterine or post-natal infection; and immunity after one vaccination should be long-lasting, preferably throughout the economic life span of the animal.

Many vaccines offer clinical protection against disease (level vi) above) but do not (completely) prevent virus multiplication and shedding on exposure of the animal. The protection level a vaccine must primarily provide differs according to the disease and also depends on the aim of vaccination and whether an eradication policy is to be pursued or not.

The following examples illustrate these points:

- Because porcine parvovirus is only harmful to foetuses before the seventieth day of gestation, an efficacious vaccine must prevent the transmission of parvovirus from the sow to foetuses during that period.

- Persistent infections with bovine viral diarrhoea (BVD) virus, owing to transplacental transmission, play a key role in the pathogenesis, clinical manifestation and epizootiology of BVD. Thus, an efficacious BVD vaccine must primarily prevent viraemia and, in consequence, must ensure that no congenitally BVD-infected calves are born.
- Preventing viraemia after exposure to field virus or decreasing its level below the threshold required to infect the invertebrate host must also be the primary protective requirements of all vaccines against vector transmitted diseases such as Rift Valley fever, African horse sickness and bluetongue.
- Vaccination of pigs against Aujeszky's disease (AD) has been practised widely for decades. At first, the aim was to produce high antibody titres in sows because piglets, which are the most susceptible group, had to be protected; later when clinical AD occurred in finishing herds the prime goal was to protect the fattening pig from developing severe growth retardation when infected with field virus. For these purposes, vaccines offering protection level vii) sufficed. The change of policy in some countries to a combined vaccination and eradication programme for AD not only required the use of serological "marker" vaccines but also the selection of vaccines that prevent the establishment of latency after infection (Kimman, 1992) and reduce the average number of secondary cases per infectious individual (i.e. the basic reproduction ratio R_o) below unity (De Jong and Kimman, 1994).

In general, vaccination campaigns launched to eradicate a disease, whether in combination with serological methods or otherwise, must utilize vaccines that are able to break the animal-to-animal transmission of field virus. Vaccination must, therefore, prevent or at least reduce virus shedding to the extent that the transmission of virus to contacts is impeded (levels iv) and v)). Examples of vaccines that have proved to be effective in arresting the transmission of field virus after exposure of the vaccinated host are the cell culture-attenuated Kabete O strain of rinderpest virus (Plowright, 1984) and the Chinese strain of swine fever virus (Terpstra and Wensvoort, 1988). Annual vaccination of cattle in the JP15 Rinderpest Campaign with the Plowright vaccine strain was successful in eradicating the disease in most East and West African countries (Lépissier and MacFarlane, 1966). In the Netherlands, classical swine fever has been eradicated from enzootic areas (where there is intensive pig farming) by systematic vaccination with C strain virus in combination with a "stamping out" policy (Terpstra, 1991).

BIOASSAYS TO ASSESS POTENCY

The potency of MLV vaccines can be determined *in vivo*, either in the target host or in a suitable laboratory animal model, or *in vitro*, the latter two options being derived parameters. Determination of potency *in vivo* may be based on assaying the 50 percent protective dose (PD_{50}), a titration of the virus or the serological response induced in either the target species or a laboratory animal model. To reduce the use of laboratory animals, efforts should be made to replace *in vivo* titration of vaccine virus – usually by intracerebral inoculation of baby mice – by titration in a suitable cell culture system.

PD_{50} assay on master seed virus

Production of MLV vaccines should be based on a seed lot system and, as regards efficacy, the relation between virus content of the vaccine dose and the resulting protection in the target species should be determined at least once in the history of a master seed virus. The dose-response relationship may be determined on a sample of the master seed or on a representative derivative.

For a quantitative dose-response analysis, groups of target animals are given graded doses of vaccine virus and challenged thereafter with a standard dose of virulent virus, preferably administered via a natural route. The virus dosages used for vaccination should be calculated on the basis of the geometric mean titre of at least five replicate virus titrations in a suitable cell culture system or in embryonated eggs.

To obtain meaningful results, 100 percent of the unvaccinated controls should respond to the challenge. For this reason it is common practice to use an overdose of challenge virus, usually 10^3 to 10^5 50 percent infective doses (ID_{50}). The aim of the dose-response analysis is to estimate the median protective dose (PD_{50}), the 95 percent protective dose (PD_{95}) or other aspects of the dose-response curve. The PD_{50} is the vaccine virus dose that protects 50 percent of the vaccinated animals. Using an infinite number of doses (and therefore animals), the dose-response relationship would follow approximately a symmetrical sigmoid curve. This empirical fact often leads to the so-called logistic regression or probit analysis as a satisfactory statistical method for the estimation of the PD_{50} value. For ethical as well as cost reasons, the number of target animals available for a PD_{50} experiment will be limited. It is important therefore to design the experiment in such a way that an optimal estimate of the dose-response curve is obtained.

The following aspects should be considered in designing a dose-response experiment:

- At least two doses should result in a partial response (i.e. neither 0 percent or 100 percent of the animals receiving these doses should respond to the challenge) otherwise an invalid estimate of the dose-response curve is obtained.
- Doses providing less than 50 percent and more than 50 percent protection are essential for estimating an accurate PD_{50}.
- If the requirement is to estimate the PD_{95} – the dose providing 95 percent protection which is to be aimed at in the field – care should be taken to assure that some groups receive doses high enough to ensure complete protection, otherwise the curve has to be extrapolated in the upper region, which on the basis of a sigmoid curve leads to large statistical uncertainties.
- Doses providing 0 percent protection are less critical and not strictly necessary.
- Care should be taken that the majority of the responses are not located in the extreme lower or extreme upper part of the curve as this would not be an efficient way of using the available animals.

The natural quantitative criteria to be satisfied are:

- the mean squared error of the PD_{95} should be minimal;
- the mean squared error of the PD_{50} should be minimal;
- the number of times that an unreliable estimate is found (i.e. all doses used in the experiment are smaller than that of the estimated PD_{95}) should be minimal.

The dilution range to be covered may be assessed in a pilot experiment using tenfold dilutions and one or two animals per group. The optimal design of the ultimate experiment depends on a priori knowledge of the curve and on the specific quantitative criteria aimed for. Computer simulations can be carried out, using a varying number of doses and varying numbers of animals per dose to see how well the different designs perform with regard to the quantitative criteria mentioned above. The simulations are based on the parameters of the curve as estimated in the pilot experiment. In general, it is advised to use five or six different doses and 3.2-fold (0.5 log) dilutions as this provides a compromise among different objectives and makes it possible to test the model. A useful review of the literature on the subject can be found in Chapter 8 of Morgan (1992). The best-fitting curve of a dose-response experiment can be determined by computer, using a probit or, easier to use, logit analysis. If a logistic regression model is chosen, the dose providing "100p" percent effective protection (PD_{100p}) can be calculated according to the following formula:

$$PD_{100p} = e^{a - \frac{\left[\ln\left(\frac{1}{p} - 1\right)\right]}{b}}$$

in which "a" stands for the natural logarithm of the dilution giving 50 percent protection, "b" for the slope of the curve and "p" for the protected fraction.

Parameter "a" (PD_{50}) determines the place of the curve, whereas parameter "b" determines its shape. The higher the value of "a" the higher the PD_{50} and the less potent the vaccine, while the higher the value of "b" the steeper the curve. Figure 18 illustrates a dose response function with "a" = -3.117 and "b" = 1.511. Standard deviations of "a" and "b" can also be calculated from one dose-response curve.

The above formula allows the calculation of the dose for each protection level wanted. For example the dose providing 95 percent protection in the PD_{50} experiment represented by the curve in Figure 18 equals:

$$e^{-3.117 - \frac{\left[\ln\left(\frac{1}{0.95} - 1\right)\right]}{1.511}} \qquad e^{-3.1}$$

$$= e^{-3.117 + 1.9486} = e^{-1.168} = 0.31 \qquad e^{-3.1}$$

In this example one PD_{50} ($e^{-3.117}$) equals 0.044.

The unit to be used in expressing the PD_{50} value will depend on the most reproducible titration system available for a particular pathogen, for example plaque-forming units, tissue culture infective units and egg infective units.

In principle, a dose-response curve can be determined for any of the vaccine efficacy levels i) to vii) discussed on p. 382. For reasons of easy and quantifiable measurement, physical signs of disease such as fever, viraemia or viral excretion are the parameters chosen most often in allocating individual animals to "protected" or "susceptible" categories after challenge.

The PD_{50} and the relationship between protection and vaccine virus dose obtained in a dose-response analysis are only valid for the conditions applied in that particular test. The outcome therefore may not be extrapolated to another master seed virus, another animal breed with a different susceptibility for the pathogen, a different target species or a different vaccination or challenge route. A dose response analysis is performed only occasionally, for example when the manufacturer changes to another virus strain or when a new master seed has been produced.

The protection observed in a properly performed vaccination challenge experiment in the target species should be regarded as the sole primary parameter of immunity. Any other parameter having an established correlation with the primary parameter and used to measure immunity should be regarded as secondary. Examples of secondary parameters are: protection obtained in non-target (laboratory) animals, *in vitro* infectivity titre of vaccine virus and level of antibody provoked in the target species.

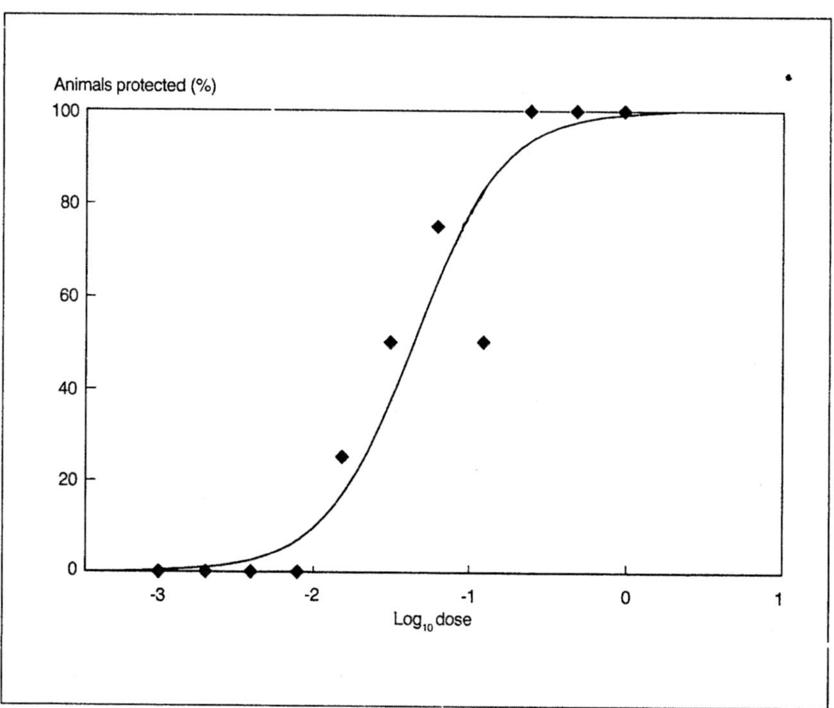

FIGURE 18
Dose-response relation using 11 groups of four animals (a = 3.117 and b = 1.511)

Calculated versus observed PD_{50}. By definition 1 PD_{50} protects 50 percent of the animals vaccinated. It follows that a vaccine containing a calculated 100 PD_{50} per dose protects 50 percent ($p = 0.5$) of "*n*" animals when used at a dilution of 1:100 ("*n*" = large number). When testing a random sample of, say, ten animals vaccinated with a 1:100 dilution, the probabilities of finding nought, one, two, etc. up to ten animals protected are binomially distributed (Table 20).

The probability of each outcome "z" can be calculated according to the formula:

$$\text{probability} = \binom{n}{z} \times p^{z} \times (1 - p)^{n-z}$$

in which: "n" = sample size (10 in the example) and "p" = protected fraction (0.5 in the example).

The probability that fewer than five animals are protected is the sum of the probabilities of finding nought, one, two, three and four protected animals, which equals 0.37695 (Table 20). The probability, therefore, that the batch fails to pass the test is 37.7 percent, despite the fact that one dose contains 1 PD_{50} in the dilution tested. A vaccine producer therefore has to incorporate more than the calculated 100 PD_{50} per dose to increase the probability that the PD_{50} as observed by the controlling authority meets the requirements.

In order to obtain, say, 90 percent confidence that the batch will pass the potency test the sum of probabilities to find fewer than four animals protected should be ≤0.1. By using the above formula in a spreadsheet model, a value of 0.1 for this sum of probabilities is obtained when "p" = 0.6458. This means that the manufacturer has to safeguard a protected fraction of 0.65 per dose instead of 0.5. The dose providing 65 percent protection depends on the shape of the dose-response curve and can be calculated with the logit formula. In the example of the dose-response curve shown in Figure 18, the PD_{65} = 0.0667, which is 1.52 times the 0.044 required for 1 PD_{50}. The producer should therefore incorporate at least 152 PD_{50} per dose in order to be 90 percent certain that the vaccine batch will pass the potency test requirements.

Potency tests on vaccine batches

Unlike inactivated vaccines, which require an *in vivo* potency test on each batch, the PD_{50} of an MLV vaccine is assessed only

TABLE 20

Calculation of the probability distribution of the number of protected animals in a random sample of ten out of a population vaccinated with 1 PD_{50} per animal

Number protected in random sample (*z*)	Possibilities	Probability
0	1	0.000977
1	10	0.009766
2	45	0.043945
3	120	0.117188
4	210	0.205078
5	252	0.246094
6	210	0.205078
7	120	0.117188
8	45	0.043945
9	10	0.009766
10	1	0.000977
Σ	**1 024**	**1.000002**

once on the master seed virus or a representative vaccine batch of the virus seed. The potency of subsequent batches prepared from the master seed can be based on the relation between virus dose and protection as observed in the dose-response curve. A titration of the vaccine virus, therefore, according to the method used in determining the dosage titre in the dose-response analysis, enables the calculation of the required infectivity per dose, thus ensuring a certain degree of protection.

Subject to the regulations of the appropriate national authority, a limited *in vivo* test may be required for each batch or may be omitted as a routine control if the final product, after reconstitution, contains per dose not less than the quantity of virus that conferred an accepted degree of protection in a potency test on the master seed. Whatever the method, a general rule is that a protection test is required for each vaccination route recommended by the manufacturer and for each strain incorporated in the vaccine when different virus strains are combined.

Tests in the target species

A commonly used procedure for estimating the potency of a vaccine batch *in vivo* involves two groups of target animals, one being vaccinated and the other serving as a control. After a certain immunization period the animals of both groups are challenged with a highly virulent virus strain by an appropriate route.

The degree of protection of the vaccinated animals is measured by comparing their reactions with those of the controls. The number of animals used, their age, the interval between vaccination and challenge, the challenge dose and the route differ from vaccine to vaccine, and so do the criteria for an acceptable degree of protection such as signs of disease, height and duration of virus excretion and growth retardation. Table 21 lists some specifications from the published monographs of the European Pharmacopoeia for potency tests of batches of MLV vaccines for farm animals.

An alternative procedure for estimating potency in the target species is based on determing the antibody titre in the serum of vaccinated animals. The response of usually neutralizing or haemagglutination-inhibiting antibody is measured according to a standard method, using positive and negative reference preparations as controls. The reliability of serological methods depends on an established correlation between humoral antibody and protection. It goes without saying that the procedure is less satisfactory as the vaccine-induced protection is more dependent on mucosal or cellular immunity.

Tests in laboratory animals

Whereas potency testing in laboratory animals is common practice in human vaccine production, it is the exception in veterinary vaccines. The use of laboratory animals, however, may be indicated when the costs of testing in the target species are prohibitive, when non-immune target animals are difficult to obtain or when alternative methods for quantifying the vaccine virus are lacking. Examples of each category are equine vaccines, vaccines against arthropod-transmitted diseases, which may be widespread in an animal population, and the C strain of swine fever virus.

Potency estimations of vaccines against vector-borne diseases may be made in mice and potency estimations of the C strain by titrating the vaccine virus in rabbits. For example 1 PD_{50} of the C strain virus for pigs corresponds to approximately 4 ID_{50} for rabbits (Biront and Leunen, 1988). The potency of rabies vaccines for domesticated animals and wildlife is also estimated in mice, which are analogous to human rabies

TABLE 21

Specifications from the European Pharmacopoeia for potency tests of MLV vaccines for farm animals

Specifications	IBR fowlpox	AD	CSF	AIB	Vaccine against AIE		IBD	NCD	MD
E.P. monograph No.	696	745	65	442	588	587	450	589	649
Year of publication	1990	1991	1983	1985	1988	1988	1989	1994	1989
Animal species	Cattle	Pigs	Pigs	Chickens	Chickens	Chickens	Chickens	Chickens	Chickens
Age/weight	2-3 mo.	15-35 kg	6 wks	min.	3 wks	min.	min.	1day	n.sp.
No. vaccinated animals	5	≥5	2 x 5	≥20	≥20	≥20	≥20	≥30	≥20
No. control animals	2	5	2	10	20	20	10	30	20
Challenge at days after vaccination	21	21	14	21	28	14	14-21	9	21
Challenge route	i.n.	i.n.	i.m.	i.tr.	i.c.	i.o.	i.m.	n.sp.	i.d./i.f.
Observation period (days)	21	7	14	7	21	10	10	70	21
Criterion	Virus excretion	Av. daily weight gain	100 PD_{50}/ dose	≤20 % no virus excretion	≥80% no signs of disease	≥90% no severe bursal lesions	≥90% no signs of disease	≥80% reduction of spec. lesions	≥90% no signs of disease

AIE = avian infectious encephalomyelitis;
AD = Aujeszky's disease;
AIB = avian infectious bronchitis;
CSF = classical swine fever;
IBD = infectious bursal disease (Gumboro);
IBR = infectious bovine rhinotracheitis;
MD = Marek's disease;
NCD = Newcastle disease;

i.c. = intracerebral;
i.d. = intradermal;
i.f. = intrafollicular;
i.o. = intraocular;
i.m. = intramuscular;
i.n. = intranasal;
n.sp. = not specified;
i.tr. = intratracheal;
min. = minimum age as specified for vaccination;
mo. = months.

vaccines (WHO, 1984). A requisite for all these tests is that a good correlation has been obtained between the response measured in laboratory animals and protection in the target species.

In vitro tests

An *in vitro* prediction of efficacy can be based on titrating the vaccine virus in a suitable cell culture system or in embryonated eggs. The relationship is partly explained by the fact that virus titre and the level of immunity induced in the target animal are both functions of virus replication. In this light, it is not surprising that the relationship between the 50 percent tissue culture infective dose ($TCID_{50}$) or the 50 percent median egg infective dose (EID_{50}), on the one hand, and PD_{50}, on the other, often approaches unity. For example, for cattle 1 PD_{50} of the cell culture-adapted Kabete O strain of rinderpest virus, at any passage level between 34 and 90, was virtually identical with 1 $TCID_{50}$ (Plowright and Ferris, 1962). Similarly, in pigs 1 PD_{50} of the cell culture-adapted C strain of swine fever virus equals 1.6 $TCID_{50}$ (Terpstra, Woortmeyer and Barteling, 1990) and 1 PD_{50} of the Turkey herpes virus strain of Marek's disease virus corresponds with four plaque-forming units (PFU) (Witter and Burmester, 1979). On the other hand, the PD_{50} of the cell-associated CVI 988 strain of Marek's disease virus was found to be about 40 PFU (De Boer *et al.*, 1981).

It is common practice, however, to use a wide safety margin to compensate for inaccuracy in titration, loss of titre during storage, inexact dosage, etc. For cell culture-adapted rinderpest and swine fever vaccines $10^{2.5}$ $TCID_{50}$ has been the norm. Each final lot of vaccine ready for use in the field should undergo a titration to verify that the infectivity contained in each dose is as expected. A standard reference virus preparation should be titrated in parallel to ensure that the *in vitro* test system employed is of uniform sensitivity.

With respect to infectivity, the European Pharmacopoeia generally requires that one dose of reconstituted vaccine contains not less than the expected amount of virus according to the minimum virus titre stated on the label or in the leaflet, and that this amount satisfies the criterion for potency acceptance of the product.

The United States Code of Federal Regulations (CFR) for animals and animal products (1993) generally requires that batches of MLV vaccines contain, at any time within the expiration period, a virus titre $10^{0.7}$ greater than the sample of master seed virus that provided an accepted level of protection in an animal potency test assessed by challenge.

The minimum requirements of the quantity of virus per dose are specified for the following vaccines:

- $10^{2.5}$ $TCID_{50}$: bovine para-influenza, infectious bovine rhinotracheitis, bovine virus diarrhoea, Aujeszky's disease, Venezuelan equine encephalitis;
- $10^{2.0}$ EID_{50}: fowl pox, avian infectious bronchitis;
- $10^{2.5}$ EID_{50}: avian infectious encephalomyelitis;
- $10^{2.5}$ EID_{50} or $10^{2.5}$ $TCID_{50}$: avian laryngotracheitis;
- $10^{5.5}$ EID_{50}: Newcastle disease;
- $10^{2.0}$ PFU or $10^{2.0}$ ID_{50}: infectious bursal disease, infectious tenosynovitis;
- $10^{3.0}$ PFU: Marek's disease.

Similar to the methods based on serology, the *in vitro* titration tests are not potency assays in the strict sense, since they merely ensure an adequate viability of the vaccine batch at a level similar to products that have been shown to be effective.

DURATION OF PROTECTION

In the previous sections, the efficacy of a MLV vaccine was determined on the basis of a vaccination challenge experiment in the target animal (i.e. a primary parameter) or on the basis of deduced (secondary) parameters. The results of a potency test are usually read two to three weeks after vaccination when immunity may be expected to be at its peak.

In principle, the endurance of protection claimed by the producer should be based on the successful outcome of a vaccination challenge experiment in the target animal made after a defined period of time. Important requisites for accepting the results are that the vaccine used in the duration experiment was of minimum potency and that a predetermined percentage of the vaccinates (usually 80 to 90 percent) passed the requirements of the challenge test.

The actual duration of immunity can be expected to be greater, since protection does not end at the time of challenge. For reasons of economy, the lack of facilities to accommodate experimental animals for prolonged periods of time or reductions in the usage of experimental animals, it may be justifiable to extend the anticipated duration of immunity by extrapolating from additional data obtained in the vaccination challenge experiment, for example the path of the antibody curve. Published data on the duration of immunity with a parent strain may also be extrapolated to an otherwise identical daughter strain of a higher passage level or a daughter strain adapted to grow on a different substrate. This is legitimate provided that the immunogenic relationship between primary and/or secondary parameters and protection remains unchanged in comparison with that of the parent strain, and that the frequency, interval and application route are also the same.

In addition to the use of a vaccine in a primary target species, a secondary related species (e.g. cattle/sheep; horse/donkey) or an unrelated species may also be involved. Age and interval of vaccination, antigen dose, PD_{50}, immune response and persistence of protection may all vary among species. As a consequence, the extrapolation of data concerning the duration of immunity in the primary species to a secondary species is not justified without a successful vaccination challenge experiment in the secondary species. However, when a positive correlation can be shown between protection – or the value of a secondary parameter such as serology – in the primary and the secondary target species, data obtained in the former species may be used to evaluate the effect of the vaccine in the latter species.

THE VALUE OF FIELD TRIALS

Veterinary vaccines are not only developed to control or eradicate a contagious disease, they should above all satisfy the farmer, who has the need to apply preventive measures against a certain agent for reasons of economy. The vaccine therefore should be efficacious not only in laboratory tests but also under field conditions.

Field trials are, however, accompanied by a number of difficulties:

- they require large numbers of animals, are difficult to monitor, are laborious and consequently expensive;
- as opposed to laboratory tests, in which only seronegative animals are used, animals vaccinated in field trials may possess, either actively or passively, acquired antibodies;
- the prevalence of the agent and, thus, the immune status may vary from farm to farm;
- other infections present on the farm may interfere with the development of immunity or may mask the clinical effects of vaccination;
- the effect of vaccination on the spread of field virus cannot be measured unless a marker vaccine with a com-

panion serological test is used to distinguish vaccine-induced antibodies from antibodies against field virus;

- the use of controls is hampered, because farmers are reluctant to accept that groups of animals should remain unprotected, and becomes virtually impossible (even with separate housing) when the vaccine virus spreads;
- a standardized challenge with a virulent strain of field virus is not acceptable.

In view of the above, field trials are often not undertaken. The omission, however, raises the question of whether it is justifiable to extrapolate from the results of laboratory tests to performance of the vaccine in the field.

The following are the conditions for a well-designed efficacy trial in the field as formulated by Pijpers and Verheijden (1991):

- a representative group of animals that remains unvaccinated or is given another vaccine must be included as a concurrent control;
- randomization, the process by which all animals are equally likely to be assigned to either the vaccination or the control group, is necessary to avoid bias;
- codification (i.e. the basis of a "blind" trial) is always desirable and is essential if subjective parameters such as the severity of clinical signs are used for evaluation;
- an adequate statistical analysis of the results is of paramount importance.

Furthermore, for a meaningful evaluation of the vaccine under field conditions it is essential that:

- the vaccine contains the minimum titre of potency per dose as specified by the producer;
- a natural challenge occurs during the observation period, preferably with a virulent virus strain.

As suggested by van Oirschot (1992), a workable compromise between assessing vaccine efficacy in the laboratory and in the field could be to vaccinate animals under field conditions, keep them with unvaccinated controls and, if they do not become infected, to subject both groups to a challenge infection in the laboratory. It should be emphasized that little value can be attached to field trials, which in essence do not comply with the requirements above.

BIBLIOGRAPHY

Biront, P. & Leunen, J. 1988. Vaccines. *In* B. Liess, ed. *Classical swine fever and related viral infections*, p. 181-200. Netherlands, M. Nijhoff.

De Boer, G.F., Orthel, F.W., Krasselt, M., Oei, H.L., Pereboom, W.J. & Barendregt, L.G. 1981. Comparative 50 percent protective dose assays (PD_{50}) of Marek's disease virus strain CVI 988. *J. Biol. Stand.*, 9: 15-22.

De Jong, M.C.M. & Kimman, T.G. 1994. Experimental quantification of vaccine-induced reduction in virus transmission. *Vaccine*, 12: 761-766.

European Pharmacopoeia Commission. 1983. Monograph 65. Sainte-Ruffine, France, Maisonneuve.

European Pharmacopoeia Commission. 1985. Monograph 442. Sainte-Ruffine, France, Maisonneuve.

European Pharmacopoeia Commission. 1988. Monograph 587. Sainte-Ruffine, France, Maisonneuve.

European Pharmacopoeia Commission. 1988. Monograph 588. Sainte-Ruffine, France, Maisonneuve.

European Pharmacopoeia Commission. 1989. Monograph 450. Sainte-Ruffine, France, Maisonneuve.

European Pharmacopoeia Commission. 1989. Monograph 649. Sainte-Ruffine, France, Maisonneuve.

European Pharmacopoeia Commission. 1990. Monograph 696. Sainte-Ruffine, France, Maisonneuve.

European Pharmacopoeia Commission. 1991. Monograph 745. Sainte-Ruffine, France, Maisonneuve.

European Pharmacopoeia Commission. 1994. Monograph 589. Sainte-Ruffine, France, Maisonneuve.

Hubbard, K.A., Baskerville, A. & Stephenson, J.R. 1991. Ability of a mutagenised virus variant to protect young lambs from Rift Valley fever. *Am. J. Vet. Res.*, 52: 50-55.

Kimman, T.G. 1992. Acceptability of Aujeszky's disease vaccines. *Develop. Biol. Stand.*, 79: 129-136.

Lépissier, H.E. & MacFarlane, I.M. 1966. Organization of African Unity. Scientific, Technical and Research Commission Joint Campaign against Rinderpest. Phase I, Final Report. *Bull. Epizoot. Dis. Afr.*, 14: 193-224.

Lin, T.T.C. & Lee, R.C.T. 1981. An overall report on the development of a highly safe and potent lapinized hog cholera virus strain for hog cholera control in Taiwan. *Nat. Sci. Council Spec. Publ.*, 5: 1-44.

Morgan, B.J.T. 1992. *Analysis of quantal response data.* London, Chapman & Hall.

Morill, J.C., Jennings, G.B., Caplen, H., Turell, M.J. & Johnson, A.J. 1987. Pathogenicity and immunogenicity of a mutagen-attenuated Rift Valley fever immunogen in pregnant ewes. *Am. J. Vet. Res.*, 48: 1042-1047.

Pijpers, A. & Verheijden, J.H.M. 1991. Guidelines for the evaluation of clinical efficacy. *Acta Vet. Scand., Suppl.*, 87: 315-317.

Plowright, W. 1984. The duration of immunity in cattle following inoculation of rinderpest cell culture vaccine. *J. Hyg. (Camb.)*, 92: 285-296.

Plowright, W. & Ferris, R.D. 1962. Studies with rinderpest virus in tissue culture. The use of attenated culture virus as a vaccine for cattle. *Res. Vet. Sci.*, 3: 172-182.

Terpstra, C. 1991. Hog cholera: an update of present knowledge. *Brit. Vet. J.*, 147: 397-406.

Terpstra, C. & Wensvoort, G. 1988. The protective value of vaccine-induced neutralizing antibody titres in swine fever. *Vet. Microbiol.*, 16: 123-128.

Terpstra, C., Woortmeyer, R. & Barteling, S.J. 1990. Development and properties of a cell culture produced vaccine for hog cholera based on the Chinese strain. *Dtsch. Tieraerztl. Wochenschr.*, 97: 77-79.

USDA. 1993. *Animals and animal products.* CFR title 9. Animal and Plant Health Inspection Service, United States Department of Agriculture.

van Oirschot, J.T. 1992. Efficacy of porcine vaccines. *Proc. 12th Int. Pig Vet. Soc. Congr.*, The Hague, 12: 15-18.

WHO. 1984. Expert Committee on Rabies, Technical report series 709, p. 18-27. Geneva, Switzerland.

Witter, R.L. & Burmester, B.R. 1979. Differential effect of maternal antibodies on efficacy of cellular and cell-free Marek's disease vaccines. *Avian Pathol.*, 8: 145-156.

Potency assessment of inactivated viral vaccines

T.R. Doel

A broad division exists between the methodologies employed to evaluate the potencies of live and inactivated viral vaccines. With live vaccines, it is common practice to assess a preparation by measuring the number of infectious particles in an *in vitro* assay, where a correlation has been established previously based on the minimum titre required to give an effective vaccine. Live vaccines may occasionally be potency tested in the target species particularly where the cost of the animals is relatively low, as with poultry.

In contrast, potency testing of inactivated vaccines is in the main done in the target species or an animal model. One reason for this is the often complex nature of formulations where potency is not caused solely by the antigen content but also the influence of the adjuvants which are invariably used in the final product. This is perhaps best illustrated by foot-and-mouth disease (FMD) vaccines where the list of regularly used adjuvants includes aluminium hydroxide gel and saponin (the efficacy of the latter may vary significantly with the source and purity), simple and complex emulsions with mineral oil and avridine.

Clearly, potency testing of inactivated vaccines can be very costly, particularly if the host is a large animal and cannot be recovered for further use. A good example is the United Kingdom potency test for FMD vaccines in which 26 cattle are challenged with live virus, after 24 of them have been vaccinated, and are subsequently destroyed.[1] Alternative tests have been devised because of this and other considerations such as the unavailability of seronegative animals and high-security large animal facilities. The complete range of tests used with inactivated vaccines may be summarized as follows:

i) vaccination and live virus challenge of the target species;
ii) vaccination and serology only of the target species;
iii) vaccination and live virus challenge of a small animal model;
iv) vaccination and serology only of a small animal model;
v) estimation by physical methods of antigenic/immunogenic content prior to formulation of the final product.

These basic test procedures are listed in Table 22 in the context of a range of important diseases for which inactivated virus vaccines exist. Frequently, of course, workers may also undertake serology with categories i) and iii) to give added confidence in the interpretation of the data. In the case of categories ii), iii) and iv) it is necessary that a firm correlation should have been established between potency in the target

[1] It should be noted that in disease-free countries such as the United Kingdom it is unacceptable for FMD-seropositive cattle to be returned to the seronegative population. This is because it is difficult to exclude the possibility that a seropositive animal is persistently infected and it is necessary to convince trading partners that there is no risk of disease if they import livestock or livestock products.

TABLE 22

List A and list B diseases of animals for which approved inactivated virus vaccines exist

Disease	Target species		Model species	
	Challenge	Serology	Challenge	Serology
FMD	+ (cattle)	+	+ (mouse and guinea pig)	+
Rift Valley fever	–	–	+ (mouse)	–
Newcastle disease	+ (chicken)	–	–	–
Rabies	–	–	+ (mouse)	–
Infectious bovine rhinotracheitis	+ (cattle)	–	–	–
Eastern and western equine encephalitis	–	–	–	+ (guinea pig)
Equine influenza	–	+ (horse)	–	+ (guinea pig)
Equine herpes (EHV-1, types 1 and 2)	+ (horse)	+	+ (hamster)	+
Japanese equine encephalitis	–	–	+ (mouse)	–
Venezuelan equine encephalitis	–	+ (horse)	–	–
Avian infectious bronchitis	+ (chicken)	–	–	–
Infectious bursal disease	–	+ (chicken)	–	–
Bovine viral diarrhoea	–	+ (cattle)	–	–

Source: OIE, 1992. Other diseases / viruses for which inactivated vaccines exist include canine parvovirus, hepatitis and distemper, swine influenza, parvovirus and enterovirus encephalomyelitis (previously Teschen disease), egg drop syndrome and African horse sickness.

species and that predicted from either protection or serology of the animal model.

For the future, ethical considerations will have an increasingly important influence on the use of animals for vaccine testing and will stimulate the development of animal-free *in vitro* assays, as indicated in category v) above (Soulebot, Milward and Prevost, 1993) and more widespread acceptance of serological alternatives to live virus challenge procedures i.e. categories ii) and iv) in the list above.

STATISTICAL ANALYSIS

Closely related to the issues of cost and logistics of potency testing in target and model species is the question of the statistical significance of the test with the numbers of animals used. The variation seen with potency tests is for the most part an expression of the individual sensitivities of the test animals which, with a large population, have been shown to obey a binomial distribution (Prigge, cited by Hendriksen, 1988). In practical terms, a quantitative assay based on a relatively small number of animals is very inaccurate. For example, the 90 percent confidence interval for the 50 percent protection dose (PD_{50}) test for FMD vaccines using three groups of five cattle lies between 45 and 220 percent of the potency (Hendriksen, 1988). Thus potency testing in small animal models or *in vitro* tests with large numbers of sera from vaccinated target species, provided a precise correlation can be made with potency in the target species, has the attractions of reduced costs while giving improved statistical significance to the data. *In vitro* tests also offer the opportunity to include a reference serum which allows inter- and intratest differences to be quantified and corrected for.

The problem of correlation between a test in the target species and a small animal model or *in vitro* assay has been debated for many years by those involved in the testing of FMD and other vaccines. Added to this there is, perhaps, an understandable preference among the users of vaccines for direct potency data from the target species despite the inherent statistical limitations. A key issue in the establishment of a correlation is that the conditions and materials being used in the two tests are clearly defined and recognized. Although this may seem obvious, there has been a tendency, with experimental FMD vaccines at least, to make the assumption that the neutralizing antibody correlates as well with protection as that induced by the conventional inactivated viral vaccines.

That this assumption is not always valid is demonstrated by work done with synthetic peptide vaccines which induced very high levels of neutralizing antibodies in cattle but gave considerably lower levels of protection than would have been predicted (DiMarchi *et al.*, 1986).

Another issue to consider here is the level of correlation desired by a national regulatory authority and what can be achieved realistically. Thus, protective immunity will, at the very least, depend on a complex and variable interaction among antibodies (which themselves have different affinities, isotypes and antigenic specificities) and phagocytic cells involved in the clearance of antigen-antibody complexes. This may be contrasted with the extreme simplicity of an *in vitro* serological assay which measures, at best, total antibody presence and may not discriminate among the more important antibodies in relation to protection. Thus, the mouse protection test for FMD vaccine sera gives the best correlation with protection in cattle, whereas the enzyme-linked immunosorbent assay (ELISA) correlates less well but has the considerable advantages of ease of use, lower cost, reproducibility, minimal use of animals (antibody reagents), etc. Progress towards replacing live virus challenge in the target species with *in vitro* assays will be greatly assisted by a general recognition of the likely deficiencies in the correlations made and a full discussion among all the interested parties.

There are two basic types of potency test. The first type is the single-dose or qualitative test in which animals are given a single dose of vaccine followed by challenge and / or the taking of blood samples. The results are amenable to simple statistics but often the only information they provide is percentage protection. Highly potent vaccines may be overlooked because more than 100 percent protection cannot be measured. While this approach ensures that the vaccines released for sale will have a minimum potency, the test results are less informative in terms of comparisons between different batches or formulations unless a good correlation between potency and a serological parameter has been established.

An alternative, but more costly, approach is to use a quantitative test in which

TABLE 23

Specimen potency data for the calculation of PD_{50} values

Dilution factor (log_{10})	Number of animals	Number protected	Proportion protected	Cumulative			Cumulative protection (%)
				Protected	Not protected	Total	
Neat (0.000)	10	10	1	23	0	23	100
3 (1.5228)	10	7	0.7	13	3	16	81
9 (1.0457)	10	4	0.4	6	9	15	40
27 (2.5686)	10	2	0.2	2	17	19	11
81 (2.0917)	10	0	0	0	27	27	0

a dilution series of the vaccine is prepared and each dilution tested in a group of animals. For proper analysis, a minimum of three dilutions is used and, if possible, these should be arranged so that the highest and lowest vaccine concentrations confer 100 and 0 percent protection respectively. This allows calculation of the dose of vaccine that protects, or is effective on, 50 percent of the population (PD_{50} or ED_{50}) and, usually, a confidence interval which gives information on the inherent variation intrinsic to the method.

There are many methods of calculating PD_{50} values including Reed-Muench, variants on Kärber, logit and probit analysis (Fontaine *et al.*, 1985) and even more opinions as to which is the most suitable method. Kärber procedures are probably the most widely used and are generally replacing Reed-Muench which, although simpler to use, was rejected by the British statistician, D.J. Finney, who considered Spearman-Kärber to be equal or superior at all times (Finney, 1971). It is clear that Reed-Muench should not be used if the 50 percent end point lies outside the dose titration series (Henderson, 1985). On the other hand, if the extreme dilutions of the titration series show 0 and 100 percent responses, and this could often be the case with assays in cell culture or small animals, then Reed-Muench is acceptable if simplicity of calculation is an important consideration. For this reason, both procedures are given below (Astudillo and Wanderley, 1976) based on a hypothetical set of protection data (Table 23), although they may equally be applied to the calculation of 50 percent end points for other assays.

Reed-Muench

Ideally, the value of the PD_{50} should fall approximately in the middle of the dose titration which should be a geometric series composed of equally sized groups of animals. No attempt should be made to calculate a PD_{50} value when the 50 percent end point lies outside the dose titration series (Henderson, 1985).

Initially, the column at the far right, which gives percentage cumulative protection, is scanned for the two values which bracket the percentage protection required and the corresponding log dilution factors are noted. Of course, this is 50 percent protection for the 50 percent lethal dose (LD_{50}) calculation but 25 and 75 percent are required for the estimation of the standard error.

The general Reed-Muench equation is given by:

$$\text{Log}_{10}\text{PD}_{\text{A\%}} =$$

$$\frac{\text{Log Inf} + \text{A\%} - \text{\%Protection at Log Inf}}{\text{\%Protection Log Sup} - \text{\%Protection Log Inf}}$$

$$\times\ (\text{Log Sup} - \text{Log Inf})$$

Where A% is the percentage protection required, i.e. 50, 25, etc; log inf is $\log_{10}$ of the dilution that gives less than A% protection; log sup is $\log_{10}$ of the dilution that gives more than A% protection; %protection log sup and % protection log inf are cumulative percentage protection at the dilutions which bracket A%. Thus:

$$\text{Log}_{10}\,\text{PD}_{50} = 1.0457 + \left[\frac{50 - 40}{81\text{-}40}\right] \times [1.5228 - 1.0467]$$

which calculates to $\text{Log}_{10}\ \text{PD}_{50}$ of 0.8380 or an arithmetic PD_{50} of 6.89, this being the dilution factor required to give 50 percent protection.

The following equation allows an approximation to the standard error of the $\log_{10}\text{PD}_{50}$ and was suggested by Pizzi (cited by Finney, 1964):

$$\text{SE}_{PD50} = \sqrt{\frac{0.79 \times h \times R}{n}}$$

Where 0.79 is a constant; n is the number of animals per dose; R is the interquartile interval ($\text{PD}_{75} - \text{PD}_{25}$) calculated using the standard Reed-Muench formula as described above; h is the $\log_{10}$ interval between doses, which is as follows, in the example given:

$$\frac{\text{Log}_{10}\text{ dilution neat vaccine-Log}_{10}\text{ dilution 1 in 81 vaccine}}{\text{number of doses - 1}}$$

i.e. $$h = \frac{0 - (2.0917)}{4} = 0.4771$$

From the Pizzi equation, the SE of the PD_{50} of the above data set calculates as follows:

$$\text{SE} = \sqrt{\frac{0.79 \times 0.4771 \times 0.6541}{10}} = 0.157$$

Therefore, the 95 percent confidence limits of the $\log_{10}\ \text{PD}_{50}$ value are $\pm 1.96 \times 0.157$ or in arithmetic form the potency of the vaccine is 6.89 PD_{50} with upper and lower 95 percent confidence limits of 13.99 and 3.39, respectively.

Spearman-Kärber

The extreme dilutions of the dose titration series should show 0 and 100 percent protection for the best use of this method although, if necessary, an assumption can be made that either of these values lies beyond the end of the series. The only important effect of making such an assumption is that it will not be possible to deduce the true PD_{50}. Rather, it will be necessary to express the calculated PD_{50} as equal to or greater than the observed value.

The basic formula for Spearman-Kärber is as follows:

$$\text{Log}_{10}\text{PD}_{50} = \sum_{i=1}^{k} \frac{(p_{i+1} - p_i)\ (x_i + x_{i+1})}{2}$$

Where k is the number of doses, p_i and p_{i+1} are the proportions protected in doses i and i+1, and x_i and x_{i+1} are $\log_{10}$ of the dilution factors for doses i and i + 1.

The calculation of

$$\frac{(p_{i+1} - p_i)\ (x_i + x_{i+1})}{2}$$

is made for each dilution in the data set given above and the products summed to give the $\log_{10}\ \text{PD}_{50}$. For comparison with Reed-Muench, the same data set gave an arithmetic PD_{50} value of 7.23.

The standard error of the $\log_{10}\ \text{PD}_{50}$ is calculated from the following expression:

$$\text{SE} = d\sqrt{\sum \frac{p_i q_i}{(n\text{-}1)}}$$

Where $d = x_i - x_{i+1}$ and x_i and x_{i+1} are $\log_{10}$ of the dilution factors for doses i and i+1, respectively; p_i is the proportion protected in dose i; q_i is $1 - p_i$; and n is the number of animals per group.

Using data from Table 22, the SE calculates as follows:

$$SE = 0.4771 \times \sqrt{\frac{0.61}{9}} = 0.124$$

Therefore, the 95 percent confidence limits of the $\log_{10}$ PD_{50} value are $\pm 1.96 \times 0.124$ or in arithmetic form the potency of the vaccine is 7.23 PD_{50} with upper and lower 95 percent confidence limits of 12.64 and 4.13, respectively.

Probit analysis

A more complete approach than the Reed-Muench and Spearman-Kärber procedures is to subject the potency data to probit analysis (Finney, 1971). Essentially, the percentage protection data are transformed into probit responses by reference to tables and weighted iterative regression analysis is performed on the resulting $\log_{10}$ dose/probit response line. For many years, the Wellcome FMD production laboratories at Pirbright, United Kingdom, used sets of probit tables calculated for all possible permutations of two versions of the European Pharmacopoeia test for FMD vaccines (Pay and Parker, 1977). In the case of the experimental protocol using three groups of five cattle, there are 216 possible sets of responses of which only 88 have positive slopes. Furthermore, it is not possible to calculate the lower 95 percent confidence on more than 20 sets. It should be emphasized, however, that less sophisticated procedures such as Spearman-Kärber cannot be relied on any more readily.

While it is extremely important to recognize that the PD_{50} value and confidence limits obtained may vary with the statistical method employed – particularly where small numbers of test animals are used (Pay and Parker, 1977) – it is also probably true to say that large differences between the statistical methods are not likely to be seen, given good data in which the PD_{50} value is bracketed by the doses tested (Henderson, 1985). This can be seen here with the two calculation methods used. In the final analysis, it requires little extra effort to submit the results of a potency test to several statistical methods provided the experimental design is compatible with each.

Finally, a further option with the quantitative test is the use of a standard or reference vaccine in parallel with the product under test. Clearly this increases the cost of potency testing but provides more information with particular respect to controlling or at least recognizing and allowing for experimental variables other than individual animal variation. In this way all batches of vaccine may be compared against the baseline of the reference preparation so that trends or major fluctuations in quality can be identified. The slopes of the respective dose-response curves of the reference and test vaccines provide additional information. Thus, essentially equivalent preparations differing only in antigen content should have parallel slopes. Significant deviation from this may be indicative of problems of vaccine quality or the manner in which the potency test was performed – having made the assumption that the reference vaccine is stable and has not deteriorated with time.

POTENCY TESTING OF SOME INACTIVATED VIRAL VACCINES

The following review, which is not intended to be comprehensive, draws heavily on OIE (1992).

Foot-and-mouth disease

Numerous procedures have been developed for the testing of FMD vaccines. Some of these are direct methods involving the challenge of cattle, others are indirect methods based on correlations with protection data. *In vitro* procedures are growing in popularity.

In the case of direct methods, probably the best known is that prescribed by the 1985 version of the European Pharmacopoeia. This specifies the use of 18- to 30-month cattle obtained from FMD-free areas that are seronegative for FMD and have never been vaccinated. Vaccine is diluted in an inert diluent to give three dose levels at not more than fivefold intervals and is used to inoculate groups of at least five cattle according to the volume and route stated on the label, using one dose level per group. Three weeks after vaccination, the vaccinated animals and a control group of two non-vaccinated cattle are challenged intradermolingually with 2 × 0.1 ml of a suspension containing 10 000 ID_{50} of cattle-adapted virus that is fully virulent and appropriate to the virus type of the vaccine under test. Animals are observed for eight days. Unprotected animals show lesions at sites other than the tongue and control animals must develop lesions on at least three feet.

Occasionally, vaccinated animals may develop a lesion on one foot despite evidence to suggest that the vaccine is potent. These "one-footers" are most probably the result of virus entry via an external abrasion rather than a consequence of viraemia and are considered by some workers as protected. High-quality FMD vaccines such as those prepared from antigens stored in emergency reserves (Doel and Pullen, 1990) not only protect against generalization, even at high dilution, but can suppress the febrile response and vesicular erosion of the tongue at the sites of injection of challenge virus.

For the vaccine to pass the European Pharmacopoeia test it must contain at least 3 PD_{50} per dose.

The most recent version of the European Pharmacopoeia Monograph on FMD vaccines (1993) describes a number of important changes in procedure. First, cattle of not less than six months of age are indicated which is more consistent with the general practice of a number of European laboratories and has considerable operational and cost advantages. It is also probably more relevant to test the vaccine in animals at or closer to the age recommended for the first vaccination (four to six months).

The second change is more controversial and indicates the use of different volumes of vaccine to vary the dosage rather than using different dilutions. While this procedure may prove to be acceptable, it must be said that it is a significant departure from well-accepted practices and it does not have a large body of data to support it.

Another direct test has been used by workers at the Institute for Animal Health in which three groups, each of eight cattle, are vaccinated with a twofold, a tenfold or a fiftyfold dilution of the field dose in adjuvant. Challenge is as above except that 10 × 0.1 ml of a suspension containing 100 000 ID_{50} of cattle-adapted virus is used. The inclusion of adjuvant rather than inert diluent gives a flatter dose-response curve and, thus, higher PD_{50} values than those for vaccines tested by the United Kingdom method. This is reflected in the United Kingdom pass-mark of 6 PD_{50} and Ahl *et al.* (1990) have demonstrated that the approximate relationship is:

$$\text{The European} PD_{50} = \sqrt{\text{of the United Kingdom } PD_{50}}$$

Several procedures have been described in which protection of cattle with a single field dose of vaccine is measured. The K index procedure described by Lucam and Fedida (cited by Pay and Parker, 1977) was widely used by a number of countries to assess their FMD vaccines. Briefly, virus is titrated intradermolingually in four vaccinated cattle and compared with the titre in four susceptible control animals, the reduction in titre being proportional to the potency of the vaccine. To the author's knowledge this procedure is now rarely used.

A more popular test is the protection against generalization (PG) procedure in which each of 16 cattle is vaccinated and subsequently challenged, usually 21 days later, with 10 000 ID_{50} of virus (Vianna Filho *et al.*, 1993). For a vaccine to pass the test, it is usually necessary to protect at least 12 cattle. This test is perhaps most suited to South America, where it is applied extensively to the many batches of vaccine being produced for routine use in the subcontinent, because it provides the information required in an unambiguous form, i.e. the minimum percentage of animals that will be protected if the vaccine is used. With the PG method there is not the temptation to apply statistics to inadequate data, in particular the calculation of PD_{50} values from data lacking a dose-response relationship. According to Vianna Filho *et al.* (1993), 3 PD_{50} by the European Pharmacopoeia method corresponds to 78, 78 and 79 percent protection by the PG method for virus serotypes O, A and C, respectively.

Following recovery from challenge, cattle may be reused to test a vaccine of another serotype despite the fact that they may have high-quality immunity to the first serotype and may be persistently infected. The reuse of cattle is particularly appropriate to testing based only on serology, where there is no disease security risk involved in holding the animals for a significant period of time.

Other species are occasionally used for direct potency testing of FMD vaccines. For example, oil-adjuvanted vaccines for pigs may be tested in this species although the procedure is complicated by factors such as overchallenge which can occur because of the very high level of virus excretion by susceptible animals. With oil formulations, it is common practice to deliver a range of volumes of vaccine although it is possible to prepare a dilution series.

Guinea pigs have been used extensively as a model species for potency testing of FMD vaccines. They are less favoured now, however, owing partly to the occasional failure to correlate the results with potency in cattle and the development of serological tests to replace challenge work in animals. In the author's experience, guinea pigs are most useful with vaccines made from pure or semi-pure antigens such as those held in antigen banks (Doel and Pullen, 1990) where the correlation between cattle and guinea pig potency appears to be good. There is some evidence that the high levels of contaminating cellular proteins in conventional FMD vaccines may interfere in the immune response of guinea pigs to viral antigens (T.R. Doel, unpublished results). It is important to recognize another possible reason for the occasionally poor correlation between the two challenge tests, namely the respective passage histories of the cattle- and guinea pig-adapted challenge viruses and, indeed, the vaccine production strain, which may lead to significant antigenic divergence.

In addition to the ethical issues involved in live challenge work, there are two main disadvantages associated with direct challenge methods in cattle. The first of these is the risk of dissemination of FMD from the testing area which may have additional cost implications depending on the level of biosecurity required by the veterinary authorities. The second disadvantage is that it is not feasible to challenge test more than a single strain of virus at any one time whereas most commercial FMD vaccines are multivalent, containing two, three or even four strains of the virus.

For these and other reasons, many workers have examined the correlation between direct indices of protection and serological parameters, in particular neutralizing antibody (Stellman *et al.*, 1968; Sutmöller, Gomes and Astudillo, 1984: Ahl *et al.*, 1990; Pay and Hingley, 1986 and 1992). Pay and Hingley (1986) claimed that a good correlation could be obtained between virus neutralizing antibody and vaccine potency when both were expressed in $\log_{10}$ antigen PD_{50} units. Because the procedure required three separate regression slopes, these authors refined their method to allow the conversion of a mean titre virus neutralizing antibody titre directly into a percentage protection value using a single regression slope (Pay and Hingley, 1992). In commenting on some apparent batch-to-batch variation that was found, they stressed the necessity for each laboratory to set up its own database because of variables such as the virus neutralization test (i.e. cell sensitivity, etc.) and the relationship between the serum assay virus and the vaccine virus.

Ahl *et al.* (1990) also made a valuable contribution to this subject. Using a plaque-reduction assay with a large number of cattle sera obtained from potency tests, they concluded that their approach fulfilled the requirements to replace the official PD_{50} challenge test in Germany. They also calculated the relationships among a number of different serological and protective parameters used by various FMD laboratories including United Kingdom and European PD_{50} values.

Sutmöller, Gomes and Astudillo (1984) compared the microtitre neutralization test with a passive immunity test in mice (i.e. mouse protection test or MPT) and protection data from cattle. They derived a table of expected percentages of protection (EPP) versus the reciprocal of the log serum dilution that neutralized 50 percent of 100 ID_{50} of virus and concluded that the serum neutralization test was a useful alternative for the estimation of the potency of FMD vaccines, although it tended to underestimate the number of vaccines that would be approved compared with the mouse protection test. In the latter procedure, six- to seven-day mice are injected with cattle serum and, one hour later, challenged with a dilution series of mouse-adapted virus. The results of the test are expressed as the mouse protection index (MPI), being the difference between the $\log_{10}$ virus titres obtained in the presence and absence of test serum (Gomes and Astudillo, 1975). The MPT is in regular use for the potency assessment of FMD vaccines made at the Pan American Foot-and-Mouth Disease Center and is the only procedure capable of assessing reliably the levels of protection conferred by some synthetic FMD peptide vaccines in cattle. Thus, the virus neutralizing antibody titres of peptide vaccinated cattle give little indication of the probability of protection in contrast to the MPT titres of the same sera, which show a good correlation (Mulcahy *et al.*, 1991). The relative superiority of the MPT for the serological assessment of vaccine potency is understandable. Pure *in vitro* tests such as ELISA and the neutralization test are less able to discriminate between those sera that have the affinities / isotypes / specificities of antibodies most appropriate to protection and those sera that do not (Steward *et al.*, 1991). Furthermore, these tests take no account of *in vivo* antigen-antibody clearance mechanisms, in contrast to the MPT.

Despite these limitations, ELISA in one of its many versions has been or is being evaluated by a number of FMD laboratories as an assay to measure the protective capacity of cattle sera. A liquid phase-blocking ELISA, described by Hamblin, Barnett and Hedger (1986), is used regularly by the World Reference Laboratory for FMD as an alternative to the serum neutralization test. In addition, a similar assay is being used in a large study in

South America involving laboratories in Argentina, Brazil and Uruguay and coordinated by the Pan American Foot-and-Mouth Disease Center. The titres of almost 1 000 sera from vaccine potency tests are being determined using a liquid phase-blocking ELISA, a virus neutralizing antibody test and the MPT. The correlations achieved will be of considerable interest to manufacturers and users of FMD vaccines.

Rift Valley fever

The test for inactivated Rift Valley fever vaccine is performed in two stages. Serial fivefold dilutions of vaccine are prepared and a single dose of 0.5 ml is used to inoculate ten adult mice per dilution by the intraperitoneal route (OIE, 1992). The mice are challenged two weeks later with 10^5 to 10^6 mouse LD_{50} of an appropriate challenge strain by the subcutaneous route. The challenge strain should be different from the vaccine strain. A second assay is conducted based on the results of the first but using serial twofold dilutions to bracket the expected 50 percent end point of the test. Data from the second test are plotted on probit paper and the confidence limits of the assay determined. Thus, the two-stage procedure allows a more precise end point to be determined without using very large numbers of mice.

Rabies

It has been established that the antigenic potency in mice of inactivated rabies vaccine is a reliable indicator of efficacy in the target species. One of two tests may be used (OIE, 1992). In the case of the European Pharmacopoeia test, groups of at least ten mice, aged three to four weeks, are inoculated with single decreasing doses of vaccine, whereas the National Institute of Health (NIH) test requires two doses, separated by a period of one week. A sufficient number of dilutions must be made to permit the calculation of the dilution of vaccine at which 50 percent of the mice are protected against intracerebral challenge 14 days after the last vaccination. A WHO reference vaccine is available for testing in parallel and allows the expression of the potency of the vaccine under test in terms of international units (IU).

To be valid, the PD_{50} of each set of data should lie between the extreme points of the dilution series. Statistical analysis should show dose-response lines that are linear and parallel with significant slopes and the 95 percent confidence limits should be not less than 25 percent and not more than 400 percent of the estimated potency. Finally, the titre of the challenge virus should be not less than 10 ID_{50} per 0. 03ml. The vaccine passes the test if the estimated potency is not less than 1 IU.

There has been considerable dispute surrounding the available potency tests for rabies vaccine because of their failure to distinguish satisfactorily between different vaccine products and the widely differing results observed when the same vaccine is tested by different laboratories. As a result, *in vitro* methods such as ELISA have been investigated with the aim of replacing the problematic *in vivo* methods (Hendriksen, 1988). One of the newer methods is an antibody binding test in which a vaccine dilution is mixed with an equal volume of neutralizing antiserum followed by live rabies virus. This mixture is inoculated on to a chick embryo fibroblast culture and the infectious foci detected by fluorescent antibody techniques. The potency of the vaccine dilution is thus proportional to the number of infectious foci on the cell sheet. This test has been validated in comparison with the NIH test and gave less variable and more reproducible data.

Viruses of poultry

With inactivated virus vaccines for poultry, it is completely feasible to test all preparations in the target species. The diseases of major importance include Newcastle disease, avian infectious bronchitis and infectious bursal disease (OIE, 1992).

Newcastle disease vaccines are tested by a number of methods (OIE, 1992). The European Pharmacopoeia indicates the vaccination of 20 birds at the minimum recommended age by the route and dose given by the manufacturer. After 14 to 21 days, the vaccinated birds, along with ten control birds, are each challenged with 10^5 LD_{50} of a suitable strain of Newcastle disease virus such as the Herts 33 strain. For the vaccine to pass the test, all control birds should die within six days of challenge and 90 percent of the vaccinated birds survive at least ten days with no sign of disease.

The potency test used for avian infectious bronchitis (AIB) vaccines depends on the type of protection required (OIE, 1992). To protect laying birds, 30 or more specific pathogen-free (SPF) birds are vaccinated at the earliest possible age (not later than three weeks of age). A second group of 30 control birds are included in the test and all are housed separately until four weeks before peak egg production. At this time they are housed together and individual egg production is monitored until it is regular, at which time all birds are challenged. Egg production is monitored for a further four weeks and the challenge should be sufficiently severe to ensure a loss of at least 67 percent of production in the control group during the first three weeks of the post challenge period. The group given one dose of inactivated vaccine should show a drop of production intermediate between the control group and what is normally observed with live AIB vaccines.

In fact, it is not unusual to carry out a composite potency test with live as well as inactivated preparations. Sera are collected from all birds at vaccination, four weeks later and following challenge. None of the sera from the control group should show antibodies against the virus.

If the vaccine is required to protect against respiratory disease, groups of 20 SPF birds, aged four weeks, are vaccinated as indicated by the manufacturer. Their antibody responses, as well as those of 20 control birds, are determined four weeks later. All groups are housed together and there should be no antibody response in the control group. Finally, all birds are challenged with 10^3 ID_{50} of virulent virus and killed four to seven days later. Sections of the trachea are examined for cilial motility and at least 80 percent of the control group should display complete ciliostasis whereas the tracheal cilia of a similar percentage of vaccinated birds should remain normal.

With infectious bursal disease (IBD) vaccines, an efficacy test is performed initially and once only, using a typical batch of vaccine (OIE, 1992). In this test, 20 SPF birds, near to point of lay, are vaccinated with a single dose of vaccine by the recommended route and the antibody response measured with reference to a standard antiserum over a period of four to six weeks post vaccination. In the United Kingdom, this antiserum may be obtained from the Central Veterinary Laboratory (CVL), Weybridge, United Kingdom. Eggs are collected for hatching and 25 progeny chicks challenged at four weeks of age by installation of eye drops containing 10^2 ID_{50} of a virulent strain such as CVL 52/70. Ten control birds of the same breed are also challenged. After three days, the bursa of Fabricius is removed from each bird and examined histologically or tested for the presence of virus antigen by the agar gel precipitin test. For the test to be acceptable, all control birds must show evidence of IBD infection whereas not more than three of the progeny from vaccinated hens should be affected.

For the routine vaccine potency test, 20 chicks, approximately four weeks of age, are vaccinated as above. The vaccinated birds are housed with ten control birds and the antibody responses of each bird determined with reference to a standard antiserum over a period of four to six weeks post vaccination. The mean antibody level of the vaccinated birds should not be significantly less than the level recorded in the efficacy test and the control birds should remain seronegative.

Viruses of horses

OIE (1992) describes six virus diseases of horses for which inactivated vaccines exist. These are Japanese, eastern, western and Venezuelan equine encephalomyelitis (JEE, EEE, WEE and VEE, respectively), equine influenza and equine rhinopneumonitis. The need for these vaccines relates both to the high value of bloodstock and the fact that humans are hosts for all of the equine encephalomyelitis viruses listed above, occasionally with fatal consequences.

Potency testing of both EEE and WEE is performed by inoculation of ten guinea pigs with one-half of a horse dose of vaccine on two separate occasions. The interval between the vaccinations should be 14 to 21 days and the route used with the guinea pigs should be as indicated for the horse. Two to three weeks after the second dose, sera are collected and tested by a plaque-reduction neutralization test. The EEE and WEE titres should be ≥1.4 and ≥1.32 respectively.

With JEE, a mouse protection test exists in which 30 mice, aged three to four weeks, are inoculated intraperitoneally with 0.1 ml of a tenfold dilution of vaccine in phosphate-buffered saline. The vaccine is given twice at three-day intervals. Eight days after the first inoculation the vaccinated mice, along with an equivalent uninoculated group, are challenged with graded doses of live virus and observed for 14 days. For the vaccine to pass the test, the survival rate should be more than 40 percent in the immunized group and the mortality rate in the control group should be more than 90 percent.

Inactivated VEE vaccines are tested in horses. Each of 20 susceptible animals is inoculated subcutaneously as recommended and sera taken within 21 to 28 days of vaccination. For a valid test, at least 19 of 20 horses must have haemagglutination inhibition (HI) antibody titres of at least 1 in 20 or serum neutralizing antibody titres of at least 1 in 40.

Equine influenza vaccines may be tested either in horses or in guinea pigs. For the target species, one vaccine dose is inoculated by the recommended route into each of five susceptible horses. A second dose of the same vaccine is injected after the period stated on the manufacturer's label. Blood is collected from each animal one week after the first vaccination and two weeks after the second vaccination, sera are prepared and the haemagglutinating activity (HA) determined.

For the vaccine to pass the test, the HA antibody titre of each serum taken after the second vaccination should not be less than 1 in 64 and the serology after the first vaccination must not show evidence of an anamnestic response. The latter safeguards against the use of horses that have pre-existing low levels of immunity to the disease. Such animals may be replaced and the test repeated in fresh animals. In general, it is not necessary to carry out this test with subsequent batches of vaccine prepared from the same seed lot system. Instead, ten guinea pigs are vaccinated as specified on the label and blood samples taken 21 days later. HA antibody titres are determined and should not be less than 1 in 16.

Equine rhinopneumonitis is caused by an equine herpesvirus of which there are two antigenically, biochemically and biologically distinguishable types referred to as EHV-1 and EHV-4. The former is the more common cause of abortion and the latter is more commonly found with acute respiratory disease of young horses.

Vaccine potency is tested preferentially in horses and, in the case of anti-abortion vaccine, in pregnant mares. Challenge is by the intranasal route with a virulent strain of virus. In the case of vaccines containing inactivated EHV-1, the potency test in horses may be substituted by a protection test in which vaccinated hamsters are challenged with a lethal dose of hamster-adapted virus. Because EHV-4 does not adapt to hamsters, vaccines containing this subtype may be tested by demonstrating seroconversion of virus-neutralizing antibodies in the test animal.

CONCLUDING COMMENTS

It is worth reflecting on the role of vaccine potency testing in the overall scheme of vaccine production and usage. First and foremost it exists to ensure that the customer, often a regional or national veterinary authority in the context of the diseases reviewed here, receives a product of known minimum potency. Indeed, the same authorities may control the official potency test and naturally wish to see an increase in the minimum potency requirements so that future batches of vaccine purchased by them are more effective.

At the same time, the manufacturer obtains information from a potency test which may be of value in recognizing problems during production and/or allows either the future production of more potent vaccine or an increased output of the minimum potency product. The latter option is particularly attractive because of the potential for increased profitability in an area where profit margins are relatively small.

Thus, the control authority and the manufacturer are occasionally in conflict over the most appropriate passmark for a vaccine. It is clear, however, that excessive demands for more potent veterinary vaccines may persuade the manufacturer to change to more lucrative products or result in very costly vaccines. The net consequence will often be the same. The customer may not be able to maintain a programme of vaccination either because the producer no longer makes the vaccine or because the cost of the vaccine is too high. The latter is particularly relevant to developing countries where the funds available for the purchase of animal vaccines are extremely limited.

With diseases of great economic importance such as FMD the consequences of a reduction in the level of vaccination for the agricultural economy of a country may be disastrous. There is a need, therefore, for a mutual understanding between the vaccine manufacturer and the control authority. In other words, control authorities should consult fully with vaccine manufacturers so that all concerned appreciate the consequences of a requirement for higher potency vaccine.

In the same vein, the move towards replacing official challenge tests in animals with *in vitro* assays will be greatly facilitated by full and proper discussion between the interested parties at all stages of the process.

BIBLIOGRAPHY

Ahl, R., Haas, B., Lorenz, R.J. & Wittman, G. 1990. Alternative potency test of FMD vaccines and results of comparative antibody assays in different cell systems and ELISA. *Report of the Session of the Research Group of the Standing Technical Committee of the European Commission for the Control of Foot-and-Mouth Disease*, Lindholm, Denmark. Rome, FAO.

Astudillo, V. & Wanderley, M. 1976. *Métodos estadísticos para ensayos biológicos*. Serie de Manuales Didácticos, No 8. Centro Panamericano de Fiebre Aftosa.

DiMarchi, R., Brooke, G., Gale, C., Cracknell, V., Doel, T. & Mowat, N. 1986. Protection of cattle against foot-and-mouth disease by a synthetic peptide. *Science*, 232: 639-641.

Doel, T.R. & Pullen, L. 1990. International bank for foot-and-mouth disease vaccine: stability studies with virus concentrates and vaccines prepared from them. *Vaccine*, 8: 473-478.

European Pharmacopoeia Commission. 1993. European Pharmacopoeia (Veterinary) Monograph 63. Sainte-Ruffine, France, Maisonneuve.

Finney, D.J. 1964. *Statistical method in biological assay.* London, Charles Griffin and Co.

Finney, D.J. 1971. *Probit analysis.* Cambridge, UK, Cambridge University Press.

Fontaine, J., Brun, A., Camand, R., Chappuis, G., Duret, C., Lombard, M., Moreau, Y., Precausta, P., Riviere, M., Roulet, C., Soulebot, J.P. & Stellman, C. 1985. Product testing: an introduction. *In* R.E. Spier and J.B. Griffiths, eds. *Animal cell biotechnology*, Vol II, p. 312-314. London, Academic Press.

Gomes, I. & Astudillo, V. 1975. Foot-and-mouth disease: evaluation of mouse protection test results in relation to cattle immunity. *Bol. Cent. Panam. Fiebre Aftosa*, 17-18: 9-16.

Hamblin, C., Barnett, I.T.R. & Hedger, R.S. 1986. A new enzyme-linked immunosorbent assay (ELISA) for the detection of antibodies against foot and-mouth disease virus. I. Development and method of ELISA. *J. Immunol. Methods*, 93: 115-121.

Henderson, W. 1985. *A personal history of the testing of foot-and-mouth disease vaccines in cattle.* The Massey Ferguson Papers.

Hendriksen, C.F.M. 1988. *Laboratory animals in vaccine production and control: replacement, reduction and refinement.* Kluwer Academic Publishers.

Mulcahy, G., Pullen, L.A., Gale, C., DiMarchi, R.D. & Doel, T.R. 1991. Mouse protection test as a predictor of the protective capacity of synthetic foot-and-mouth disease vaccines. *Vaccine*, 9: 19-24.

OIE. 1992. *Manual of standards for diagnostic tests and vaccines.* Paris, Office Internationale des Epizooties.

Pay, T.W.F. & Hingley, P.J. 1986. The use of serum neutralizing antibody assay for the determination of the potency of foot-and-mouth disease (FMD) vaccines in cattle. *Dev. Biol. Stand.*, 64: 153-161.

Pay, T.W.F. & Hingley, P.J. 1992. A potency test method for foot-and-mouth disease vaccine based on the serum neutralizing antibody response produced in cattle. *Vaccine*, 10: 707-713.

Pay, T.W.F. & Parker, M.J. 1977. Some statistical and experimental design problems in the assessment of FMD vaccine potency. *In* International Symposium on Foot-and-Mouth Disease, Lyon, France, 1976. *Dev. Biol. Stand.*, 35: 369-383.

Soulebot, J.P., Milward, F. & Prevost, P. 1993. *In vitro* potency testing of inactivated biologics: current situation in the EC. *Vet. Microbiol.*, 37: 241-251.

Stellman, C., Bornarel, P., Lang, R. & Terré, J. 1968. Contrôle quantitatif du vaccin antiaphteux. Analyse statistique de la relation liant les titres d'anticorps neutralisants au pourcentage de protection bovine. *Rec. Méd. Vét.*, 144: 325-331.

Steward, M.W., Stanley, C.M., DiMarchi, R., Mulcahy, G. & Doel, T.R. 1991. High-affinity antibody induced by immunization with a synthetic peptide is associated with protection of cattle against foot-and-mouth disease. *Immunol.*, 72: 99-103.

Sutmöller, P., Gomes, I. & Astudillo, V. 1984. Potency estimation of foot-and-mouth disease vaccines according to antibody assay results. *Bol. Cent. Panam. Fiebre Aftosa,* 49-50: 31-34.

Vianna Filho, Y.L., Astudillo, V., Gomes, I., Fernandez, G., Rozas, C.E.E., Ravison, J.A. & Alonso, A. 1993. Potency control of foot-and-mouth disease vaccine in cattle. Comparison of the 50 percent protective dose and the protection against generalization. *Vaccine,* 11: 1424-1428.

In vitro potency testing of inactivated biologics: current situation in the European Union

J.P. Soulebot, F. Milward and P. Prevost[1]

The EEC Council Directive 90/677 (EC, 1990) defines an immunological veterinary medicinal product (IVMP) as: "a veterinary medicinal product administered to animals in order to produce active or passive immunity"; and: "the quantitative particulars of an IVMP shall be expressed by mass or by international units, or by units of biological activity or by the number of germs or by specific protein content where possible, as appropriate to the product concerned". The mass, number of germs or specific protein content are not determined *in vivo* but rather *in vitro*. This definition would allow, in principle, for the replacement of potency tests performed in animals by *in vitro* tests. Such a change would not only save animal lives (which is an ethical requirement) but also save costs (animal tests are particularly costly and often of long duration) and solve some practical difficulties – certain tests can adequately be performed only in specific pathogen-free (SPF) animals, animals that are free of specific antibodies or animals that have never previously encountered the specific organism and, in many cases, such animals are not available. Both industry and official laboratories should obviously be in favour of such changes.

The directive cited above is part of a whole series of regulations, which are implemented throughout the European Union (EU), in the field of IVMPs. These regulations complement the monographs of the European Pharmacopoeia which is itself widening its field of application. The object of these regulations is to ensure a very high level of safety and efficacy but, unfortunately, they often lead to the increased use of animals in test procedures, especially target animals for routine safety tests and, for ethical, economic and practical reasons, this is undesirable.

Although in the past the assessment of biological products – particularly tests of potency of vaccines – were mainly carried out in animals, either laboratory species or domestic livestock, such tests could be expensive, time-consuming and, in the case of some products, of only limited value. The advent of modern physico-chemical, immunological or molecular biological methods of measuring with considerable precision the essential immunizing component of antigens destined for the preparation of vaccines, offers significant advantages to those involved with developing in-process quality control tests. Not only are there advantages in terms of precision and the saving of time and financial costs, there is also no need for the use of animals – a not inconsiderable factor from the viewpoint of those concerned with animal welfare.

[1] This paper is reproduced by kind permission of Elsevier Science Publishers BV, Amsterdam, the Netherlands.

REGULATIONS

In the EU, three levels of rules must be considered. At the most general level, recently published Commission Directive 92/18/EEC (EC, 1992c) modifying the annex to Council Directive 81/852, indicates that potency tests may be: "based upon *in vitro* or *in vivo* methods,... (and) in exceptional circumstances, potency testing may be carried out at an intermediate stage, as late as possible in the production process". This represents a significant opportunity, allowing for instance to move the control test to a stage upstream of the addition of adjuvants, thus avoiding all the difficulties related to the need to separate the active ingredients from the adjuvants and other ingredients for testing. However, the term "in exceptional circumstances" considerably limits the scope of this opportunity.

The directive is supplemented by guidelines including "General requirements for the production and control of inactivated mammalian bacterial and viral vaccines for veterinary use" (EC, 1992a) which, however, does not give any further precision concerning potency tests and merely states: "the vaccine shall be shown to be of satisfactory potency using validated methods".

In the meantime, some countries have already adopted species-specific guidelines. In the United Kingdom, for example, guidelines are available for the production and control of avian virus vaccines, veterinary bacterial vaccines, porcine virus vaccines, canine virus vaccines, equine virus vaccines and bovine virus vaccines. These documents do not include any particular indication concerning *in vitro* or *in vivo* potency tests – it is only stated that: "each batch of vaccine shall be shown to be of satisfactory potency using an approved method" (Veterinary Medicines Directorate, 1991) – except in the avian guidelines where the use of serological tests for four specific vaccines (Newcastle disease, egg drop syndrome, infectious bronchitis and infectious bursal disease vaccines) are planned (Veterinary Medicines Directorate, 1990).

The final level of rules within the EU are the national pharmacopoeias, which include IVMP monographs (for example British Pharmacopoeia Commission, 1985; Commission Nationale de Pharmacopée, 1992). It should be noted that national pharmacopoeias must use the European Pharmacopoeia monographs where they exist, but may include monographs that are not in the European Pharmacopoeia.

THE EUROPEAN PHARMACOPOEIA

The European Pharmacopoeia extends its domain of application beyond the EU, since it concerns at least all the member countries of the Council of Europe, 19 nations in all. The Pharmacopoeia consists of monographs, general notices and analytical methods.

Monographs

The European Pharmacopoeia includes 12 monographs for killed vaccines and a general monograph for "veterinary vaccines". None of these specifies the use of *in vitro* tests. Five other monographs for killed vaccines are at the level of projects published for public appraisal (European Pharmacopoeia Commission, 1991a, 1991b, 1991c, 1991d and 1991e). None of these projects plans for *in vitro* tests, with the exception of the document concerning foot-and-mouth disease (FMD) vaccine. The chapter pertaining to in-process control of antigenicity states: "the content of antigen is determined by an *in vitro* method (e.g. 146S-particle measurement by sucrose density gradient centrifugation and ultraviolet spectrophotometry at 259 nanometres)". This test may be used for the release of vaccine but only in cases of extreme urgency. The section reads: "If the test for potency has been carried out with satisfactory results on a representative batch of vaccine prepared from a given batch of antigen, then a batch of vaccine prepared from the same batch of antigen may, in cases of extreme urgency and subject to agreement by the national authority, be released before completion of testing if it has been shown that the batch has an antigen content not less than that of the representative batch, determined in an in-process control by an *in vitro* method."

It may seem that the European Pharmacopoeia excludes the use of *in vitro* tests and refers exclusively to challenge tests or vaccination followed by antibody titration. However, certain monographs allow that: "if the test for potency (in animals) has been carried out with satisfactory results on a representative batch of vaccine, this test may be replaced by a manufacturer as a routine test on other batches of vaccine prepared from the same seed lot by an alternative test for which satisfactory correlation of the results with those of the Pharmacopoeia method has been established by a statistical evaluation, subject to agreement by the national authority."

General Notices. The preamble to Part IV-1, General Notices (European Pharmacopoeia Commission, 1985) states that the monographs are official standards applicable within countries of the Contracting Parties (countries of the Council of Europe) and that: "statements under the headings Identification, Tests, Assay and Potency are mandatory requirements", but that: "with the agreement of the national authority, alternative methods of analysis may be used for control purposes, provided that the methods used enable an unequivocal decision to be made as to whether compliance with the standards of the monographs would be achieved if the official methods were used".

Analytical methods

An opening in favour of substituting *in vitro* test for *in vivo* assay seems to appear. The fifteenth fascicle (European Pharmacopoeia Commission, 1991f) introduces in its chapter on analytical methods, under heading V 2.1.10, the important paragraph concerning immunochemical methods: "These methods are employed to detect or quantify either antigens or antibodies". Of course, it is underlined that: "the results of immunochemical methods depend on the experimental conditions and the nature and quality of the reagents used. It is essential to standardize the components of an immunoassay and to use, wherever available, international reference preparations for immunoassays".

Two main types of methods are quoted as quantitative methods for determining antigens. These are methods in which a labelled antigen or a labelled antibody is used and methods in which an unlabelled antigen or antibody is used. The latter group is divided into immunoprecipitation methods such as single radial immunodiffusion (SRID) and immunoelectrophoretic methods such as crossed immunoelectrophoresis, electroimmunoassay (often referred to as rocket immunoelectrophoresis) and counter-immunoelectrophoresis.

No technical details are described. However, validation criteria and validation methods are detailed. It is stated that a quantitative immunochemical method is not valid unless:

- the antibody or antigen does not significantly discriminate between test and standard. For a labelled reactant, the corresponding reactant does not significantly discriminate between labelled and unlabelled compound;
- the method is not affected by the assay matrix, i.e. any component of the test sample or its excipients, which can vary from sample to sample and may

include high concentrations of other proteins, salts, preservatives or contaminating proteolytic activity;

- the limit of quantification is below the acceptance criteria stated in the individual monograph;
- the precision of the assay is such that the variance of the results meets the requirements stated in the individual monographs;
- the order in which the assay is performed does not give rise to systematic errors.

In order to verify these criteria, the validation design includes the following elements:

- the assay is performed in at least triplicate;
- the assay includes at least three different dilutions of the standard preparation and three dilutions of sample preparations of activity presumed to be similar to the standard preparation;
- the assay layout is randomized:
- if the test sample is presented in serum or formulated with other components, the standard is likewise prepared;
- the test includes measurement of non-specific binding of the labelled reactant;
- for displacement immunoassay maximum binding (zero displacement) is determined and dilutions cover the complete response range from values close to non-specific binding to maximum binding, preferably for both standard and test preparations.

The following is provided on the statistical calculation of results: "to analyse the results, response curves for test and standard (must be) analysed.... Significant non-parallelism indicates that the antibody or antigen discriminates between test and standard and the results are not valid. In displacement immunoassays, the values for non-specific binding and maximum displacement at high test or standard concentration must not be significantly different. Differences may indicate effects due to the matrix, either inhibition of binding or degradation of tracer".

From all that has been said about regulations in the EU, it can be concluded that *in vitro* potency testing on final products is almost never proposed but is not excluded and that *in vitro* antigen quantification methods are indicated but with no technical details. Validation criteria and methods are more detailed, but no or few data are available for statistical calculations. Reference preparations, which would be particularly useful, are not available. Thus, *in vitro* tests are essentially used for in-process controls. Methods are generally internal to the different laboratories and may be part of the industrial expertise – under such conditions, it is understandable that few methods have been standardized. The following are examples of widely used methods.

Foot-and-mouth disease. The antigenic content of FMD vaccine (Fargeaud, Fayet and Roumiantzeff, 1969) is determined by first preparing sucrose density gradients. Samples clarified by centrifugation are then loaded on the gradients, ultracentrifugation is performed and ultraviolet spectrophotometric results are plotted. The area under the peak is proportional to the concentration of 146S particles of the sample. Using a standard curve established with different dilutions of a purified viral suspension containing a known concentration of 146S particles, the concentration of 146S particles in the test sample can be calculated.

Rabies and pseudorabies. Antigenic glycoprotein content is determined using a single radial immunodiffusion test, derived from Ferguson's method (Ferguson and Schild, 1982). A concentration gradient is established for the antigen diffusing from an external source into the gel medium containing the corresponding antibody at a comparatively low concentration. When the equilibrium between the external and the internal reactants has been established, the circular precipitation area, originating from the site of the external reactant, is directly proportional to the amount of the antigen applied and inversely proportional to the concentration of the antibody in the gel. Various dilutions of the test glycoprotein and standard glycoprotein solutions are used. The formula for the linear response can be established as d2 = ac + b where: "d" is the diameter of the circular precipitation area; "a" is the slope; "c" is the dilution rate; and "b" is the original intercept.

The titre of the test suspension is expressed by the ratio of the slopes multiplied by the concentration of the standard expressed in micrograms per millilitre. For rabies, many other methods have been proposed, from enzyme-linked immunosorbent assay (ELISA) tests (Bruckner *et al.*, 1988) to antibody binding tests (Barth *et al.*, 1985) or even determination of the *in vitro* production of specific interleukin-2 (Joffret *et al.*, 1991).

Tetanus vaccine and other clostridial vaccines. Current pharmacopoeia requirements for tetanus vaccines for veterinary use specify a final product potency test based on direct challenge of mice or titration of antibodies from vaccinated guinea pigs or rabbits. The titration of antibodies is performed by a serum neutralization method against a standard toxin in mice. In all cases, these tests require the use of animals. Although variations of these standard methods have been proposed to reduce the number of animals (Knight and Roberts, 1987; Huet, Relyveld and Camps, 1990), *in vitro* tests should be considered as alternatives. One of the first objectives could be to replace the existing toxin neutralizing tests performed in mice by an *in vitro* antibody assay method. Numerous test systems have been proposed: gel diffusion, nephelometry, immunoelectrophoresis and ELISA (Calmels *et al.*, 1981). The present availability of reagents, high standards of quality and widespread use of the technique would make the ELISA test a good candidate to replace *in vivo* testing. Many other researchers have developed such a test and correlation with *in vivo* methods has often been found to be good (Cox *et al.*, 1983; Gentilli, Pini and Collotti, 1985).

Complete *in vitro* potency testing would require the direct titration of tetanus toxoid in the final product. Such methods have been proposed (Melville-Smith, 1985) and are currently in use for the identity testing of tetanus vaccines. The earliest test for direct quantification of the tetanus toxoid is Ramon's flocculation test. Although cumbersome, it has the advantage of referring to an international standard and is used to quantify the tetanus toxoid prior to vaccine formulation (i.e. 100 Lf/dose). Toxoid measurement in the final product is more easily performed by gel diffusion or ELISA. When run against a standard, a quantitative estimation can be obtained.

While tetanus vaccines have been the most widely studied, all that has been said could also be applicable to veterinary clostridial vaccines. *In vitro* antibody titration methods have already been proposed (Knight *et al.*, 1990). The main problem connected with these approaches remains the reliability of measurement on adjuvanted vaccines and is discussed in Conditions for the development of *in vitro* tests (p. 416).

Pasteurella multocida. In this example, *in vitro* tests for the determination of dermonecrotoxin content (DNT) have been made possible owing to the much better knowledge that now exists of the pathogenesis of the disease. Research has moved on from a situation where the etiology of atrophic rhinitis (AR) was ascribed to many infectious and non-infectious causes, through the narrowing of the cause to two bacteria, *P. multocida* and *Bordetella bronchiseptica,* to the discovery and proof through challenge models of the role of the dermonecrotic toxin (DNT) of *P. multocida*. This has allowed the preparation of vaccines of progressively better-defined content. Current modern vaccines are based on purified DNT toxoid which gives an opportunity to apply several *in vitro* tests.

Toxin determination, initially tested by intradermal injection in guinea pigs can now be performed *in vitro* in embryonic bovine lung cells or Vero cells. This assay can then be used to determine the neutralizing antibody level.

An ELISA test has been designed to measure toxoid content in the active ingredient and the final vaccine. Using a sandwich technique, the test has been successfully used to titrate toxoid content in adjuvanted vaccine. As in previous examples, the critical point is the quality (purity and stability) of the standard. This test is used to standardize batch formulation and could be used as a release method provided that a reference vaccine from the same production process with the same amount of toxoid has been shown to be protective.

CONDITIONS FOR THE DEVELOPMENT OF *IN VITRO* TESTS

Most vaccines are adjuvanted, either as aluminium hydroxide-adsorbed formulations or as oil emulsions. This makes testing more difficult and is a source of variability.

It is necessary either to separate the antigen in the vaccine, taking into account the loss or denaturation of antigen, or to adapt the test to use on the finished product with possible interference from other vaccine constituents.

Two ways around this difficulty would be either to estimate the average amount in the final product and the variability of a given process without attempting to retrieve the exact amount introduced in the formulation (as seen for DNT) or to accept the in-process testing upstream of formulation provided that all steps in formulation are correctly described, validated and performed. The second approach is preferable because it allows a precise determination of the amount of antigen that will be introduced in the vaccine and thus constitutes a guarantee, provided that quality is ensured and the final steps of formulation are reproducible. This is why the possibility provided by Directive 92/18/EEC (EC, 1992c) to carry out potency tests upstream in the process, even if limited to "exceptional circumstances", is particularly important. This approach is only acceptable under the following three conditions, however:

- batch-to-batch consistency must be formerly validated;
- a quality assurance system must be implemented;
- the system must be properly maintained and regularly subjected to a suitable inspection procedure.

The first condition is obvious. It may, however, be useful to remember that: "validation is the action of proving, in accordance with the good manufacturing practice (GMP) principles, that any procedure, process, equipment, material, activity or system actually leads to the expected results" (EC, 1992b) and that: "total validation of manufacturing processes, in order to ensure continuous conformity of batches" is required for IVMPs (EC, 1990).

Concerning the second condition, it is not only necessary to validate batch-to-batch consistency, but it must also be shown that this batch-to-batch consistency will last indefinitely – the defect detection and reaction system must be replaced by a defect prevention system. This will consist of developing an overall quality assurance system.

The International Organization for Standardization (ISO, 1991) defines quality assurance as: "all those planned and systematic actions nécessary provide adequate confidence that a product or service will satisfy given requirements for quality". EU good manufacturing practice (GMP) (EC, 1992b) adds: "Quality assurance is a wide-ranging concept which covers all matters which individually or collectively influence the quality of a product. It is the total sum of the organized arrangements made with the object of ensuring that medicinal products are of the quality required for their intended use. Quality Assurance, therefore, incorporates Good Manufacturing Practice plus other factors outside the scope of this Guide."

Regarding GMP, principles and guidelines were laid down for veterinary medicinal products (VMPs) by Directive 91/412/EEC (EC, 1991) and are explained in detail in the 162 pages of EC, 1992b, in which 16 pages are dedicated to the specific requirements of IVMPs. GMP deals with that part of quality assurance that ensures that products are consistently produced and controlled to the quality standards appropriate to their intended use. GMP refers to "personnel, premises, equipment, documentation, production, quality control, contract manufacture and analysis, complaints and product recall as well as self-inspection". Its implementation is compulsory and subject to inspection.

What would be the use of applying GMP, implementing a rigorous quality assurance system, if this did not ensure quality, especially in the final blending stages of vaccine formulation, and thus allow the limiting of final product testing? The last steps at least should be subject to a parametric release system, i.e. they should be based on documented production data rather than on control data.

The third condition concerns the quality assurance system maintenance (Soulebot, 1992). Once implemented, the quality assurance system, like any other system, can be maintained and avoid drifting only under the influence of a double set of pressures – internal and external. Internal pressure is represented by verifications, such as self-inspections, as recommended by GMP, but also the continuous attention of top management, etc. External pressures are those exerted by competition and customers. The latter exercise direct pressure (by placing orders or not) or indirect pressure through legal authorities, audits and other official inspections. Such inspections are, in all circumstances, of the greatest importance as controls alone have proved to be insufficient (nevertheless, controls should be submitted to GMP). The application of GMP is then of prime importance. Consequently, it is particularly important that an efficient inspection system be implemented for IVMPs. The new inspection system, concerning specifically quality assurance and quality control implemented by the United Kingdom (Lee, 1992) besides GMP general inspection, is a big step towards making this evolution easier by increasing the necessary confidence of all.

CONCLUSION

By following the suggestions made in this chapter, *in vivo* potency tests could be progressively replaced by *in vitro* tests. *In vivo* tests would be used only for product development, establishment and validation of correlations and exceptional verifications. A last point must be emphasized; there are no standardized *in vitro* techniques or reference preparations in the EU, in spite of the fact that many tests are used or being developed. In order to avoid future problems, it is particularly important that, as of now, efforts be made among Europe, the United States and other countries for the harmonization of new techniques and standard preparations.

BIBLIOGRAPHY

Barth, R., Gruschkau, H., Milcke, L., Jaeger, O. & Weinmann, E. 1985. Validation of an *in vitro* assay for the determination of rabies antigen. *Develop. Biol. Stand.*, 64: 87-92.

British Pharmacopoeia Commission. 1985. *British Pharmacopoeia (Veterinary)*. London, Her Majesty's Stationery Office.

Bruckner, L., Palatini, M., Ackermann, M., Muller, H.K. & Kihm, U. 1988. Reduction of the number of mice used for potency testing of human and animal rabies vaccines. *Experientia*, 44: 853-857.

Calmels, D., Audonnet, J.C., Tixier, G. & Desmettre, P. 1981. Etude comparative de différentes méthodes de titrage des antitoxines tétaniques, p. 439-450. 6th Int. Conf. Tetanus, Fondation Mérieux, Lyons, France.

Commission Nationale de Pharmacopée. 1992. *Pharmacopée Française*, 10th edition, Sainte-Ruffine, France, Maisonneuve.

Cox, J.C., Premier, R.R., Finger, W. & Hurrel, J.G.R. 1983. A comparison of enzyme immunoassay and bioassay for the quantitative determination of antibodies to tetanus toxin. *J. Biol. Stand.*, 11: 123-127.

European Pharmacopoeia Commission. 1985. *European Pharmacopoeia*, 2nd edition. Sainte-Ruffine, France, Maisonneuve.

European Pharmacopoeia Commission. 1991a. Vaccinum Influenzae ad suem inactivatum. *Pharmeuropa*, 3: 15.

European Pharmacopoeia Commission. 1991b. Vaccinum Parvovirosis ad suem inactivatum. *Pharmeuropa*, 3: 81.

European Pharmacopoeia Commission. 1991c. Vaccinum Aphtharum epizooticarum inactivatum pro ruminantibus. *Pharmeuropa*, 3: 82.

European Pharmacopoeia Commission. 1991d. Vaccinum Bursitidis infectivae aviariae inactivatum. *Pharmeuropa*, 3: 100.

European Pharmacopoeia Commission. 1991e. Vaccinum Pseudopestis aviariae inactivatum. *Pharmeuropa*, 3: 102.

European Pharmacopoeia Commission. 1991f. *European Pharmacopoeia*, 15 fascicle, Chapter V. Sainte-Ruffine, France, Maisonneuve.

EC. 1990. Council Directive 90/677/EEC of 13 December 1990. *Off. J. Eur. Comm.*, L 373: 26-28 (31 December 1990).

EC. 1991. Commission Directive 91/412/EEC of 23 July 1991. *Off. J. Eur. Comm.*, L 228: 70-73.

EC. 1992a. *Guidelines for the production and control of inactivated mammalian vaccines for veterinary use*, Draft No. 5, III/3181/91 (March 1992).

EC. 1992b. *Good manufacturing practice for medicinal products in the European Community*. The Rules Governing Medicinal Products in the European Community (EEC/III/3093/92-EN), January 1992, Vol. IV, p. 1-163.

EC. 1992c. Commission Directive 92/18 of 20 March 1992, modifying the annex to Council Directive 81/852/EEC in respect to the testing of veterinary medicinal products. *Off. J. Eur. Comm.*, L 97: 1-23 (10 April 1992).

Fargeaud, D., Fayet, M.T. & Roumiantzeff, M. 1969. Analyse par centrifugation zonale en gradient de saccharose des particules virales contenues dans une préparation du virus de la Fièvre Aphteuse. *Revue d'Immunol.*, 3: 335-344.

Ferguson, M. & Schild, G.C. 1982. A single radial immunodiffusion technique for the assay of rabies glycoprotein antigen: application for potency test of vaccine against rabies. *J. Gen. Virol.*, 59: 197-201.

Gentilli, G., Pini, C. & Collotti, C. 1985.

The use of an immunoenzymatic assay for the estimation of tetanus antitoxin in human sera; a comparison with seroneutralization. *J. Biol. Stand.*, 13: 53-59.

Huet, M., Relyveld, E. & Camps, S. 1990. Méthode simple de contrôle de l'activité des anatoxines tétaniques adsorbées. *Biologicals,* 18: 16-67.

ISO. 1991. *Quality management and quality assurance vocabulary,* ISO 8402. Geneva, Switzerland, International Organization for Standardization.

Joffret, M.L., Zanetti, C., Morgeaux, S., Leclerc, C., Sureau, P. & Perrin, P. 1991. Appraisal of rabies vaccine potency by determination of *in vitro,* specific interleukin-2 production. *Biologicals,* 19: 113-123.

Knight, P.A. & Roberts, P.A.G. 1987. An evaluation of some proposals for a reduction in the number of animals used for the potency testing of diptheria and tetanus vaccines. *J. Biol. Stand.,* 15: 165-175.

Knight, P.A., Queminet, J., Blanchard, J.H. & Tilleray, J.H. 1990. *In vitro* tests for the measurement of clostridial toxins, toxoids and antisera. II. Titration of *Clostridium perfringens* toxins and antitoxins in cell culture. *Biologicals,* 18: 263-270.

Lee, A. 1992. Control of product batches (before and after registration). The British approach. *Develop. Biol. Stand.,* 79: 175-177.

Melville-Smith, M.E. 1985. Single radial immunodiffusion as a method for the identification and quantification of diptheria and tetanus toxoids in adsorbed vaccines. *J. Biol. Stand.,* 13: 77-86.

Soulebot, J.P. 1992. FEDESA's point of view: quality, application to IVMPs. *Develop. Biol. Stand.,* 79: 201-211.

Veterinary Medicines Directorate. 1990. *Guidelines for the production and control of avian virus vaccines.* MAL 74. Weybridge, UK, Central Veterinary Laboratory.

Veterinary Medicines Directorate. 1991. *Guidelines for the production and control of veterinary bacterial vaccines.* MAL 76. Weybridge, UK, Central Veterinary Laboratory.

Sterility management and testing of vaccines and raw materials for adventitious agents

G. Blocks

Sterility management is the system that combines the continuous efforts of research and development (R&D), production, quality control (QC) and quality assurance (QA) in reducing and controlling the level of microbiological contamination of products. The principal sources of microbiological contamination are personnel, air and equipment. Therefore, to maintain the sterility of a product, the "bioburden" of the premises has also to be controlled.

The risk of infection during the production, storage, sampling and testing of a batch of product has to be controlled, monitored and documented. Production has therefore to be in accordance with current good manufacturing practice (GMP) and QC has to be in accordance with both GMP and good laboratory practice (GLP).

An important factor is that in R&D, production, QC and QA, all actions, results, findings and observations should be properly documented, i.e. clear descriptions, which are dated, signed and easily retrievable should be given.

Sterility is a built-in characteristic of the production process. During R&D of a product, special attention has to be given to minimize the risk of contamination in the production process. Special consideration should also be given to the number of aseptic handlings, the production process must be designed in accordance with the premises and utilities available and, if there are incompatabilities between the designed process and the production facilities, these should be addressed before starting production. Changes in the process or in the production facilities after the start of production are less time-effective and cost-effective than establishing a well-designed process before starting production. There is also an increased risk when producing outside the boundaries of the product licence if adaptations are made after the start of production.

One essential component of a sterility management system is the assurance that the necessary samples are collected, stored, tested and interpreted in the proper manner. Trend analyses can be performed to determine consistent problem factors but corrective actions need to be immediate and cannot wait for a trend analysis timetable.

Products that have to be sampled include: starting materials, intermediate products and final product. Utilities that must be sampled are: water systems, steam systems and the compressed air system. Premises that need to be monitored are those critical working areas where the product is in direct contact with the environment, including: surfaces, air, fingertips and the laboratories that are the background for the critical working areas. For each sampling point, test requirements have to be defined, including the sampling method, the frequency of sampling, alert levels and action levels.

Sterility is defined as the absence of microbial agents in a product. Microbial agents can be bacteria, mycoplasmata, moulds, yeasts and viruses. An indication of sterility can be obtained by performing the appropriate tests for the absence of microbial agents on a representative sample of the batch of product.

The selection criteria for tests to demonstrate sterility have to be based on the origin and properties of the product, the possible contaminants and the species for which the product is destined.

Tests of sterility may be limited in their ability to detect live and/or inactivated microbial agents and their residues. During interpretation of test results, the following points should be considered:

- the range of species of microbial agents detected;
- minimum detection levels of live microbial agents;
- minimum detection levels of inactivated microbial agents;
- minimum detection levels of sub-lethally damaged microbial agents;
- sampling and storing procedures;
- QC laboratory procedures;
- the activity of antimicrobial agents.

The interpretation of test results therefore has to be based on the validity of the test procedures available for the particular product. Test results have to be compared with the results of positive and negative control samples, which should be an integral part of every test that is performed.

Special consideration should be given to metabolites of killed microbial agents such as endotoxins. These can be the cause of adverse effects in the target species and can also influence the production process.

References are given at the end of this chapter for further details of guidelines and appropriate tests.

SAMPLES

Samples can be taken from different sources. The origin of the sample influences the sampling method. It is therefore necessary to have standard operating procedures (SOPs) in which each sampling method is described. The sample should be representative of the product from which it is taken. It will be obvious that, before a sample is taken, the contents of the container must be homogenous.

Furthermore, special consideration should be given to the prevention of contamination of the sample at the time of sampling. Samples should only be taken by properly trained personnel.

GENERAL RECOMMENDATIONS ON CONTROL TESTS

For non-biological starting materials and sterilized biological starting materials tests should be made for bacterial and fungal sterility.

For biological starting materials tests should be made for: bacterial and fungal sterility; the absence of *Mycoplasma* spp.; and the viral sterility of product on sensitive cell cultures including primary cells from the species of origin.

For cell substrates tests should be made for: bacterial and fungal sterility; the absence of *Mycoplasma* spp.; and the viral sterility of the product (i.e. tests for cytopathogenic viruses, haemadsorbent viruses, specific viruses of the species of origin and specific viruses of the intended species).

For bacterial seeds tests should be made for: bacterial monoculture; and the absence of *Mycoplasma* spp.

For mycoplasmal seeds tests should be made for: bacterial and fungal sterility; and mycoplasma monoculture.

For viral seeds tests should made for: bacterial and fungal sterility; and the absence of *Mycoplasma* spp. Tests should also be performed on: primary cells of the species of origin of the virus; cells that are sensitive to viruses pathogenic for the species for which the vaccine is intended; and cells that are sensitive to pestiviruses.

On the final product to be administered parenterally tests should be made for: bacterial and fungal sterility (in the case of a live bacterial vaccine the test for bacterial monocultures should be used); and the absence of *Mycoplasma* spp.

For the final product to be administered non-parenterally tests should be made for bacterial and fungal sterility (if the test fails, a viable bacterial count may be performed – the maximum acceptance level is one non-pathogenic organism per dose – and, in the case of a live bacterial vaccine, the test for bacterial monocultures should be used); and the absence of *Mycoplasma* spp.

TESTS FOR BACTERIOLOGICAL AND FUNGAL STERILITY OF A PRODUCT

Tests of sterility are necessary for assessing samples from a product that should be bacteriologically or fungally sterile, since they give information on the presence of viable aerobic or anaerobic bacteria and of viable fungi. Tests for sterility are described in detail in various pharmacopoeias. Based on the regulations that are in force in the country of production and in the country of destination of the product, a suitable pharmacopoeia should be selected to be used as a reference for the preferred test method.

Where sterilization is the final step in production, the validation of the sterilization process for a particular product and the documentation on the actual sterilization run give the greatest assurance of sterility.

In the case of aseptically filled products, the results of tests for bacteriological and fungal sterility must be combined with the validation of the production processes, such as filling, lyophilization and capping, and the actual batch record.

The working area in which control tests are performed should be protected against contamination at the same level as the production areas. Assurance that tests are performed under suitable conditions is derived from the validation of the tests (i.e. negative control samples) and from microbiological monitoring of the critical working areas (surface swabs, air samples and fingertips) and also from the additional negative control samples included in every test. The results of such negative control samples should be that no growth is observed.

Test methods

Two test methods – membrane filtration and direct inoculation – are described in the European Pharmacopoeia. Whenever it is possible, based on the nature of the product and on the capacities of the QC laboratory, the membrane filtration technique should be used. The membrane filtration method is preferred over the direct inoculation method because of the lower sensitivity to anti-microbial agents in the product and because it involves fewer aseptic handlings.

The suitability of a test for a particular product is derived from the validation of that test and from the positive control samples included in every test. Preparations that are used as positive control samples should consist of 100 viable microorganisms (aerobes, anaerobes and fungi).

The results of the test on the positive control samples should be that early and copious growth is observed.

Interpretation of results

Test media are observed at intervals throughout the incubation period. They are examined for macroscopic evidence of microbiological growth.

The test results can be accepted if the test is validated by the appropriate controls, i.e. if the negative control samples do not show evidence of microbiological growth and if the positive control samples do show evidence of microbiological growth.

If a product fails a test that has been

shown to be valid, an investigation must be undertaken by the QA section into the causes of the contamination. Microscopic examination of the contaminating organism should be undertaken by means of Gram's-stained slides. In the case of a product that contains inactivated bacteria, special attention must be given to the possibility of failure of the inactivation process. Only when it can be shown that the probable cause of contamination occurred during sampling or testing are the results of the re-testing acceptable, otherwise the entire batch of product must be rejected.

If a product fails a re-test that is declared valid, all the previously mentioned points regarding the reasons for failing a test should be considered. A second re-test is only acceptable if the microorganism identified is without doubt different from that isolated in the first test; if it is not, the entire batch of affected product must be rejected.

If tests on negative control samples frequently (>1 percent of the samples) show microbial growth, the test should be revalidated with special attention given to possible sources of contamination (culture media, glassware, critical working area and laboratory technique).

If tests on positive control samples frequently (>1 percent of the samples) show no growth, the test should be revalidated with special attention given to the possibility of the presence of growth-inhibiting substances in the product.

If trend analysis of the results of tests of a product show a rise in positive results, while the control samples give the expected results, investigations should be made into the cause of the contamination of the product. Special attention should be given to the production process, sample taking techniques and the quality of the containers used to fill the product and for the taking of samples.

TESTS TO DEMONSTRATE FREEDOM FROM CONTAMINATION IN PRODUCTS CONTAINING LIVE BACTERIAL OR MYCOPLASMAL STRAINS

With bacterial seeds or products containing a live bacterial strain, the standard tests to demonstrate bacterial and fungal sterility cannot be used since microbial growth will always result. The same applies to sterility tests on products containing live strains of mycoplasmata. Nevertheless, it is as important to demonstrate freedom from contamination with such products as it is with products containing inactivated organisms.

The tests used for this type of product are likely to be less sensitive than those used with inactivated preparations, making it even more important to ensure that the production conditions fully meet the requirements of GMP/GLP, that all control tests are completely validated and that attention is given to the need for microbial monitoring of the production process and the associated sampling methods.

The tests to be used need to exclude as much as possible the presence of microbiological strains other than the intended one. Such tests are based on biochemical, serological or morphological properties.

Examples of tests

Plating of samples on solid agar medium. Media to be used can be those that have general growth-promoting properties, such as blood agar in Petri dishes, or specific media, which have growth-promoting properties for a selected range of microbiological organisms.

The result of this type of test must be an early and copious growth of only one type of colony, which has the macroscopic properties of the production strain. At least five colonies should be sampled individually and fixed and stained according to Gram's method. The microscopic examination of these Gram's-stained preparations should show only one type of microorganism that has the characteristics of the production strain. Where appropriate, other staining techniques can also be applied.

Serological tests. Suitable laboratory test animals are inoculated with the test sample. During the test no clinical signs of disease may be observed other than those signs that normally occur after inoculation of the tested product.

At the time of inoculation and after an interval of three weeks (usually), blood samples are taken for serological testing. The paired blood samples should only show a rise in the level of antibodies that are correlated to the microbiological strain of the product. If evidence is found of other types of antibodies, the test should be repeated. If in the repeat test the same antibodies are detected, the product must be rejected.

The test should always include at least two animals that are not inoculated. Their paired sera are used as negative controls and, if in the sera from the control animals or from the test animals an unexpected antibody increase is observed, there is a high probability that these animals were infected during the test. Such a situation does not constitute evidence of contamination of the sample.

Biochemical tests. There are several biochemical test kits available commercially. When using one of these kits, a negative control sample consisting of a "blank product" should always be included. A blank product is similar to the product under test but does not contain the essential microbiological strain. If possible it should be sterile.

If there are consistent results with the control blank at the time of validation of the test, these values can be disregarded as background "noise". The results of the test should always be in accordance with the biochemical properties of the production strain.

If unexpected results are obtained, it will be necessary to undertake a re-test and, if in the re-test similar results are obtained, the product should be rejected.

TEST FOR THE PRESENCE OF BACTERIAL ENDOTOXINS

If a batch of starting, intermediate or finished product is negative in tests for bacterial sterility (i.e. no viable bacteria are detected) it is still possible that there are residues of inactivated bacteria. Among these inactivated bacteria are bacterial endotoxins, which can give rise to adverse reactions in vaccinated animals or can cause undesirable effects during the production process.

In some cases it is not possible to remove all of these bacterial endotoxins. In such a situation a limited amount of endotoxin may be acceptable. In all other cases, the presence of bacterial endotoxins is the result of bacterial infection and the product is therefore not acceptable. Products that should give a negative result in this test but prove positive must be re-tested and, if the re-test confirms the finding of the first test, the batch of product should be rejected.

TESTS FOR THE ABSENCE OF MYCOPLASMATA IN PRODUCT

Two tests are described in the European Pharmacopoeia. The first detects the avian strains *Mycoplasma gallisepticum* and *M. synoviae* using two different media. The other test detects the non-avian strains *M. hyopneumoniae* and *M. urealyticum.* During validation of the test, it is necessary to demonstrate the sensitivity of the test system to neutralizing agents, which may be part of the tested product. If neutralizing agents are present, a suitable inhibitory substance should be used. This inhibitory substance must not interfere with the sensitivity of the test.

Positive controls are used to show that the test system is capable of detecting small numbers of mycoplasmata. Negative controls are included to show whether contamination has occurred during the course of the test or during other laboratory manipulations.

Special attention has to be given to products that normally contain live mycoplasmal strains. By using these tests and, where appropiate, tests capable of giving serological evidence of the presence of other strains, assurance can be given that the product is not contaminated with other strains of mycoplasmata.

For the interpretation of test results together with the results of positive and negative controls, refer to Tests for bacteriological and fungal sterility of a product (p. 423).

TESTS FOR VIRAL STERILITY OF PRODUCTS

Tests should be conducted on starting materials that contain material of animal origin and on the final product. Starting materials of animal origin include the master seed virus, the production cell system and the serum and trypsin used during the production process.

Samples that contain the master seed virus or the live virus vaccine require to be inactivated in such a manner that the vaccine strain is inactivated – without affecting any contaminating viruses that are present. Inactivation can be achieved by the use of serum with a high titre of neutralizing antibodies specific to the seed virus used to prepare the vaccine. Care has to be taken in the preparation of the antiserum that the virus used is well characterized and possibly purified by cloning. If not there is the possibility that, should there be a contaminating virus or viruses present in the original master seed, they may also be present in the antiserum prepared with the latter. If possible the antiserum should have a different source and history than the master seed.

If this method of producing neutralizing antibodies is not possible, other methods of selectively removing contaminants from the seed virus may be used.

Tests can be categorized as general tests that demonstrate the presence of large groups of viruses and tests that demonstrate the presence of a specific virus or group of viruses. Tests may also be described in terms of their ability to demonstrate the presence of live viruses or to show that the sample under test can induce the production of antibodies in test animals against the specific virus or group of viruses under consideration.

Tests for viral sterility are described in detail in several pharmacopoeias and guidelines. Based on the regulations that are in force in the country of production and in the country of destination of the product, the applicable set of guidelines and tests should be selected.

The suitability of a test for any particular product will be indicated by the original validation of the test (i.e. the results from positive control samples) and also from the positive control samples included in every subsequent test. In tests that give evidence of the presence of live viral agents, the test cultures are observed at intervals during the incubation period and at its conclusion. Test cultures are observed for both macroscopic and microscopic evidence of viral growth. The test is valid and the results can be accepted if the negative control samples do not show evidence of viral growth and if the positive controls do show evidence of typical viral growth.

If a product fails a test that is declared valid, an investigation must be made by the QA section into the causes of the product failure. Identification of the virus strain isolated should be made using a suitable method. Only when it can be shown that the probable cause of contamination occurred during sampling or testing, is a re-test acceptable, otherwise the batch of product must be rejected.

If a product fails a valid re-test, the batch of product must be rejected.

If tests of negative control samples frequently (>1 percent of the samples) show the presence of virus, the test should be revalidated with special attention given to possible contamination sources (i.e. starting materials, critical working areas and laboratory techniques).

If tests of positive control samples frequently (>1 percent of the samples) indicate the absence of virus growth, the test should be revalidated.

If trend analysis of the tests of a product show a rise in positive results, while the control samples give the expected results, investigations should be made into the cause of the contamination of the product. Special attention should be given to the production process, sample taking techniques and the quality of the containers used to fill the product and for the taking of samples.

BACTERIOLOGICAL MONITORING OF SERVICES

Only the minimum microbiological monitoring of services is described here. All other types of analyses on these systems are not included. Depending on the production site and on the regulations that are in force, an extended programme of bacteriological monitoring may be advisable.

In the case of production problems related to bacteriological sterility or the validation of a new or modified production process, an extended programme is also advisable. Such programmes may consist of a higher frequency of sampling, the sampling of additional work areas and the use of other specific culture media, etc.

Some services provide basic requirements or elements of the process and, with respect to the clean steam and compressed air systems, their end products may come in direct contact with the biologicals that are produced, up to the final stages of production.

The services that have to be monitored for microbiological contamination include the main water supply system, the purified water (PUW) system, the water for injection (WFI) system, the main steam system, the clean steam system and the compressed air system.

Services should be checked on a regular basis, preferably every week, for the number of viable microorganisms present and for the level of degradation products of microorganisms such as endotoxins.

The standards for PUW and WFI are defined in various pharmacopoeias. Condensates of clean steam and compressed air have to be in accordance with the requirements for WFI.

Tests should be made on samples taken from sampling points that are close to the point of usage in the system.

If a sample does not fulfil the requirements, another sample should be tested. If this sample also fails to fulfil the requirements, an investigation should be made into the cause of the contamination. From the results of this investigation corrective measures such as sterilization and/or maintenance of the system should be instituted.

BACTERIOLOGICAL MONITORING OF PREMISES

Effective SOPs should be written to describe the rooms that are sampled, the sampling points, the sampling techniques, the frequency of sampling and the time at which samples are taken. For air samples, the volume of air sampled should be prescribed and for surface swabs the number of square inches/centimetres of surface to be sampled should be prescribed.

The reasons for the bacteriological monitoring of premises are:

- to check on the effectivenesss of previously validated sanitary, disinfection and sterilization procedures – samples should be collected by using surface swabs or contact agar plates and air samplers. The frequency of testing should be once a month for clean rooms and once every two months for other areas that are microbiologically monitored;
- to check on contamination levels during production.

Samples should be taken at critical working points such as: air (settle plates), surfaces (swabs or contact plates) and fingertips (contact plates). Furthermore, samples (swabs or contact plates) should be taken from the environment of critical working areas (e.g. clean rooms and QC laboratories).

The following are recommended frequency levels for testing:

- *critical working areas* (usually a laminar airflow cabinet) using settle plates should be tested continuously during production. (It is recommended that plates should be changed every two hours, depending on how fast they dry out which is mainly dependent on the composition and thickness of the medium in the plate);
- *surfaces* should be tested once per production day;
- *fingertips* should be tested once per working day for every laboratory technician.
- surfaces in *the critical working area environment* should be tested once every week.

Sampling methods should be validated and special attention should be given to the detergents, disinfectants and sterilizing agents used in the production process since residues of these can decrease the viability of microorganisms in the various samples taken for testing. Where this is the case, neutralizing agents for these residues should be used.

BIBLIOGRAPHY

European Pharmacopoeia Commission. 1985. *European Pharmacopoeia,* second edition. Sainte-Ruffine, France, Maisonneuve.

EC. 1981. Council Directive 81/851/EEC of 28 September 1981 on the application of the laws of the Member States relating to veterinary medical products.

EC. 1981. Council Directive 81/852/EEC of 28 September 1981 on the application of the laws of the Member States relating to analytical, pharmaco-toxicological and clinical standards and protocols in respect to the testing of veterinary medicinal products.

EC. 1990. Council Directive 90/677/EEC of 13 December 1990 on the application of the laws of the Member States relating to veterinary medicinal products and laying down additional provisions for immunological veterinary medicinal products.

EC. 1991. General Requirements for the production and Control of Live Mammalian Bacterial and Viral Vaccines for Veterinary Use, ref. 111/3182/91-EN.

EC. 1991b. General Requirements for the Production and Control of Inactivated Mammalian Bacterial and Viral Vaccines for Veterinary Use, ref. 111/3181/91-EN.

EC. 1992. Requirements for the production and control of porcine live and inactivated vaccines, ref. 111/3362/92-EN.

EC. 1992. Requirements for the production and control of bovine live and inactivated viral and bacterial vaccines, ref. 111/3487/92-EN.

EC. 1992. Requirements for the production and control of ovine and caprine live and inactivated viral and bacterial vaccines, ref. 111/3618/92-EN.

EC. 1993. Requirements for the production and control of equine live and inactivated viral and bacterial vaccines, ref. 111/3001/93-EN.

EC. 1993. Requirements for the production and control of fish live and inactivated viral and bacterial vaccines.

USDA. 1994. *Animals and animal products.* CFR title 90. Animal and Plant Health Inspection Service, United States Department of Agriculture.

Contributors

Contributors

Alexandra Adams
Institute of Aquaculture
University of Stirling
Stirling FK9 4LA
United Kingdom

V. Astudillo
Pan American Foot and Mouth Disease Center
Rio de Janeiro
Brazil

H.G. Bahnemann
Postfach 1358
46452 REES
Germany

P.B.V.P. Bangar Raju
Indian Immunologicals
Gachibowli
Hyderabad 500133
India

J. Blancou
Office International des Épizooties
12 rue de Prony
F-75017 Paris
France

G. Blocks
Veterinary Medicines Directorate
Woodham Lane
New Haw
Addlestone
Surrey KT15 3NB
United Kingdom

R. Bomford
Institut Pasteur
28 rue du Dr Roux
75724 Paris, Cedex 15
France

F. Bover
CSL Limited
45 Poplar Road
Parkville
Victoria 3052
Australia

F. Brown
Plum Island Animal Disease Center
P.O. Box 848
Greenport, Long Island
New York 11944-0848
United States

P. Chartier
Ministère de la Coopération
Direction du Développement
Bureau de la Production agricole, industrielle et Échanges
1 bis avenue de Villars
75700 Paris
France

P. De Greve
Internationaal Agrarisch Centrum
Post Box 88
6700 AB Wageningen
The Netherlands

J.M. de Ree
Solvay-Duphar B.V.
Post Box 900
1380 DA WEESP
The Netherlands

A.J. de Vos
c/o Tick Fever Research Centre
280 Grindle Road
Wacol
Queensland 4076
Australia

T.R. Doel
Pan American Foot and Mouth Disease Center
Post Box 589
20001-970 Rio de Janeiro
Brazil

A.I. Donaldson
Institute for Animal Health, Pirbright Laboratory
Woking
Surrey GU24 0NF
United Kingdom

J. Estefanell de Maria
CZ Veterinaria S L
Ap. C.16, Porriño, 36400
P.O. Pontevedra, Spain

A.J.B. Haigh
18 Smarts Heath Road
Woking
Surrey GU22 0NP
United Kingdom
It is with great regret that the death of Barry Haigh in early 1995 has to be recorded here.

Pamela Hunter
Foot and Mouth Disease Laboratory
Private Bag X6
0110 Onderstepoort
Republic of South Africa

W.K. Jorgensen
c/o Tick Fever Research Centre
280 Grindle Road
Wacol
Queensland 4076
Australia

A.P. Kariath
Indian Immunologicals
Gachibowli
Hyderabad 500133
India

P.A. Knight
81 High Street
Shoreham, Sevenoaks
Kent TN14 7TB
United Kingdom

D.P. Knox
Moredun Research Institute
408 Gilmerton Road
Edinburgh EH17 7JH
United Kingdom

B.W.J. Mahy
Division of Viral and Rickettsial Diseases
National Center for Infectious Diseases
Centers for Disease Control and Prevention
1600 Clifton Road
Atlanta, GA 30333
United States

J.C. Mariner
Pan African Rinderpest Campaign
Thermostable Rinderpest Vaccine Transfer of Technology Project
OAU/IBAR/PARC
Post Box 30786
Nairobi
Kenya

J.B. McFerran
19 Knocktern Gardens
Belfast BT4 3LZ
United Kingdom

Jacqueline B. McKeand
Department of Veterinary Parasitology
University of Glasgow
Bearsden Road
Glasgow G61 1QH
United Kingdom

C.A. Mebus
USDA Animal and Plant Health Inspection Service
Veterinary Services, National Veterinary Services Laboratories
Foreign Animal Disease Diagnostic Laboratory
Post Box 848
Greenport, NY 11944
United States

L.O. Mesopir
Kenya Veterinary Vaccines Production Institute
Post Box 53260
Nairobi
Kenya

W.I. Morrison
Institute for Animal Health
Compton, Nr Newbury
Berkshire RG16 0NN
United Kingdom

F. Musisi
c/o Tick Fever Research Centre
280 Grindle Road
Wacol
Queensland 4076
Australia

V. Palya
Pan African Veterinary Vaccine Centre (PANVAC)
c/o FAO, Post Box 5536
Addis Ababa
Ethiopia

E. Pipano
c/o Tick Fever Research Centre
280 Grindle Road
Wacol
Queensland 4076
Australia

A. Provost
CIRAD-EMVT
10 rue Pierre Curie
94704 Maison-Alfort CEDX
France

P.J. Radlett
Poacher's Cottage
Stockley Hamlet
Okehampton
Devon EX20 1QH
United Kingdom

R.J. Roberts
Institute of Aquaculture
University of Stirling
Stirling FK9 4LA
United Kingdom

M. Rweyemamu
Pan African Veterinary Vaccine Centre (PANVAC)
c/o FAO, Post Box 5536
Addis Ababa
Ethiopia

J.P. Soulebot
59 bis boulevard des Belges
Lyon, France

P.B. Spradbrow
Department of Veterinary Pathology
University of Queensland
Post Box 125, Kenmore
Brisbane 4069
Australia

V.A. Srinivasan
Indian Immunologicals
Gachibowli
Hyderabad 500133
India

C. Stellmann
Laboratoire IFFA
254 rue Marcel Mérieux
B.P. 7009 – 69342 Lyon, Cedex 07
France

D. Sylla
Pan African Veterinary Vaccine Centre (PANVAC)
c/o FAO, Post Box 5536
Addis Ababa
Ethiopia

C. Terpstra
Institute for Animal Science and Health
Houtribweg 39
Post Box 365
NL-8200 AJ Lelystad
The Netherlands

K.D. Thompson
Institute of Aquaculture
University of Stirling
Stirling FK9 4LA
United Kingdom

M. Truszczynski
Office International des Épizooties
12 rue de Prony
F-75017 Paris
France

Sandra E. Ullah
c/o American Red Cross Blood Services
Fort Wayne Region
1212 E. California
Fort Wayne, IN 46825
United States

B. Vallat
Ministére de la Coopération
Direction du Développement
Bureau de la Production agricole, industrielle et Echanges
1 bis avenue de Villars
75700 Paris
France

P. Vannier
CNEVA Ploufragan
LCRAP UR Station de Pathologie Porcine
B.P. 53
22440 Ploufragan
France

P.D. Walker
Peter Walker Associates
37 Aperfield Road
Biggin Hill, Westerham
Kent TN16 3LU
United Kingdom

E.E. Worrall
Tymawr, Trefilan, Talsarn
Lampeter
Dyfed SA48 8RD
United Kingdom

Editors

G.N. Mowat
46 Boxgrove Avenue
Guildford
Surrey GU1 1XQ
United Kingdom

M. Rweyemamu
Animal Health Service
Animal Production and Health Division
Food and Agriculture Organization
Viale delle Terme di Caracalla
00100 Rome
Italy